Skull Base Imaging

F. Allan Midyett • Suresh K. Mukherji

Skull Base Imaging

The Essentials

Springer

F. Allan Midyett
Fayetteville, AR
USA

Suresh K. Mukherji
Marian University
Carmel, IN
USA

ISBN 978-3-030-46446-2 ISBN 978-3-030-46447-9 (eBook)
https://doi.org/10.1007/978-3-030-46447-9

This Springer imprint is published by the registered company Springer Nature Switzerland AG
The registered company address is: Gewerbestrasse 11, 6330 Cham, Switzerland

To my parents, whom I miss even more with each passing day.

To my wife, Rita Patel. You are the strongest and kindest person I have ever met. Thanks for putting up with me for all these years.

To my children, Anika and Janak. Although I helped raise you, both of you have turned into my role models!

Suresh K. Mukherji

Foreword

Let's be honest, how many of us really understand the anatomy of the skull base and know of all the lesions that arise there? I dare to say that if you are not dedicated to head and neck imaging, the answer is: very few. Skull base anatomy and pathology are something that is taught in medical school and the process of learning those stretches throughout our entire professional lives. The reason for this may be the way in which it is taught. This book tries to do this in a different way. Instead of the conventional details of all structures and lesions found there, the present book approaches the skull base on a case by case basis. Although the list of cases is not all inclusive, the lesions presented here are those most commonly found in this region. I would wage, that after reading this entertaining book, any radiologist will gain tremendous confidence when encountering a skull base lesion.

Both authors, Drs. Midyett and Mukherji, have been colleagues of mine here at the University of North Carolina. Based on their dedication and knowledge, it comes as no surprise that they have managed to publish two excellent books so far (this one being one of them). So, dear reader, you should not be surprised if after reading this book once you keep coming back to it just the fun of it!

Mauricio Castillo, MD, FACR
James H Scatliff Distinguished Professor of Radiology
Chief, Division of Neuroradiology
University of North Carolina School of Medicine
Chapel Hill, NC, USA

Acknowledgments

As I look back on a long exciting Radiology career, I recall the impressive radiology showman David S. Carroll who caused me to say "Wow, I can't believe he can see all that in an image!" And, I just *had* to pursue Radiology. Then, I realized that while Dr. Carroll really was a great Radiologist, he was first and foremost a gifted entertainer! While Dr. Carroll's list of accomplishments is longer than this acknowledgment, it was his showmanship which moved me and many others to become radiologists. And then, I settled down to truly train under the thoughtful tutelage of C. Allen Good. While no one ever accused Dr. Good of being an entertainer, no one ever doubted he was an exceptional Radiologist. Dr. Good set superb standards for radiology practices both at the Mayo Clinic and in fact for the entire country during the more than quarter century he led the American Board of Radiology as its president and secretary.

My mentors are truly "too numerous to count." Many, including Bob Scanlon, Dave Reese, Colin Holman, and Hillier L. "Bud" Baker, have relocated and are currently consulting with us from above.

And, if these impressive individuals were not enough, I had the outstanding opportunity to have a Neuroradiology Fellowship with Mauricio Castillo and Suresh Mukherji where I saw a vision of Academic Neuroradiology I had never seen before. Their level of expertise blew my mind, and in this transformative process I developed a love for Head & Neck Radiology, and in specific Skull Base Imaging.

And, while my half century in Radiology has taught me that we can't constantly be like Dave Carroll dazzling people all the time, I will submit that these are truly some of my most memorable motivational moments in Radiology. Specifically, for *Skull Base Imaging: The Essentials*, I want to thank Drs. Suresh Mukherji, C. Douglas Phillips, and James G. Smirniotopoulos.

Dr. Mukherji has been a marvelous mentor and invaluable Co-Author for *Orbital Imaging* and now its subsequent successor, *Skull Base Imaging: The Essentials.*

Dr. Phillips provided plain film images of Paget's disease. Chief Editor of *MedPix*, Dr. Smirniotopoulos, graciously contributed extraordinary color images of a colossal clivus cordoma of the skull base.

I do hope you enjoy the book and startle someone with something you learn from *Skull Base Imaging: The Essentials.*

F. Allan Midyett, MD

Contents

About the Authors

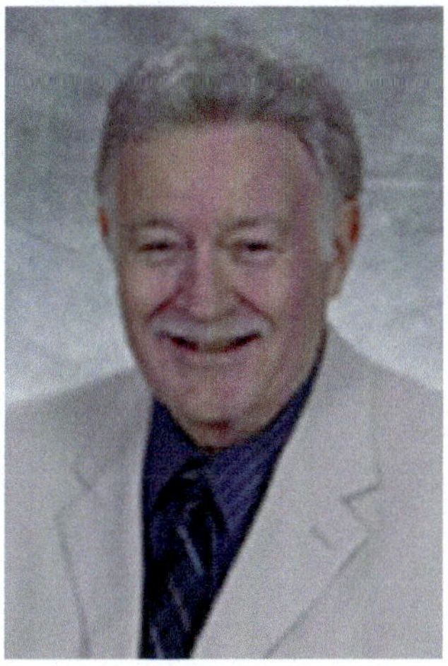

F. Allan Midyett, MD received his M.D. in Medicine and Surgery from the University of Tennessee, College of Medicine, in 1965. Following a rotating internship at the Baptist Memorial Hospital in Memphis he completed his residency in Diagnostic Radiology at the Mayo Clinic in Rochester, Minnesota, in 1970 and for three decades practiced diagnostic radiology with a special interest in Neuroradiology. While practicing in Australia, Dr. Midyett's interests turned toward teaching and academic radiology so he returned to the USA to complete a formal two-year Neuroradiology fellowship in 1999. While at the University of North Carolina, Chapel Hill, he trained with Drs. Mauricio Castillo and Suresh Mukherji.

Dr. Midyett's primary passion is teaching neuroradiology, and he has been involved in teaching residents and fellows for the last two decades at large teaching hospitals including Howard University Hospital in DC. He is a senior member of the ASNR and holds a current Certificate of Added Qualification in Neuroradiology by the American Board of Radiology.

Dr. Midyett has authored more than 100 scientific publications including book chapters and peer-reviewed articles. His first book *Orbital Imaging*, co-authored by Dr. Mukherji, has been well received and is currently published in English, Spanish, and Portuguese. *Skull Base Imaging: The Essentials* follows the same general format as its predecessing publication and continues to depict imaging for the complex anatomy and pathology of the skull base.

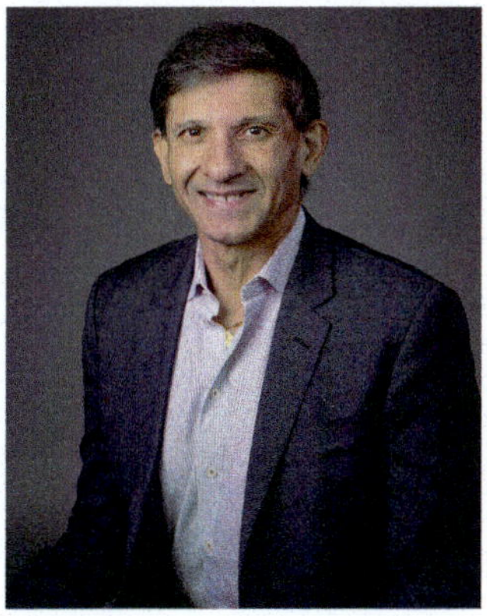

Suresh K. Mukherji, MD, MBA, FACR received his M. D. degree from Georgetown University (1987) and M.B.A. from the University of Michigan (2013). He completed his Radiology residency at the Brigham and Women's Hospital, Harvard Medical School, in 1992. He was a Neuroradiology Fellow, with emphasis on head and neck imaging, at the University of Florida in Gainesville, Florida, from 1992 to 1994. Dr. Mukherji is a recognized authority in Head & Neck and Neuroradiology and has been an active contributor to the neuroradiology literature by authoring over 400 scientific manuscripts and book chapters and has written or edited 13 textbooks. He has been an invited speaker on nearly 400 occasions. Dr. Mukherji's primary interests have been focused on investigating emerging metabolic and physiologic imaging techniques to evaluate head and neck cancer and to differentiate recurrent tumor from post-therapeutic changes in previously treated patients. These technologies include imaging with fluorodeoxyglucose analogues imaged with prototype Single Photon Emission Computed Tomography, Gamma Cameras, standard PET, and CT-PET. Other metabolic and physiologic imaging techniques he has investigated include Thallium-201, magnetic resonance spectroscopy, CT perfusion, and CT spectral imaging.

Quick Decoder for Acronyms and Abbreviations

A	"Aunt Minnie"	Common radiology term for
		a familiar face we know
		because it looks that way
	ABC	Aneurysmal Bone Cyst
	AC	Arachnoid Cyst
	ACC	Adenoid Cystic Carcinoma,
	ACF	Anterior Cranial Fossa
	ADC	Apparent Diffusion Coefficient
	ADF	Anisotropic Diffusion Filtering
	AFM	Anterior Fossa Meningioma
	AFRS	Allergic Fungal Rhinosinusitis
	AFS	Allergic Fungal Sinusitis
	AIFS	Acute Invasive Fungal Sinusitis
	AKA	Also Known As
	AP	Anterior to Posterior; Antrochoanal Polyp
	APC	Adenomatous Polyposis Coli
	AR	Androgen Receptor
	AV	Arteriovenous
	AVF	Arteriovenous Fistula
	AVM	Arteriovenous Malformation
	Ax	Axial or Transverse
B	BBB	Blood Brain Barrier
	BC	Before Christ
	BCC	Basal Cell Carcinoma
	BMT	Bone Marrow Transplant
	BMT	Benign Mixed Tumor
	BOLD	Blood-Oxygen-Level-Dependent
	BP	Blood Pressure
	BRAF OR B-Raf	BRAF Gene encodes B-Raf Protein
	β	Beta
	β2 transferrin	CSF protein
C	cm	Centimeter
	Ca^{++}	Calcification, Calcifications
	CC	Clivus Chordoma or Craniocaudal
	CCA	Carotid Cavernous Aneurysm
	CCC	Cylindrical Cell Carcinoma
	CCF	Carotid-Cavernous Fistula
	CCP	Convoluted Cerebriform Pattern
	CD	Choroidal Detachment
	CDC	Centers for Disease Control and Prevention
	CECT	Contrast Enhanced Computed Tomography
	CG	Cholesterol Granuloma
	CGPA	Cholesterol Granuloma of the Petrous Apex
	cGy	Centigray radiation dose measurement
	CHARGE Syndrome	Coloboma, Heart anomalies, Choanal Atresia, Retardation of growth and development Genital and Ear Abnormalities
	CHF	Congestive Heart Failure
	CISS	Chaos in the Steady State (Imaging Protocol)

	CLL	Chronic Lymphocytic Leukemia	
	CML	Chronic Myeloid Leukemia	
	CMV	Cytomegalovirus	
	CN	Cranial Nerve	
	CN I	Cranial Nerve I	Olfactory Nerve
	CN II	Cranial Nerve II	Optic Nerve
	CN III	Cranial Nerve III	Ophthalmic Nerve
	CN IV	Cranial Nerve IV	Trochlear Nerve
	CN IX	Cranial Nerve IX	Glossopharyngeal Nerve
	CN V	Cranial Nerve V	Trigeminal Nerve
	CN V1	Ophthalmic Branch of Trigeminal Nerve	
	CN V2	Maxillary Branch of Trigeminal Nerve	
	CN V3	Mandibular Branch of Trigeminal Nerve	
	CN VI	Cranial Nerve VI	Abducens Nerve
	CN VII	Cranial Nerve VII	Facial Nerve
	CN VIII	Cranial Nerve VIII	Vestibulocochlear Nerve
	CN X	Cranial Nerve X	Vagus Nerve
	CN XI	Cranial Nerve XI	Spinal Accessory Nerve
	CN XII	Cranial Nerve XII	Hypoglossal Nerve
	CNS	Central Nervous System	
	COACH Syndrome	Cerebellar vermis hypoplasia, Oligophrenia, Congenital ataxia, Coloboma, Hepatic Fibrosis	
	CPA	CerebelloPontine Angle	
	CPA-IAC	CerebelloPontine Angle- Internal Auditory Canal	
	CR	Craniopharyngioma	
	CRP	C-Reactive Protein	
	CS	Cavernous Sinus, Chondrosarcoma, Cervical Spine	
	CSA	Cavernous Sinus Aneurysm	
	CSF	CerebroSpinal Fluid	
	CST	Cavernous Sinus Thrombosis	
	CT	Computed Tomography	
	CTA	CT Angiography	
	CTC	CT Cisternography	
	CTD	CT Dacrocystography	
	CTV	CT Venography	
	CVJ	Cranio Vertebral Junction	
	CVT	Cerebral Venous Thrombosis	
D	DCC	Deleted in Colon Cancer	
	DDR	Distal Dural Ring	
	DDx	Differential Diagnosis	
	DFS	Disease Free Survival	
	DI	Diabetes Insipidus	
	DNA	DeoxyriboNucleic Acid	
	DSA	Digital Subtraction Angiography	
	DTI	Diffusion Tensor Imaging	
	DTPA	Diethylene Triamine Penta Acetic Acid	
	DWI	Diffusion Weighted Imaging	
	DWM	Dandy-Walker Malformation	
E	EAC	External Auditory Canal	
	EBRT	Electron Beam Radiation Therapy	
	EBV	Epstein-Barr Virus	
	EC	Epidermoid Cyst	
	ECA	External Carotid Artery	
	ECD	Erdheim-Chester Disease	
	ED	Emergency Department	
	EH	Extramedullary Hematopoiesis	
	EMP	Extramedullary Plasmacytoma	
	EN	Ectopic Neurohypophysis	
	ENB	Esthesioneuroblastoma	
	ENT	Ear, Nose, Throat	

	EOM	Extraocular Muscle or Extra-Ocular Motion
	EPP	Ectopic Posterior Pituitary
	↓EOM	Decreased Extra-ocular Motion
	ES	Ewing's Sarcoma
	ESR	Eyrthrocyte Sedimentation Rate
	EWS Gene	RNA binding gene associated with Ewing's Sarcoma
F	^{18}F FDG PET /CT	Fluoride 18, fluorodexyglucose
		Positron Emission Tomography/CT
	FAP	Familial Adenomatous Polyposis
	Fat-Sat	Fat Saturation Technique in MRI
	FB	Foreign Body
	FD	Fibrous Dysplasia
	FDG	FluDeoxyGlucose
	FDG-PET	Fludeoxyglucose Positron Emmission
		Tomography
	FDG-PET CT	Fludeoxyglucose Positron Emmission
		Tomography with Computed Tomography
	FH	Family History
	FIESTA	fast imaging employing steady state acquisition (by GE)
	FLAIR	Fluid Attenuated Inversion Recovery
	fMRI	Functional MRI
	FOM	Floor of Mouth
	FS	FibroSarcoma
G	Ga^{67}	Radioisotope of Gallium 67
	GCG	Giant Cell Granuloma
	GCT	Giant Cell Tumor
	Gd	Gadolinium
	GDC	Gugliemi Detachable Coils
	GFAP Stain	A Stain performed for glial fibrillary acidic
		protein, found in glial cells
	GH	Growth Hormone
	GI	Gastrointestinal
	GJ	Glomus Jugulare
	GJP	Glomus Jugulare Paraganglioma
	GKS	Gamma Knife Surgery
	GNAS	G Subunit-regulatory protein
		gene at locus at 20q13.2-q13.3
	GO	Graves Orbitopathy
	GRE	GRadient Echo
	GS	Granulocytic Sarcoma
	G-subS G	Protein receptors
	GSW	Gunshot Wound
	GU	GenitoUrinary

H	H&E	Hematoxylin & Eosin
	H&N	Head and Neck
	HA	Headache
	HAART	Highly Active AntiRetroviral Therapy
	HASH1	gene involved in olfactory neuronal differentiation
	HB	HemangioBlastoma
	HBO	HyperBaric Oxygen
	HCMV	Human CytoMegaloVirus
	HESX1	Mutations in this gene are associated with septooptic dysplasia
	HH	Hypothalamic Hamartoma
	HIV/AIDS	Human immunodeficiency virus/ Acquired immunodeficiency syndrome
	HLA-DQB1	gene providing instructions for producing a protein Several alleles associated with increased risk for type II diabetes
	HPC	Hemangiopericytoma
	HPT	Hyperparathyroidism
	HPV	Human Papilloma Virus
	HRCT	High Resolution Computed Tomography
	HSD	Hypertrophic Sinus Disease
	HU	Hounsfield Units
	Hyams	Hyams Histologic Grading System
	hypoglobus	inferior globe displacement
I	I^{125}	Radioisotope of Iodine 125
	I^{131}	Radioisotope of Iodine 131
	IAC	Internal Auditory Canal
	ICA	Internal Carotid Artery
	ICH	Intracranial Hemorrhage
	ICP	Intra Cranial Pressure
	IFS	Invasive Fungal Sinusitis
	IIP	Increased Intracranial Pressure
	ILS	Intralabyrinthine Schwannoma
	IM	Intraosseous Meningiomas
	IMRT	Intensity Modulated Radiotherapy
	INH	Infundibular NeuroHypophysitis
	IOI	Idiopathic Orbital Inflammation or Idiopathic Orbital Pseudotumor
	IOP	Idiopathic Orbital Pseudotumor
	IOP or ↑ OP	Increased Orbital Pressure
	IP	Inverted Papilloma
	iso-	isointense
	ISSVA	International Society for the Study of Vascular Anomalies
	IV	IntraVenous
J	JAF	Juvenile Angiofibroma
	JFP	Jugular Foramen Paraganglioma
	JNA	Juvenile Nasopharyngeal Angiofibroma
	JNAAR	Juvenile Nasopharyngeal Angiofibroma Androgen Receptor Genetic receptor pathway encoding transcription factors SOX4 and AP-2a and members the Wnt/Beta-catenin signaling pathway
	JPA	Juvenile Pilocytic Astrocytoma
K	KIT	Gene abnormal in mucosal melanoma patients
L	LCH	Langerhans Cell Histiocytosis
	LM	Lymphatic Malformation
	LOH	Loss of Heterozygosity

M	M:F	Male to Female Ratio
	M:F= 1:1	Male to Female Ratio is 1 to 1
	MA	Mycotic aneurysm
	MALT	Mucosa Associated Lymphoid Tissue
	MCA	Middle Cerebral Artery
	MCF	Middle Cranial Fossa
	MCM	Mega Cisterna Magna
	MDCT	Multidetector CT
	MEC	MucoEpidermoid Carcinoma
	MEN	Multiple Endocrine Neoplasia
	MEN 1	Multiple Endocrine Neoplasia Type 1
	MEN 2	Multiple Endocrine Neoplasia Type 2
	MGS	Morning Glory Syndrome
	MIBG	MetaIodoBenzylGuanidine
	MM	Multiple Myeloma
	MMF	Mycophenolic acid, AKA: mycophenolate
	MOG	Malignant optic glioma
	MPR	Multiplanar Reconstruction
	MR	Magnetic Resonance
	MRA	Magnetic Resonance Angiography
	MRD	Magnetic Resonance Dacrocystography
	MRI	Magnetic Resonance Imaging
	MRS	Magnetic Resonance Spectroscopy
	MRSA	Methicillin Resistant Staphylococcus Aureus
	MRV	Magnetic Resonance Venogram
	MS	Multiple Sclerosis
	MTHFR	Gene involved in Folic Acid metabolism
	myopia	nearsightedness
N	NAA	N-acetyl-aspartate is an amino acid
		Neural osmolyte involved in brain fluid balance
		Source of acetate for lipid an myelin synthysis
		Surrogate marker of neuronal damage
	NB	Note Well
	NCAM	Neural Cell Adhesion Molecule
	NCC	Neurocysticercosis
	NE	Neurenteric Cyst
	NEC	Neuroendocrine Carcinoma
	NECs	Neuroendocrine Carcinomas
	NECT	Non Enhanced Computed Tomography
	NET	NeuroEndocrine Tumor
	NF	Neurofibromatosis, Neurofibroma
	NF- I	Neurofibromatosis Type I
	NF1	Neurofibromatosis Type I
	NF2	Neurofibromatosis Type II
	NFE	Nasofrontal Encephalocele
	NF-II	Neurofibromatosis Type II
	NG	Nasal Glioma
	NHL	Non-Hodgkin's Lymphoma
	NK/T Cell Lymphoma	rare type of non-Hodgkin lymphoma
	NKSCC	Nonkeratinizing squamous cell carcinoma
	NPC	Nasopharyngeal Carcinoma
	NPTC	Nasopharyngeal Type Undifferentiated Ca
	NRAS	gene providing instructions for making
		a protein called N-Ras that is involved
		primarily in regulating cell division
	NS	Neurosarcoidosis
	NSGCT	Non-seminomatous germ cell tumors
	NTD	Neural Tube Defects

O	OCH	Orbital Cavernous Hemangioma, Ocular Cavernous Hemangioma
	OGM	Olfactory Groove Meningioma
	OGS	Osteogenic Sarcoma
	ON	Optic Nerve
	OS	OsteoSarcoma
	OSA	OsteoSarcoma
	OVV	Orbital Venous Varix
P	P32	Phosphorus-32 is a radioactive isotope of phosphorus
	PA	Petrous Apex; Pituitary Adenoma
	PAS	Periodic acid-Schiff (PAS) stain
	PAX2 gene	Paired box gene 2
	PAX3 gene	Paired box gene 3 Involved in neural tube closure
	PCF	Posterior Cranial Fossa
	PCNSL	Primary CNS Lymphoma
	PD	Proton Density
	PDR	Proximal Dural Ring
	PE	Physical Examination
	PES	Partially Empty Sella
	PET	Positron Emission Tomography
	PFAC	Posterior Fossa Arachnoid Cyst
	PFM	Posterior Fossa Meningioma
	PMMA	Polymethylmethacrylate
	PNET	Primitive Neuroectodermal Tumor
	PNF	Plexiform NeuroFibroma
	PNS	Paranasal Sinus; Perineural Spread; Perineural Tumor Spread
	POF	Petro-Occipital Fissure
	post-Gd	post Gadolinium
	PPF	PterygoPalatine Fossa
	pPNETs-ETs	Primitive peripheral neuroectodermal tumor-Ewing's Tumor
	pRb	Retinoblastoma Protein
	PRN	Latin "pro re nata" when needed
	PSIS	Pituitary Stalk Interruption Syndrome
	PTC	Pseudotumor Cerebri
	Pts	Patients
	PVA	Polyvinyl Alcohol
R	R/O	Rule Out
	RANK	Receptor Activator of Nuclear factor Kappa B
	RANK/RANKL	Signaling pathway producing extraordinarily exuberant osteoclastic proliferation
	RANKL	Receptor Activator of Nuclear factor Kappa B Ligand
	RB	RetinoBlastoma
	RB1	Retinoblastoma Tumor Suppressor Gene
	RB-1	Retinoblastoma Tumor Suppressor Gene
	rCBV	Relative Cerebral Blood Volume
	RCC	Rathke's Cleft Cyst
	RIOS	Radiation Induced OsteoSarcomas
	RIS	Radiation Induced Sarcoma
	RLF	RetroLental Fibroplasia
	RMS	RhabdoMyoSarcoma
	RNC	Radionuclide Cisternography
	RPLN	Retropharyngeal Lymph Nodes
	RPN	Retropharyngeal Nodes
	RT, RöRx	Radiation Therapy

S	S100	Family of low-molecular weight proteins encoded by a family of genes
	SAH	Subarachnoid Hemorrhage
	SBC	Skull Base Chondrosarcoma
	SBL	Skull Base Lymphoma
	SBO	Skull Base Osteomyelitis
	SBP	Solitary Bone Plasmacytoma
	SBRT1	Stereotactic Radiation Therapy for Pediatric Sarcomas
	SCC	Squamous Cell Carcinoma
	SCC LG	Squamous Cell Carcinoma of Lacrimal Gland
	SCCA	Squamous Cell Carcinoma
	SCRT	Stereotatic Conformal Radiotherapy
	SD	Standard Deviation
	SDH	Subdural Hemorrhage
	SHMT1	Gene involved in Folic Acid metabolism
	SI	Signal Intensity
	SJGD2	Monoclonal Antibody Therapy in Younger Patients
	SMARCB1	A Protein Coding Gene
	SMARCE1	A core subunit predicted to mediate the interaction between the SWI/SNF complex and transcriptional activators/ repressors, as well as DNA binding.
	SNHL	Sensoneural Hearing Loss
	SNM	Sinonasal Melanoma
	SNR	Signal to noise ratio
	SNUC	Sinonasal Undifferentiated Carcinoma
	SOD	Septo-Optic Dysplasia
	Sonic Hedgehog	A secreted protein called "SONIC HEDGEHOG" (SHH [MIM 600725]), which sets off a chain of events in target cells, leading to the activation and repression of target genes by transcription factors in the Gli family
	SOV	Superior Ophthalmic Vein
	SQ	Subcutaneous
	STD	Sexually Transmitted Disease
	STIR	Short Tau Inversion Recovery, Special MRI Sequence
	SUFU	Negative regulator of hedgehog signaling
	SWI	Susceptibility Weighted Imaging
T	T1	Basic MRI pulse sequence
	T1 + Gd	Gadolinium Enhanced T1 Imaging
	T1 Gd	Gadolinium Enhanced T1 Imaging
	T1 WI	T1 Weighted Images
	T2	Basic MRI pulse sequence
	T2 WI	T2 Weighted Images
	Tc^{99m}	Radioactive Isotope of Technicium, 99 m
	TCA	Traumatic Cerebral aneurysm
	TCC	Transitional Cell Carcinoms
	TED	Thyroid Eye Disease
	TEs	Time to Echos (s)
	THS	Tolosa-Hunt Syndrome
	TM	Tympanic Membrane
	TMN	Tumor Node Metastasis Classification System
	TO	Telangiectatic Osteosarcoma
	TOF	Time-of-Flight
	TOF-MRA	Time-of-Flight MRA
	TS	Tuberous Sclerosis, Trigeminal Schwannoma
	TSH-R	Thyroid Stimulating Hormone - R (An Antigen)

U	U.S.	United States
	UCLA	University of California Los Angeles
	URI	Upper Respiratory Infection
	US	Ultrasound
V	VANGL1	Gene which encodes for glucose metabolism
	VHL	Von Hippel-Lindau Syndrome
	VLM	Venous Lymphatic Malformation
	VS	Vestibular Schwannoma
W	WG	Wegener's Granulomatosis
	WHO	World Health Organization
	WI	Weighted Images
	1^0	Primary
1		
	2^0	Secondary
2	2D-TOF	Two Dimensional Time-of-Flight
	3D-CRT	Three Dimensional Conformal Radiation Therapy
3	3D TOF	Three Dimensional Time-of-Flight
	3D	Three Dimension
	+	plus
	−	minus
	±	plus or minus, more or less
	~	about, approximately
	>	Greater Than, More Than
	<	Less Than
	≤	Less Than or equal to
	≥	More than or equal to
	↑	Increased 1+
	↑↑	Mildly Increased 2+
	↑↑↑	Moderately Increased 3+
	↑↑↑↑	Highly Increased 4+
	↓	Decreased

Overview

All agree that the skull base forms the cranial cavity's floor separating brain from facial structures below. Aficionados affirm its intricate anatomy and plethora of pathology combined to create diagnostic and therapeutic dilemmas best addressed by a team of dedicated professionals.

Traditionally the skull base is divided into anterior, middle, and posterior sections. Much like real estate where the most important thing is location, location, and location, we can clearly do better by being more specific about location. So, we elected to further divide the anatomy and pathology as follows:

Pituitary Region
Cerebellopontine Angle
Anterior Cranial Fossa/Anterior Skull Base
Middle Cranial Fossa
Posterior Cranial Fossa
Craniovertebral Junction
Inflammatory Disease
Sarcomas
Skull Base and Facial Foramina

While we are aware that this volume cannot consider every skull base abnormality in 50 cases (and their differentials), we believe this is a significant start toward a case-based approach for this complex subject. And in the process, we emphasize essential concepts useful for interpreting cases which may not appear in this treatise. For those who wish to review anatomy, Chap. 51 on skull base and facial foramina is undoubtedly as much (and probably more) than you ever wanted to know. But it is there as a handy reference when needed. And, when all is said and done, you will probably thank us less for what we put into the textbook, and more for what we left out. In fact, the temporal bone has been largely ignored as it has been more completely covered by other excellent dedicated monographs. This thesis looks at the "rest of the story" and hopefully will provide *essentials* you need to know.

Part I

Pituitary Region

1 Rathke's Cleft Cyst

Pertinent Points

- *Definition:* A Rathke's cleft cyst (RCC) arises from faulty development of Rathke's pouch, resulting in a fluid-filled cyst in the posterior portion of the anterior pituitary.
- Rathke's cleft cysts can range from 2 to 40 mm in diameter.
- Gender preference: F:M = 2:1
- The most common theory about the origin of RCCs is that they are derived from true remnants of the embryologic Rathke's pouch [1].
- *Classic Clue*: A pack of clinicians come to confront you about a cystic sellar mass which seems to be confined to the pituitary. A middle-aged female patient has been having headaches and is now very upset about her neurosurgical referral and seems certain she's "going to die from a brain tumor."

Imaging

General Imaging Features

- RCCs are sharply marginated and discretely defined on CT and MRI [2].
- Most RCCs *do not* enlarge the sella [2].

CT Features

- Well-circumscribed, cystic sellar mass sometimes showing suprasellar extension [3].
- CT attenuation varies with content and while more often hypo-, can be iso- or hyper-attenuating [2, 3].
- Complex cysts can contain septations.
- CT has one advantage over MRI with its sensitivity to small amounts of calcium.
- Although some RCCs contain calcifications, the presence of calcifications implies an alternative diagnosis such as craniopharyngioma [4].
- CT shows superiority to MRI in demonstrating adjacent bony remodeling [4].
- Enhancement is usually not a feature unless leakage of cyst contents causes inflammation of adjacent structures.
- Because of variability in findings, CT alone cannot establish a definitive diagnosis. Clinical, biochemical, pathologic, and MRI findings must be considered.

MRI Features

- Although frequently not the first examination to encounter RCC, MRI is clearly the modality of choice for its evaluation.
- MRI signal is variable on both T1 and T2 because of variations in content of cholesterol, protein, and blood products each of which may demonstrate different MRI signals [2].
- T1 typically shows homogeneous low signal similar to CSF (Fig. 1.1a).
- T2 is ↑ similar to CSF (Fig. 1.1b).
- T1 Gd sometimes shows a thin rim of normally enhancing pituitary [2] (Fig. 1.1d).

F. A. Midyett, S. K. Mukherji, *Skull Base Imaging*, https://doi.org/10.1007/978-3-030-46447-9_1

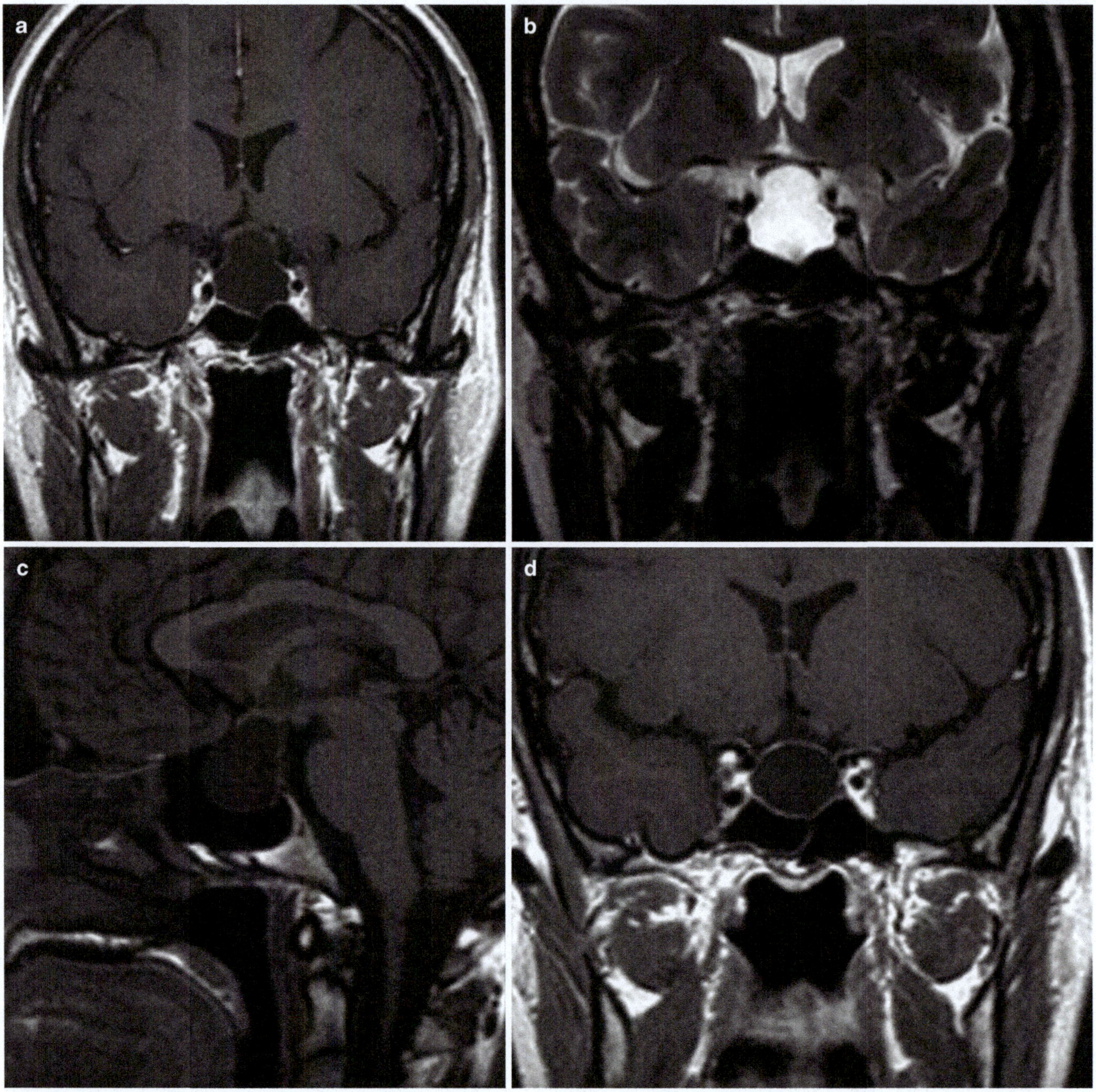

Fig. 1.1 (**a**) Coronal T1 shows large sellar and suprasellar mass with "waist" at the sellar diaphragm, extending cranially to displace the chiasm. The mass has a homogeneous low T1 signal similar to CSF. (**b**) Coronal T2 shows large sellar and suprasellar mass with "waist" at the sellar diaphragm, extending cranially to displace the chiasm. The mass has a homogeneous high T2 signal similar to CSF suggesting it is a fluid-filled cyst. (**c**) Sagittal T1 shows large sellar and suprasellar mass with "waist" at the sellar diaphragm, elevating the chiasm cranially. The mass has a homogeneous low T1 signal similar to CSF. (**d**) Coronal T1 Gd shows large sellar and suprasellar mass. The contents of the mass show a homogeneous low T1 signal similar to CSF. No enhancement within the mass, although close comparison shows the thin enhancing rim of normal pituitary surrounding lesion

Clinical Issues

Presentation

- Asymptomatic Rathke's cleft cysts are common, being found in up to 1/4 of autopsies.
- Patients with symptomatic Rathke's cleft cysts may have hypo-functioning pituitaries with multiple endocrinopathies [1].
- Younger patients having hypopituitarism from an early age generally have growth retardation [1].
- The second most common expression is visual field defects caused by chiasmatic compression.
- The third most common complaint is headache with >50% being frontal.
- RCCs can also cause low libido or impotence in men and hyperprolactinemia in women.
- RCCs may be associated with pituitary adenomas [5].

Epidemiology and Pathology

- The most common theory for the origin of RCC is that they are derived from true remnants of the embryologic Rathke's pouch [1].
- Rathke's pouch typically reverts to a narrow Rathke's cleft which usually regresses.
- Persistence and enlargement of Rathke's cleft are considered to cause RCC.
- RCCs are benign, pseudostratified epithelium-lined intrasellar cysts [2].
- RCCs are usually round, ovoid, or dumbbell shaped.
- Most are <2 cm but can vary in size from 2 mm to 40 mm.
- Its cystic capsule can vary from transparent to tan, pink, gray, red, white, blue, yellow, or green.
- The cystic fluid is usually yellow but can be clear, white, gray, or green.
- The presence of ciliated epithelial and mucous-secreting cells in a pituitary gland is pathognomonic for RCC [5].

Treatment and Prognosis

- The most common treatment for symptomatic cysts is transsphenoidal surgery with biopsy, partial excision, and drainage [6, 7].
- Complete excision is problematic because of potential bleeding and unnecessary damage to vital structures.
- Patients requiring a craniotomy approach face a recurrence rate which is twice that accompanying transsphenoidal surgery [8].
- High-dose steroid therapy has been shown to reduce the size of cysts showing inflammatory changes.
- Endoscopic endonasal approaches show some signs of improved outcomes.
- Post treatment prognosis is usually excellent with recurrence in <10% of cases.

Differential Diagnosis

The differential of sellar cysts includes:

A. Craniopharyngioma (CR)
- Craniopharyngiomas commonly contain mixed cystic and enhancing solid components.
- Craniopharyngiomas are commonly calcified.
- Like liquid products in your automobile, the varying viscosity of craniopharyngioma's cystic fluid fluctuates from yellowish proteinaceous fluid to classic "crank-case oil" containing cholesterol and blood products.
- Craniopharyngiomas infiltrate adjacent structures on MRI, not a feature of RCC.
- CRs can occasionally enlarge and/or erode the sella. Most RCC's *do not* enlarge the sella [2].
- RCCs are usually smaller, less heterogeneous, and nonenhancing with *no* solid components.
- See Chap. 3, Craniopharyngioma.

B. Arachnoid cyst (AC)
- Contains fluid identical to CSF.
- See Chap. 7, Intrasellar Arachnoid Cyst.

C. Epidermoid cyst
- Often slightly hyperintense to CSF.
- Sometimes shows a bumpy border.
- Restricted diffusion with bright DWI and corresponding dark defect on ADC.
- See Chap. 9, Epidermoid Cyst.

D. Cystic pituitary adenoma
- Rarely pituitary adenomas can occur concomitantly with RCC.
- Having both cystic and solid components could cause confusion regarding a craniopharyngioma.
- See Chap. 2, Pituitary Adenoma.

E. Abscess
- Abscesses show thick enhancing rims. RCCs have a thin capsule which does not enhance, but they may have a thin rim of normally enhancing pituitary.
- Abscesses show shaggy irregular margins. RCCs are sharply marginated and discretely defined on CT and MRI related to their thin capsule [2].

A Closer Look

I. Fast Facts

- The rare group of solely suprasellar RCCs may require craniotomy and/or stereotactic aspiration.
- Some suggest that RCCs develop as the rostral out-pouching of the primitive oral cavity during the third to fourth gestational weeks. Failure to fully obliterate the out-pouching results in RCCs.

II. Historic Highlights

- 1913 Goldzieher first described RCC as an incidental autopsy finding.

Selected References

1. Voelker JL, Campbell RL, Muller J. Clinical, radiographic, and pathological features of symptomatic Rathke's cleft cysts. J Neurosurg. 1991;74(4):535–44.
2. Fischbein NJ, Dillon WP, Barkovich AJ. Teaching atlas of brain imaging. New York: Thieme; 2000. p. 55–7.
3. Nakasu Y, Isozumi T, Nakasu S, et al. Rathke's cleft cyst: computed tomographic scan and magnetic resonance imaging. Acta Neurochir. 1990;103(3–4):99–104.
4. Le BH, Towfighi J, Kapadia SB, et al. Comparative immunohistochemical assessment of craniopharyngioma and related lesions. Endocr Pathol. 2007;18(1):23–30.
5. Shin JL, Asa SL, Woodhouse LJ, et al. Cystic lesions of the pituitary: clinicopathological features distinguishing craniopharyngioma, Rathke's cleft cyst, and arachnoid cyst. J Clin Endocrinol Metab. 1999;84(11):3972–82.
6. Frank G, Sciarretta V, Mazzatenta D, Farneti G, Modugno GC, Pasquini E. Transsphenoidal endoscopic approach in the treatment of Rathke's cleft cyst. Neurosurgery. 2005;56(1):124–8; discussion 129.
7. Cavallo LM, Prevedello D, Esposito F, Laws ER Jr, Dusick JR, Messina A, et al. The role of the endoscope in the transsphenoidal management of cystic lesions of the sellar region. Neurosurg Rev. 2008;31(1):55–64; discussion 64.
8. Fager CA, Carter H. Intrasellar epithelial cysts. J Neurosurg. 1966;24(1):77–81.

Pituitary Adenoma

2

Pertinent Points

- Definition: Abnormal growth of pituitary cells cause pituitary tumors which comprise 10% of all brain tumors. Differences in biologic function can divide pituitary tumors into three convenient categories: benign adenoma, invasive adenoma, or carcinoma. By definition adenomas <10 mm are microadenomas, and adenomas >10 mm are macroadenomas.
- *Classic Clue*: Abrupt onset and progression of severe headache, visual field defects, ophthalmoplegia, and altered mental status in a patient who has a sellar mass. Clinicians can be concerned that the patient may have subarachnoid hemorrhage.
- AKA: Pituitary macroadenoma [by definition including those pituitary adenomas >10 mm]

Imaging

General Imaging Features

- Characteristic "figure of eight" or "Biker on a Harley" appearance on coronal imaging.
- The "waist" corresponds to the sellar diaphragm.
- Typically see both sellar and suprasellar components with sellar enlargement.
- Radiologic anatomic classification of pituitary adenomas [11]:
  - Stage I: Microadenomas <1 cm with no sellar expansion
  - Stage II: Macroadenomas ≥1 cm and may extend above sella
  - Stage III: Macroadenomas with sellar enlargement and invasion of the sellar floor or suprasellar extension
  - Stage IV: Sellar destruction (Fig. 2.1a–d)
- *Pituitary apoplexy* – general.
  - Clinically, pituitary apoplexy is caused by sudden pituitary infarction and may be hemorrhagic or "bland" (without hemorrhage).
  - This may occur within a normal or neoplastic gland but is more frequently found with pituitary adenoma where the gland outgrows its blood supply.
  - Clinical symptoms include severe headache, sudden loss of visual acuity, oculomotor palsies, ↓ sensorium, hypopituitarism, and subarachnoid irritation.

CT Features

- Typically exhibits expansion, erosion, and remodeling of sella.
- Tumor usually displays intermediate density.
- Hyperdensity suggests hemorrhage with "pituitary apoplexy."
- Pituitary apoplexy – CT
  - See pituitary apoplexy in *General Imaging Features*.
  - CT can show ↑ attenuation in the acute phase (approximately 3 days).
  - Subacute (4–30 days) and chronic (> 1 month) can be confused on CT with cystic degeneration, abscess, and non-hemorrhagic "bland" infarction [2].
  - MRI is usually more helpful in evaluation of subacute and chronic pituitary apoplexy cases.

MRI Features

- Combined sellar and suprasellar mass with "waist" at sellar diaphragm.
- Characteristic "figure of eight" or "Biker on Harley" appearance on coronal or sagittal imaging. (See Fig. 2.5a)
- Usually homogeneously isointense on both T1 and T2 (see below for pituitary apoplexy)

F. A. Midyett, S. K. Mukherji, *Skull Base Imaging*, https://doi.org/10.1007/978-3-030-46447-9_2

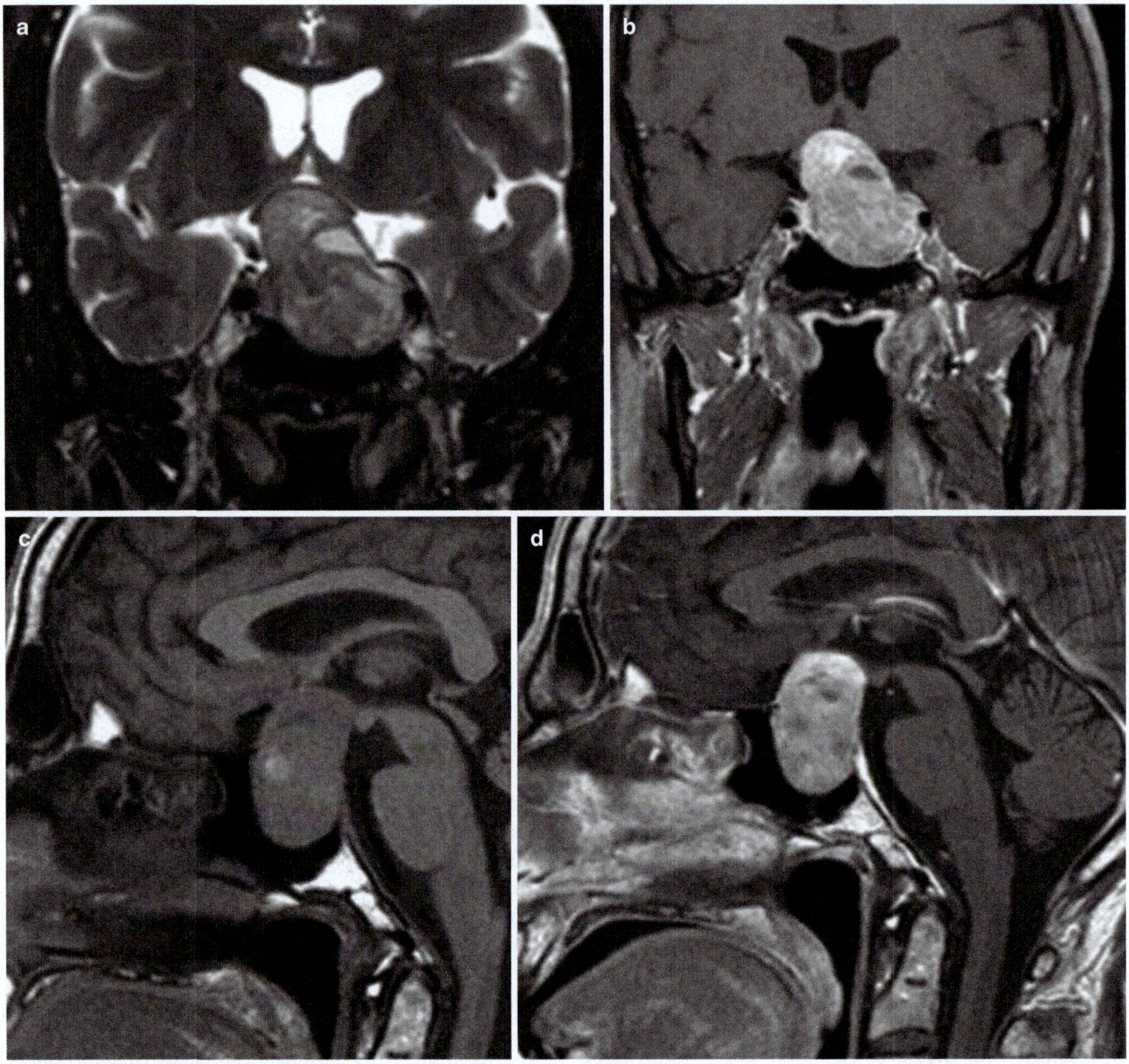

Fig. 2.1 (**a**) Coronal T2 shows large sellar and suprasellar mass extending cranially to displace the chiasm. The mass extends laterally into the left cavernous sinus, displacing and narrowing the left internal carotid artery. The mass is mildly heterogeneous with an area of necrosis superiorly on the left containing high signal fluid. (**b**) Coronal T1 Gd shows large sellar and suprasellar mass extending cranially to displace the chiasm and laterally displacing the cavernous sinuses and carotid arteries. The mass is mildly heterogeneous with an area of non-enhancing necrosis superiorly on the left. Tumor appears to incompletely encase the carotids on this image. This sequence better demonstrates extension into the left cavernous sinus narrowing the left internal carotid artery. (**c**) Sagittal T1 shows large sellar and suprasellar mass elevating chiasm cranially. The mass is relatively homogeneous except for small area of signal ↑ near its midportion anteriorly probably related to blood products in a small area of necrosis. The patient showed no sign of pituitary apoplexy. (**d**) Sagittal T1 Gd shows large sellar and suprasellar mass elevating the chiasm cranially. The mass has heterogeneous enhancement with multiple areas of ↓ enhancement, probably related to areas with marginal blood supply

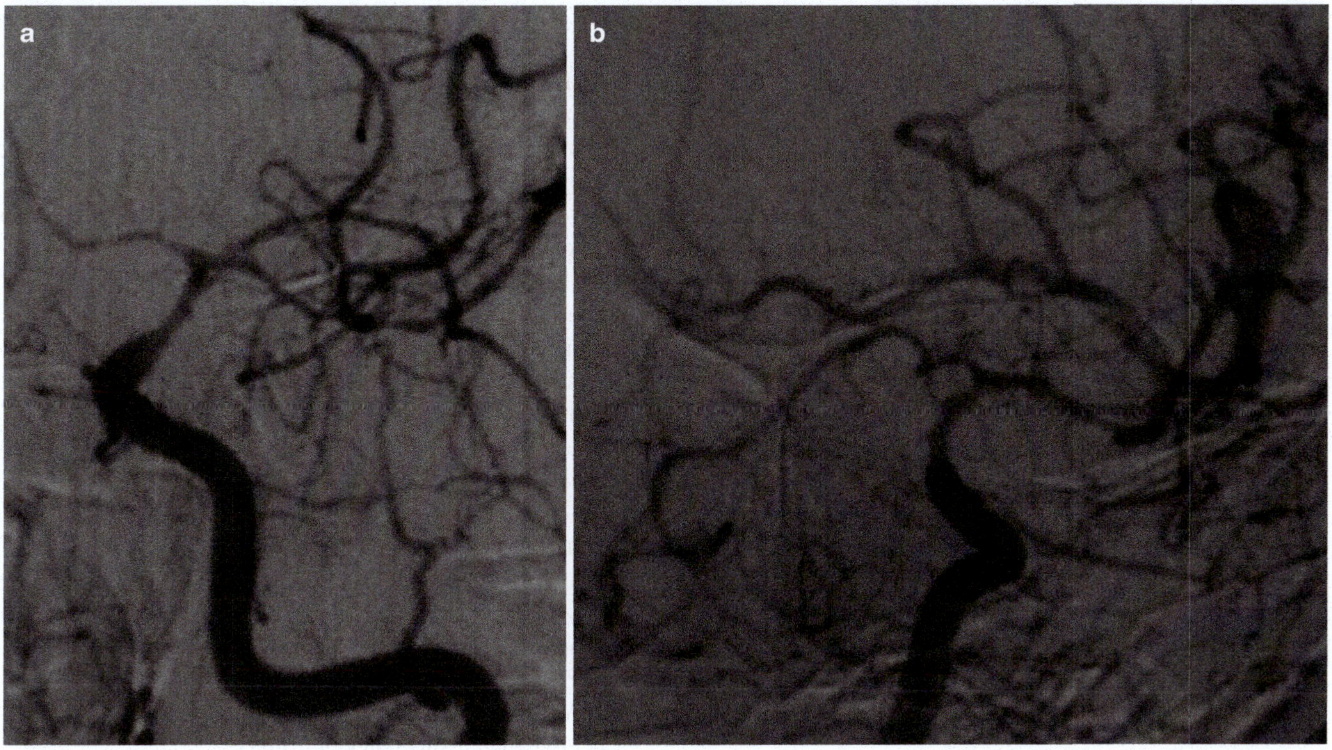

Fig. 2.2 (a, b) AP (a) and lateral (b) left ICA angiogram shows abrupt smooth tapered narrowing of cavernous ICA extending distally to involve the ICA bifurcation and proximal anterior and middle cerebral arteries. The narrowing is directly related to a pituitary adenoma which surrounded and narrowed these arteries

- Solid mass shows moderate homogeneous enhancement on T1 Gd.
- Typically displaces, encases, or invades cavernous sinus structures.
- Necrosis, hemorrhage, or cyst formation can cause significant signal alterations and aberrations.
- Pituitary adenomas if left unchecked often encase the carotid arteries, and the degree of encasement should be reported by the interpreting radiologist.
- Narrowing of the carotid arteries by pituitary adenomas is less frequent but clearly can be clinically problematic (see Fig. 2.2a, b Angiogram).
- If carotid artery narrowing is present and the diagnosis is not clear and/or established, meningioma should be considered.
- Postoperative pituitary images can be confusing.
  - Packing the sphenoid sinus with fat is common and causes signal which parallels that of fat.
  - This fat usually necroses over time and adopts a signal which more closely parallels that of residual or recurrent tumor.
- Pituitary apoplexy
  - See pituitary apoplexy – general (above).
  - Subacute hemorrhage (4 days to 1 month) shows significant hyperintensity on T1 images.
  - Like other intracranial infarctions, pituitary apoplexy can cause restricted diffusion, providing valuable early diagnostic information [3].
  - DWI show bright ↑ signal, and ADC map show corresponding ↓ signal "black hole."
  - No contrast enhancement.
- MR spectroscopy (MRS)
  - MRS has been suggested as a useful and safe noninvasive option for characterizing pituitary lesions, enabling patients to embark on proper medical care avoiding an invasive procedure as in the case of pituitary tuberculoma [10].

Clinical Issues

Presentation

- Visual field defects comprise some of the most common complaints from badly behaved macroadenomas by directly compressing the optic chiasm.
- The most common complaints comprise bitemporal hemianopsia.
- Invasion into the cavernous sinus can cause cranial nerve palsies.

- And the big thing that gets men to take that trip to the doctor:
  ↓ libido from hypopituitarism.
- And then there's "pituitary apoplexy."
  – This pathologic process is quite capable of getting anyone's attention!
  – It is related to sudden infarction with/without hemorrhage.
  – It occurs in ~10% of patients with pituitary adenomas.
  – The gland suddenly swells compressing adjacent structures (including but not limited to the optic chiasm).
  – Patients complain of sudden severe headache, loss of vision, ↓ sensorium, oculomotor palsies, or Addisonian crisis [5].
  – Patients may have subarachnoid hemorrhage (SAH) or have symptoms which mimic SAH.
  – A couple of thousand years ago, it may have taken a burning bush to get someone's attention, but in this day and age, pituitary apoplexy can still do the trick real fast!

Epidemiology and Pathology

- Differences in biologic function can divide pituitary tumors into three convenient categories: benign adenoma, invasive adenoma, or carcinoma.
- ~65% are benign adenomas, and ~35% are invasive adenomas. Pituitary carcinomas comprise ~0.1% (1 in 1000) [9].
- By definition adenomas ≤10 mm are microadenomas, and adenomas ≥10 mm are macroadenomas.
- Noninvasive and non-secreting pituitary adenomas are assumed to be benign.
- The prevalence of microadenomas varies from 15% to almost 25% when comparing autopsy to radiologic studies [7, 8].
- Most microadenomas are found as incidental findings (incidentalomas).
- Most macroadenomas are non-secreting and are the most common cause of hypopituitarism.
- 90% of patients with pituitary apoplexy have pituitary macroadenomas.
- 10% of patients with pituitary apoplexy occur in patients with otherwise "healthy" glands.
- Other predisposing factors for pituitary apoplexy include:
  – Medical treatment of a prolactinoma, particularly with bromocriptine [4]
  – Prior radiation therapy
  – Anticoagulation
  – Pregnancy (Sheehan syndrome)
  – Cerebral angiography
  – Trauma and surgery
  – Fluctuation of intracranial pressure (Fig. 2.3a, b)

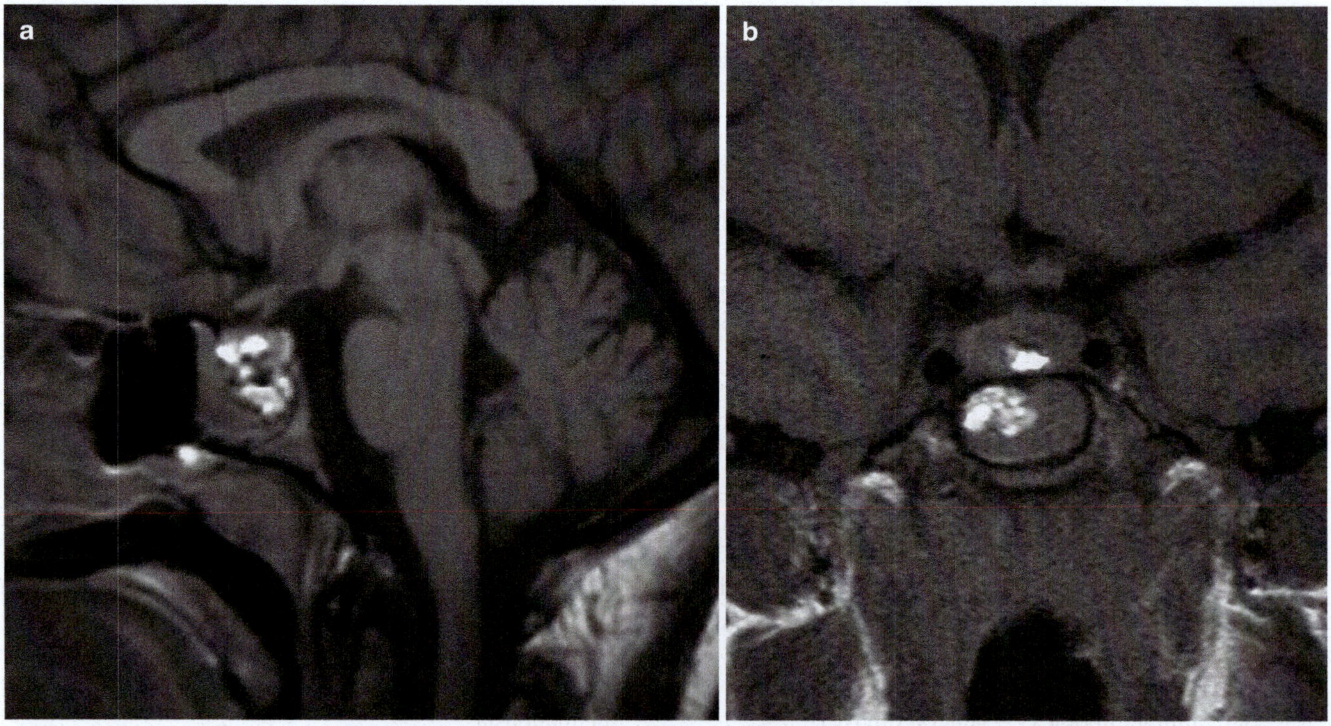

Fig. 2.3 (**a**, **b**) Sagittal (**a**) and coronal (**b**) T1 images show abnormal bright high signal located within the sella and in the adjacent sphenoid sinus. This high signal is from "fat packing" from prior a transsphenoidal approach for the patient's pituitary adenoma. While smaller than prior to surgery, the pituitary remains enlarged. Note dark areas adjacent fat from "chemical shift" artifact particularly in image (**a**)

Treatment and Prognosis

- Patients with pituitary adenomas frequently face watchful waiting as well as medical, surgical, or radiation therapy.
- Pituitary apoplexy is an emergency usually treated by steroids and prompt surgical decompression if there are significant neuro-ophthalmic signs or ↓ consciousness.
- Hormonally active prolactinomas may be treated with bromocriptine.
- Radiation therapy is usually reserved for incompletely resected and/or aggressive tumors.
- Prognosis for pituitary apoplexy is usually good with early diagnosis and aggressive treatment.
- Not all of the neurologic defects are reversible, so "time is of the essence."

Differential Diagnosis (DDx)

A. Craniopharyngioma

- Like liquids in your automobile, the varying viscosity of craniopharyngioma's cystic fluid fluctuates from yellowish proteinaceous fluid to classic "crank-case oil" containing cholesterol and blood byproducts.
- Craniopharyngiomas often have mixed cystic and enhancing solid components.
- Craniopharyngiomas are often calcified.
- Craniopharyngiomas infiltrate adjacent structures on MRI.
- Craniopharyngiomas can occasionally enlarge and/or erode the sella.
- See Chap. 3, Craniopharyngioma.

B. Rathke's Cleft Cyst (RCC)

- RCC usually does not erode sella.
- Cystic pituitary adenoma may be difficult to distinguish from RCC (see Figs. 2.4a–f).
- See Chap. 1, Rathke's Cleft Cyst.

C. Pituitary Metastasis

- Pituitary metastasis is rare, most commonly from lung and breast carcinoma.
- They less commonly have been reported from prostate, renal cell, lymphoma, leukemia, thyroid, plasmocytoma, and GI cancer [12].
- Metastasis usually does not enlarge the sella.
- Not surprisingly, metastases are more irregular than pituitary adenomas.
- Amazingly, some series show 6–29% of breast cancer patients develop pituitary metastasis [12].

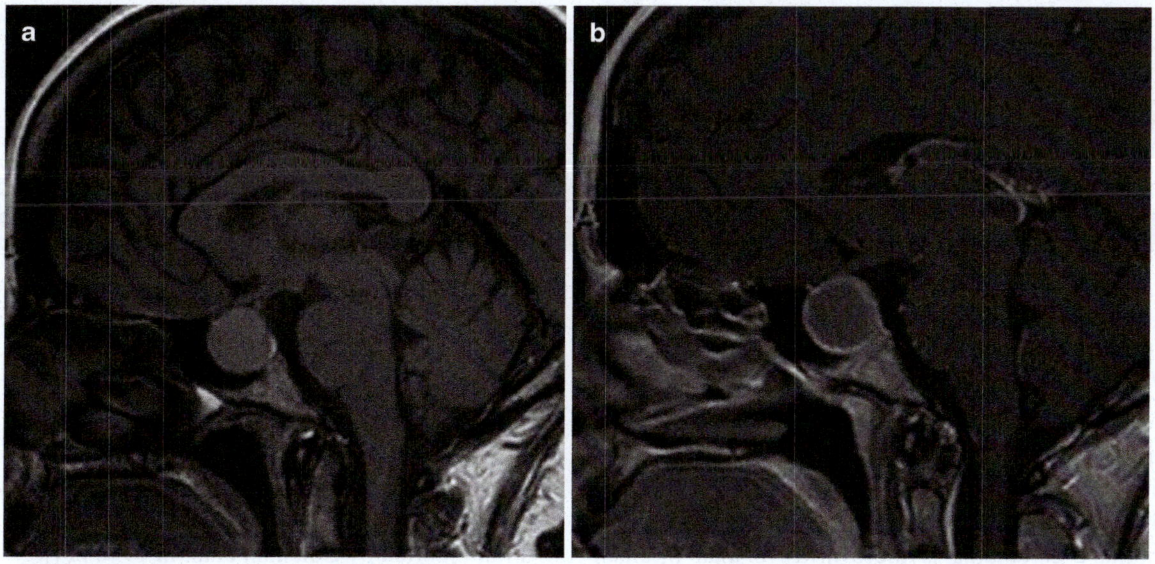

Fig. 2.4 (**a**, **b**) Sagittal (**a**) T1 and (**b**) T1 Gd images show low signal sellar and suprasellar mass extending superiorly to abut the chiasm. Avid rim enhancement

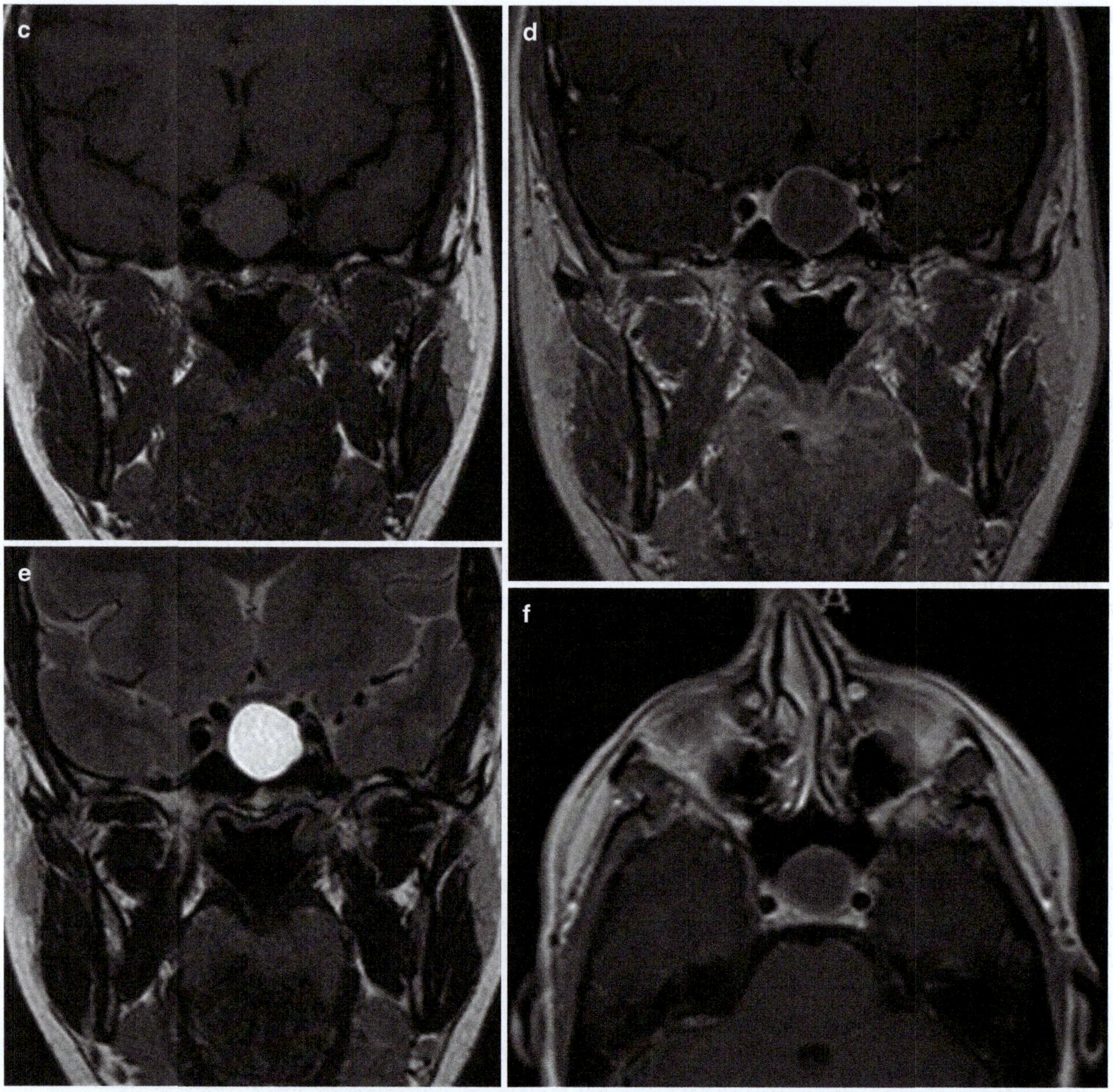

Fig. 2.4 (continued) (**c, d**) Coronal (**c**) T1 and (**d**) T1 Gd images show low signal sellar and suprasellar mass extending superiorly to abut and elevate the chiasm. Avid rim enhancement. (**e**) Coronal T2 image shows bright homogeneous signal sellar and suprasellar mass extending superiorly to abut and elevate the chiasm. (**f**) Axial T1 Gd shows cystic pituitary mass with slightly irregular enhancing rim. This was a cystic pituitary adenoma. This lesion appears similar to the RCC case (see Chap. 1) but shows several subtle differences

D. Pituitary Carcinoma

- Pituitary carcinoma is rare comprising ~0.1% (1 in 1000 primary pituitary tumors) [9].
  - Pituitary carcinoma is more invasive than pituitary adenoma.

E. Pituitary Abscess

- Abscesses show shaggy irregular margins [8].
- Abscesses show a thick enhancing rim.
  - Abscesses are often associated with sphenoid sinusitis.
  - Abscesses are usually void of hemorrhage.

F. Pituitary Tuberculoma

- Extremely rare entity even in regions endemic for TB.
- First reported by Coleman et al. in 1940 [14].
- Since the initial report in 1940, only 81 cases have been documented in the world's literature up to 2015 [13].
- Usually found in developing countries and/or immunocompromised individuals [10].
- Magnetic resonance spectroscopy is sometimes helpful in establishing the diagnosis [10].

A Closer Look

I. Fast Facts

- Non-hormone-secreting adenomas are frequently found as larger lesions than their more biologically boisterous hormone-secreting cousins.
- Macroadenomas account for 1/2 of suprasellar masses.
- Approximately 25% of patients with intrasellar hemorrhage have pituitary apoplexy [2].
- Sure, they say pituitary apoplexy is a *clinical diagnosis.* Hemorrhage can occur without apoplexy, and apoplexy can occur without hemorrhage.
- But, be sure and don't miss it. Otherwise, you may need a good malpractice lawyer!

II. Historic Highlights

- 1898 Bailey reported a fatal case of hemorrhagic pituitary tumor.
- 1905 German physician Bleibtreu documented pituitary apoplexy as a pathologic entity.
- 1950 Brougham, et al. described this pathology in detail in five post-mortem cases [6].

III. Genetics

- While 95% of pituitary adenomas are seemingly sporadic, only 5% are flagrantly familial.
- Familial pituitary adenomas are associated with multiple endocrine neoplasia type 1 (MEN1), the Carney complex (CNC), MEN4, and familial isolated pituitary adenomas (FIPA).
- These familial frequencies of pituitary adenomas should be identified as they are often more aggressive than their sporadic although more copious counterparts.
- Currently complicit genes include AIR, PRKAR1A, and CDKN1B (Fig. 2.5a–c) [15].

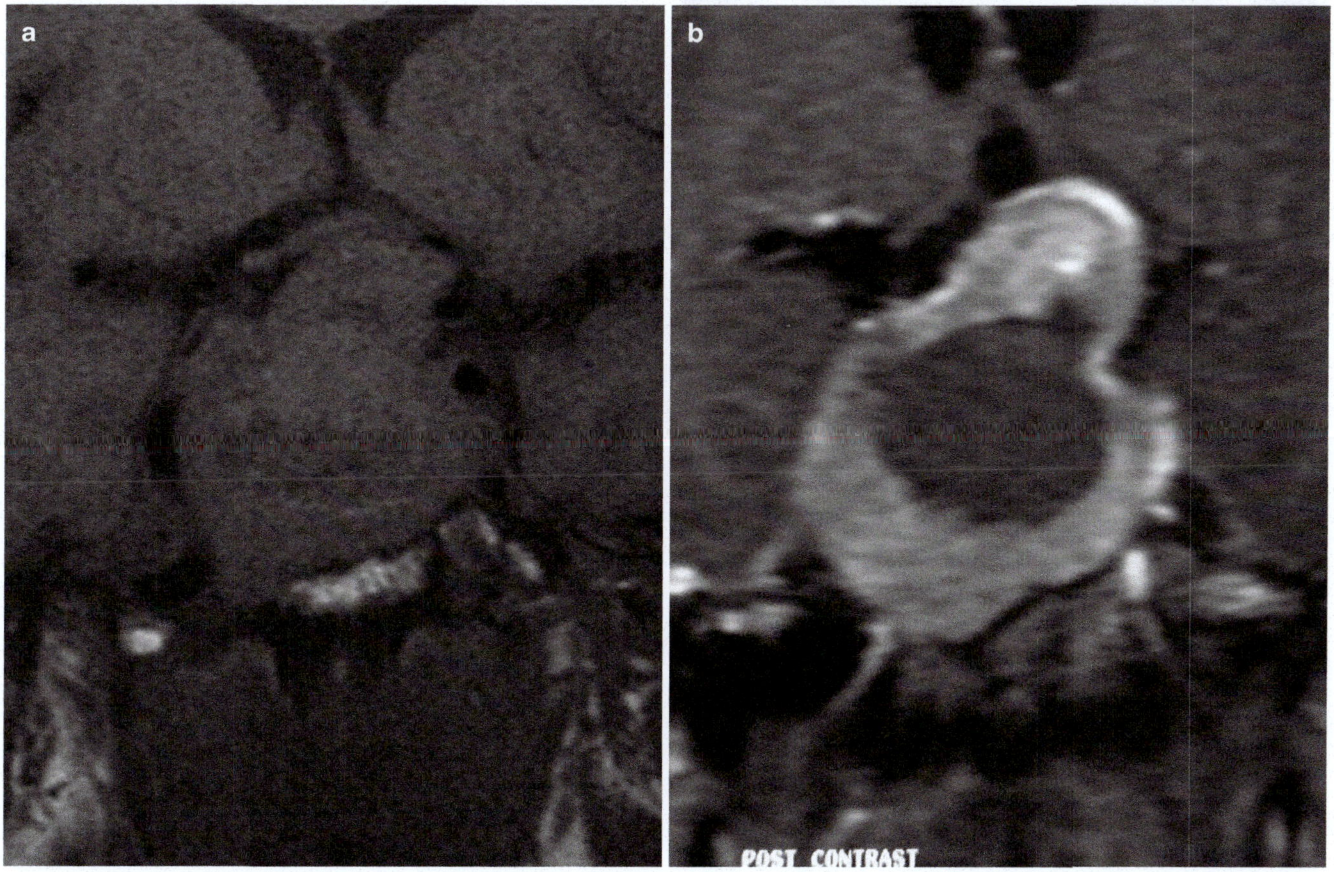

Fig. 2.5 (**a**) Coronal T1 shows huge sellar and suprasellar mass with "figure of eight" configuration abuts and elevates optic chiasm. Large area of heterogeneous signal in center of mass. (**b**) Coronal T1 Gd shows avid enhancement of sellar and suprasellar mass with "figure of eight" configuration abuts and elevates optic chiasm. Large non-enhancing area in center of mass related to prior debulking within this huge pituitary adenoma. The mass extends laterally to displace and partially encircle the carotid siphons

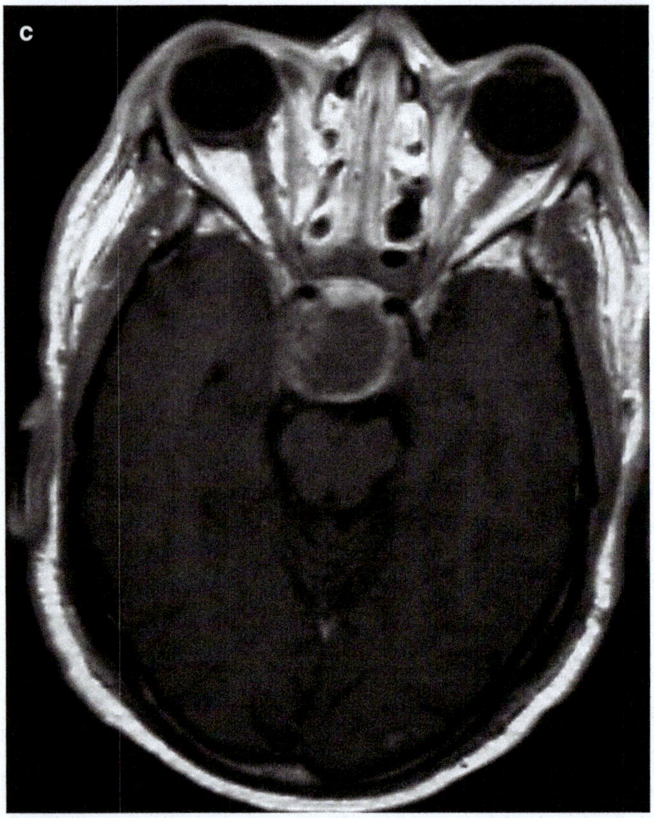

Fig. 2.5 (continued) (c) Axial T1 Gd shows avid enhancing periphery of pituitary mass. Large non-enhancing area in center of mass related to prior debulking within this pituitary adenoma

Selected References

1. Fischbein NJ, Dillon WP, Barkovich AJ. Teaching atlas of brain imaging. New York: Thieme; 2000. p. 52–4.
2. Ostrov SG, Quencer RM, Hoffman JC, et al. Hemorrhage within pituitary adenomas: how often associated with pituitary apoplexy syndrome? AJNR. 1989;10:503–10.
3. Rogg JM, Tung GA, Anderson G, et al. Pituitary apoplexy: early detection with diffusion-weighted MR imaging. AJNR. 2002;23:1240–5.
4. Lazaro CM, Guo WY, Sami M, et al. Haemorrhagic pituitary tumours. Neuroradiology. 1994;36(2):111–4.
5. Mattke AF, Vender JR, Andstadt MR. Pituitary apoplexy presenting as Addisonian crisis after coronary artery bypass grafting. Tex Heart Inst J. 2002;29(3):139.
6. Turgut M, Seyithanoglu MH. Rathke's Cleft Cysts Mimicking Pituitary Apoplexy, Fuminari Komatsu. Turgut DM, Mahapatra AK, Powell M, Muthukumar N (Eds) 2014 Springer-Verlag Berlin Heidelberg, pp 3–4.
7. Ezzat S, Asa SL, Couldwell WT, et al. The prevalence of pituitary adenomas. Cancer. 2004;101(3):613–9.
8. Asa SL. Practical pituitary pathology: what does the pathologist need to know? Arch Pathol Lab Med. 2008;132(8):1231–40.
9. Daly AF, Rixhon M, Adam C, et al. High prevalence of pituitary adenomas: a cross-sectional study in the province of Liege, Belgium. J Clin Endocrinol Metabol. 2006;91(12):1765–75.
10. Saini KS, Patel AL, Shaikh WA, et al. Magnetic resonance spectroscopy in pituitary tuberculoma. Singap Med J. 2007;48(8):783–6.
11. Asa SL, Ezzat S. The cytogenesis and pathogenesis of pituitary adenomas. Endocr Rev. 1998;19(6):798–827.
12. Fassett DR, Couldwell WT. Metastasis to the Pituitary gland. Neurosurg Focus. 2004;16(4).
13. Srisukh S, Tanpaibule T, Kiertiburanakul S, et al. Pituitary tuberculoma: a consideration in the Differential diagnosis in patient manifesting with pituitary apoplexy-like syndrome. Science Direct, Elsevier. 2016;5:63–6. https://doi.org/10.1016/j.idcr.2016.07.012. Accessed 2 Oct 2018.
14. Coleman CC, Meredith JM. Diffuse tuberculoma of the pituitary gland simulating tumour with post operative recovery. Arch Neuro Psy. 1940;44:1076–85.
15. Vandeva S, Jaffrain-Rea ML, Daly AF, et al. The genetics of pituitary adenomas. Best Pract Res Clin Endocrinol Metab. 2010;24(3):461–76.

3 Craniopharyngioma

Pertinent Points

- Definition: Craniopharyngiomas are relatively benign (WHO grade I) sellar/suprasellar neoplasms comprising ~3% of all brain tumors. They can occur anywhere along the infundibulum from the floor of the third ventricle to the pituitary gland.
- *Classic Clue*: Teen or middle-aged adult patient presenting with variable CNS complaints is found to have a complex sellar/suprasellar mass showing enhancement of solid components with varying MRI signals from cystic components. CT depicts curvilinear calcification along the rim of cystic components and coarse calcification of solid elements.
- Gender Preference: M = F
- AKA: No synonyms

Imaging

General Imaging Features

- 90% rule: 90% of childhood craniopharyngiomas are cystic and 90% are calcified.
- 95% of craniopharyngiomas have a significant suprasellar component.
- 75% involve suprasellar and intrasellar spaces.
- 20% are purely suprasellar.
- 5% are purely intrasellar and sometimes show sellar expansion [1].
- ↑ T1 signal in a suprasellar mass suggests craniopharyngioma.
- Like liquids in your automobile, the varying viscosity of craniopharyngioma's cystic fluid fluctuates from yellowish proteinaceous fluid to classic "crank-case oil" containing cholesterol and blood byproducts.
- Craniopharyngiomas often have mixed cystic and enhancing solid components.
- Craniopharyngiomas often infiltrate adjacent structures on MRI.
- Craniopharyngiomas may occasionally enlarge and/or erode the sella.

Plain Films

A. Calcifications in the suprasellar region ↑ specificity for the diagnosis of craniopharyngioma.
B. Plain films are not usually obtained when a higher level of imaging is available.

CT Features

- Cystic components
  - Typically large
  - Near CSF attenuation (see Fig. 3.1a)
- Solid components
  - Soft tissue attenuation
  - Exhibit avid enhancement
- Calcifications
  - Confirmed in 90%
  - Often coarse in solid components and curvilinear along cyst's periphery (see Fig. 3.1a, b)

F. A. Midyett, S. K. Mukherji, *Skull Base Imaging*, https://doi.org/10.1007/978-3-030-46447-9_3

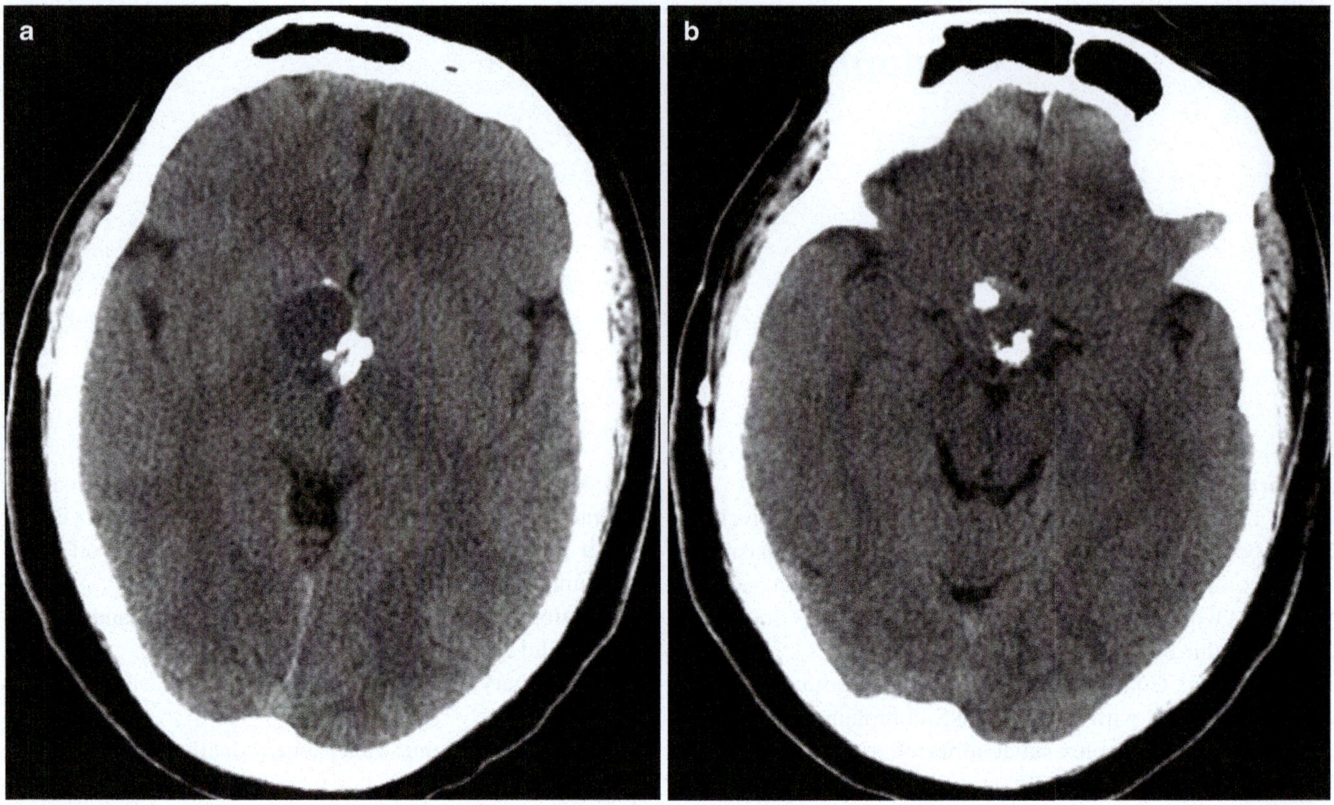

Fig. 3.1 (**a**, **b**) NECT brain algorithm shows homogeneous cystic low attenuation suprasellar mass with calcification of the cyst wall and coarse calcifications involving solid tumor components

MRI Features [2, 3]

- Cystic components
  - Great variability of enhancement pattern for cyst, depending on content [as discussed in general imaging features]. See Fig. 3.4a, b.
  - T2 signal variable: 80% are hyperintense on T2 (see Figs. 3.3d and 3.4d).
  - T1 signal is variable depending on protein content: occasionally hyperintense on T1 (see Fig. 3.4e).
  - FLAIR (fluid-attenuated inversion recovery) sequences may be helpful in depiction of a craniopharyngioma and adjacent enlarged ventricles (see Fig. 3.3e, f).
  - Tumor typically enclosed by an enhancing cystic rim (see Figs. 3.2a, b, 3.3a–c, and 3.4c).
- Solid components
  - T1: iso- to slightly hypointense to brain
  - T2: variable to mixed correlating with amount of Ca^{++} on CT.
  - T1 Gd: an avidly enhancing solid component is present in most cases (see Fig. 3.2a, b).
  - Consistently compromise adjacent structures with chiasmatic and hypothalamic infiltration.
- Calcifications
  - Calcifications can be more difficult to detect on MRI than CT.
  - Susceptible sequences may better show calcifications.
- MRA [magnetic resonance angiography]
  - MRA may demonstrate displacement of A1 segment of ACA (anterior cerebral artery).
- MRS [magnetic resonance spectroscopy]
  - Cyst contents contain broad lipid spectrum on a flat baseline [4].

Clinical Issues

Presentation

- Symptoms are routinely related to mass effect.
- Pressure on the chiasm can cause visual disturbances.
- Mass effect on the frontal lobes leads to headache and behavioral change.

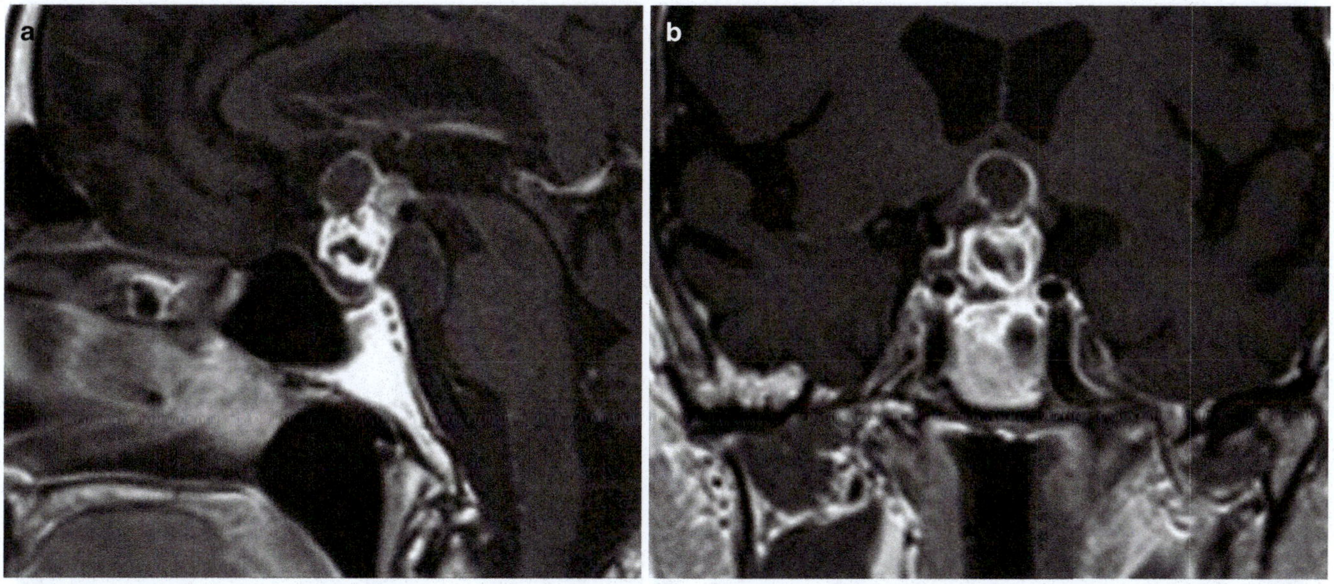

Fig. 3.2 (**a**, **b**) T1 Gd sagittal (**a**) and coronal (**b**) images show sellar and suprasellar mass with cystic and solid components. Enhancement of solid components and cyst rims. Large cystic component extends along the clivus displacing the pons posteriorly

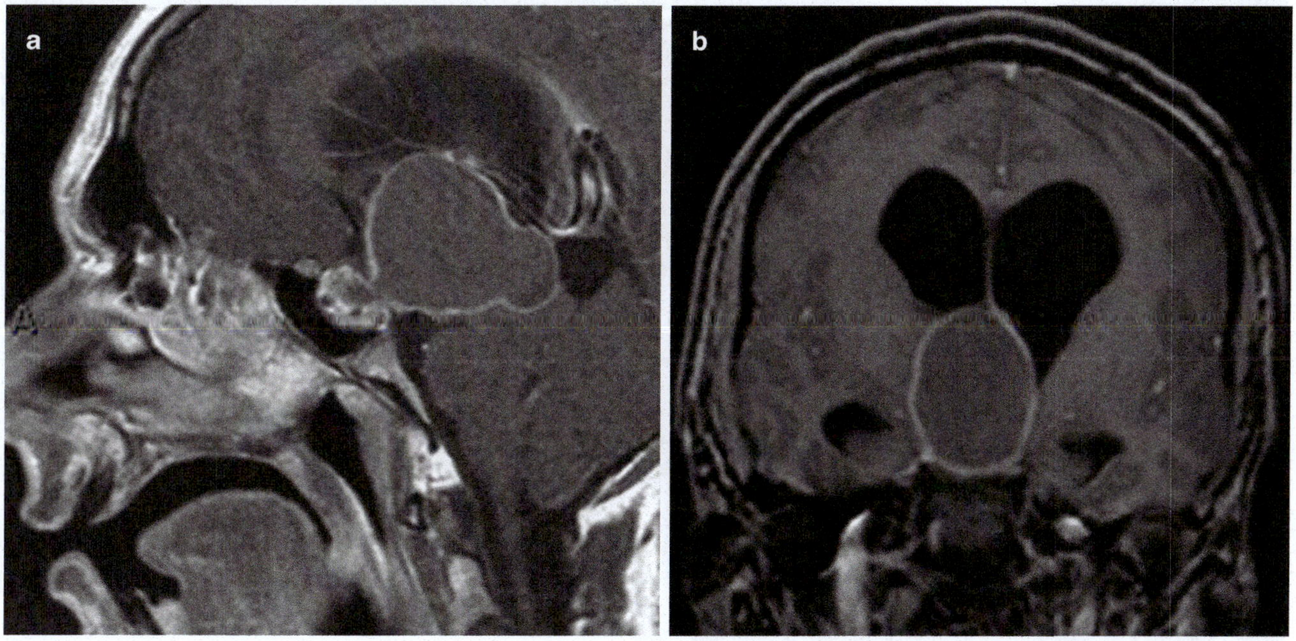

Fig. 3.3 (**a–b**) T1 Gd sagittal (**a**), coronal (**b**)

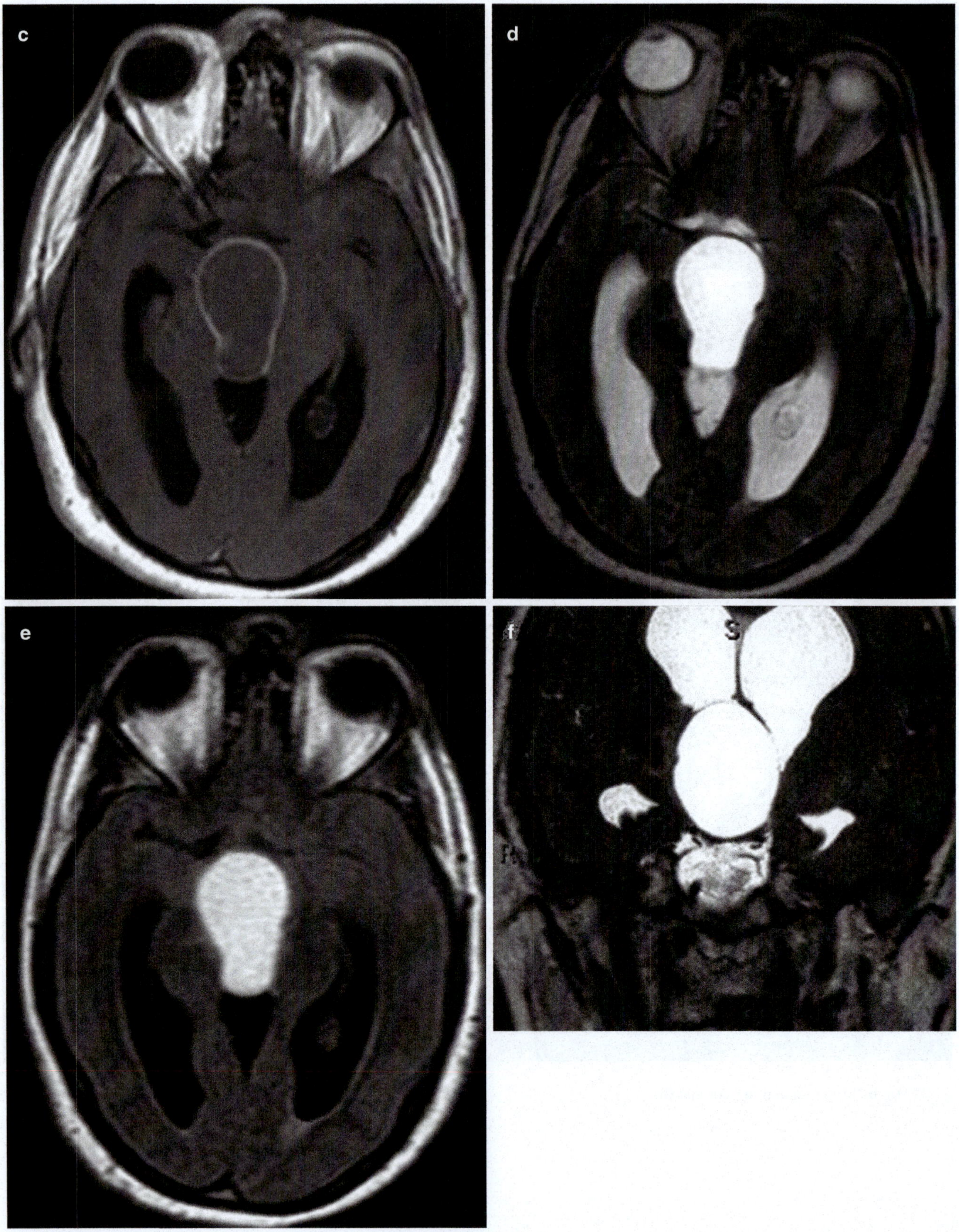

Fig. 3.3 (continued) Axial (**c**) images show large mass filling sella with even larger suprasellar component which is predominately cystic. Enhancement of the solid sellar components and the cyst rim. Homogeneous but non-enhancing cyst contents. Hydrocephalus with shunt tube in place. (**d, e**) Axial T2 (**d**) and FLAIR (**e**) show that the fluid-filled craniopharyngioma appears bright on T2 and FLAIR and is dramatically distinguished from the hydrocephalic ventricles on the FLAIR where the CSF is depicted as dark. (**f**) T2 coronal. Yes, the dilated ventricles and the fluid-filled tumor do combine to look like "Mickey Mouse"! But do we really need to saddle Mickey with yet another medical sign? Maybe we should just let him enjoy the magic kingdom

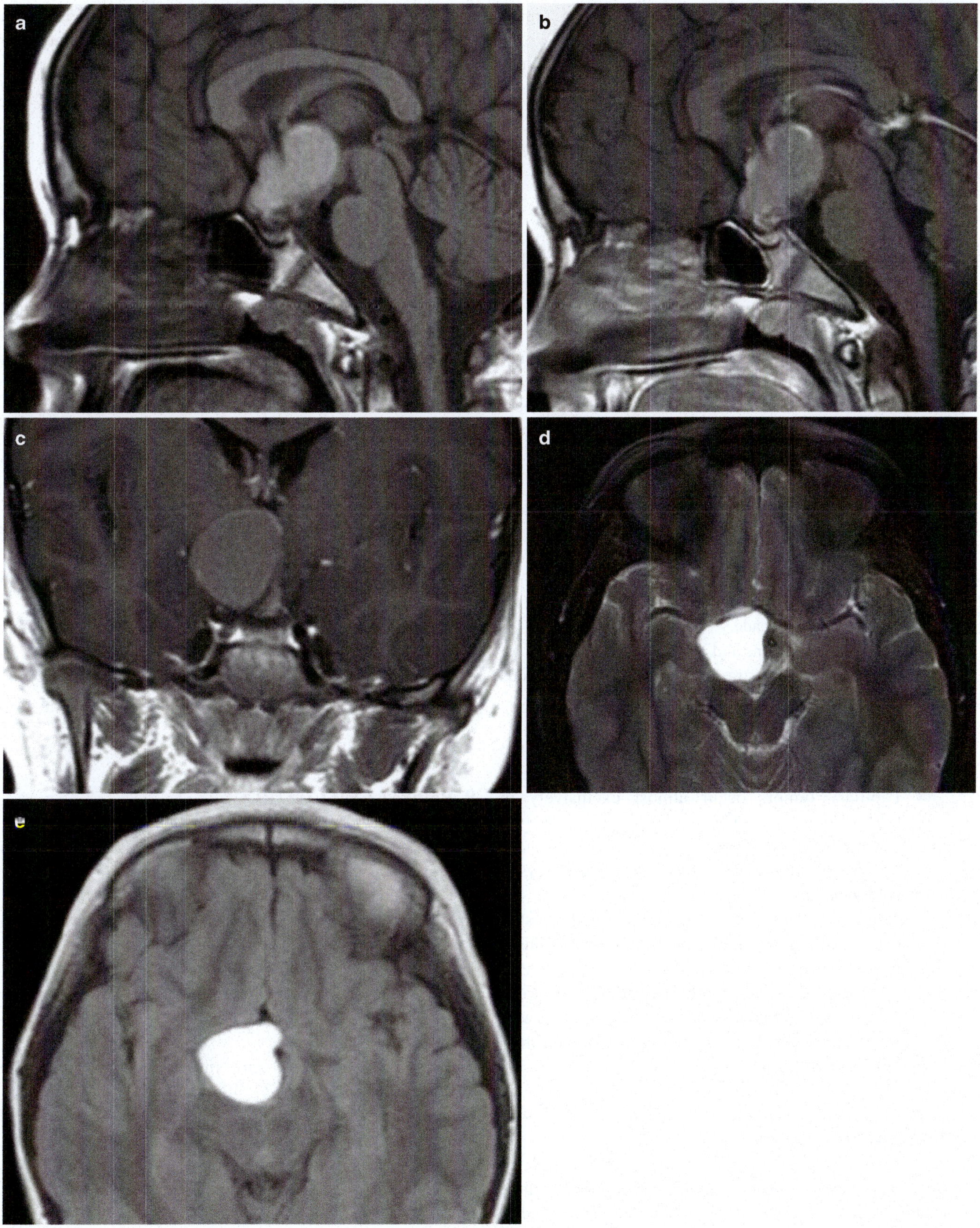

Fig. 3.4 (**a**, **b**) T1 Sag without (**a**) and with (**b**) Gd show large sellar and suprasellar mass predominately cystic with "lumpy" internal margins secondary to solid components which have some elevated T1 signal before and after contrast. (**c**) Coronal T1 Gd shows the mass to have an enhancing rim. (**d**, **e**) Axial T2 (**d**) and T1 (**e**) shows the cystic component of the craniopharyngioma to be bright on both T1 and T2 imaging. T1 shortening varies depending on the tumor's content

- Constriction of the critical the hypothalamic region engenders endocrine dysfunction.
- Confinement of critical CSF drainage conduits can cause hydrocephalus.

Epidemiology and Pathology

- ~3% of intracranial tumors [2].
- 50% occur in children and young adults [2].
- Usually suprasellar. Occasionally purely intrasellar [2].
- Intrasellar extension is common, causing sellar enlargement and erosion of dorsum.
  - Craniopharyngiomas are typically subdivided into types. Some scholars feel that they fall into a spectrum ranging from adamantinomatous to squamous epithelium with transitional and mixed types in between. Some of the "types" typically listed in the literature include the following [2, 3, 5]:
  - Type I: childhood type
    Typical peak 10–14 years of age
    Frequent calcification and cyst formation
    Adamantinomatous microscopic appearance
    Portends poor prognosis
  - Type II: adult type
    Peaks in sixth decade.
    Fewer calcifications and cysts.
    Microscopic portrays papillary squamous epithelium.
  - Type III: papillary craniopharyngiomas
    Truly the *black sheep* which tries to violate all the imaging rules!
    Papillary tumors occur almost exclusively in *adults* [6].
    More spherical in shape.
    These usually lack the customary cystic components.
    Most are *solid* or contain only a few smaller cysts.
    Calcification is *rare* in the papillary subtype. This is a fact frequently forgotten by imagers [7].
    There is probably no significant difference between the adamantinomatous and papillary variants with respect to resectability, response to radiation therapy, or overall survival [6].

Treatment and Prognosis

- Surgery is the treatment of choice but is unfortunately usually subtotal because of the tumor's tendency to affix to critical adjacent structures.
- Options for residual or recurrent tumor include radiation therapy, cyst aspiration, or intracystic instillation of P_{32} or sclerosing agents.
- Prognosis varies with age, tumor type, tumor size, and extent of tumor resection.
- Radiation therapy appears to ↓ recurrence rates after subtotal resection [2, 5, 8].

Differential Diagnosis (DDx)

A. Pituitary Adenoma

- CT typically shows sellar expansion, erosion, and remodeling.
- Pituitary adenomas usually display intermediate attenuation on CT.
- Combined sellar and suprasellar mass with "waist" at sellar diaphragm creating characteristic "figure of eight" or "Biker on Harley" appearance on coronal imaging.
- Usually homogeneously isointense on both T1 and T2 (pituitary apoplexy has hemorrhage which changes with age of blood products.)
- Solid mass shows moderate homogeneous enhancement on T1 Gd.
- Typically displaces, encases, or invades cavernous sinus structures.
- Cystic and/or hemorrhagic pituitary adenomas may be difficult to distinguish from a craniopharyngioma (see Fig. 3.4a–f).
- See Chap. 2, Pituitary Adenoma.

B. Rathke's Cleft Cyst (RCC)

- RCCs are often smaller than craniopharyngiomas.
- RCCs are usually more homogeneous than craniopharyngiomas.
- Craniopharyngiomas have enhancing solid components. RCCs are non- enhancing except for a small surrounding rim of normal pituitary.
- RCC usually does not erode the sella.
- See Chap. 1, Rathke's Cleft Cyst.

C. Pituitary Metastasis

- Pituitary metastasis is *rare*, most commonly from lung and breast carcinoma.
- Pituitary metastasis has less commonly been reported from prostate, renal cell, lymphoma, leukemia, thyroid, plasmocytoma, and GI cancer [9].
- Metastasis usually does not enlarge the sella.
- Some series show 6–29% of breast cancer patients develop pituitary metastasis [9].

D. Pituitary Carcinoma

- Pituitary carcinoma is *rare* comprising 1 in 1000 (0.1%) of primary pituitary tumors [10].
- Pituitary carcinoma is typically more invasive than craniopharyngioma which is WHO grade I.

E. Pituitary Abscess

- Pituitary abscess shows a thick enhancing rim and/or shaggy irregular margins [11].
- Pituitary abscess is often associated with sphenoid sinusitis.
- Pituitary abscess is usually void of hemorrhage.

F. Pituitary Tuberculoma

- Frequently found in developing countries and/or immunocomprised individuals [12].
- Magnetic resonance spectroscopy can clearly be helpful in diagnosis, avoiding an invasive procedure [12].

G. Aneurysms

- Typically show lamellated thrombus calcifications.
- May see phase artifact from flow if aneurysm is still patent.
- It is important to keep aneurysm in this differential.

A Closer Look

I. Embryology

- Embryologists tender two chief conjectures as to the cause of craniopharyngioma.
- Theory ONE is that they remain from the remnants of the craniopharyngeal duct [which connects the stomodeal ectoderm with Rathke's pouch]
- Theory TWO is that they start from squamous epithelial cells in the pars tuberalis of the adenohypophysis.
- Current thinking favors "Theory One" and classifies "Theory Two" as the "old" theory [1].
- If these are the sorts of questions which keep you awake at night, you probably should get a new embryology text or pursue professional help.

II. Fast Facts

- Ectopic craniopharyngiomas have been found in the third ventricle, nasopharynx, sphenoid bone, cerebellopontine angle, pineal region, and very rarely the lateral ventricle [13].

III. Historic Highlights

- 1857 Friedrich Albert von Zenker was the first pathologist to characterize what we now call craniopharyngioma [14]. Yes, this is the SAME Zenker whose name is associated with a pharyngeal diverticulum. How many Zenkers could there have been in medicine in those days?
- 1904 Jacob Erdheim was the first pathologist to accurately describe the histopathology of what he called "hypophyseal duct tumors," and Cushing later gave these the name "craniopharyngioma."
- Joseph Babinski (1857–1932) was the first neurologist to characterize the clinical presentation of a patient with craniopharyngioma. And yes, this is the same Babinski we associate with the abnormal plantar reflex.
- 1910 A.E. Halstead performed in a Chicago Hospital the first successful resection of a craniopharyngioma using an infranasal approach.
- 1923 Cushing operated on a patient with craniopharyngioma who lived another 50 years, becoming the longest recorded survivor of craniopharyngioma. Harvey Cushing (1869–1939) reported 92 craniopharyngiomas in his series of 2000 brain tumors. He favored the transsphenoidal approach for the majority of his pituitary surgeries but favored the transcranial approach for craniopharyngiomas [15].
- The introduction of antibiotics, steroids, and surgical microscopes significantly improved outcomes. Stereotactic radiosurgery, brachytherapy, and intracapsular chemotherapy have improved tumor control and have ↓ complications [16].
- Advances in neuroradiology have been monumental during the 100 years since Halstead successfully resected that first craniopharyngioma which was called by Cushing as "the most formidable of intracranial tumors." Let's all see what we can contribute in the next 100 years.

IV. Genetics

- *BRAF:* Almost all papillary craniopharyngiomas commonly associated with adults contain mutations in *BRAF* genes.
- *CTNNB1*: Almost all adamantinomatous craniopharyngiomas, frequently found in children, contain mutations in *CTNNB1* (β-catenin) [17].

Selected References

1. Bernstein M. Neuro-Oncology. The Essentials. Second Edition. By Mark Bernstein, Mitchel S. Berger. New York, NY: Published by Thieme Medical Publishers; 2007. p. 496.
2. Fischbein NJ, Dillon WP, Barkovich AJ. Teaching atlas of brain imaging: Thieme, New York; 2000. p. 58–61.
3. Sartorett-Schefer S, Wichman W, et al. MR differentiation of adamantinomatous and squamous-papillary Craniopharyngiomas. AJNR. 1997;18:77–87.
4. Keating RF, Goodrich JT, Packer RJ. Tumors of the pediatric central nervous system: George Thieme Verlag; 2001.
5. Ekdevik OP, Blaivas M, Gabrielsen TO, et al. Craniopharyngioma: radiologic and histologic findings and recurrence. AJNR Am J Neuroradiol. 1996;17:1427–39.
6. Crotty TB, Scheithauer BW, Young WF Jr, et al. Papillary Craniopharyngioma: a clinicopathological study of 48 cases. J Neurosurg. 1995;83(2):206–14.
7. Eldevik OP, Blaivas M, Gabrielsen TO, et al. Craniopharyngioma: radiologic and histologic findings and recurrence. AJNR. 1996;17:1427–39.
8. Yasargil MG, Curcic M, Kis M, et al. Total removal of Craniopharyngiomas. Approaches and long-term results in 144 patients. J Neurosurg. 1990;73:3–1.
9. Fassett DR, Couldwell WT. Metastasis to the Pituitary gland. Neurosurg Focus. 2004;16(4).
10. Daly AF, Rixhon M, Adam C, et al. High prevalence of pituitary adenomas: a cross-sectional study in the province of Liege, Belgium. J Clin Endocrinol Metabol. 2006;91(12):1765–75.
11. Asa SL. Practical pituitary pathology: what does the pathologist need to know? Arch Pathol Lab Med. 2008;132(8):1231–40.
12. Saini KS, Patel AL, Shaikh WA, et al. Magnetic resonance spectroscopy in pituitary tuberculoma. Singap Med J. 2007;48(8):783–6.
13. Singh J, Ganesan K, Desai SB, et al. Lateral ventricle Craniopharyngioma – MRI demonstration of migratory nature of ectopic Craniopharyngioma from the suprasellar region. Indian J Radiol Imaging. 2003;13:427–9.
14. Barkhoudarian G, Laws ER. Craniopharyngioma: history. Pituitary. 2013;16(1):1–8.
15. Roderick E, Karavitaki N, Wass JAH. Craniopharyngiomas. Historical aspects of their management. Hormones. 2008;7(3):271–4.
16. Lindholm J, Nielsen EH. Craniopharyngioma: historical notes. Pituitary. 2009;12(4):352–9.
17. Brastianos PK, Taylor-Weiner A, Manley PE, et al. Exome sequencing identifies BRAF mutations in papillary craniopharyngiomas. Nat Genet. 2014;46(2):161–5.

Ectopic Neurohypophysis

4

Pertinent Points

- Definition: Ectopic neurohypophysis (EN) is a congenital abnormality related to faulty embryogenesis causing incomplete caudal extension of the infundibulum and is one of the more common causes of pituitary dwarfism.
- *Classic Clue*: Patient presenting with short stature is shown to have small anterior pituitary. The pituitary "bright spot" is not seen in the sella and seems to be sited near the median eminence.
- *AKA*: Ectopic posterior pituitary, posterior pituitary ectopia, pituitary stalk interruption syndrome (PSIS).
- It is clinically important to determine whether the pituitary stalk can (or cannot) be identified with thin slice T1 Gd imaging [1].
- It is important for the neuroradiologist to look for and identify associated abnormalities. *Don't settle* for "low hanging fruit." Keep looking for other abnormalities which may be numerous.

Imaging

General Imaging Features

- Tiny bright T1 posterior pituitary located near the median eminence instead of in the sella.
- The ectopic neurohypophysis migration abnormality may be complete or partial [1].

Plain Films

- Bone age studies show patients to have delayed bone maturation.

CT Features

- Not an appropriate imaging technique for this entity.

MRI Features [2, 3]

- MRI is the modality most capable of correctly identifying EN.
- Sagittal midline T1 images show:
  - Bright ↑ T1 signal 3–8 mm soft tissue protuberance at the median eminence of the third ventricular floor in up to 90% of patients (see Fig. 4.1a, b)
  - Absence of the "normal" intrasellar posterior pituitary "bright spot."
  - Hypoplasia of the anterior hypophysis [1].
  - Cases in which the pituitary stalk is visible tend to have an isolated growth hormone deficiency [1].
  - Patients with visualization of *no* pituitary stalk after the injection of Gd have a more severe childhood disease form with multiple anterior pituitary hormone deficiencies [1].
- Neuroradiology associations:
  - SOD (septo-optic dysplasia)
  - Optic nerve hypoplasia
  - ACC (agenesis of the corpus callosum) (see Fig. 4.2a–d)
  - Chiari I malformation (see Fig. 4.1a)
  - Heterotopic periventricular gray matter
  - Vermian dysplasia
  - Medial ICA deviation
  - Basilar impression
  - Kallman syndrome
  - Persistent craniopharyngeal canal

F. A. Midyett, S. K. Mukherji, *Skull Base Imaging*, https://doi.org/10.1007/978-3-030-46447-9_4

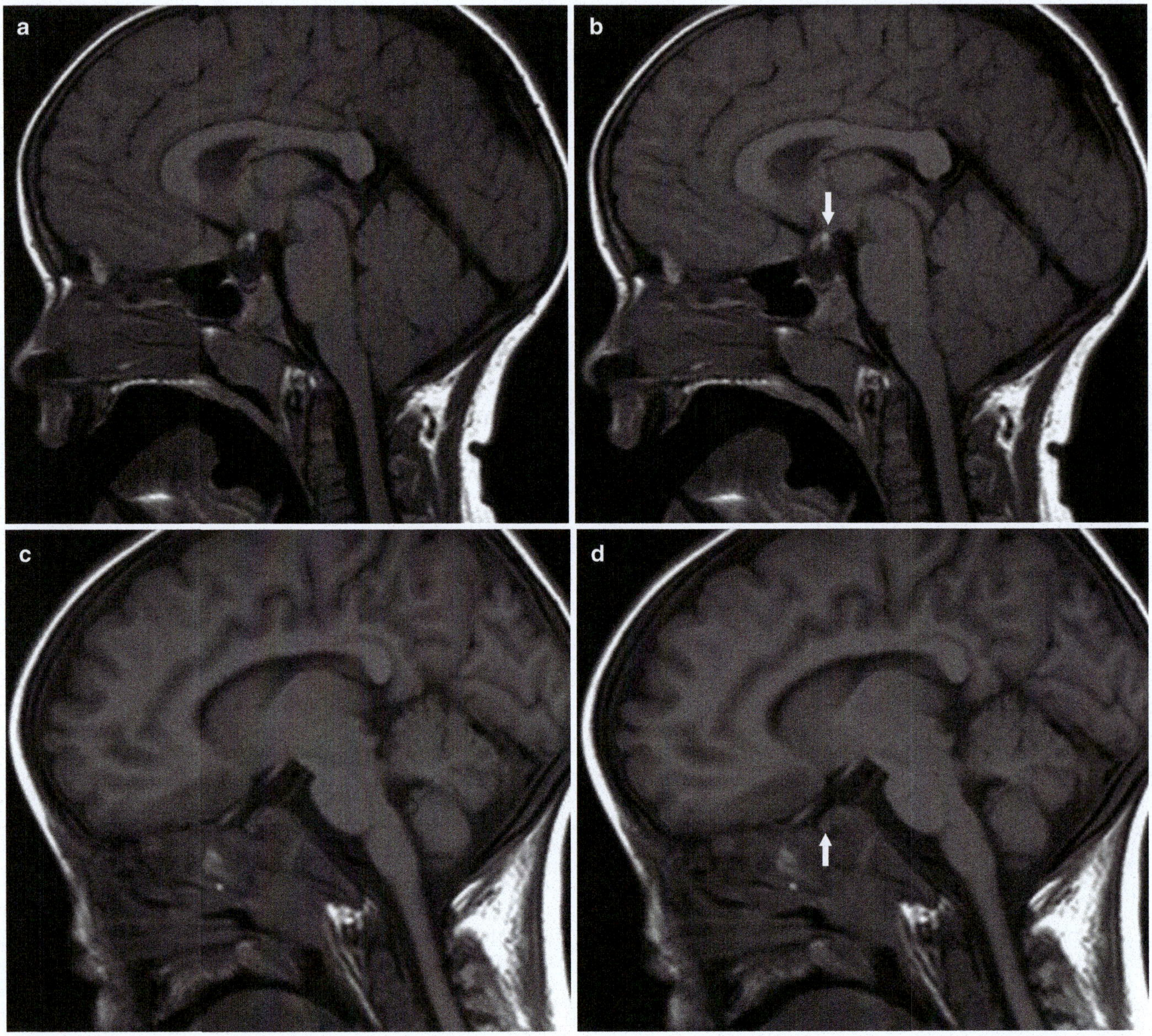

Fig. 4.1 Midline sagittal T1 without (**a**) and with (**b**) arrow shows tiny bright "dot" of the posterior pituitary located multiple millimeters cranial to its usual location, outside the sella in the suprasellar region near the median eminence. Arrowhead on (**b**) is larger than the EN. And, in the reading room, many of us may have focused on the more obvious finding of low hanging tonsils and posterior fossa crowding in this patient with Chiari I malformation, one of the many associated abnormalities. (**c, d**) Parasagittal T1 without (**c**) and with (**d**) arrow shows the anterior pituitary located within the sella. No adjacent bright posterior pituitary within sella on this [or any other images]

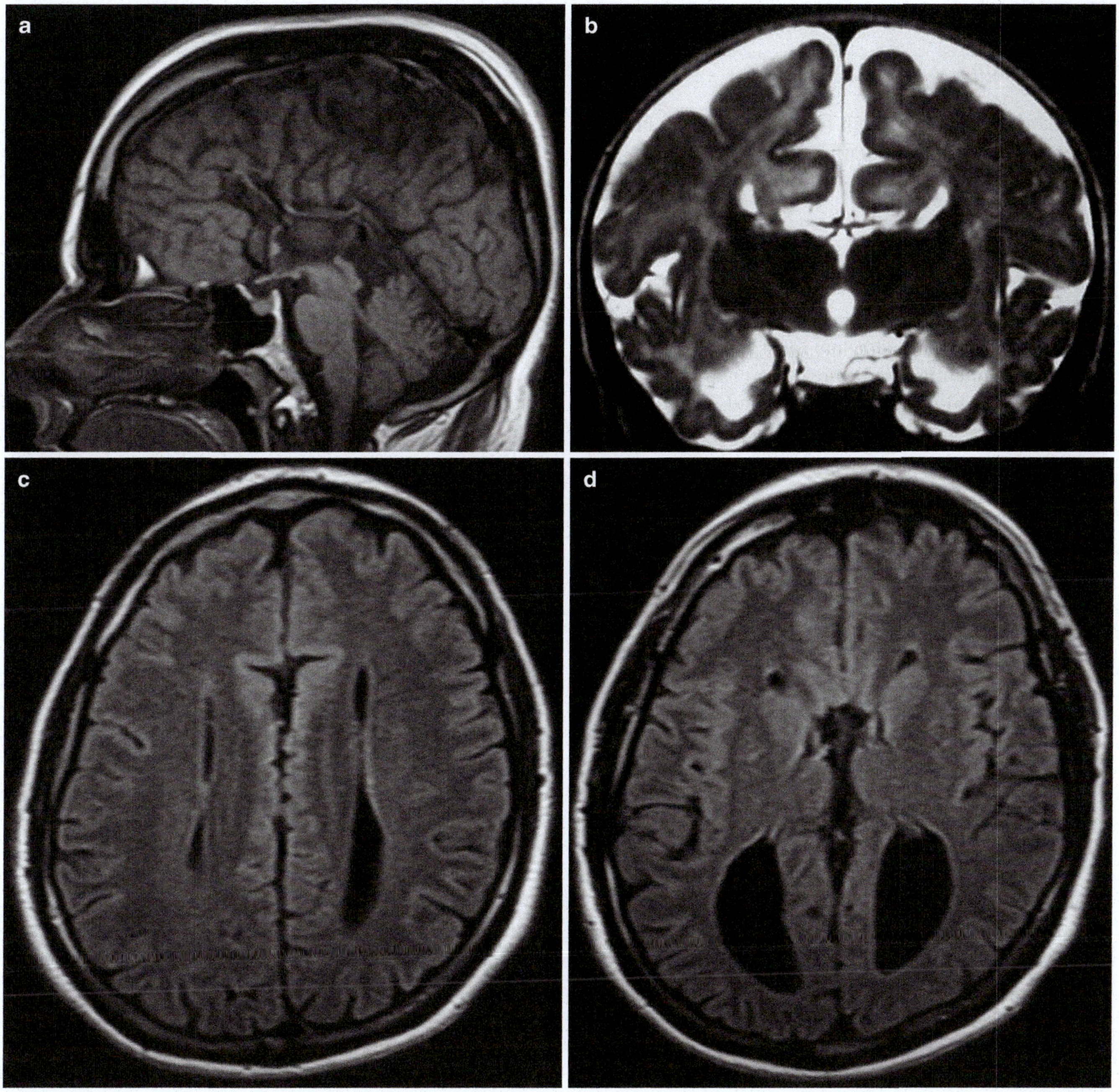

Fig. 4.2 Agenesis of Corpus Callosum (AGC) is another intracranial abnormality associated with EN and is depicted in a second patient by Figures 4.2a–d (**a**) Midline sagittal T1 MRI shows complete AGC with medial hemispheric sulci extending in "radial" fashion to the third ventricle. (**b**) Coronal T2 WI shows "Texas Longhorn" or "Viking" appearance of upturned lateral ventricles bordered medially by Probst bundles. The hippocampi are more vertical than usual. (**c**) Axial FLAIR MRI shows interdigitating gyri between unusually positioned parallel lateral ventricles. (**d**) Axial FLAIR MRI shows small widely separated frontal horns. Large occipital horns. High, prominent third ventricle

Clinical Issues

Presentation

- Patients may present with features of growth hormone deficiency (pituitary dwarfism) or neonatal hypoglycemia [2].

Epidemiology and Pathology

- Ectopic neurohypophysis results from incomplete caudal extension of the infundibulum (diencephalon).
- The median eminence is one of seven areas which can bypass the blood-brain barrier, and is the primary point for releasing hypothalamic regulatory hormones.
- The posterior pituitary's pars nervosa is usually contiguous with the median eminence connecting through the infundibular stalk.
- That connection through the hypophyseal portal system is interrupted with EN halting the direct flow of hypophysiotropic hormones from the hypothalamus to the anterior pituitary.
- Hormones released by the hypothalamus which usually traverse the hypothalamic-hypophyseal portal system to the anterior pituitary must try to take the long way around via the general circulation.
- Ectopic neurohypophysis is commonly coupled to growth hormone deficiency and tied periodically to panhypopituitarism [4].
- Recent reports suggest that EN and SOD (septo-optic dysplasia) share a similar pathogenesis with HESX1 gene implicated by both [2].

Treatment and Prognosis

- Ectopic neurohypophysis itself requires no specific treatment. However, patients regularly require treatment for associated growth hormone deficiency or panhypopituitarism [4].
- When children who have severe growth hormone deficiencies are treated, results are dramatic. With proper treatment, a child who has fallen far behind may grow into the normal height range.
- Treatment of growth hormone deficient adults can confer clear compensations including improved bone density and enhanced energy and strength.
- Adult's blood lipid levels do improve, but the murky mortality rates from cardiovascular disease do not clear concurrently.

Differential Diagnosis

A. Craniopharyngioma
- Craniopharyngiomas are usually larger than EN.
- 90% of craniopharyngiomas have Ca^{++}. EN does not have Ca^{++}.
- Usually adamantinomatous type.
- See Chap. 3, Craniopharyngioma.

B. Lipoma, Dermoid, or Teratoma
- Fatty masses show chemical shift artifact.
- Fat saturation sequences suppress these fatty tumors.

C. Aneurysm
- Aneurysms typically show lamellated thrombus calcification.
- Patent aneurysms sometimes show phase artifact.
- It is important to always keep aneurysm in this differential.

A Closer Look

I. Embryology
- The pituitary gland can clearly trace its family tree to two different developmental parts with the anterior pituitary (or adenohypophysis) arising from ectoderm and the posterior pituitary (neurohypophysis) arising from neuroectoderm.
- The anterior pituitary evolves from invagination of Rathke's cleft (stomodeum).
- The posterior pituitary develops from a downward extension of the infundibulum (diencephalon).
- The anterior and posterior pituitary are capable of functioning as separate endocrine organs, although it is clear that separation by EN can carry untoward consequences.

II. Fast Facts
- While the cause of the increased T1 signal in the posterior pituitary continues to be controversial, it most likely is secondary to lipid in posterior lobe pituicytes [5] or neurosecretory granules [3].

III. Historic Highlights
- 1920 German pathologist Priesel first described EN later publishing these findings in 1927, but the entity lay largely unnoticed for over a half century.
- 1987 Fujisawa et al. rediscovered EN with MRI [3].

IV. Genetics
- The overall spectrum of congenital pituitary stalk abnormalities is currently called "pituitary stalk interruption syndrome" (PSIS). This syndrome can cause pituitary deficiency commonly characterized by the following triad: (1) hypoplastic or

interrupted pituitary stalk, (2) ectopic (or absent) posterior pituitary (EPP), and (3) anterior pituitary aplasia. When confined to an interrupted pituitary stalk, we encounter ectopic neurohypophysis (EN) as portrayed in Fig. 4.1a–d.

- While most affected individuals show no discernible genetic cause, familial forms and congenital anomalies associated with PSIS and microphallus support prenatal factors.
- Mutations in transcription factor HESX1 (3p21.2-p21.1) and in the LHX4 gene (1q25) have been implicated in certain cases [6].

Selected References

1. Chen S, Leger J, Garel C, et al. Growth hormone deficiency with ectopic Neurohypophysis: anatomical variations and relationship between the visibility of pituitary the stalk asserted by magnetic resonance imaging and anterior pituitary function. JECM. 1999;84(7):2408–13.
2. Maintz D, Benz-Bohm G, Gindele A, et al. Posterior pituitary ectopia: another hint toward a genetic etiology. AJNR Am J Neuroradiol. 2000;21(6):1116–8.
3. Fujisawa I, Asato R, Nishimura K, et al. Anterior and posterior lobes of the pituitary gland: assessment by 1.5 T MR imaging. J Comput Assist Tomogr. 1987;11:214–20.
4. Sartor K. Diagnostic and interventional neuroradiology, a multimodality approach: Georg Thieme Verlag. Stutgart, Germany; 2002.
5. Kucharczyk W, Lenkinski R, Kucharczyk J, et al. The effect of phospholipid vesicles on the NMR relaxation of water: an explanation for the appearance of the Neurohypophysis? AJNR Am J Neuroradiol. 1990;11:693–700A.
6. Bar C, Zadro C, Diene G, et al. Pituitary stalk interruption syndrome from infancy to adulthood: clinical, hormonal, and radiological assessment according to the initial presentation. PLoS One. 2015;10(11):e9142354; Accessed on line 1/27/2020.

5 Hypothalamic Hamartoma

Pertinent Points

- Definition: Hypothalamic hamartomas are rare congenital, non-neoplastic heterotopic malformative masses comprised of normal neuronal tissue arising from the tuber cinereum which may be symptomatic early associated with precocious puberty or present later when associated with those very unusual gelastic seizures.
- *Classic Clue*: Patient presents with a history of seizures and is found to have a small *non-enhancing* hypothalamic mass. Observers often thought patient was kidding around because of the appearance of smiling or laughing during seizure episodes.
- *AKA*: Hamartoma of the tuber cinereum.
- Incidence: M > F
- *Sessile* lesions are associated with *seizures*. *Pedunculated* lesions are associated with *precocious puberty* [1].

Imaging

General Imaging Features

The third ventricular floor should be smooth from the infundibulum to the mamillary bodies with any nodularity sparking suspicion for a hamartoma in the correct clinical context (see Fig. 5.2a–c).

- Pedunculated or sessile hypothalamic mass.
- Pedunculated
  - Attached to the tuber cinereum.
  - Project into the suprasellar cistern.
  - Pedunculated lesions are associated with precocious puberty [1].
  - Displace columns of the fornix anterolaterally.
  - May displace and/or distort mamillary bodies.
  - Extension below the third ventricle is variable [2].
- Sessile lesions associated with seizures [1].
- In the axial plane, the mass may appear to lie within suprasellar/interpeduncular cisterns (see Fig. 5.1b).
- These typically do not enhance or grow!
- Classically 1–2 cm in size but rarely range up to 4–5 cm [3].

CT Features

- See General Imaging Features.
- Pedunculated or sessile mass which is isodense to the brain.
- *No enhancement!*
- *No hemorrhage*.
- Sometimes see calcifications or cystic components.
- Modern volumetric scans with coronal and sagittal reconstructions are especially effective.

MRI Features

* See General Imaging Features

- T1 *isointense* to *gray matter* (see Fig. 5.2a–c).
- T2 iso- to hyperintense with gray matter.
- The posterior pituitary bright spot is usually present.
- T1 Gd exhibits *no enhancement.*
- T2 signal is directly proportional to the number of glial cells. I.e., the more glial cells, the higher the T2 signal [4].
- MRS (magnetic resonance spectroscopy)
  - May be helpful in distinguishing between hypothalamic hamartoma and glioma using the following features [4]:
  - ↓ NAA/creatine ratio
  - ↑ myoinositol
  - ↑ choline/creatine ratio (compared to amygdala) [4]

F. A. Midyett, S. K. Mukherji, *Skull Base Imaging*, https://doi.org/10.1007/978-3-030-46447-9_5

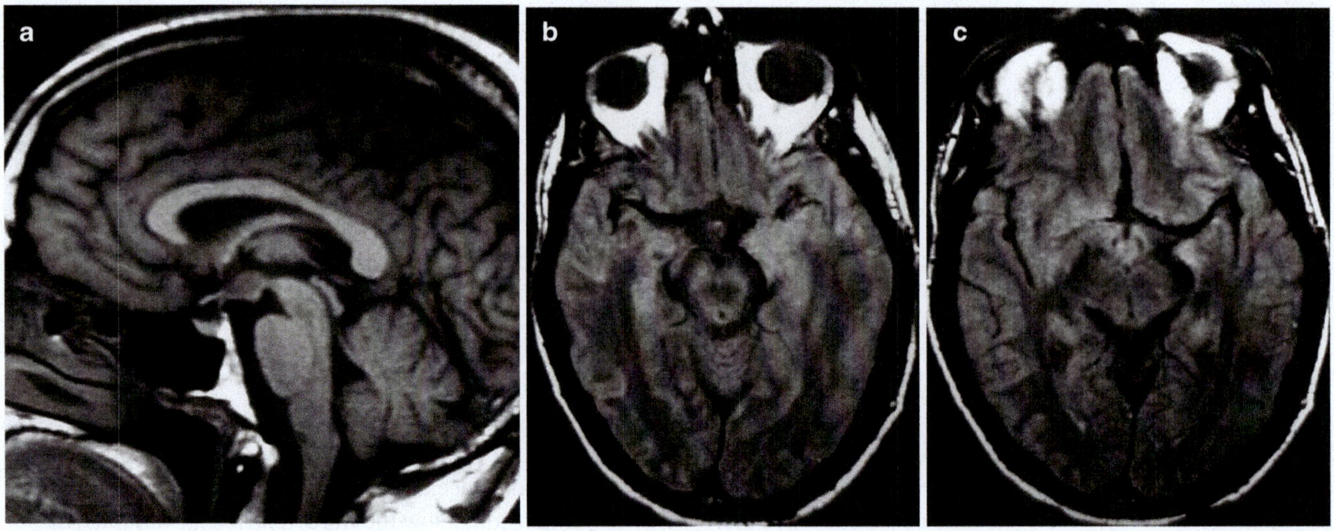

Fig. 5.1 (**a**) Sag T1 shows 1 cm oval sessile hypothalamic mass arising near the floor of the third ventricle from the tuber cinereum. The mass shows a signal which is isointense to cortical gray matter. (**b**) Axial T1 shows 1 cm oval hypothalamic mass arising projecting into the suprasellar cistern. The signal is isointense to cortical gray matter. (**c**) Axial T1 shows 1 cm oval hypothalamic with signal isointense to cortical gray matter. Subsequent T1 Gd images showed *no* enhancement

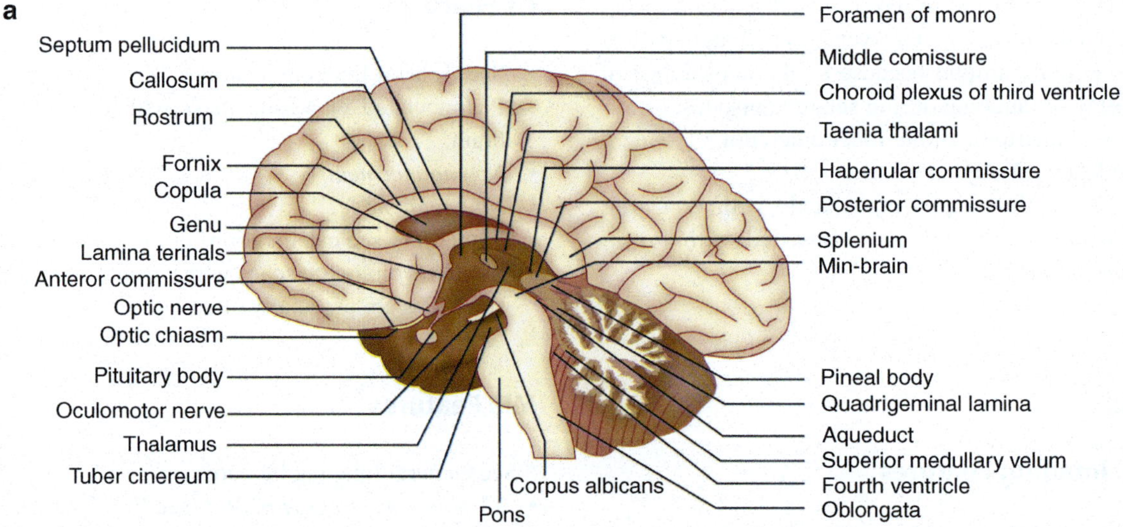

Fig. 5.2 (**a**) Sagittal midline drawing by Gray shows that the floor of the third ventricle is normally flat from the infundibulum posteriorly to the mamillary bodies located just anterior to the midbrain. Compare that to the sagittal MR image 1A, and the abnormality sticks out like a proverbial "sore thumb." (**b**) Gray's axial anatomic drawing depicts the relationship of mamillary bodies (corpora mammillaria) to the tuber cinereum. (**c**) Gray's anatomic drawing of the inferior brain surface shows the mamillary bodies as paired circular structures just posterior to the pituitary infundibulum

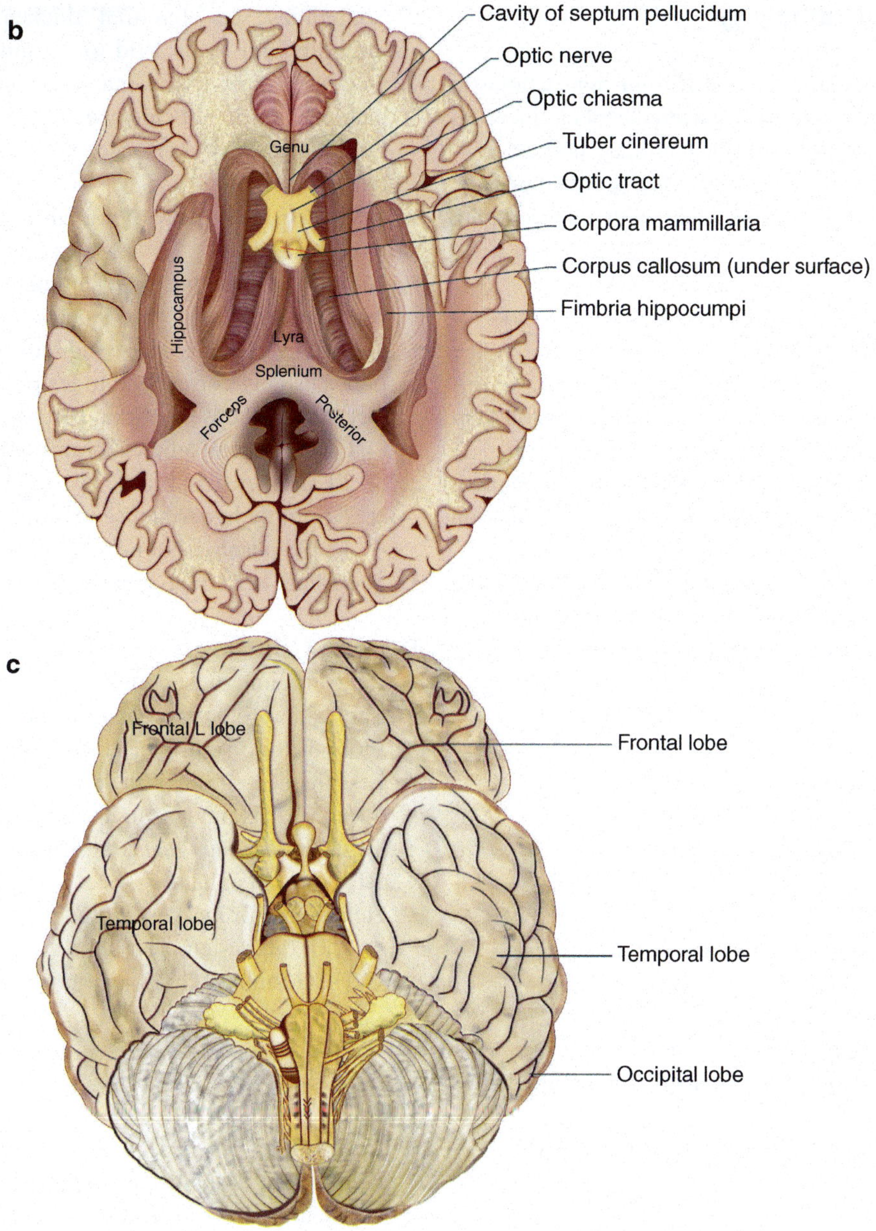

Fig. 5.2 (continue)

Clinical Issues

Presentation

- Patients may present with precocious puberty, usually beginning <2 years of age.
- Patients may present with seizures. The classic patient presenting with "gelastic" seizures exhibits spasmodic laughter. The patient associated with images (Fig. 5.1a–c) did not laugh but was observed to occasionally show a small smile during seizure activity.
- HH can cause visual or behavioral problems, early-onset puberty, or gelastic seizures [4].
- Gelastic seizures:
  - Typically are short duration of 2–30 seconds.
  - These patients may exhibit uncontrollable laughter.
  - Most manifest no loss of consciousness.
  - Sometimes show status gelasticus [5].

Epidemiology and Pathology

- A hypothalamic hamartoma is a benign non-neoplastic mass of heterotopic tissue arising from the tuber cinereum between the optic chiasm and the mamillary bodies.
- Gray's graphic drawing (Fig. 5.2) clearly illustrates the intricate normal anatomy associated with this complex region of interest.

Treatment and Prognosis

- Medical therapy is recommended for sessile lesions but can be very expensive over the course of many years.
- Surgical treatment is suggested for patients with pedunculated lesions showing symptoms refractory to medication [6, 7].
- While surgery seems successful with pedunculated lesions, it often proves problematic for sessile masses.
- Medical treatment involves luteinizing hormone receptor agonists.

Differential Diagnosis

A. Hypothalamic/Chiasmatic Glioma
- Infiltrative
- Associated with NF-1
- Most are JPAs [juvenile pilocytic astrocytomas]
- T1: Typically hypointense.
- T2: Habitually hyperintense.
- T1 Gd: Solid components usually enhance.
- MRS (MR spectroscopy) may be helpful in distinguishing between HH and glioma [4].
- See preceding section Imaging/MRI Features/MRS.

B. Other Gliomas
- The hypothalamic region would be an unusual location for other gliomas.
- Other gliomas are usually brighter on T2.
- MRS (MR spectroscopy) may be helpful in distinguishing between HH and glioma [4].

C. Langerhans Cell Histiocytosis
- LCH may present with diabetes insipidus when involving the infundibulum or hypothalamus.
- Orbital involvement often causes patients to present with proptosis.
- Temporal bone involvement may elucidate emergence of hearing loss and chronic ear drainage.
- Dural involvement can cause headache.
- Cerebellar involvement may activate ataxia and dysmetria.
- Sometimes see abnormal thickening of the pituitary infundibulum with avid postcontrast enhancement of associated soft tissue mass. By contrast hypothalamic hamartomas do not enhance.
- Sometimes shows absence of the normal posterior pituitary bright spot.
- May see mass involving the optic chiasm and/or hypothalamus.
- Nodular enhancing thickening of the dura and/or leptomeninges.
- Destructive lesions involving calvarium and/or temporal bones usually correspond to lesions demonstrated on CT.
- Occasionally observe brain parenchyma lesions:
  - Cerebral hemispheres, brainstem, or cerebellum.
  - T1 isointense to brain.
  - T2 mildly hyperintense to brain.
  - T1 Gd usually (but not always) enhances.
- See Chap. 8, LCH, Langerhans Cell Histiocytosis.

D. Germ Cell Tumors
- Pineal region: most common site.
- Suprasellar region: second most common location.
- Floor of third ventricle: third most common site.
- Less frequent sites: fourth ventricle, basal ganglia, thalamus.
- T1 and T2: isointense to gray matter
- T1 Gd*: exhibit enthusiastic enhancement*. By comparison HH does not enhance.
- Helpful tumor markers include:
  - AFP (alpha-fetoprotein)
  - HCG (human chorionic gonadotropin)

A Closer Look

I. Embryology
- Hypothalamic hamartomas probably develop from deviant neural migration materializing during the in utero time frame of 35–40 days [4].

II. Fast Facts
- Hamartoma comes from the Greek *hamartia* meaning error of judgment or unintended faux pas. In medicine a hamartoma is a developmental defect.
- Gelastic originates from the Greek *galaein* meaning "to laugh." In medicine *gelastic* indicates the association of a symptom or syndrome with laughter.
- Tuber cinereum comes from the Latin *cinereum* "ash or gray" and *tuber* "mass-like," i.e., gray mass.
- Hypothalamic hamartomas have a prevalence of 1 in 200,000.
- Pallister-Hall syndrome:
  - HH is associated with Pallister-Hall Syndrome in 5% of cases [8].

  - Multiple malformations include facial anomalies, imperforate anus, polydactyly, and large hypothalamic hamartomas.
  - Pallister-Hall syndrome patients experience less severe neurologic symptoms [3].
- 40% of hypothalamic hamartoma patients with epilepsy also have precocious puberty.

III. Historic Highlights

- Late nineteenth century: Laughter was first recognized as an uncommon manifestation of seizure activity.
- Late twentieth century: The specific association between gelastic seizures and HH appreciated with the introduction and general use of MRI.

IV. Genetics

- So, the *sonic hedgehog* rears its horrid head again.
- *GLI3*: Mutations of *GLI3* have been incriminated during development. The GLI family of DNA-binding transcription factors mediate sonic hedgehog (SHH) signaling.
- *GLI3* genetic mutations have been associated with multiple abnormalities including the Pallister-Hall syndrome which has multiple abnormalities, with pituitary insufficiently frequently fatal for undiagnosed infants [9].

Selected References

1. Boyko OB, Curnes JT, Oakes WJ, et al. Hamartomas of the tuber cinereum: CT, MR, and pathologic findings. AJNR Am J Neuroradiol. 1991;12(2):309–14.
2. Tonn J, Westphal M, Rutka JT. Oncology of CNS tumors. New York: Springer Berlin Heidelberg; 2009.
3. Arita K, Ikawa F, Kurisu K, et al. The relationship between magnetic resonance imaging findings and clinical manifestations of hypothalamic hamartoma. J Neurosurg. 1999;91(2):212–20.
4. Amstutz DR, Coons SW, Kerrigan JF, et al. Hypothalamic hamartomas: correlation of MR imaging and spectroscopic findings with glial content. AJNR Am J Neuroradiol. 2006;27(4):794–8.
5. Engel J, Pedley TA, Aicardi J. Epilepsy, a comprehensive textbook. Philadelphia: Wolters Kluwer Health/Lippincott Williams & Wilkins; 2007.
6. Fischbein NJ, Dillon WP, Barkovich AJ. Teaching atlas of brain imaging. New York: Thieme; 2000. p. 39–41.
7. Albright AL, Lee PA. Neurosurgical treatment of hypothalamic hamartomas causing precocious puberty. J Neurosurg. 1992;78:77–82.
8. Craig DW, Itty A, Panganiban C, et al. Identification of somatic chromosomal abnormalities in hypothalamic hamartoma tissue at the GLI3 locus. Am J Hum Genet. 2008;82:366–74.
9. Biesecker LG. Pallister-Hall syndrome. In Adam MP, Aringer HH, Pagon RA, et al, editors. GeneReviews [Internet]. Seattle (WA); University of Washington, Seattle; 1993–2020; Initial Posting: 5/25/2000; Accessed on internet 1/31/2020.

6 Neurohypophyseal Sarcoidosis

Pertinent Points

- Definition: Neurosarcoidosis with pituitary and hypothalamic involvement is relatively common in patients with systemic sarcoidosis and is more frequently found in cases with largely leptomeningeal involvement, but findings are occasionally confined to the infundibulum.
- *Classic Clue*: Middle-aged African-American female patient presents to ED with excessive urination, extreme thirst, vomiting, diarrhea, fever, and blurred vision. Urinalysis shows ↓ specific gravity, ↓ osmolarity, and ↓ electrolytes. Urine glucose is *not* increased. Serum shows ↑ sodium and potassium. Neuroradiology fellow is trying to transfer the CT request to MRI.
- *AKA*: Sarcoidosis of pituitary stalk.
- Incidence: F > M; Blacks > Whites.
- While it is very rare to see neurosarcoidosis without systemic disease, patients with CNS disease are frequently first to show symptoms.
- The spectrum of disease involving the pituitary infundibulum is broad but distinctly different from that affecting the sella and parasellar regions [26].
- The pituitary stalk normally tapers inferiorly and superiorly spreads out into the infundibular recess of the third ventricle.
- Enlargement of the pituitary stalk is pathologic.
  - Published measurements for the infundibular diameter are:

    3.25 mm +/− 0.56 (SD) mm at the level of the optic chiasm

    1.91 mm +/− 0.40 (SD) mm at the level where the stalk enters the pituitary
  - 95% of people fall within 2 SD and stalk measures:

    ≤4.4 mm at the level of the optic chiasm, and

    ≤2.7 mm where stalk enters the pituitary. [27]
- Remember, the pituitary and its stalk are largely ***outside*** the ***blood-brain barrier*** and ***normally enhance*** with Gd.

Imaging

General Imaging Features

- CT is clearly not as sensitive or specific as MRI, but it is frequently the first imaging modality used in patients with neurosarcoidosis.
- Up to 60% of patients with neurosarcoidosis have "negative" CT scans [20].

CT Features

- Infundibular enlargement with enhancement.
- May demonstrate mass-like or plaque-like dural thickening.
- ↑ attenuation.
- Has no hemorrhage or calcifications.

MRI Features

- Infundibular enlargement with enhancement.
- T1: Usually is isointense to the brain (see Fig. 6.1a).
- *T2: Sarcoid is often hypointense* [19]. This is a **key** feature!
- T1 Gd: Avid enhancement which varies from homogeneous to heterogeneous (see Fig. 6.1b, c).
- Sometimes shows associated cerebral edema.

F. A. Midyett, S. K. Mukherji, *Skull Base Imaging*, https://doi.org/10.1007/978-3-030-46447-9_6

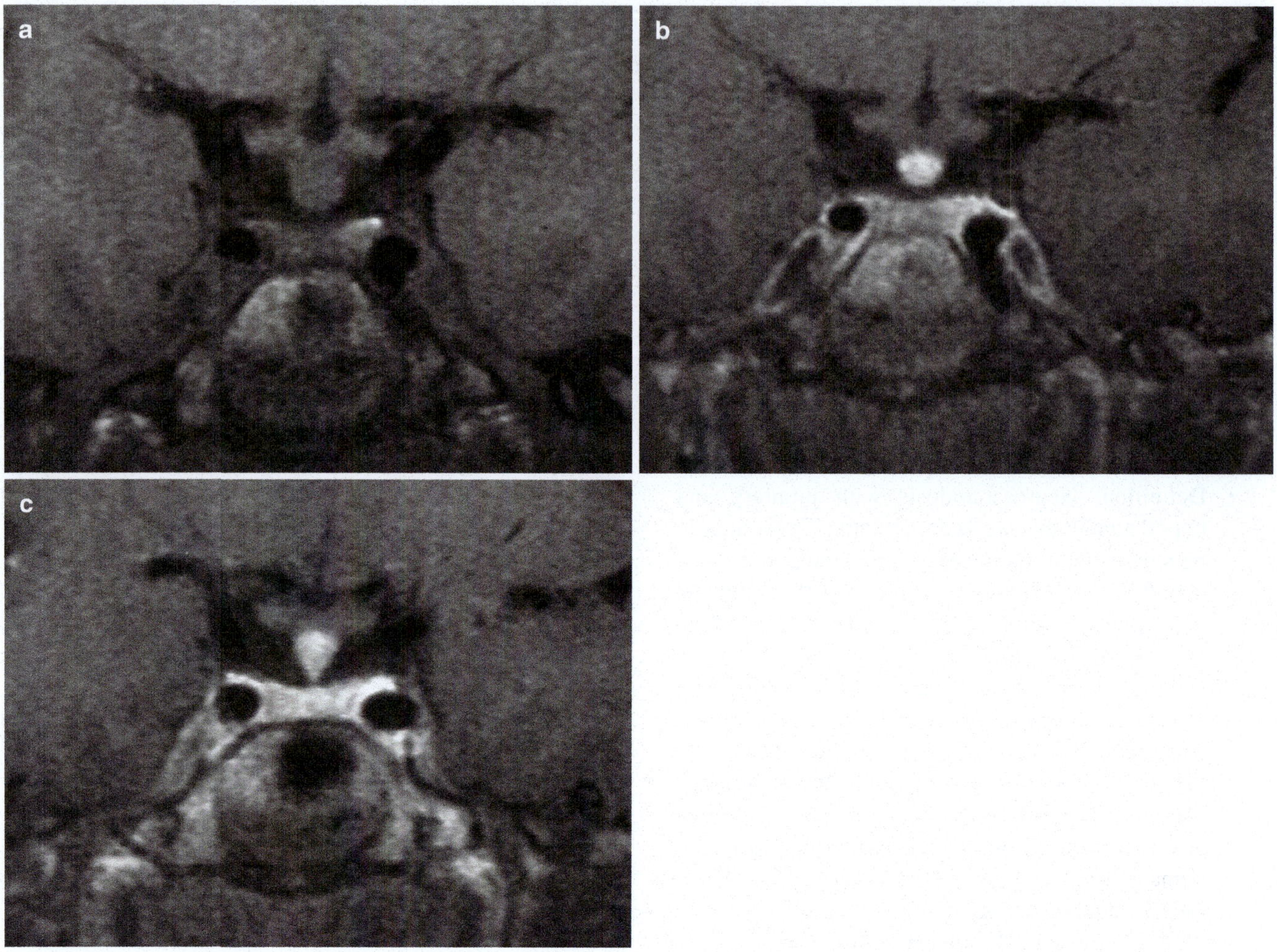

Fig. 6.1 (**a**) Coronal T1 shows oval infundibular mass with signal isointense to the brain. (**b**, **c**) Coronal T1 Gd exhibits avid enhancement of oval infundibular mass extending cranially to level of optic chiasm. The lesion resembles a "spinning top" in image (**c**)

Clinical Issues

Presentation [1, 2]

- Diabetes Insipidus
  - Patient presents to ED with excessive urination, extreme thirst, vomiting, diarrhea, fever, and blurred vision. Urinalysis shows ↓ specific gravity, ↓ osmolarity, and ↓ electrolytes. Urine glucose is *not* increased.
- Generalized symptoms: fever, fatigue, weakness, weight loss, and malaise.
- Orbital symptoms: discomfort, diplopia, proptosis, ptosis, and eyelid swelling.
- Pulmonary symptoms: cough, chest pain, and dyspnea.
- Enlargement and/or irritation of affected organs [5].
- Sarcoidosis is repeatedly referred to as an impersonator or "snowflake" disease because patients predictably present with several symptoms.

Natural History

- Usually presents at 20–40 years old with a second peak between 50 and 60 years old.
- Gender Preference: F > M.
- Overall incidence in Caucasians ~20 per 100,000.
- May affect any organ system [15, 16, 21].
- One half of sarcoidosis patients are asymptomatic.
- African-Americans, Irish, and Scandinavians are most commonly affected [4, 6, 7, 11].
- Lacrimal gland involvement in >50% of patients with sarcoidosis causing "dry eye" symptoms [16].
- Other ocular involvement includes anterior uveitis, vitritis, vasculitis, and choroiditis [14].
- Neurologic involvement of the cranial nerves [including ON], pituitary, spinal cord, and leptomeninges.
- 90% of sarcoidosis patients have pulmonary involvement including interstitial infiltrates with pulmonary fibrosis,

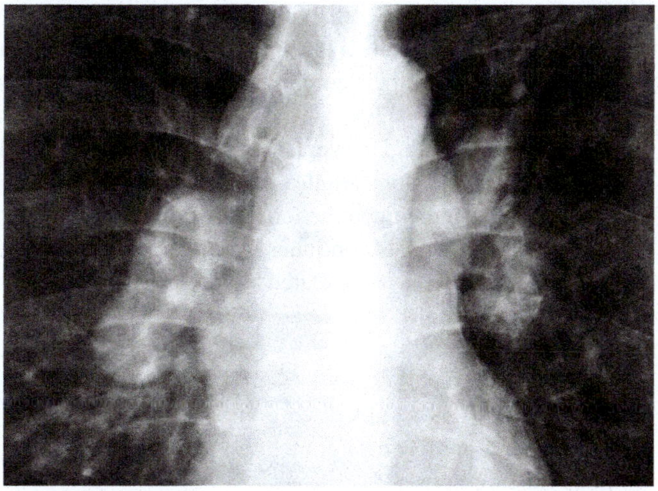

Fig. 6.2 Coned PA chest shows enlargement of bilateral hilar and right paratracheal nodes secondary to sarcoidosis

hypertension, and restrictive pulmonary disease as well as the familiar hilar adenopathy (see Fig. 6.2).

- 30% of patients have dermatologic involvement including cutaneous sarcoidosis and erythema nodosum.
- 25% of patients have cardiac involvement including dysrhythmias and cardiomyopathy.
- Workup may show splenomegaly or reveal renal failure.
- Lofgren syndrome: Hilar adenopathy, polyarthralgia, and erythema nodosum.
- Remember also to look elsewhere for signs of sarcoidosis (see Fig. 6.2 showing classic adenopathy in the chest radiograph).

Epidemiology and Pathology

- Sarcoidosis is a multisystem granulomatous disease with infiltrating T lymphocytes distorting the micro architecture, causing noncaseating granulomas.
- Despite decades of delving into this dire disease, its etiology remains elusive.
- Some suggest it represents an immune illness [12, 13].

Treatment

I. Corticosteroids
   - Mainstay of medical treatment [9].
   - High dose for 2 weeks, followed by gradual tapering after inflammation is controlled.
   - May require maintenance doses for weeks to months.
   - Steroid responsive cases remain at risk for relapse [3, 5, 8].

II. Methotrexate
   - Second line of medical treatment [9].
   - May use to "spare steroids" [5].
   - Methotrexate can cause life-threatening pneumonitis and meningitis after only a few doses in *some* patients.

III. Some patients with systemic sarcoidosis many ***not*** require treatment. However, sarcoidosis is usually treated if the orbit [5] or neurohypophysis is involved [10].

Differential Diagnosis (DDx)

- For the differential of pituitary infundibulum involvement, consider in addition to sarcoidosis [26]:

A. Infundibular Neurohypophysitis (INH)

- Most common cause (>25%) of adult infundibular disease
  - Causes enhancing, mass-like thickening of the pituitary infundibulum [26]

B. Metastasis

- Ties with Whipple's disease for third most frequent (11%) cause of infundibular disease in adults [26]
- Causes enhancing mass-like thickening of pituitary infundibulum [26]

C. Whipple's Disease

- Ties with metastatic disease for third most frequent (11%) cause of infundibular disease in adults.
- Other granulomatous diseases which can involve the pituitary stalk include Wegener's disease and tuberculosis [26].

D. Langerhans Cell Histiocytosis

- Second most common cause of pediatric infundibular disease at almost 20%, second only to hypoplasia accounting for >60%.
- Predominately pediatric population, age 1–5.
- M: F = 2:1 [18]
- See Chap. 8, Langerhans Cell Histiocytosis.

E. Pituicytomas/Infundibuloma

- 5% of adult infundibular disease tied in frequency with duplication, Rathke's cleft cyst, leukemia, and germinoma.
- Rare, arising from specialized glial cells in the neurohypophysis and infundibulum [17].
- Peak incidence in the fifth decade. All cases >20 years old.
- Gender preference: M < F = 1:2.
- WHO Grade I, histologically fibrillary astrocytomas.

- T1: isointense solid mass.
- T1 Gd: avid enhancement.
- T2: heterogeneous. Iso- to hypointense.
- Often observe absent pituitary bright spot [17].

F. Granular Cell Tumor of Pituitary

- AKA: Pituitary choristomas
- Previously believed to be the same as pituicytoma but now felt to be a separate entity.

G. Lymphoma

- Lymphoma infiltrating pituitary is difficult to differentiate from an adenoma, meningioma, or other sellar lesion.
- When T1 and T2 show iso-hypointense mass lesions in an immunocompromised older patient, lymphoma must be considered [25].

H. Leukemia

- Causes 5% of adult infundibular disease.

A Closer Look

I. Fast Facts

- One half of sarcoidosis patients achieve remission within 3 years.
- Two thirds of sarcoidosis patients achieve remission within 10 years.
- One third of sarcoidosis patients have persistent disease.
- 5% of sarcoidosis patients die from cardiac, respiratory, or neurologic disease with pulmonary fibrosis the most common cause of death [4, 5].
- 10% of patients with sarcoidosis have clinically symptomatic CNS involvement. 25% of patients with sarcoidosis have CNS involvement at autopsy [19, 22].
- Pituitary, hypothalamic, or optic chiasmatic sarcoidosis occurs in only 0.5% of all patients with sarcoidosis [24].
- Sarcoidosis is the second most frequent cause (14%) of adult infundibular disease second to INH (infundibular neurohypophysitis) [26].

II. Historic Highlights

- 1869 Sir Jonathan Hutchinson, English surgeon, ophthalmologist, dermatologist, venereologist, and pathologist, first described skin lesions associated with sarcoidosis. In his day sarcoidosis was considered a dermatological curiosity [29].
- Some suggest noted Scottish physician and writer Arthur Conan Doyle and English Physician Jonathan Hutchinson connected through their common interest in ophthalmology and sarcoidosis [30].
- 1897 Caesar Boeck, Norwegian dermatologist, described (in a policeman) skin nodules which he thought resembled sarcoma and coined the term "sarcoid."
- Interest in sarcoidosis continues to remain high. To date, more than 5000 sarcoid related articles have been published [22, 23, 28].

III. Genetics

- Familial clusters coupled with inconstant ethnic incidences lend credence to contentions of genetic connections for sarcoidosis.
- Nearly a century after Martensen showed sarcoidosis in siblings, few environmental connections have been established [31, 32].
- However, numerous HLA and non-HLA genetic candidates have been connected to sarcoidosis susceptibility.
- In summary, sarcoidosis is currently considered to be a consequence of complex interactions between various environmental agents and assorted alleles [32].

Selected References

1. Weinreb RN, Tessler H. Laboratory diagnosis of ophthalmic sarcoidosis. Surv Ophthalmol. 1984;28:653–64.
2. Morgenthau AS, Iannuzzi MC. Recent advances in sarcoidosis. Chest. 2011;139:174–82.
3. Yarnardag H, Pamuk ON. Lacrimal gland involvement in sarcoidosis. Swiss Med Wkly. 2003;133:388–91.
4. Iannuzzi MC, Fontana JR. Sarcoidosis: clinical presentation, immunopathogenesis, and therapeutics. JAMA. 2011;305(4):391–9.
5. Tsui J, Allen R. Sarcoidosis affecting the lacrimal gland. Eye Rounds.org. July 14, 2011.
6. Bresnitz EA, Strom EB. Epidemiology of sarcoidosis. Epidemiol Rev. 1983;5:124–56.
7. Mavrikakis I, Rootman J. Diverse clinical presentations of orbital Sarcoid. Am J Ophthalmol. 2007;144:769–75.
8. Prabhakaran VC, et al. Orbital and adnexal sarcoidosis. Arch Ophthalmol. 2007;125(12):1657–62.
9. Smith JK, Matheus MG, Castillo M. Imaging manifestations of neurosarcoidosis. AJR Am J Roentgenol. 2004;182(2):289–95.
10. Johns CJ, Michele TM. The clinical Management of Sarcoidosis: a 50-year experience at the Johns Hopkins Hospital. Medicine. 1999;78:65–111.
11. Koyama T, Ueda H, Togashi K, et al. Radiologic manifestations of sarcoidosis in various organs. Radiographics. 2004;24:87–104.
12. Weerakkody Y, Gillard F, et al. Sarcoidosis. Radiopaedia.org.

13. Miller BH, Rosado-deChristenson ML, Mcadams HP, et al. Thoracic sarcoidosis: radiologic-pathologic correlation. Radiographics. 1995;15(2):421–37.
14. Baughman RP, Lower EE, Kaufman AH. Ocular sarcoidosis. Semin Respir Crit Care Med. 2010;31(4):452–62.
15. Hunninghake GW, Costabel U, Ando M, et al. ATS/ERS.WASOG statement on Sarcoidosis. American Thoracic Society/European Respiratory Society/World Association of Sarcoidosis and other Granulomatous Disorders. Sarcoidosis Vasc Diffuse Lung Dis. 1999;15:149–73.
16. Boukes RJ, de Vries-Knoppert WA. Lacrimal gland enlargement as one of the ocular manifestations of Wegener's granulomatosis. Documenta Ophthalmlogica. 1985;59(1):21–6.
17. Gibbs WN, Monuki ES, Linskey ME, et al. Pituicytoma: diagnostic features on selective carotid angiogram and MR imaging. AJNR Am J Neuroradiol. 2006;27(8):1639–42.
18. Hann IM, Smith OP. Pediatric hematology: Wiley-Blackwell; 2006.
19. Fischbein NJ, Dillon WP, Barkovich AJ. Teaching atlas of brain imaging. Thieme New York 2000; 213–215.
20. Kornienko VN, Pronin IN. Diagnostic neuroradiology: Springer Verlag; 2008.
21. Katzman GL, Langford CA, Sneller MC, et al. Pituitary involvement by Wegener's granulomatosis: a report of two cases. AJNR Am J Neuroradiol. 1999;20:519–23.
22. Iannuzzi MC, Rybicki BA, Teirstein AS. Sarcoidosis. N Engl J Med. 2007;357:2153–65.
23. Sharma OP. Definition and history of sarcoidosis. European Respiratory Monograph; ISSN 1025-448x. ISBN 1–904097–22-7.
24. Athyal RP, Sellar SS. Sellar and Parasellar Neurosarcoidosis: magnetic resonance imaging features. Indian J Radiol Imaging. 2002;12:487–9.
25. Tamer G, Kartal I, Aral F. Pituitary infiltration by non-Hodgkin's lymphoma: a case report. J Med Case Rep. 2009;3:9293.
26. Hamilton BE, Salzman KL, Osborn AG. Anatomic and pathologic spectrum of pituitary infundibulum lesions. AJR 2007;188(3).
27. Simmons G, et al. MR Imaging of the pituitary Stalk. AJR. 1992;159
28. Boeck C. Multiple benign sarcoid of the skin. J Cutan Gen Urin Dis. 1899;17:543–50.
29. James GD, Sharma OP. From Hutchinson to now: a historical glimpse. Current opin Pulm Med. 2002;8:416–23.
30. Arthur Conan Doyle and Jonathan Hutchinson: the sarcoidosis connection. Sarcoidosis. 2003;10(1):69–70.
31. Martenstein H. Knochveranderungen bei lupus pernio. Zentralbl Haut Geschlechtskr Grenzeb. 1923;7:308.
32. Annuzzi MC, Rybicki BA. Genetics of sarcoidosis: candidate genes and genome scans. Proc Am Thorac Soc. 2007;4(1):108–16. https://doi.org/10.1513/pats.200607-141JG.

Intrasellar Arachnoid Cyst

7

Pertinent Points

- Definition: True intrasellar arachnoid cysts are very rare arising from unexplained tearing or splitting of the already spider-like arachnoid membrane [1].
- *Classic Clue*: Patient having a long history of headache, menstrual irregularity, and dizziness developed recent onset ↓ visual acuity. Non-enhancing fluid-filled mass fills and expands the sella displacing the pituitary posteriorly and inferiorly.
- Synonyms: Intracranial arachnoid cyst, subarachnoid cyst.
- Incidence: M > F [2, 3].
- Intracranial arachnoid cysts occur most frequently in the middle cranial fossa with <10% seen in sellar and parasellar regions [1, 4–6].
- Though rare, intrasellar arachnoid cysts represent an important cause of reversible visual loss [7].

Imaging

General Imaging Features

- Cystic intrasellar mass often showing suprasellar extension [8].
- Characteristic arachnoid-like, thin transparent, cyst walls are just barely seen on imaging.

CT Features

- CT attenuation in Hounsfield units is identical to CSF.
- No postcontrast enhancement.
- Often shows suprasellar extension [1, 8–10].
- Has no hemorrhage or calcifications.

MRI Features

- T1: Usually isointense to CSF (see Fig. 7.1a–c).
- T2: Usually isointense to CSF (see Fig. 7.1d).
- T1 Gd: *No enhancement.*
- Cystic intrasellar mass often shows suprasellar extension [8].

Clinical Issues

Presentation

- 20% of patients are asymptomatic at the time of diagnosis and may not require surgery [1, 9].
- Generalized symptoms: resemble that of patient with nonfunctional pituitary adenoma, craniopharyngioma, Rathke's cleft cyst, epidermoid, and empty sella. Symptoms include headache, visual symptoms, menstrual irregularities, ↓ libido, rapid weight gain, vertigo, confusion, and impotence [8, 11, 12].

Natural History

- *Prevalence:* The prevalence of intracranial arachnoid cysts in patients with prior MRIs at a large university was 1.4% in adults [3] and 2.6% in children [2].
- Gender preference: M > F in adults and children [2, 3].
- Arachnoid cysts are symptomatic in only a small number of patients. Those who present without symptoms usually show a benign natural history [3].

F. A. Midyett, S. K. Mukherji, *Skull Base Imaging*, https://doi.org/10.1007/978-3-030-46447-9_7

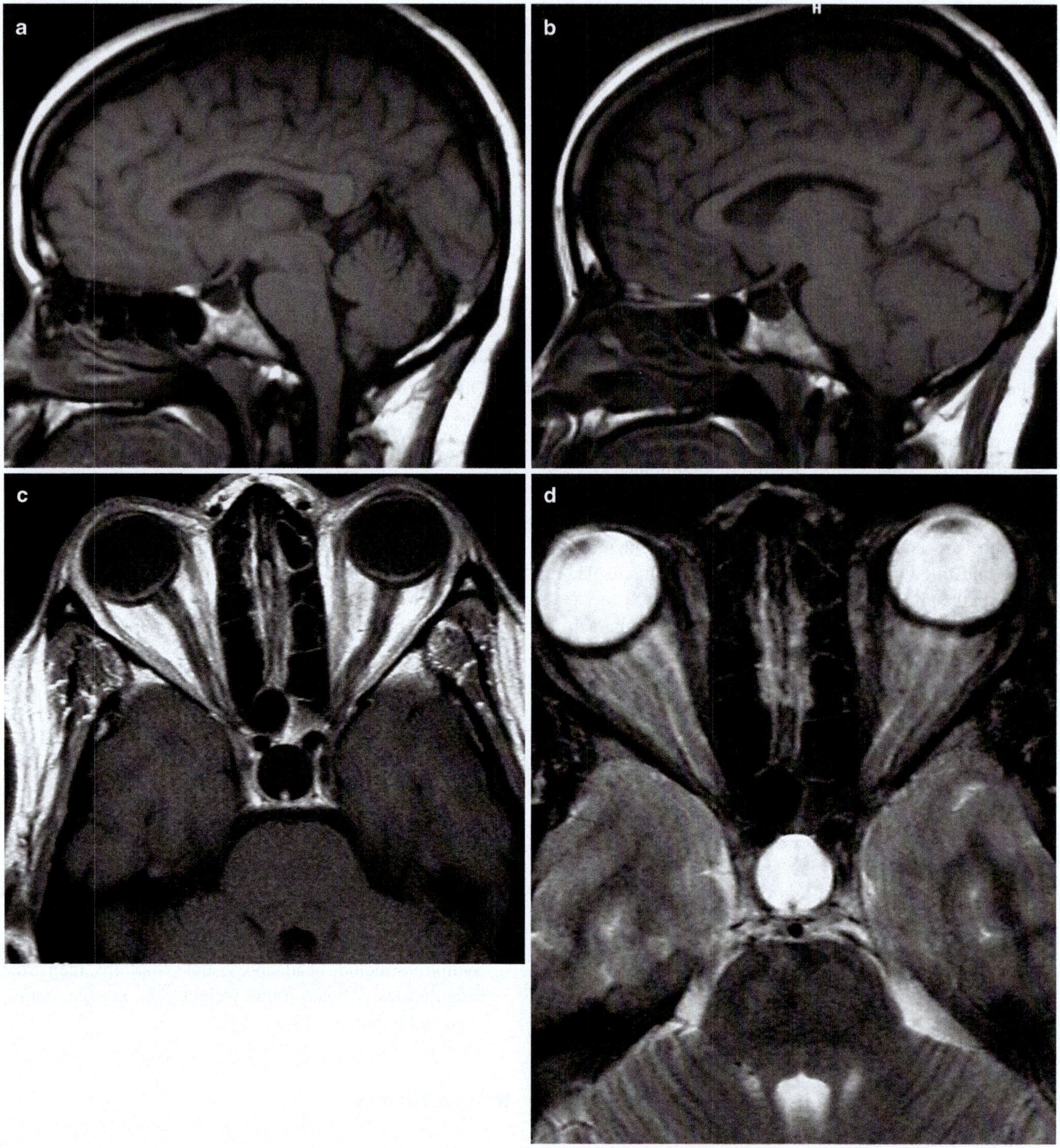

Fig. 7.1 (**a**, **b**) Sagittal T1 depicts intrasellar mass showing signal slightly hyperintense to adjacent CSF. The normal pituitary is not seen on these images. Intrasellar arachnoid cyst. (**c**) Axial T1 shows low signal of fluid-filled intrasellar mass with bright signal from infundibulum located posteriorly. (**d**) Axial T2 shows bright signal of fluid-filled intrasellar mass with "filling defect" of low signal infundibulum located posteriorly

Epidemiology and Pathology

- Intracranial arachnoid cysts develop in the arachnoid mater [located between the superficial dura mater covering the skull and the deeper pia mater covering the brain] and appear to arise from some strange splitting of this spindly shroud.
- Arachnoid cysts are benign CSF-filled masses enclosed by thin, transparent cyst walls.
- The cyst fluid is usually clear and colorless but can occasionally be hemorrhagic or proteinaceous.
- Arachnoid cysts can be congenital or acquired usually beginning in infancy although often not showing symptoms until adolescence or adulthood.
- Microscopically the cyst wall has a vascular collagenous membrane lined by arachnoid cells [13] appearing histologically indistinguishable from the normal arachnoid membrane [14].
- Progressive enlargement of arachnoid cysts has prompted theories of (1) active cyst wall secretion of fluid, (2) osmotic gradient diffusion of fluid into cyst, and (3) "ball-valve" mechanism.

Treatment

- 20% of intrasellar arachnoid cysts are asymptomatic and may not require surgery [1, 9].
- Symptomatic intrasellar arachnoid cysts are probably best treated by transsphenoidal microsurgery with decompression and fenestration to restore lost vision and pituitary function [7].
- CSF rhinorrhea is the major complication of transsphenoidal surgery [1, 15, 16].

Differential Diagnosis (DDx)

- The differential of an intrasellar cystic lesion (in addition to AC arachnoid cyst) includes:

A. Rathke's Cleft Cyst (RCC)

- Most RCCs do *not* enlarge the sella. ACs sometimes enlarge the sella.
- RCCs sometimes show septations. Not a feature of AC.
- RCC's with CSF intensity fluid is common in up to 44% [1, 5, 9, 17].
- Cyst walls often do not enhance with either RCC or AC (arachnoid cyst).
- Asymptomatic RCCs are common, being found in 1/4 of autopsies. By contrast, the prevalence of intracerebral ACs is closer to 2–3% [2, 3] with only 10% of those being intrasellar [12].
- See Chap. 1, Rathke's Cleft Cyst.

B. Cystic Pituitary Adenoma

- Pituitary adenoma usually shows solid components, but a totally cystic pituitary adenoma may be a problematic differential.
- See Chap. 2, Pituitary Adenoma.

C. Craniopharyngioma (CR)

- Craniopharyngiomas often have mixed cystic and enhancing solid components. Not a feature for arachnoid cysts.
- Craniopharyngiomas are often calcified. Not a feature of AC.
- Like liquid products in your automobile, the varying viscosity of craniopharyngioma's cystic fluid fluctuates from yellowish proteinaceous fluid to classic "crank-case oil" containing cholesterol and blood products. *Not a feature of AC.*
- Craniopharyngiomas infiltrate adjacent structures on MRI. *Not a feature of AC.*
- Craniopharyngiomas occasionally enlarge and/or erode the sella. *Not a feature of AC.*
- See Chap. 3, Craniopharyngioma.

D. Epidermoid Cyst

- Epidermoids exhibit restricted diffusion and are bright on DWI with corresponding dark signal on ADC map. Not a feature for arachnoid cysts which follow CSF on all imaging sequences.
- Epidermoids are rare in children [13].
- See Chap. 9, Epidermoid Cyst.

E. Empty Sella

- Does not have a discrete intrasellar mass.
- Fluid filling sella has a signal which follows CSF on all imaging sequences.
- See Fig. 7.2a–c.

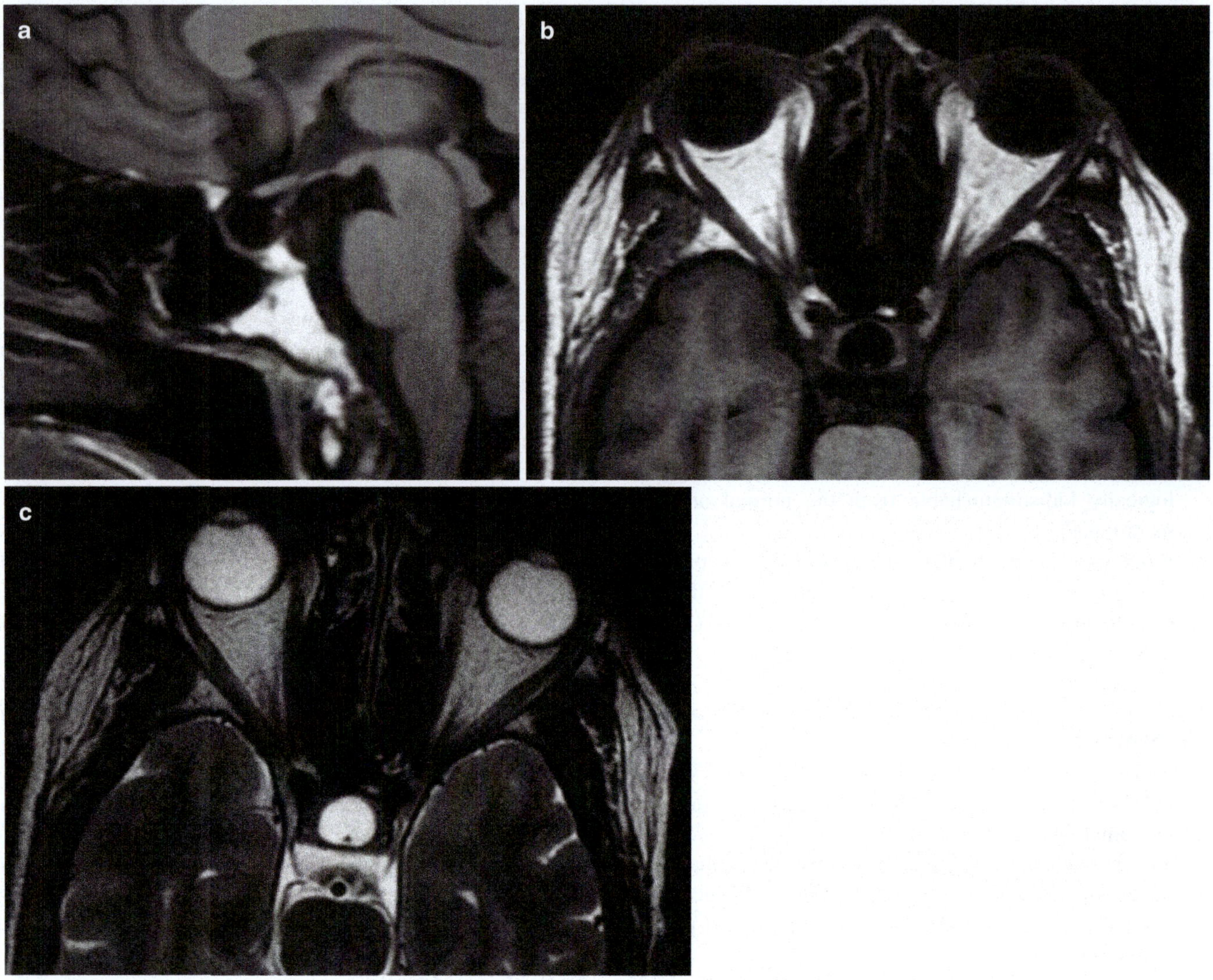

Fig. 7.2 (**a**) Sagittal T1 FLAIR shows sella filled predominately by CSF. The infundibulum and pituitary are displaced posteriorly in this case of "empty sella." (**b**) Axial T1 shows low signal of fluid-filled sella with tiny bright signal from infundibulum located posteriorly in this case of "empty sella." (**c**) Axial T2 shows bright signal of fluid-filled sella with tiny "filling defect" from low signal infundibulum located posteriorly in this case of "empty sella"

A Closer Look

I. Fast Facts

- The long-standing pulsatile pressure produced by arachnoid cysts probably causes more damage to adjacent structures than other types of cysts [1, 15].
- Arachnoid cysts cause 1% of intracranial space-occupying lesions [12].
- 10% of symptomatic intracranial arachnoid cysts are intrasellar [12].

II. Historic Highlights

- 1831 Richard Bright first described arachnoid cysts [18]. Yes, this is the same Bright we remember for "albuminuric nephritis" as Bright's disease. The brilliance of Bright's pioneering descriptions appear even more amazing when you consider he didn't have the help of a microscope or formaldehyde to preserve tissue.
- 1935 Barlow published the first case of a suprasellar arachnoid cyst [19].

- 1958 Starkman reported ACs lie between two membranes of normal arachnoid and described them as "intra-arachnoid" cysts.
- 1907 Placzek and Krause successfully surgically treated an arachnoid cyst.
- 1981 Stein advocated shunting for primary treatment of AC.
- 2000 German Air Force began head and spine MRI screening for ACs. Kriebel and Maxon (2002) suggested ACs are "time bombs" in pilot's head which should render them "unfit to fly" [20].
- Many may debate whether ACs are problematic for pilots or passengers, but most nations do not pre-screen their pilots with MRI and those pilots presumably have a prevalence of intracranial arachnoid cysts of about 2%.

III. Genetics and Associations

- The current consensus continues to counsel that arachnoid cysts arise from "unexplained tearing" of arachnoid membranes.
- The precise primary elemental etiology enigmatically endures. Acknowledged associations include agenesis of the corpus callosum, arachnoiditis, mucopolysaccharidosis, and, of course, Chudley-McCollough and Marfan's syndromes.
- Reports of intracranial arachnoid cysts in siblings suggest some familial cases where inheritance is influenced by an autosomal recessive or polygenic pattern [21–24].

Selected References

1. Gok B, Kapanoglu E, Solaroglu O. Intrasellar arachnoid cyst: a case report. Neuroanatomy. 2003;2:22–4.
2. Al-Holou WN, Yew AY, Boomsaad ZE, et al. Prevalence and natural history of arachnoid cysts in children clinical article. J Neurosurg Pediatr. 2010;5(6):578–85.
3. Al-Holou WN, Terman S, Kilburg C. Prevalence and natural history of arachnoid cysts in adults. J Neurosurg. 2013;118(2):222–31.
4. Hasegawa M, Yamashima T, Yamashita J, et al. Symptomatic intrasellar arachnoid cyst: case report. Surg Neurol. 1991;35:355–9.
5. Kucharczyk W, Peck WW, Kelly WM, et al. Rathke cleft cysts: CT, MR imaging and pathologic features. Radiology. 1987;165:491–5.
6. Rengacharry SS, Watanabe I, Brackett CE. Pathogenesis of intracranial arachnoid cysts. Surg Neurol. 1978;9:139–44.
7. Weil RJ. Rapidly progressive visual loss caused by a sellar arachnoid cyst: reversal with transsphenoidal microsurgery. South Med J. 2001;94(11). Lippincott Williams & Wilkins.
8. Dubuisson AS, Stevenaert A, Martin DH, et al. Intrasellar arachnoid cysts. Neurosurgery. 2007;61(3):505–13.
9. Myer FB, Carpenter SM, Laws ER Jr. Intrasellar arachnoid cysts. Surg Neurol. 1987;28:105–10.
10. Iqbal J, Kanaan I, Al HM. Non-neoplastic cystic lesions of the sellar region presentation, diagnosis and management of eight cases and review of the literature. Acta Neurochir. 1999(141):389–97.
11. Tanaka Y, Hayashi S, Nakai M, et al. Intrasellar arachnoid cyst: a case report. No Shinkei Geka. 1995;23(9):801–6.
12. Chang CW, Lin JH, Won JGS. Intrasellar arachnoid cyst with Panhypopituitarism: a case report. Formos J Endocrin Metab. 2012;3(3):57–60.
13. Fischbein NJ, Dillon WP, Barkovich AJ. Teaching atlas of brain imaging. New York: Thieme; 2000. p. 78–81.
14. Miyagami M. Tsunokawa: histological and ultrastructural findings of benign intracranial cysts. Noshuyo Byori. 1993;10:151–60.
15. Baskin DS, Wilson CB. Transsphenoidal treatment of non-neoplastic intrasellar cysts. A report of 38 cases. J Neurosurg. 1984;60:8–13.
16. Sumida M, Uozumi T, Yamanaka M, et al. Displacement of the normal pituitary gland by sellar and juxtasellar tumours: surgical-MRI correlation and use in differential diagnosis. Neuroradiology. 1994;36:372–5.
17. Ross DA, Norman D, Wilson CB. Radiologic characteristics and results of surgical management of Rathke's cysts in 43 patients. Neurosurgery. 1992;30:173–8.
18. Bright R. Serous cysts in the arachnoid. In: Rees O, Brown G, editors. Diseases of the brain and nervous system. Part I. London: Longman Group Ltd; 1831. p. 437–9.
19. Barlow A. Suprasellar arachnoid cyst. Arch Ophthalmol. 1935;14:53–60.
20. Lueling F, Zschommler Y. Intracranial arachnoid cysts in German military aircraft pilots. Flugmedizinisches Institut der Luftwaffe. German Air Force Institute of Aviation Medicine. 2017.
21. Handa J, Okamoto K, Sato M. Arachnoid cyst of the middle cranial fossa: report of bilateral cysts in siblings. Surg Neurol 1981;16:127–30. [PubMed: 7280984, related citations] [Full Text].
22. Helland CA, Wester K. Monozygotic twins with mirror image cysts: indication of a genetic mechanism in arachnoid cysts? Neurology. 2007;69:110–1. [PubMed: 17606888, related citations] [Full Text].
23. Pomeranz S, Constantini S, Lubetzki-Korn I, Amir N. Familial intracranial arachnoid cysts. Childs Nerv Syst. 1991;7:100–2. [PubMed: 1863926, related citations] [Full Text].
24. Wilson WG, Deponte KA, McIlhenny J, Dreifuss FE. Arachnoid cysts in a brother and sister. J Med Genet. 1988;25:714–5. [PubMed: 3225827, related citations] [Full Text].

8 Langerhans Cell Histiocytosis

Pertinent Points

- Definition: Langerhans cell histiocytosis (LCH) is the modern moniker bestowed on a rare, ill understood but significant, pathologic process related to proliferation of macrophages and dendrites [formerly hailed as histiocytes].
- *Classic Clue*: Pediatrics refer for MRI a child with a history of diabetes insipidus who is found to have an avidly enhancing infundibular stalk enlargement and an absent posterior pituitary bright spot.
- AKA: Hand-Schüller-Christian disease, Abt-Letterer-Siwe disease, histiocytosis X, histiocytosis X syndrome, eosinophilic granulomatosis [misnomer].
- Gender preference: M > F = 2:1; rare in African-Americans [1].
- LCH predominately involves age 1–5 pediatric population, typically appearing during the first decade.
- LCH is the most common cause of an abnormal enhancing infundibular mass in the pediatric population.

Imaging

General Imaging Features

- See Chap. 6, Neurohypophyseal Sarcoidosis\Imaging\General Imaging Features, for discussion on pituitary stalk enlargement.

MRI Features

- Abnormal thickening of the pituitary infundibulum (see Fig. 8.1a) with avid postcontrast enhancement of associated soft tissue mass (see Figs. 8.1b and 8.2b, d).
- Absence of the normal posterior pituitary bright spot (see Fig. 8.1a).
- Mass involving the optic chiasm and/or hypothalamus.
- Nodular enhancing thickening of the dura and/or leptomeninges.
- Destructive lesions involving the calvarium and/or temporal bones usually correspond to lesions demonstrated on CT (see Fig. 8.2a, c).
- Brain parenchymal lesions include:
  - Cerebral hemispheres, brainstem, or cerebellum.
  - T1 isointense to brain.
  - T2 mildly hyperintense to brain.
  - T1 Gd usually (but not always) enhances.

CT and Plain Film Features

- Lytic lesions are sometimes seen involving the calvarium and/or temporal bones (see Fig. 8.3).
- MRI is superior for demonstrating dural and brain parenchymal disease.

Clinical Issues

Presentation

- Diabetes insipidus (DI) is a common presentation for patients with involvement of the infundibulum or hypothalamus.
- 5% of patients with LCH present with DI.
- One third of patients with LCH develop DI.
- Different disease sites cause diverse symptoms:
  - Orbital involvement often causes presentation with proptosis.
  - Temporal bone involvement may elucidate emergence of hearing loss and chronic ear drainage.

F. A. Midyett, S. K. Mukherji, *Skull Base Imaging*, https://doi.org/10.1007/978-3-030-46447-9_8

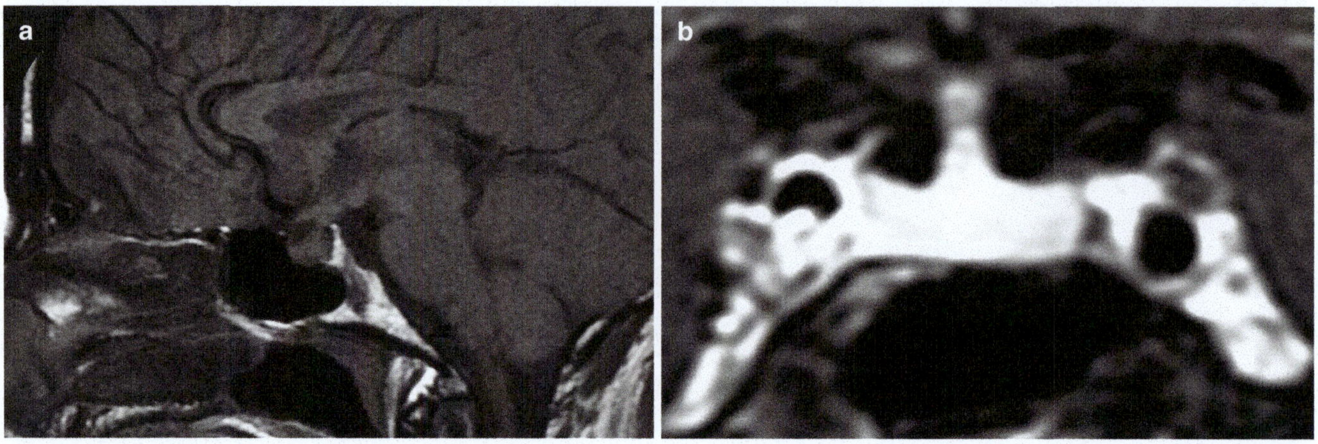

Fig. 8.1 (**a**) Sagittal T1 shows abnormal thickening of the pituitary infundibulum with conspicuous absence of the normally seen posterior pituitary bright spot. (**b**) Coronal T1 Gd shows enhancement of conspicuously enlarged infundibulum from the pituitary to the hypothalamus

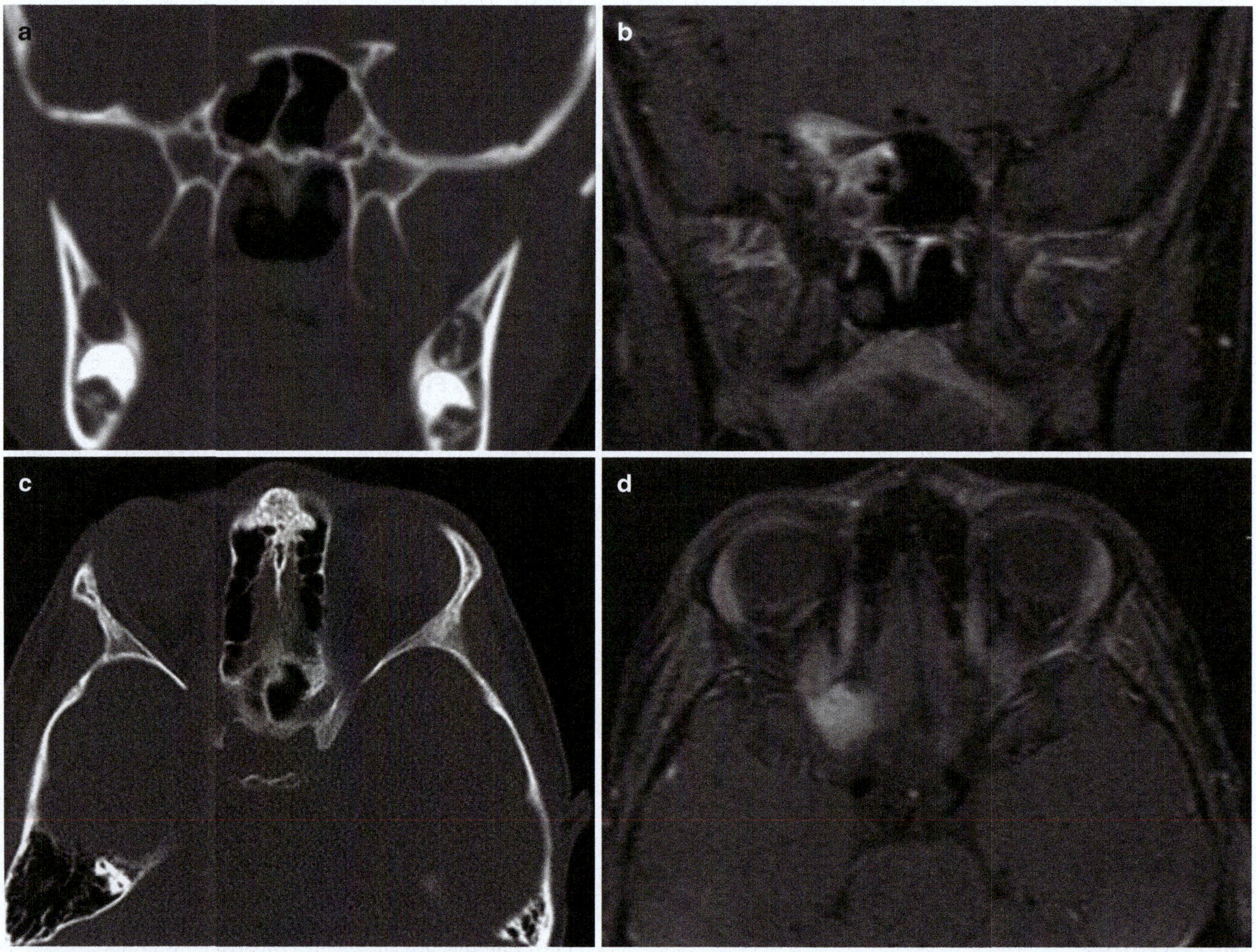

Fig. 8.2 (**a**) Coronal NECT bone algorithm shows seemingly surgically sharp bony defect involving the roof of the right sphenoid sinus with soft tissue extending into the sinus. There is conspicuous absence of the right anterior clinoid process. Soft tissue density in the left sphenoid may be post-inflammatory in origin. (**b**) Coronal T1 Gd shows avidly enhancing mass involving the right lesser sphenoid wing extending through bony defect [demonstrated on **a**] involving the roof of the right sphenoid sinus with enhancing soft tissue extending into the sinus. (**c**) Axial bone algorithm CT shows truncation of the posterior aspect of right lateral orbital wall. There is sharp and conspicuous absence of most of the right anterior clinoid with destruction sparing a portion of its tip. (**d**) Axial T1 Gd shows avidly enhancing mass involving the right lesser sphenoid wing extending through the orbital apex into the retrobulbar region. The enhancing mass accounts for the destructive lesion on the CT (**c**). Low signal soft tissue mass in the sphenoid sinus

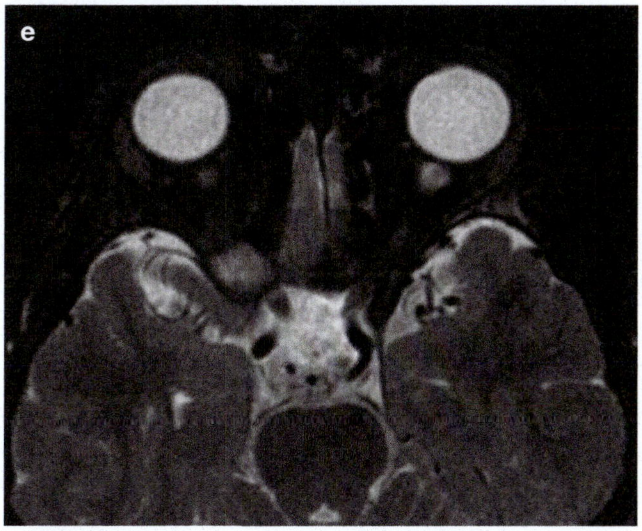

Fig. 8.2 (continued) (**e**) Axial T2 shows hyperintense mass involving the right lesser sphenoid wing extending into the orbital apex. High signal soft tissue LCH mass involves sphenoid sinus

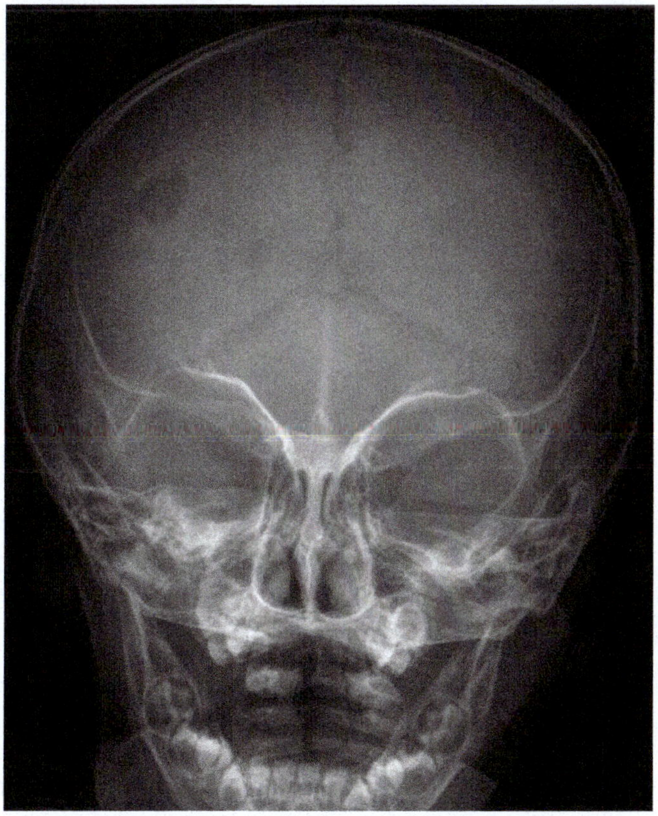

Fig. 8.3 Frontal plain film of skull shows a well-demarcated lytic lesion which typically involves the frontal or parietal bones

  - Dural involvement can cause headache.
  - Cerebellar involvement may activate ataxia and dysmetria [1].
- Patients *rarely* present with solely CNS involvement [1], so a thorough search for other lesions is imperative.
- Search sites should include the skull, spine, cord, and brain specifically including areas mentioned above.

Natural History

- The cause of LCH continues to be unknown.
- LCH is typically treated as a neoplasm, although most feel it is an immune disorder.
- LCH continues to be confusing, presenting in several modes from mild solitary "eosinophilic granuloma" to more severe forms with both bone and soft tissue involvement.

Epidemiology and Pathology

- Gross: Soft supple mass.
- Microscopic: Periadventitial granulomas contain various inflammatory cells with Langerhans' histiocytes [1].

Treatment and Prognosis

I. Chemotherapy

- Chemotherapy is currently considered to be the primary treatment for LCH.
- Clinicians are hoping for new targeted chemotherapy tied to specific gene therapy.

II. Radiation Therapy (RT)

- Some consider radiotherapy to be a safe and effective treatment option for LCH and feel that low RT doses show sufficient local control [10].

III. Surgery

- Some favor complete microsurgical resection of hypothalamic granulomas as well as other CNS lesions.
- Surgery may be required to acutely treat mass effect or to remove isolated bony lesions [1].
- Prognosis is worse in patients presenting early with extensive disease.
- Although survival rates are high for up to 15 years, event free survival at 15 years is 30% [1].
- Surgery conveys an adverse associated mortality of ≤10% [5].

Differential Diagnosis

For the differential of pituitary infundibulum involvement, consider the following in addition to LCH:

A. Neurohypophyseal Sarcoidosis

- Neurohypophyseal sarcoidosis is more frequent in middle-aged black females. LCH is more frequent in male children, reportedly *rare* in African-Americans.
- Sarcoidosis is often *hypointense* on T2 [1]. Not a feature of LCH.
- 90% of sarcoidosis patients have pulmonary involvement. Not a feature of LCH.
- 30% of sarcoidosis patients demonstrate dermatologic involvement. Not a feature of LCH.

B. Infundibular Neurohypophysitis (INH)

- INH is the most common cause (>25%) of ADULT infundibular disease. LCH is usually present in children [but 90% survive and recurrences can continue into adulthood].
- INH causes enhancing mass-like thickening of the pituitary infundibulum [2].
- INH may be indistinguishable from LCH if only imaging the neurohypophysis, but LCH is usually associated with disease elsewhere.

C. Metastasis

- Ties with Whipple's disease for third most frequent (11%) cause of infundibular disease in adults [2, 6]
- Causes enhancing mass-like thickening of pituitary infundibulum [2]
- Look for metastatic disease elsewhere

D. Whipple's Disease

- Ties with metastatic disease for third most frequent (11%) cause of infundibular disease in adults.
- Other granulomatous diseases which can involve the pituitary stalk include Wegener's disease and tuberculosis [2].

E. Pituicytomas/Infundibuloma

- 5% of adult infundibular disease tied in frequency with duplication, Rathke's cleft cyst, leukemia, and germinoma.
- Rare, arising from specialized glial cells in the neurohypophysis and infundibulum [1, 7].
- Peak incidence in the fifth decade. All cases >20 years old.
- Gender preference: M < F = 1:2.
- WHO Grade I, histologically fibrillary astrocytomas.
- T1: isointense solid mass.
- T1 Gd: exhibit avid enhancement.
- T2: heterogeneous. Iso- to hypointense.
- Pituitary bright spot [3].

F. Granular Cell Tumor of Pituitary

- AKA: Pituitary choristomas.
- Previously believed to be the same as pituicytoma but now felt to be a separate entity.
- Granular cell tumors are glial tumors arising in the posterior pituitary or pituitary stalk.
- Usually incidental tumors in adults at autopsy [8].
- Granular cell tumors of the pituitary stalk are rare, comprising <0.1% of primary brain tumors.
- They present with insidious development of HA, ↓ visual acuity, and bitemporal visual field defects.

G. Lymphoma

- Lymphoma infiltrating the pituitary can be difficult to differentiate from adenoma, meningioma, and other sellar lesions.
- When T1 and T2 show iso-hypointense mass lesions in an immunocompromised older patient, lymphoma must be considered [4].

H. Leukemia

- Leukemia causes 5% of infundibular disease in adults.
- Showing nonspecific stalk thickening, the cases are not usually diagnostic dilemmas, since the leukemic diagnosis typically precedes this postponed problem [2].

I. Hypophyseal Tuberculoma

- Extremely rare lesions.
- May occur in the absence of systemic tuberculosis.
- The finding of a thickened pituitary stalk is useful in separating them from pituitary adenomas.
- Surgery is not an appropriate primary treatment for these lesions [6].
- Accurate diagnosis is important as antituberculous chemotherapy is curative [7].

J. Rhabdomyosarcoma (RMS)

- Rare lesion of pediatric skull base temporal bone.
- Imaging characteristics are similar to LCH.
- Lesion location may be helpful in making the correct diagnosis.
- LCH more frequently involves the mastoid.
- Rhabdomyosarcoma is classically confined to the anterior temporal bone [2, 6, 11].
- See Chap. 49, Rhabdomyosarcoma.

A Closer Look

I. Genetics

- Recent studies show the majority of LCH biopsy specimens demonstrate a V600 BRAF oncogene mutation, regardless of the involved organ or development stage.
- With this mutation already found in other tumors ranging from benign nevi to malignant melanoma, it appears that more mutations are necessary to render these cells malignant.
- This discovery has, however, raised the possibility for targeted therapy [9].

II. Fast Facts

- CNS manifestations of LCH occur in ≤50% and are more frequent in patients with multisystem disease [1].
- Patients *rarely* present with isolated CNS involvement [1].

III. Historic Highlights

- Pathologists previously used the term histiocytosis X lumping both benign and severe disease forms together including [the already lumped] Hand-Schüller-Christian and Abt-Letterer-Siwe diseases.
- When a pathologic process carries this much confusion [not to mention this many eponymous names], Ricky Ricardo [Dezi Arnaz] would say someone's still "got a lot of 'splainin' to do."

Selected References

1. Fischbein NJ, Dillon WP, Barkovich AJ. Teaching atlas of brain imaging, vol. 381-5. New York: Thieme; 2000. p. 213–5.
2. Hamilton BE, Salzman KL, Osborn AG. Anatomic and pathologic spectrum of pituitary infundibulum lesions. AJ. 2007:188(3).
3. Gibbs WN, Monuki ES, Linskey ME, et al. Pituicytoma: diagnostic features on selective carotid angiogram and MR imaging. AJNR Am J Neuroradiol. 2006;27(8):1639–42.
4. Tamer G, Kartal I, Aral F. Pituitary infiltration by non-Hodgkin's lymphoma: a case report. J Med Case Rep. 2009;3:9293.
5. Komp D, El Mahdi A, Starling K. Quality of survival in histiocytosis X: a southwest oncology group study. Med Pediatr Oncol, 1980. 8(1):35–40.
6. Sinah S, Singh AK, Tatke M, et al. Hypophyseal Tuberculoma: direct radiosurgery is contraindicated for a lesion with a thickened pituitary stalk: case report. Neurosurgery. 2000;46(3):735–8; discussion 738–9.
7. Patankar T, Patkar D, Bunting T, Castillo M, Mukherji SK. Imaging in pituitary tuberculosis. Clin Imaging. 2000;24(2):89–92.
8. Lopes MBS, Scheithauer BW, Saeger W. Granular cell tumor. In: RA LL, Lloyd RV, Heitz PU, Eng C, editors. World health organization classification of tumours. Pathology and genetics of tumors of endocrine organs. France: Lyon; 2004.
9. Badalian-Very G, Vergilio JA, Fleming M, et al. Pathogenesis of Langerhans cell histiocytosis. Annu Rev Pathol. 2013;8:1–20.
10. Kriz J, Eich HT, Bruns F, et al. Radiotherapy in Langerhans cell histiocytosis – a rare indication in a rare disease. Radiat Oncol. 2013;8:233. https://doi.org/10.1186/1748-717X-8-233. ccessed 6 Feb 2016.
11. Chevallier KM, Wigging RH, Quinn NA, Gurgel RK. Differentiating pediatric rhabdomyosarcoma and Langerhans cell histiocytosis of the temporal bone by imaging appearance. AJNR Am J Neuroradiol. 2016;37:1185–9.

Part II

Cerebellopontine Angle

9 Epidermoid Cyst

Pertinent Points

- *Definition*: Epidermoids are benign, congenital cysts arising from the inclusion of ectodermal epithelial elements which gradually grow for years before regularly revealing their presence in adulthood causing symptoms of cranial nerve dysfunction or brainstem compression [1, 8].
- *Classic Clue*: Cisternal CPA lesion showing signal similar to CSF but demonstrating definitive "dirty CSF" and representative restricted diffusion demonstrating light bulb bright DWI and dark ADC map insinuating itself by creeping into the cisternal recesses.
- AKA: Epidermoid tumor, pearly tumor, congenital CPA cistern cholesteatoma, non-neoplastic inclusion cyst.
- Incidence: Epidermoid cysts comprise <2% of intracranial tumors and 5% of CPA tumors [12].
- Locations: 40% occur in the CPA. Other common locations include the para- and suprasellar regions, as well as the middle cranial fossa.
- Epidermoid cysts comprise the third most common cause of CPA masses.

Imaging

General Imaging Features

- The tiny thin wall of a CPA epidermoid cyst cleverly creeps into cisternal recesses around adjacent structures including CN VII, CN VIII, and AICA [anterior inferior cerebellar artery].
- This ability aptly illustrates its irregular, scalloped margins.

CT Features

- See General Imaging Features.
- Usually non-enhancing hypodense masses.
- One fourth show patchy peripheral calcifications.
- Attenuation resembles CSF in most cases.
- The "dense epidermoid" is a really *rare* variant which may be related to hemorrhage, saponification, or ↑ protein content [4].

MRI Features

- See General Imaging Features
- T1 and PD are usually mildly hyperintense to CSF causing the "dirty CSF" appearance which is most conspicuous on T1 (see Fig. 9.1a, b).

T1 Signal

- Hemorrhage, triglycerides, and fatty acids can cause very hyperintense T1 signal creating a *rare* "white epidermoid" [4, 7, 8].
- T1 Gd confirms that the bulk of the mass does not enhance. It may occasionally show rim enhancement related to inflammatory reaction (see Fig. 9.2a).

T2 Signal

- T2 is iso- or hyperintense to CSF but habitually has heterogeneous signal suggesting solid components (see Fig. 9.2b).

F. A. Midyett, S. K. Mukherji, *Skull Base Imaging*, https://doi.org/10.1007/978-3-030-46447-9_9

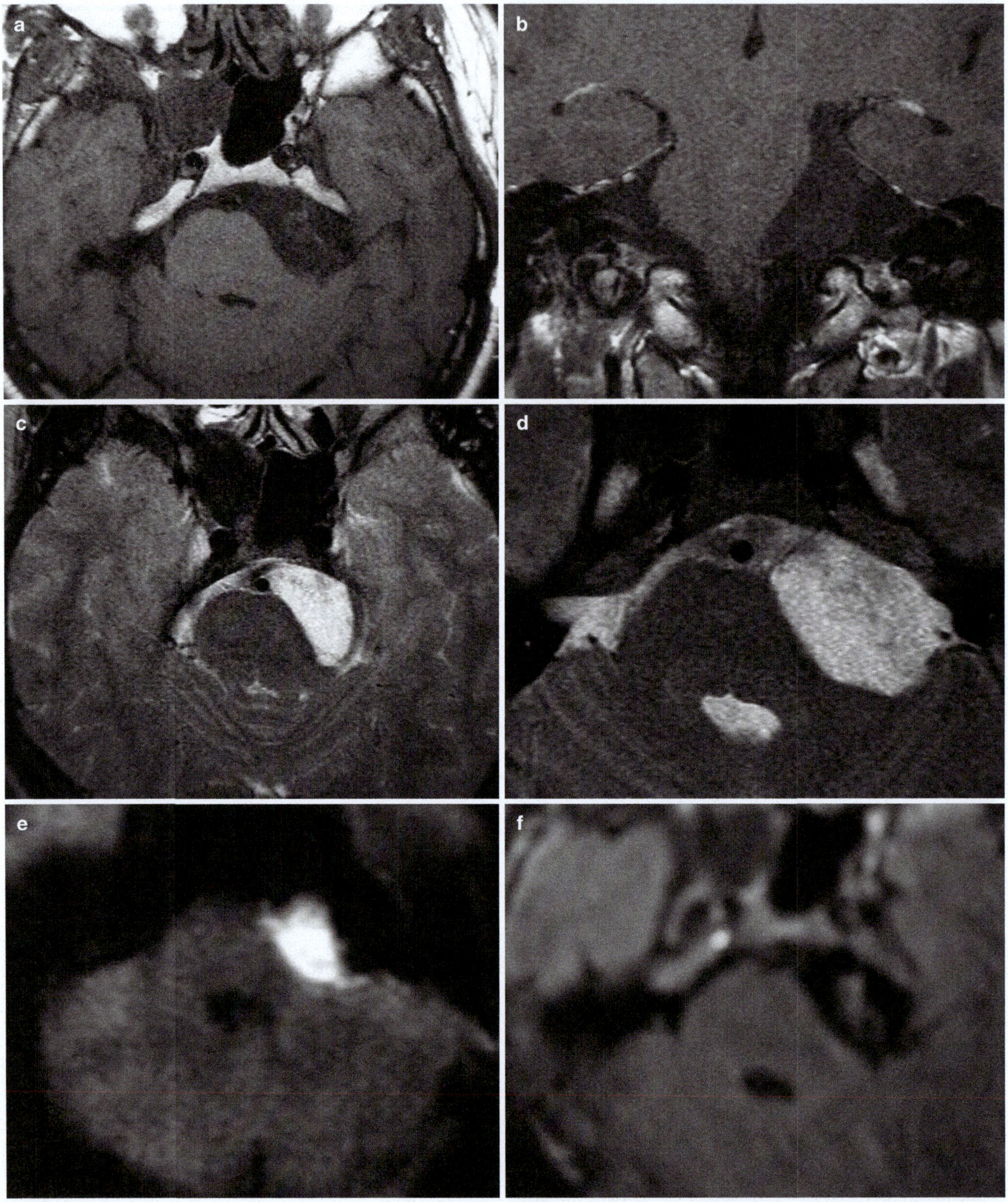

Fig. 9.1 (**a**) T1 Axial shows enlargement of the left CPA by a low signal ovoid mass which resembles "dirty CSF." The cerebellum is displaced posteriorly, and the pons is displaced contralaterally causing mass effect on the IV ventricle. (**b**) T1 coronal shows displacement of the pons by a CPA epidermoid exhibiting an emblematic "dirty CSF" appearance. (**c, d**) T2 axial shows enlargement of left CPA by a mass which is isointense to CSF. Mass effect deforms the IV ventricle. (**e**) Axial DWI shows "light bulb bright" signal from an epidermoid in the CPA. The IV ventricle is distorted from mass effect. Nearby CSF is dark. (**f**) Axial ADC shows most of the CPA tumor is discernibly dark. It still shows some higher signal in its center corresponding to higher signal seen on T1 (**a**) blood products?

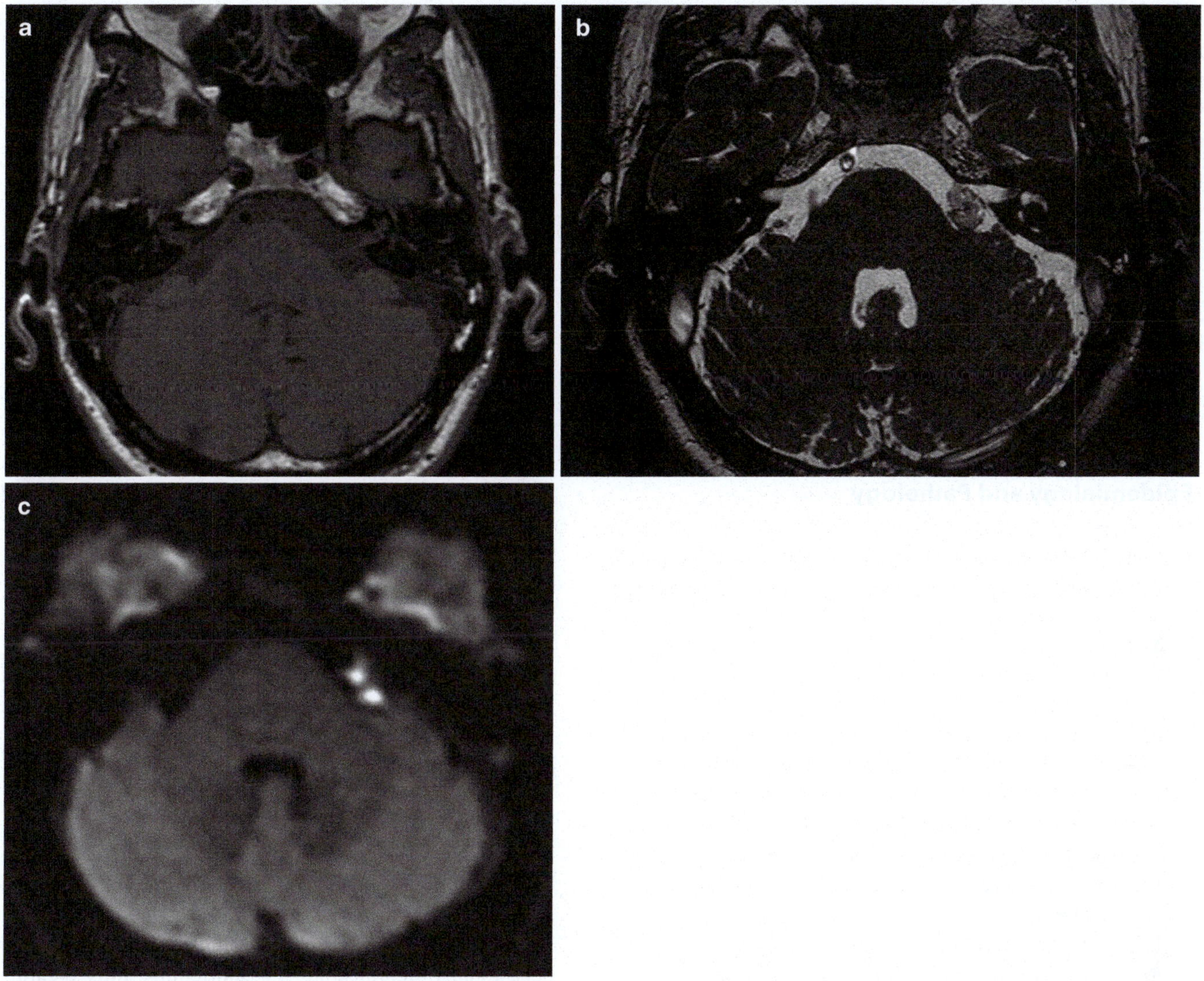

Fig. 9.2 (**a**) Axial T1 through the level of the seventh and eighth nerves is relatively unremarkable as were the T1 post-Gd images. (**b**) Axial T2 through the level of the seventh and eighth nerves shows an abnormality in the left CPA which again gives the appearance of "dirty CSF." (**c**) Axial DWI through the level of the CPAs demonstrate "light bulb bright" signal from a small epidermoid in the left CPA

DWI

- The most important and classic feature is restricted diffusion with bright signal on DWI and corresponding dark signal on the ADC map [2, 3] (see Figs. 9.1e, f and 9.2c).
- Some suggest the hyperintensity of epidermoids on echo-planar DWI is caused by T2 shine-through effect rather than diffusion restriction [8].
- The bright signal on DWI may be due a combination of "T2 shine through" and true restricted diffusion.

CISS and FLAIR

- FLAIR [fluid-attenuated inversion recovery] is an inversion recovery sequence designed to null or greatly reduce CSF signal.
- Epidermoid cysts show incomplete attenuation as they do not null CSF signal on CISS [constructive interference in steady state for motion sensitivity reduction] and FLAIR sequences.
- CISS is superior to FLAIR in elucidating the exact extent of an epidermoid's extension [3, 5].

Clinical Issues and Natural History

Presentation

- Epidermoids are benign lesions which generally grow gradually for many years before regularly revealing their presence in adulthood causing symptoms which include:
  - Headaches
  - Cranial nerve dysfunction
    - Diplopia, hearing loss, and facial pain/palsy
  - Brainstem compression and cerebellar symptoms
  - Seizures
  - Increased intracranial pressure [6]

Epidemiology and Pathology

- Epidermoids probably arise from incomplete cleavage of neural and cutaneous ectoderm at 3-5 weeks gestation causing inclusion of gestational elements.
- Slow growth is related to the rate of skin turnover, and they rarely present before the third or fourth decades.
- Epidermoids can encase rather than displace adjacent neurovascular structures [sometimes seeming somewhat similar to "the creeping blob from the black lagoon"].
- Gross: Well-defined, lobulated, cauliflower-like lesions showing shiny "mother of pearl" appearance [8, 9].
- Microscopic: Cyst wall lined by squamous epithelium filled with cholesterol crystals, lipids, and desquamated keratin [1].
- Intracranial epidermoid cysts are pathologically identical to petrous apex and middle ear cholesteatomas.

Differential Diagnosis

A. Meningioma
- Meningiomas account for 10% of CPA masses.
- Meningiomas are usually found in an older age group.
- Meningiomas are often broad-based dural masses, arising from dura, which habitually have a "tail."
- 75% show hyperdense mass on NECT.
- 25% are calcified with sand-like to chunky calcifications.
- T1 hypo- or isointense to brain parenchyma.
- T2 iso- or hyperintense to brain parenchyma.
- T1 Gd: 95% exhibit avid enhancement.
- Can cause permeative or hyperostotic bone changes.
- Meningiomas usually do not enlarge the IAC.
- 75% are isointense to gray matter.
- 25% have hemorrhage, necrosis, or cyst formation.
- See Chap. 10, CPA Meningioma.

B. Vestibular Schwannoma (VS)
- 3/4 of CPA masses.
- Usually more solid than epidermoids.
- Solid components exhibit postcontrast enhancement.
- Hypodense to brain parenchyma on NECT.
- T1 hypointense to brain parenchyma.
- T2 hyperintense to brain parenchyma.
- T1 Gd exhibits avid enhancement.
- Can contain cysts, calcifications, or hemorrhage.
- See Chap. 11, Vestibular Schwannoma.

C. Arachnoid Cyst (AC)
- Arachnoid cysts account for 1% of all CPA masses.
- Arachnoid cysts are *isodense* to CSF on CT.
- Epidermoids exhibit *restricted diffusion* and/or T2 shine through. Arachnoid cysts *do not* show restricted diffusion.
- Arachnoid cysts are isointense to CSF on T1, T2, PD, and FLAIR.
- Arachnoid cysts are *non-enhancing* on T1 Gd.
- Arachnoid cysts do not contain calcifications or hemorrhage.
- Arachnoid cysts have a spider-like thin but distinct capsule which creates a sharp margin as it pushes against adjacent structures. The epidermoids flimsy wall allows it to insinuate itself in between adjacent neurovascular structures like a growing "glob" of silly putty.
- See Chap. 12, CPA Arachnoid Cyst.

D. Dermoid
- Frequently fatty with low Hounsfield attenuation on CT and fatty signal intensity on MRI.
- Dermoids demonstrate T1 shortening. Epidermoids may occasionally demonstrate T1 shortening, thus creating confusion.
- Epidermoids demonstrate restricted diffusion. Dermoids do not.
- Dermoids may demonstrate chemical shift artifact. Epidermoids do not.
- Fat saturation pulses suppress signal in dermoids. Not a feature of epidermoids.
- The ratio of intracranial epidermoids/dermoids = 4:1.
- See Chap. 19, Nasal Dermoid.

E. Neurenteric Cyst
- Neurenteric cysts are relatively rare.
- Neurenteric cysts are frequently found in a midline location.
- Epidermoids demonstrate restricted diffusion, while neurenteric cysts do not.

F. Astrocytomas
- 1% of CPA masses are astrocytomas. Epidermoids comprise 5% of CPA tumors.

- Astrocytomas exhibit moderate postcontrast enhancement. Epidermoids do not enhance.
- Astrocytomas are exophytic. Epidermoids are cistern based.
- Astrocytomas can appear cystic. Epidermoids are cystic.

G. Ependymoma

- Ependymomas can appear cystic. Epidermoids are cystic.
- Ependymomas exhibit enhancing foci. Epidermoids do not enhance.
- Ependymomas pedunculate from brainstem. Epidermoids are clearly cistern based.

Treatment and Prognosis

- Surgical removal is offered to symptomatic patients.
- Adherence of the cyst capsule to the brainstem and cranial nerves is potentially problematic.
- Post-surgical prognosis is excellent, but patients with subtotal resection may experience recurrence. [10–12].

A Closer Look

I. Fast Facts

- Primary concerns for intracranial epidermoid cyst management remain misdiagnosis, incomplete removal at first operation, and delayed detection of recurrences [11].
- Two out of those three concerns fall into the field of neuroradiology.
- The ratio of intracranial epidermoids/dermoids= 4:1.

II. Historic Highlights

- 1829 First find reports of intraspinal epidermoids.
- 1935 Cushing reported epidermoids to be 0.6% of his surgical cases.
- 1937 Foerster reported epidermoids to be 0.7% of surgical cases.
- 1937 Tönnis reported epidermoids to be 1.8% of surgical cases.
- 1939 Zülch reported epidermoids to be 1.5% of surgical cases [12].

III. Genetics and Associations

- Most epidermoid cysts are sporadic, but congenital syndromes should be suspected when encountering multiple or early onset lesions, particularly before puberty.
- Several syndromes are currently connected to epidermoids including *pachyonychia congenita*, as well as *Gardner's* and *Gorlin's* basal cell nevus syndromes.
- Gardner's syndrome is an autosomal dominant disease related to mutation of a tumor suppression APC gene on chromosome 5q22. Affected individuals have a 50% chance of passing the perturbed gene to their offspring.
- *PTCH-1 and sonic hedgehog* function as hand and glove (or key in lock) and are essential to early embryology. PTCH-1 provides instruction for making a protein called patched-1 which retards rapid or uncontrolled cell proliferation. The sonic hedgehog protein is the key (ligand) which fits into the lock (patched-1 receptor). Normally functioning patched-1 blocks cell proliferation until sonic hedgehog's appropriate attachment.
- *PTCH1:* The chief cause of Gorlin's syndrome is mutation of the PTCH1 gene. Gorlin's syndrome is specifically related to microdeletion at 9q22.3.
- *Pachyonychia congenita* is another autosomal dominant frequently triggered by a keratin gene mutation at KRT6A, KRT6B, KRT6C, KRT16, or KRT17 [13].

Selected References

1. Fischbein NJ, Dillon WP, Barkovich AJ. Teaching atlas of brain imaging. New York: Thieme; 2000. p. 118–20.
2. Dechambre S, Duprez T, Lecouvet F, et al. Diffusion-weighted MRI postoperative assessment of an epidermoid tumour in the cerebellopontine angle. Neuroradiology. 1999 Nov;41(11):829–31.
3. Ikushima I, Korogi Y, Hirai T, et al. MR of epidermoids with a variety of pulse sequences. AJNR Am J Neuroradiol. 1997;18:1259–63.
4. Ochi M, Hayashi K, Hayashi T, et al. Unusual CT and MR appearance of an epidermoid tumor of the cerebellopontine angle. AJNR Am J Neuroradiol. 1998;19:1113–5.
5. Chen S, Ikawa F, Kurlsu, et al. Quantitative MR evaluation of intracranial epidermoid tumors by fast fluid-attenuated inversion recovery imaging and Echo-planar diffusion-weighted imaging. AJNR Am J Neuroradiol. 2001;22:1089–96.
6. deSouza CE, deSouza R, da Costa S, et al. Cerebellopontine angle epidermoid cysts: a report on 30 cases. J Neurol Neurosurg Psychiatry. 1989;52(8):986–90.
7. Chen CY, Wong JS, Hsieh SC, et al. Intracranial epidermoid cyst with hemorrhage: MR imaging findings. AJNR Am J Neuroradiol. 2006;27:427–9.
8. Gao PY, Osborn AG, Smirniotopolus JG, et al. Radiologic-pathologic correlation: epidermoid tumor of the cerebellopontine angle. AJNR Am J Neuroradiol. 1992;13:865–72.
9. DeMonte F, Gilbert MR, Mahajan A. Tumors of the brain and spine: Springer Verlag; 2007.
10. Chowdhury FH, Haque MR, Sarker MH. Intracranial epidermoid tumor; microneurosurgical management: An experience of 23 cases. Asian J Neurosurg. 2013;8(1):21–8.
11. Sekhar LN, Fessler RG. Atlas of neurosurgical techniques: Thieme; 2016. p. 711–23.
12. Sindou M. Practical handbook of neurosurgery: from leading neurosurgeons, vol. 1: Springer; 2009. p. 301.
13. Smith FJD, Hansen CD, Hull PR, et al. Pachyonychia congenita. 2006 Jan 27 [Updated 2017 Nov 30]. In: Adam MP, Ardinger HH, Pagon RA, et al., editors. GeneReviews [Internet]. Seattle (WA): University of Washington, Seattle; 1993–2018. www.ncbi.nlm.nih.gov/books/NBK1280/. Accessed on 2 Feb 2020.

10 CPA Meningioma

Pertinent Points

- Definition: Unencapsulated neoplasm arising from cap cells of arachnoid villa in the CPA-IAC cistern, usually benign although occasionally malignant.
- *Classic Clue*: Hyperdense solid CPA angle mass in middle-aged asymptomatic female is asymmetric to the IAC and avidly enhances with a *mushroom cap* and a *dural tail*.
- Meningioma is the most common CPA tumor after vestibular schwannoma, and together they comprise the majority of CPA tumors.
- < 5% of meningiomas arise in the CPA.
- Gender Preference: F > M = 3:1 Usually found in middle-aged patients with most found incidentally.
- When seen in children, think NF2!
- Meningioma + schwannoma = NF2
- Multiple meningiomas occur in 10% of sporadic cases.
- Tumor Size Classification [2]:
  - Type I
    Confined to the IAC
  - Type II
    ≤ 2.5 cm
  - Type III
    > 2.5 cm
  - Originally described for CPA vestibular schwannomas but often useful for CPA meningiomas as well [2]

Imaging

General Imaging Features

- Meningiomas comprise 10% of CPA (cerebellopontine angle) masses.
- Enhancing extra axial mass with a *mushroom cap* and a *dural tail*.
- While most meningiomas tend to be typical, considering their prevalence, statistics suggest we can probably predict a pretty large amount of "atypical" cases.
- Some unusual features can be misleading and include "ring enhancement," large cysts, and fatty transformation [1].

CT Features

- 75% show a hyperdense mass on NECT.
- 25% calcify with sand-like chunks.
- 90% exhibit avid enhancement.
- Meningiomas can cause characteristic permeative or hyperostotic bony changes.
- Usually arise from the posterior surface of the petrous bone or along the sigmoid sinus and usually do not extend into or enlarge the IAC.

MRI Features

I. T1 Signal
  - T1: Extra-axial mass, with 75% isointense [25% hypointense] to the brain parenchyma (see Fig. 10.1a, c).
  - 25% have hemorrhage, necrosis, or cyst formation.
  - T1 Gd: 95% exhibit *avid* enhancement (see Fig. 10.1g, h).

F. A. Midyett, S. K. Mukherji, *Skull Base Imaging*, https://doi.org/10.1007/978-3-030-46447-9_10

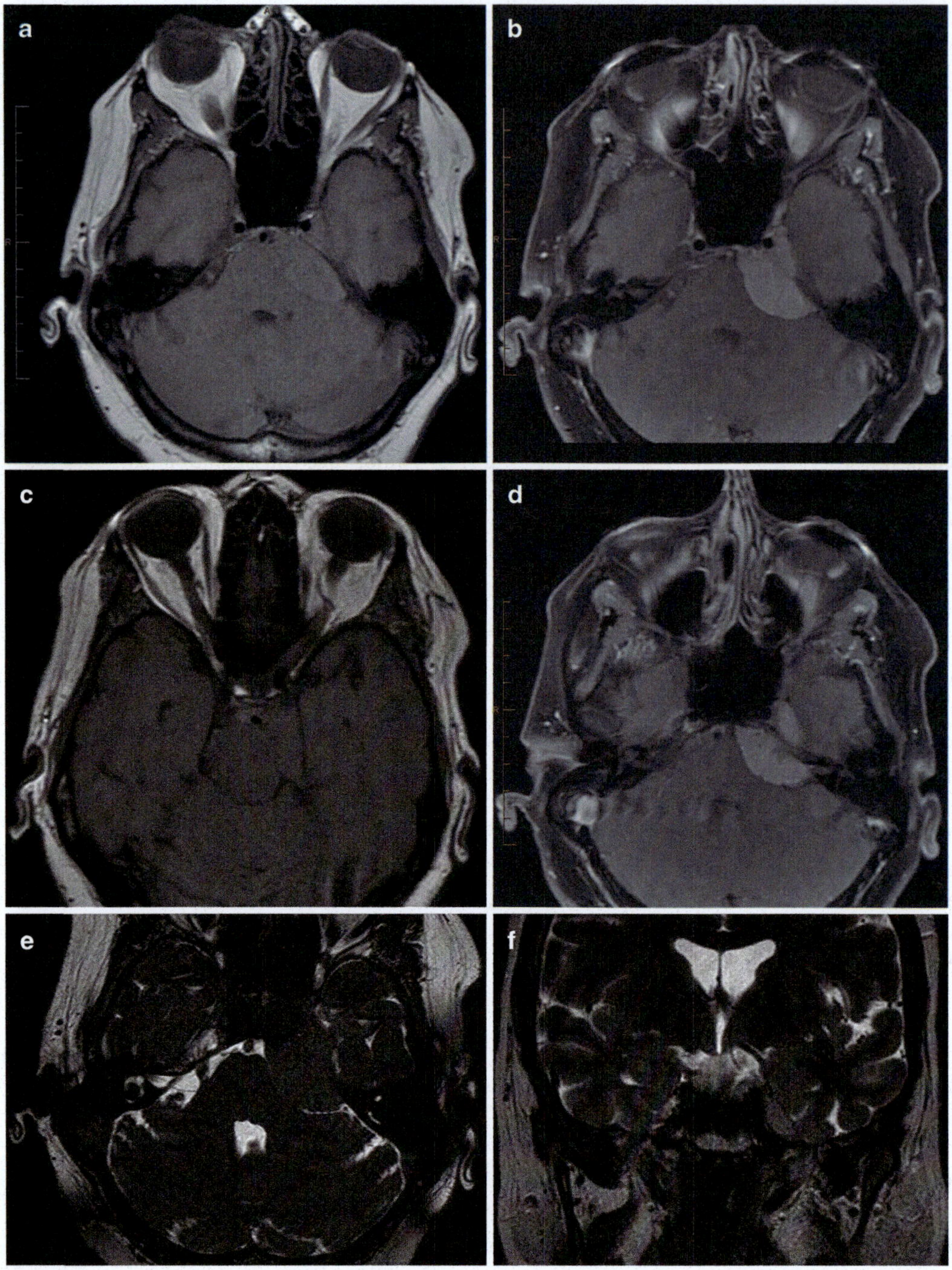

Fig. 10.1 (**a**) Axial T1 shows large left CPA mass which is isointense to brain and causes moderate mass effect on the pons. Asymmetric signal suggests anterior tumor extension into the cavernous sinus. (**b**) Axial T1 with Gd and FS confirms large left CPA mass extends anteriorly into Meckel's cave and the cavernous sinus adjacent to the left ICA. (**c**) Axial T1 shows large left CPA mass, isointense to brain causing mass effect on the pons. (**d**) Axial T1 Gd FS shows moderately enhancing left CPA mass, causing moderate mass effect on the cerebellum and pons. A separate enhancing mass anteriorly is tumor involving Meckel's cave. (**e**) Axial T2 shows large left CPA mass, causing mass effect on the cerebellum and pons. Signal is isointense to adjacent cerebellum with CSF surrounding some of its margins. (**f**) Coronal T2 shows oval abnormality isointense to brain involving Meckel's cave on the left

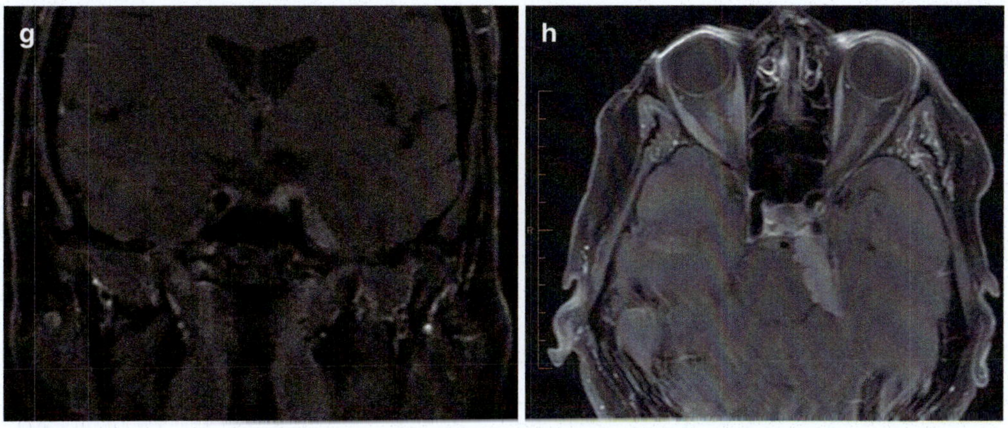

Fig. 10.1 (continued) (**g**) Coronal T1 Gd FS shows enhancing oval abnormality involving Meckel's cave extending into the left cavernous sinus adjacent to the left ICA. (**h**) Axial T1 Gd FS shows enhancing left CPA meningioma extending into the left cavernous sinus adjacent the left ICA

- The "dural tail" sign is frequent (≤75%) but not specific.
  - The "dural tail" sign may be seen with any tumor which invades the dura or causes a dural reaction.
  - The "dural tail" usually represents a hypervascular reaction rather than true tumor incursion.
- Axial and coronal T1 Gd with fat saturation best delineate the degree of disease (see Fig. 10.1b, d, g, h).

II. T2 Signal
- T2: Extra-axial mass iso- or hyperintense to the brain parenchyma (see Fig. 10.1e, f)
- Sometimes shows a CSF vascular cleft between the brain and tumor

III. DWI (Diffusion Weighted Imaging)
- Restricted diffusion appears to be a useful feature for distinguishing atypical/malignant meningioma from benign meningioma (present in the former and not the later) [3].

IV. MRS (Magnetic Resonance Spectroscopy)
- Occasionally useful in evaluating anaplastic meningiomas by measuring lipids and the choline/creatine ratio.

Angiographic Features

- The "sunburst" pattern is frequently formed from enlarged dural feeders.
- The vascular stain stays around for the venous phase. This is the Smirniotopoulos' "mother-in-law sign," like a mother in law who comes early and stays late.
- Meningiomas can cause arteriovenous shunting.
- Pial feeders nourish the rim. Dural feeders contribute to the core.

Clinical Issues and Natural History

Presentation

- CPA meningiomas are often large before becoming symptomatic.
- Symptoms are usually related to mass effect on CN III, V, VII, and VIII.
- Symptoms include ataxia, nystagmus, and facial hypesthesia. Audiologic findings may be normal or reveal a retro-cochlear pattern.
- Vestibular schwannomas (VSs) classically cause hearing loss more frequently than do CPA meningiomas [4].

Epidemiology and Pathology

- Meningiomas are the most common nonglial primary intracranial tumors and the most common extra-axial neoplasms and account for ~15% of all primary intracranial tumors [1].
- Meningiomas arise from arachnoid villi cap cells and are classified by WHO as typical, atypical, or malignant.
- Atypical and malignant meningiomas have frequent chromosome abnormalities involving 14, 1, 3, and 6.
- While unencapsulated, they are still sharply circumscribed often displaying "en plaque" or "mushroom cap" configurations in the CPAs.
- Dural thickening is usually reactive rather than infiltrative.
- The WHO classifies meningiomas as follows [5]:

  I. Grade I typical meningioma (90%)
  - Benign: meningothelial, fibrous, transitional, psammomatous, and angioblastic

   II. Grade II atypical meningioma (8%)
      - Chordoid, clear cell, and atypical.
      - Recurrence rate is between Grades I and III
   III. Grade III malignant meningioma (2%)
      - Malignant: papillary, rhabdoid, and anaplastic
- The Helsinki group classifies meningiomas into four grades:
   I. Grade I Benign
   II. Grade II Atypical
   III. Grade III Anaplastic
   IV. Grade IV Sarcomatous

Treatment

I. Surgically Resectable Lesions
- Surgical removal is treatment of choice, if resectable.

II. Lesions in Surgically Inaccessible Locations
- External beam radiation.
- Gamma knife radiosurgery.
- 95% control for 5 years with benign lesions.
- Postoperative radiotherapy is used for incomplete resections.

Prognosis

I. Typical Meningioma (90%)
   - Excellent prognosis
II. Atypical Meningioma (8%)
   - ↑ Recurrence rate = ↓ survival rate (10-year survival = 79%)
III. Malignant Meningioma (2%)
   - 10-year survival = 35% [4]

Differential Diagnosis of Solid CPA Masses

A. Vestibular Schwannoma (VS)
- Vestibular schwannomas comprise ¾ of CPA masses.
- VS exhibit enhancing solid components.
- VS are hypodense to the brain parenchyma on NECT.
- VS have T1 signal hypointense to brain parenchyma.
- VS have T2 signal hyperintense to brain parenchyma.
- VS exhibit avid enhancement on T1 Gd.
- VS can contain cysts, calcifications, or hemorrhage.
- VS is first intracanalicular before CPA extension. Rarely an intracanalicular meningioma may mimic a VS.
- CPA meningiomas compared to VS [vestibular schwannoma].
   – CPA meningiomas tend to be larger than schwannomas.
   – CPA meningiomas are more hemispheric than round.
   – CPA meningiomas show a wide dural base.
   – CPA meningiomas tend to be flatter.
   – CPA meningiomas may have hyperostosis (not a feature of VS).
   – CPA meningiomas rarely extend into or widen IAC.
   – CPA meningiomas have statistically significant very high rCBV (relative cerebral blood volume) ratios compared to schwannomas [6].

B. Neurosarcoidosis
- Usually exhibit multiple dural-based foci.
- Look for involvement of the pituitary infundibulum.
- See Chap. 6, Neurohypophyseal Sarcoidosis.

C. Lymphoma and Metastasis
- Both may be bilateral.
- Lymphoma and metastasis often manifest multifocal meningeal involvement.

D. Astrocytomas
- Astrocytomas comprise 1% of CPA masses.
- Astrocytomas are exophytic with moderate postcontrast enhancement.
- Astrocytomas can appear cystic.

E. Ependymoma
- Ependymomas usually show some focus of enhancement.
- Ependymomas pedunculate from the brainstem.
- Ependymomas can appear cystic.

A Closer Look

I. Fast Facts
- Presurgical predictors of outcome include [7]:
   – T2 hyperintensity.
   – Cortical penetration by tumor.
   – Peritumoral edema.
   – Pial vascularity on angiography.
   – Simpson grade.
   – Tumor size.
   – Osteolysis.
   – Mushroom shape.
   – All the above predict ↓ odds for favorable resectability (good surgical outcome), and most are available to neuroradiologists.

II. Historic Highlights
- 1614 Early clinical description of meningioma [in a deceased patient] [8].
- 1902 Pfahler first diagnosed a meningioma in a *living patient* by interpreting findings on conventional radiographs [8]. This was a mere 7 years after the discovery of Roentgen's ray, and we subsequently strive daily to improve our techniques.

- 1947 Hodges first described the characteristic angiographic features for meningiomas.
- 1973 Hounsfield's introduction of CT fundamentally and forever changed the way we see meningiomas.
- 1989 Wilms described dural tails associated with meningiomas on MRI [9].

III. Genetics and Environment

- Ionizing radiation exposure is the environmental risk factor most frequently found with meningiomas although <1% of irradiated individuals develop meningiomas [10].
- Endogenous and exogenous hormones have been implicated in meningioma development, although their precise role requires further study.
- The code for tumor suppressor Merlin resides in the NF2 gene and is disrupted in 1/2 of all patients with meningiomas [11].
- Mutation of the NF2 gene with resultant neurofibromatosis type 2 (NF2) is a dominantly inherited disorder where patients commonly present with bilateral vestibular schwannomas, multiple meningiomas, as well as other CNS tumors [11, 12].
- There is hereditary susceptibility for meningioma involving mutations involving multiple other genes in addition to the more commonly recognized NF2 gene.
- Currently impugned genes and locations associated with meningiomas read like an alphabet soup and include chromosomes 1, 9, 10, 14, 17, 18, and 22 and SWI/SNF with subunits SMARCB1 and SMARCE1, and the list grows daily.
- The sonic hedgehog (SHH)-GLI1 signaling pathway gene, SUFU, is clearly the causal culprit for hereditary multiple meningiomas in a Finnish family.

Selected References

1. Buetow MP, Buetow PC, Smirniotopoulos JG. Typical, atypical, and misleading features in meningioma. Radiographics. 1991;11(6):1087–106.
2. Wigand ME, Rettinger G, Haid T, et al. The removal of VIIIth nerve neurinomas from the cerebellopontine angle by enlarged middle fossa approach. HNO. 1985;33:11–6.
3. Nagar VA, Ye JR, Ng WH, et al. Diffusion-weighted MR imaging: diagnosing atypical or malignant Meningiomas and detecting tumor dedifferentiation. AJNR Am J Neuroradiol. 2008;29:1147–52.
4. Fischbein NJ, Dillon WP, Barkovich AJ. Teaching atlas of brain imaging. New York: Thieme; 2000. p. 115–7.
5. Wrobel G, Roerig P, Kokocinski F, et al. Microarray-based gene expression profiling of benign, atypical and anaplastic meningiomas identifies novel genes associated with meningioma progression. Int J Cancer. 2005;114(2):249–56.
6. Hakyemez B, Erdogan C, Bolca N, et al. Evaluation of different cerebral mass lesions by perfusion-weighted MR imaging. J Magn Reson Imaging. 2006;24:817–24.
7. Ildan F, Erman T, Göcer AI, et al. Predicting the probability of meningioma recurrence in the preoperative and early postoperative period: a multivariate analysis in the midterm follow-up. Skull Base. 2007;17(3):157–71.
8. Siegelman ES, Mischkin MM, Tavaras JM. Past, present, and future of radiology of meningioma. Radiographics. 1991;11:899–910.
9. Wilms G, Lammens M, Marchal G, et al. Thickening of dura surrounding meningiomas: MR features. J Comput Assist Tomogr. 1989;13:763–8.
10. Claus EB, Calvocoressi L, Bondy ML, et al. Clinical Article. Family and personal medical history and risk of meningioma. J Neurosurg. 2011. https://doi.org/10.3171/2011.JNS11129. Accessed 1 Sept 2016.
11. Choy W, et al. The molecular genetics and tumor pathogenesis of meningiomas and the future directions of meningioma treatments. Neurosurg Focus. 2011;30:E6.
12. Liu Y, Pang JC, Dong S, Mao B, Poon WS, Ng HK. Aberrant CpG island hypermethylation profile is associated with atypical and anaplastic meningiomas. Hum Pathol. 2005;36:416–25.

11 Vestibular Schwannoma

Pertinent Points

- Definition: Vestibular schwannoma is a slow-growing, benign, encapsulated tumor arising from Schwann cells surrounding the vestibulocochlear nerve usually in the CPA/IAC cistern.
- *Classic Clue*: Frequently found as a well-circumscribed ovoid "filling defect" in the CSF of CPA/IAC cistern or an avidly enhancing mass in a patient presenting with unilateral sensorineural hearing loss, tinnitus, or occasionally hydrocephalus.
- *AKA*: Acoustic neuroma, acoustic schwannoma.
- Vestibular schwannomas are the most common CPA tumor comprising 85% of CPA masses.
- Vestibular schwannomas are the second most common extra-axial tumor in adults.
- They usually present in the fifth to sixth decades.
- Together with meningiomas, they comprise the majority of CPA tumors.
- 95% are unilateral and when bilateral should arouse suspicion for neurofibromatosis.
- Bilateral vestibular schwannomas are characteristic of NF2 being present in >90% cases.
- Finding vestibular schwannomas [VS] in children should suggest NF2.

Imaging

General Imaging Features

- Most vestibular schwannomas arise in the IAC, but they can occasionally be intracochlear or intravestibular [1]. See discussion on ILS [intralabyrinthine schwannoma] in "Fast Facts."
- When larger, VS may contain cysts, calcification, or hemorrhage, but they usually do not calcify.
- Vestibular schwannomas are first intracanalicular before extending into the CPA. Rarely an intracanalicular meningioma may mimic VS.
- Vestibular schwannomas show associated arachnoid cysts in 0.5%.
- Tumor Size Classification [2]:
  - Type I
    Confined to the IAC
  - Type II
    ≤2.5 cm
  - Type III
    >2.5 cm

CT Features

- See Section General Imaging Features.
- Smaller lesions are usually isodense to the brain and enhance homogeneously.
- Larger lesions can contain cysts, hemorrhage, or fatty degeneration
- Enhancing extra axial CPA/IAC mass.
- Flaring of IAC by larger lesions (>8–10 mm) (see Fig. 11.1a, b).
- *No calcifications*. (Think meningioma if you see calcifications).

MRI Features

I. T1 Signal
   - T1 signal is slightly hypointense to brain parenchyma in ~2/3 and isointense in ~1/3 [3].
   - T1 Gd: 100% show *avid* enhancement (see Figs. 11.1c, and 11.2c, d).
   - May have hemorrhage (0.5%), cyst formation (15%), or necrosis.
   - T1 Gd may demonstrate relative signal void in areas of cysts or cystic necrosis especially after gamma knife.

II. T2 Signal

F. A. Midyett, S. K. Mukherji, *Skull Base Imaging*, https://doi.org/10.1007/978-3-030-46447-9_11

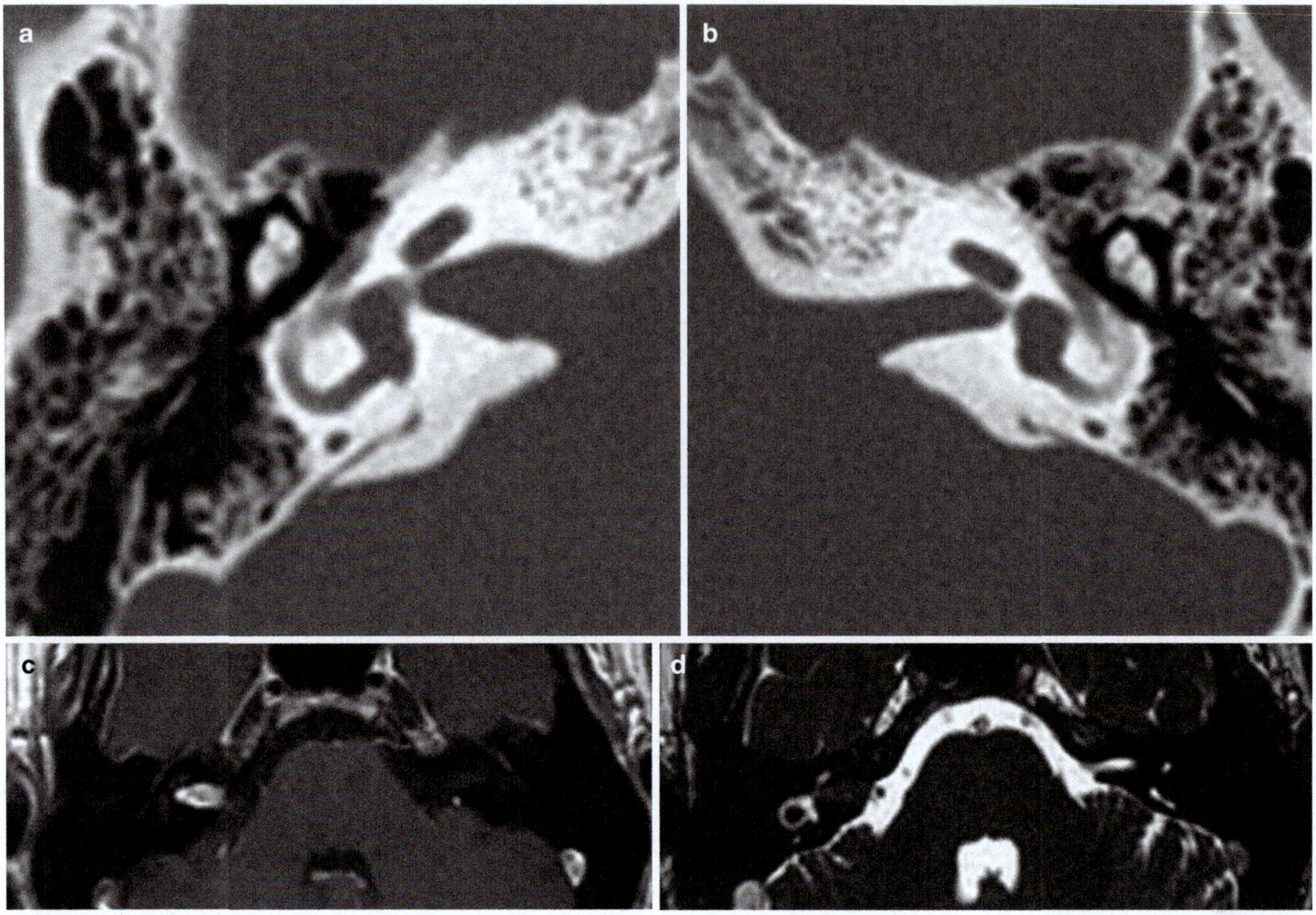

Fig. 11.1 (**a**) Axial NECT right temporal bone shows conspicuous funnel-shaped IAC widening, particularly compared to normal comparison contralateral side image 1B on left. (**c**) T1 Gd axial shows fusiform right IAC mass exhibiting avid "light bulb bright" enhancement. The tiny tumor conforms to the shape of the enlarged IAC on Fig.11.1a. (**d**) T2 axial shows low signal soft tissue mass filling the right IAC. The mass is isointense with the brain and appears totally intracanalicular. The right IAC is clearly much larger than the left

- T2: Ovoid "filling defect" in high signal CSF of the CPA/IAC cistern (see Fig. 11.1a).
- When small and intracanalicular, they appear ovoid to tubular.
- When small, it is often possible to identify the exact nerve of origin on MRI. The order of involvement (from most to least frequent) is inferior vestibular > superior vestibular > cochlear.
- Large lesions take on an "ice cream cone" appearance [with the "cone" predominately in the IAC and the "ice cream" in the CPA].
- Larger lesions are habitually more heterogeneous than smaller lesions.
- Dedicated IAC T2 sequences are useful as a screening study or as additional sequences to supplement a full brain MRI.
- Vestibular schwannomas T2 signal iso- to hyperintense to brain parenchyma (see Fig. 11.1d).
- T2 may well demonstrate cystic change with high T2 signal from fluid often related to necrosis (see Fig. 11.3a).
- Special dedicated imaging sequences like FIESTA are particularly useful in showing a tiny *filling defect* surrounded by high T2 signal [see Figs. 11.4a–f and 11.2a, b].
- FIESTA
  - FIESTA = fast imaging employing steady-state acquisition (by GE).
  - Provides images of fluid-filled structures with very short acquisition times which are shorter than FSE (fast spin echo).
  - Uses the T2 steady-state contrast mechanism to provide high SNR (signal to noise ratio).
  - It takes advantage of strong signal from fluid while suppressing background, thereby achieving exquisite contrast and small structure anatomic detail.
  - See Fig. 11.4a–f.

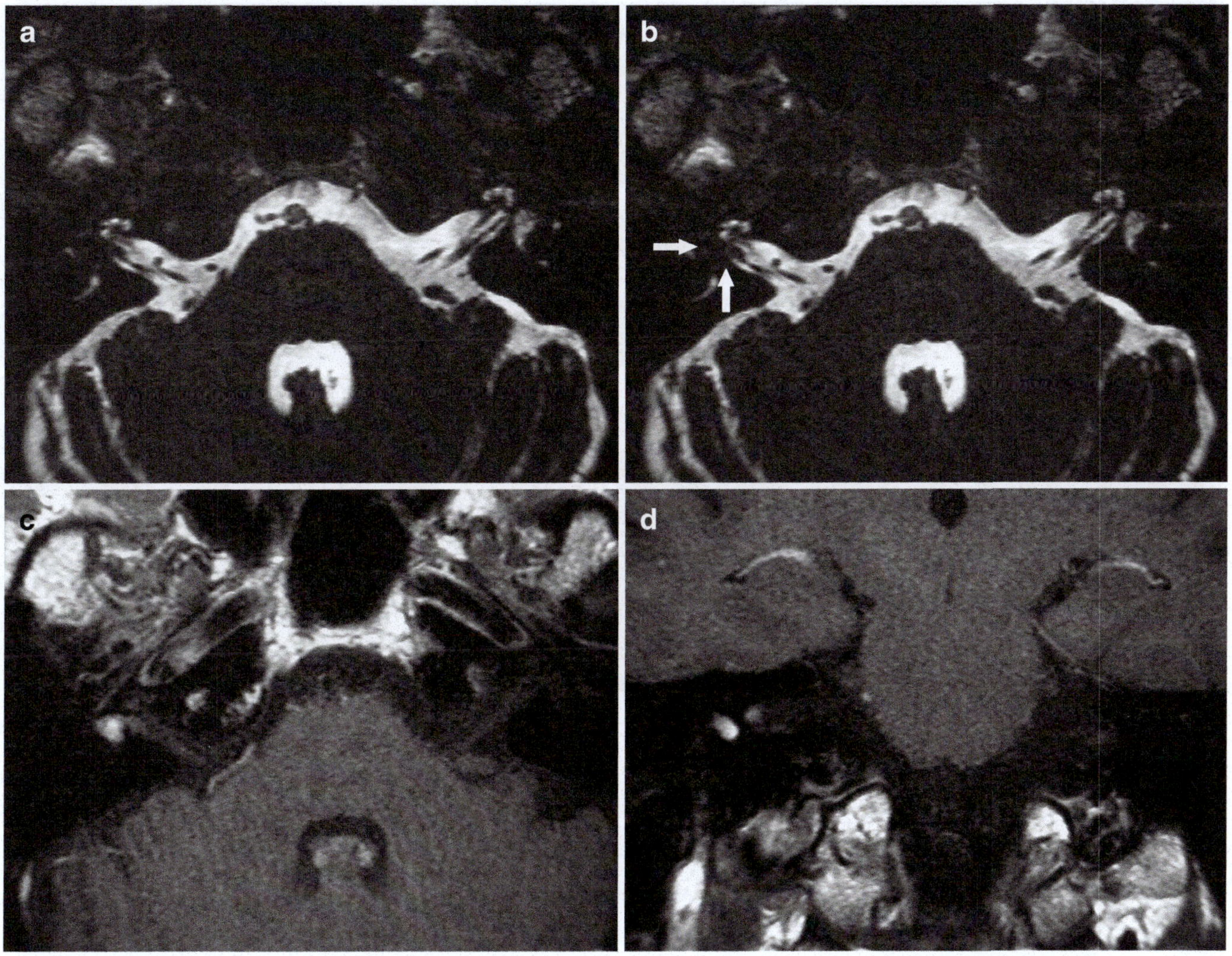

Fig. 11.2 (**a**, **b**) T2 axial thin slice image through the IAC shows small filling defect involving right intravestibular region, better appreciated with arrows (**b**) and subsequent enhanced images (**c**, **d**) T1 Gd thin slice images through level of IAC shows avidly enhancing intravestibular schwannoma on axial (**c**) and coronal (**d**) planes

Clinical Issues and Natural History

1. Presentation
   - Patients present with unilateral SNHL (sensorineural hearing loss) and/or tinnitus.
   - Large lesions can compress brainstem causing hydrocephalus.
   - Complications include intratumoral hemorrhage with CN V or VII palsies as well as SAH [1].
2. Epidemiology and Pathology
   - Slow-growing benign encapsulated tumors arising eccentrically along a nerve.
   - Most (>90%) arise from the inferior division of the vestibular nerve [4].
   - Commonly contain cystic degeneration with occasional hemorrhage [1].
   - Demonstrate two distinct tissue types:
     - Antoni A: Dense mature collagen with ↑ cellularity
     - Antoni B: Looser mucoid matrix with ↓ cellularity [1]
     - Ovoid, tan, encapsulated mass arising asymmetrically from nerve.
     - Untreated they usually demonstrate no necrosis but habitually have hemorrhage and intramural cysts.
     - Post gamma knife surgery, they show necrosis with cystic change.

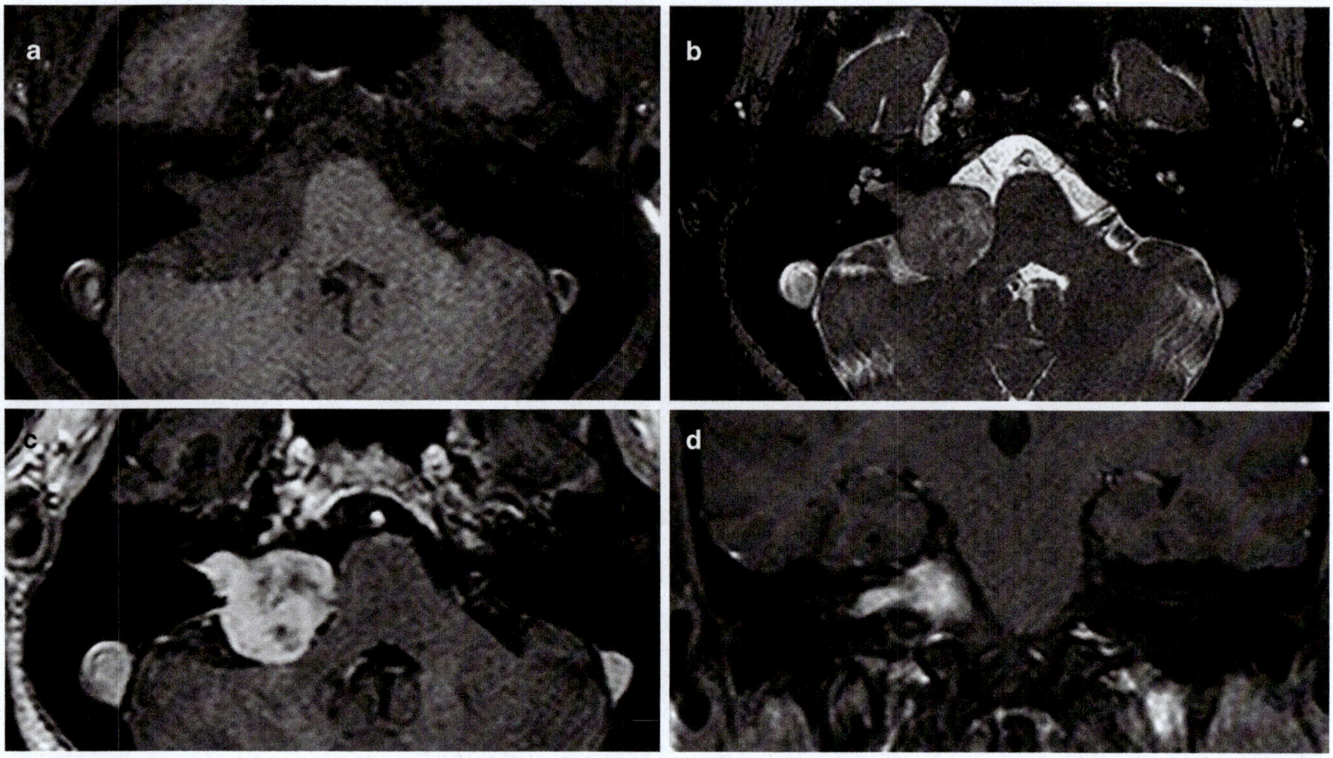

Fig. 11.3 (**a**) T1 Axial shows large right CPA abnormality causing considerable mass effect on the adjacent cerebellum and pons enlarging the IAC. (**b**) T2 Axial confirms large heterogeneous CPA mass containing a few focal fluid collections. Low signal periphery of the mass defines margins adjacent to CSF. (**c**) T1 Gd Axial confirms large 'ice cream cone' shaped right CPA mass which avidly enhances but contains conspicuous areas of internal nonenhancing necrosis. (**d**) T1 Gd Coronal shows the 'cone' of enhancing tumor extends into and enlarging the right IAC. The patient is post gamma knife surgery for treatment of a VS and exhibited progressive intratumoral necrosis and cystic change on follow up imaging

Treatment and Prognosis

- 10% of vestibular schwannomas show rapid growth, suggesting the need for treatment. Most, however, grow only 1–2 mm/year.
- The patient's options are based on tumor size, hearing status, patient age, and personal preferences.
- Options include close clinical observation with serial imaging, surgical resection, and gamma knife radiosurgery.
- Prognosis is excellent when they are totally resected; but, they can recur when resection is partial.
- No known malignant degeneration [1].
- Patients who were postoperative and/or post gamma knife treatment often have interesting imaging studies.
- Hearing preservation improves with tumors <2 cm without involvement of cochlear aperture or IAC fundus.
- Successful surgical removal does not restore previously poor or absent hearing.

Differential Diagnosis of Solid CPA Masses

A. CPA Meningiomas

- CPA meningiomas compared to VS [vestibular schwannoma]
  - CPA meningiomas tend to be larger.
  - CPA meningiomas are more hemispheric than round.
  - CPA meningiomas show a wide dural base.
  - CPA meningiomas tend to be flatter.
  - CPA meningiomas may have hyperostosis (not a feature of VS).
  - CPA meningiomas rarely extend into or widen IAC.
  - CPA meningiomas have statistically significant very high rCBV (relative cerebral blood volume) ratios compared to schwannomas [5].
  - Meningiomas comprise 10% of CPA [cerebellopontine angle] masses.
  - Enhancing extra-axial mass often displaying a *dural tail* and a *mushroom cap*.

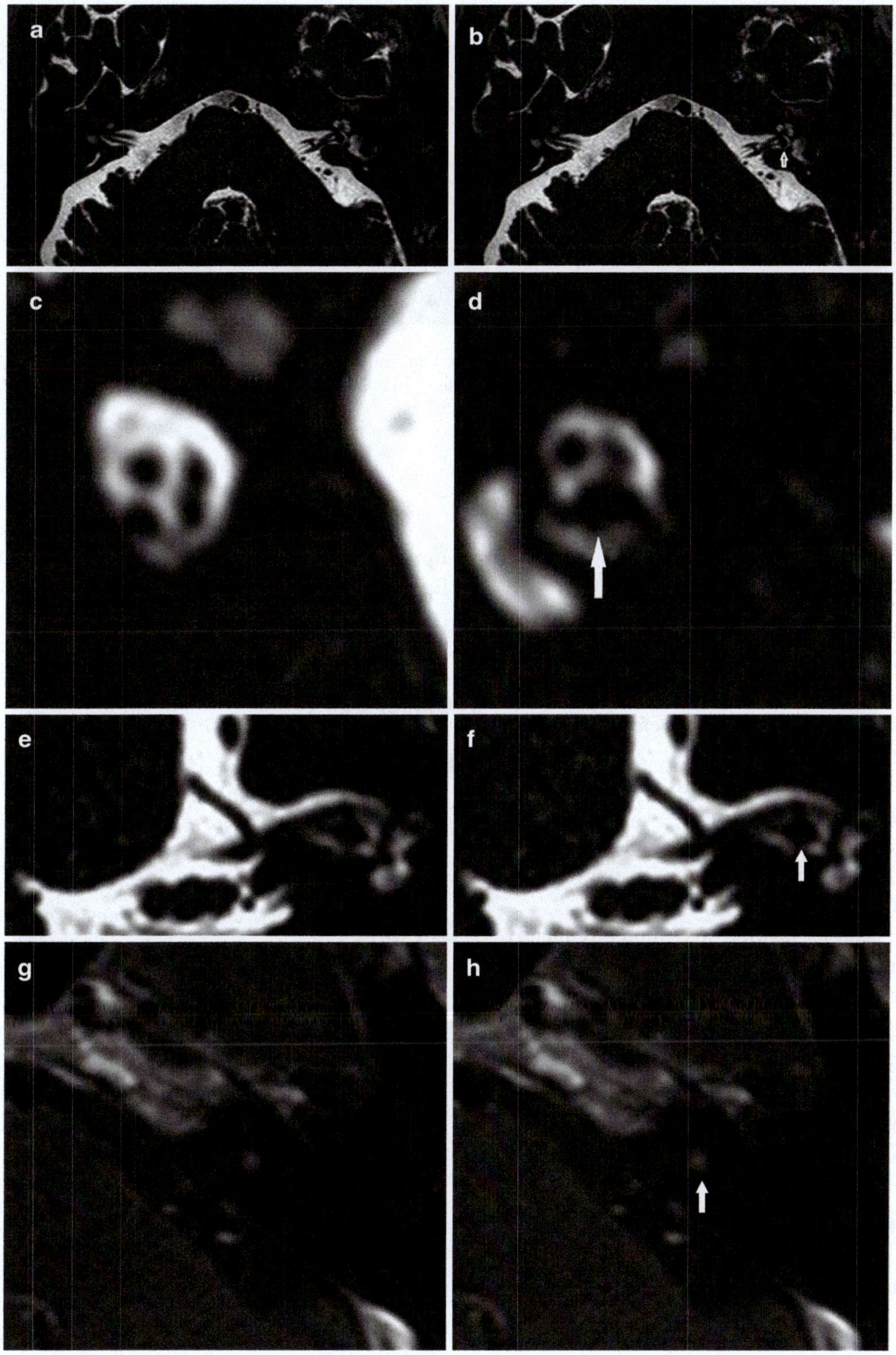

Fig. 11.4 (**a**, **b**) Axial T2 FIESTA without (**a**) and with (**b**) helper arrow shows a tiny "filling defect" in the peripheral left IAC. (**c**, **d**) Sagittal T2 FIESTA shows cross section of the IAC depicting four normal nerves on the right (**c**) compared to the tiny tumor (arrow ↑) involving the left vestibular nerve (**d**). Remember, those four demonstrated nerves include CN VII, cochlear division of CN VIII, as well as superior and inferior vestibular branches of VIII. (**e**, **f**) Coronal T2 FIESTA shows section through IAC exhibiting an "en face" look at the tiny tumor involving the left vestibular nerve without (**e**) and with (**f**) arrow (↑). Axial (**g**, **h**) and

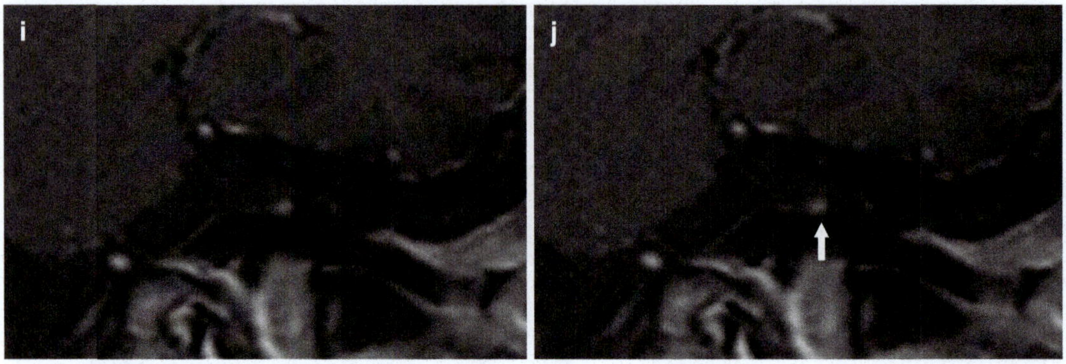

Fig. 11.4 (continued) Sagittal (**i**, **j**) T1 Gd axial shows the tiny tumor enhancement corresponds to the "filling defect" depicted by beautiful T2 FIESTA images. No matter how much this tiny tumor tries to attract attention by Gd enhancement, its FIESTA images clearly do a better job. One can appreciate that having only enhanced images (**g**, **i**), this little "fella" could have been missed without having "helper arrows (↑)' (**h**, **j**)

- While most meningiomas tend to be typical, considering their prevalence, statistics suggest we can probably predict a noteworthy number of "atypical" cases.
- Some unusual features which can be misleading include "ring" enhancement, large cysts, and fatty transformation [6].
- CPA meningiomas are often large before becoming symptomatic.
- Symptoms are usually related to mass effect on CN III, V, VII, and VIII.
- Symptoms include ataxia, nystagmus, and facial hypesthesia. Audiologic findings may be normal or show retro-cochlear pattern.
- VS classically causes hearing loss more frequently than do CPA meningiomas.
- See Chap. 10, CPA 2, CPA Meningioma.

B. Neurosarcoidosis
- Most cases manifest multiple dural-based foci.
- Look for involvement of the pituitary infundibulum.
- See Chap. 6, Neurohypophyseal Sarcoidosis.

C. Lymphoma and Metastasis
- May be bilateral.
- Often manifest as multifocal meningeal involvement.

D. Astrocytomas
- Comprise 1% of CPA masses.
- Exhibit moderate postcontrast enhancement.
- Astrocytomas are exophytic.
- Astrocytomas can appear cystic.

E. Ependymoma
- Ependymomas show some focus of enhancement.
- Ependymomas pedunculate from the brainstem.
- Ependymomas can appear cystic.

A Closer Look

I. Fast Facts
- Intralabyrinthine schwannoma (ILS) is an underreported cause of sensorineural hearing loss. It is often diagnosed long after the onset of hearing loss and surgery is usually avoided as long as possible because surgery invariably causes deafness on the involved side [7].
- ILS encompasses a rare group of lesions which, while having similar pathology to vestibular schwannomas, appears to demand different management.
- ILS currently encompasses intracochlear schwannomas, intravestibular schwannomas, vestibulocochlear schwannoma, transmacular schwannomas, transmodiolar schwannoma, and transotic schwannoma [7] (see Fig. 11.4 – Intravestibular Schwannoma).
- Vestibular schwannomas show a prevalence of 1 in 50,000.

II. Historic Highlights
- 1777 Eduard Sandifort, Netherlands anatomy professor, first described at autopsy a unilateral acoustic tumor [8].
- 1822 Wishart reported the first known case of bilateral acoustic neuromas [9].
- 1833 Sir Charles Bell documented a Meckel's cave neuroma demonstrating its relationship to the CPA [10].
- 1894 British surgeon Sir Charles Ballance, who popularized mastoidectomy for major middle ear infections, performed the first successful CPA surgery for surgical

resection of a vestibular schwannoma in which the patient survived [4, 8].

- 1917 Harvey Cushing described 30 cases suggesting intracapsular removal had ↓ perioperative fatality rate to 15%.
- 1925 Walter E. Dandy, a pupil of Cushing, described a technique for complete tumor removal which he reported in 1941 to have an 11% mortality rate. He, however, had managed to preserve the facial nerve in only 1 of ceb 46 cases.
- The journey to current surgical success has certainly been long and laborious leaving a trail of high morbidity and mortality. This journey continues today.
- Today's recurrence rate is currently <1% [11].

III. Genetics and Associations

- *Sporadic:* Most schwannomas are sporadic and not inherited showing a single tumor seemingly developing by chance.
- *Genetic:* However, some schwannomas are clearly caused by underlying genetic disorders like neurofibromatosis 2 (NF2) or Carney complex. Individuals showing multiple schwannomas probably have underlying genetic disorders.
- *PRKAR1A gene*: The Carney complex is inherited as an autosomal dominant affecting protein kinase A (PKA) through the PRKAR1A gene.
- *Other mutations:* In addition to well-known associations with NF2, lesser known players include recurrent DNA mutations in ARID1A, ARID1B, and DDR1. RNA sequencing has shown frequent SH3PXD2A-HTRA1 fusion in some sporadic cases [12].

Selected References

1. Fischbein NJ, Dillon WP, Barkovich AJ. Teaching atlas of brain imaging. New York: Thieme; 2000. p. 111–3.
2. Wigand ME, Rettinger G, Haid T, et al. The removal of VIIIth nerve neurinomas from the cerebellopontine angle by enlarged middle fossa approach. HNO. 1985;33:11–6.
3. Mulkens TH, Parizel PM, Martin JJ, et al. Acoustic schwannoma: MR findings in 84 tumors. AJR Am J Roentgenol. 1993;160(2):395–8.
4. Silk PS, JI L, Driscoll CL. Surgical approaches to vestibular schwannomas: what the radiologist needs to know. Radiographics. 2009;29(7):1955–70.
5. Hakyemez B, Erdogan C, Bolca N, et al. Evaluation of different cerebral mass lesions by perfusion-weighted MR imaging. J Magn Reson Imaging. 2006;24:817–24.
6. Buetow MP, Buetow PC, Smirniotopoulos JG. Typical, atypical, and misleading features in meningioma. Radiographics. 1991;11(6):1087–106.
7. Salzman KL, Childs AM, Davidson HC, et al. Intralabyrinthine schwannomas: imaging diagnosis and classification. AJNR Am J Neuroradiol. 2012;33:104–9.
8. Koerbel A, Gharabaghi A, Safavi-Abasi S, et al. Evolution of vestibular schwannoma surgery: the long journey to current success. Neurosurg Focus. 2005;18(4):E10.
9. Wishart JH. Case of tumours in the skull, dura mater, and brain. Edin Med Surg J. 1822;18:393.
10. Bell C. The nervous system of the human body; embracing the papers delivered to the Royal Society on the subject of the nerves. Washington, DC: Duff Green; 1833.
11. Shelton C. Unilateral acoustic tumors: how often do they recur after translabyrinthine removal? Laryngoscope. 1995;105(9 pt 1):958–66.
12. Agnihotri S, Jalali S, Wilson M, et al. The genomic landscape of schwannoma. Nat Genet. 2016;48:1339–48. https://doi.org/10.1038/ng.3688.

12 CPA Arachnoid Cyst

Pertinent Points

- Definition: Extra-axial cystic CPA mass following CSF signal on all imaging sequences with no restricted diffusion, which can cause conspicuous mass effect on adjacent structures, despite its almost imperceptible wall.
- *Classic Clue*: Often incidentally found non-enhancing fluid-filled CPA mass with an almost imperceptible wall. Fluid follows CSF CT attenuation and CSF MRI intensity with *no diffusion restriction.*
- *AKA*: Intracranial arachnoid cyst, subarachnoid cyst.
- Etiology: True arachnoid cysts arise from unexplained tearing or splitting of an already flimsy spider-like arachnoid membrane [1].
- Gender Preference: M > F: 3:1 [3, 5, 6, 12]
- Locations: Intracranial arachnoid cysts occur most frequently in the middle cranial fossa. A mere 10% occur in the posterior fossa with the CPA comprising the most common infratentorial site [4].
- Incidence: Frequently found as an incidental finding on imaging studies.

Imaging

General Imaging Features

- Cystic CPA mass which focuses to push away adjacent structures.
- Characteristic arachnoid-like, thin, transparent cyst walls barely seen on imaging (see Fig. 12.1a).

CT Features

- See General Imaging Features.
- CT attenuation in Hounsfield units usually identical to CSF. Rarely ↑ attenuation from hemorrhage or protein.
- *No postcontrast enhancement* of fluid or cyst wall.
- Shows *no calcifications* on CT.

MRI Features

- See General Imaging Features.
- T1: Usually isointense to CSF (see Fig. 12.1b–d).
- T2: Usually isointense to CSF (see Fig. 12.1a).
- T1 Gd: No enhancement.
- FLAIR: Suppresses completely.
- DWI: Shows low signal with ***no*** restricted diffusion (see Fig. 12.1e, f).

Clinical Issues

1. Presentation
   - Symptoms
     - Most cases are found as incidental findings at MRI.
     - When symptomatic see headache, dizziness, trigeminal neuralgia, hemifacial spasm, or sensorineural hearing loss (SNHL).
2. Natural History
   - A large university study showed the prevalence of MRI demonstrated intracranial arachnoid cysts to be 1.4% in adults [6] and 2.6% in children [12].
   - M > F in adults and children [6, 12].
   - Few patients with arachnoid cysts show symptoms. Those who present without symptoms usually show a benign natural history [6].
3. Epidemiology and Pathology
   - Intracranial arachnoid cysts which develop in the arachnoid mater [located between the superficial dura mater covering the skull and the deeper pia mater covering the brain] appear to arise from some strange splitting of this spindly shroud.

F. A. Midyett, S. K. Mukherji, *Skull Base Imaging*, https://doi.org/10.1007/978-3-030-46447-9_12

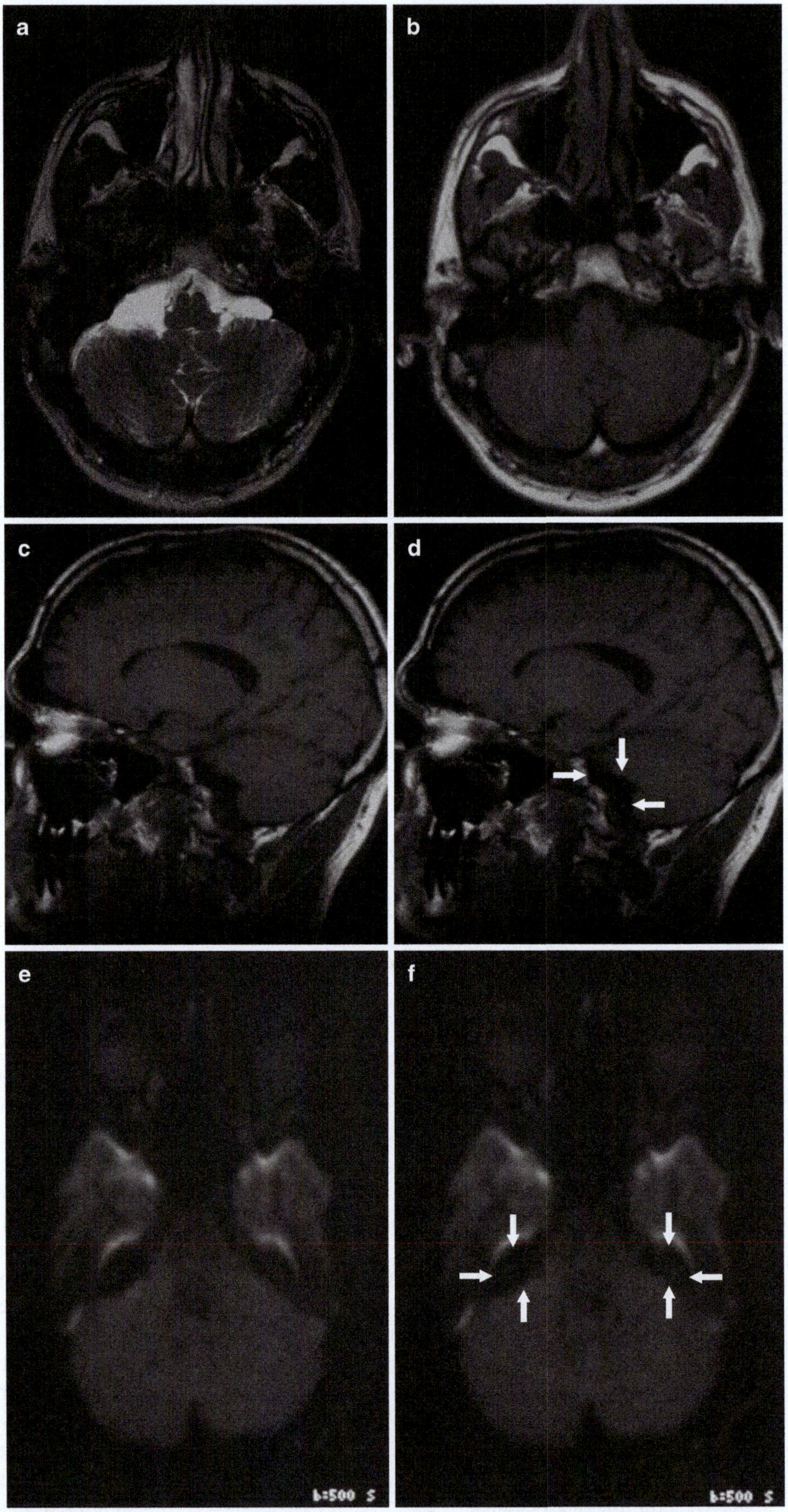

Fig. 12.1 (**a**) T2 axial shows abnormal fluid collections involving both CPAs extending across the midline through the prepontine cistern. Signal follows CSF. Some areas show super sharp margins and others reveal ultra-thin capsule. (**b**) T1 axial shows low signal abnormality involving both CPAs and the prepontine cistern. (**c**, **d**) T1 sagittal shows low signal abnormality in the CPA displacing the cerebellum posteriorly [helpful helper arrows on (**d**)]. (**e**, **f**) Axial DWI through the level of the abnormality demonstrated *no* restricted diffusion on any of the cuts or on various *b* values

- Arachnoid cysts are benign CSF-filled masses enclosed by thin, translucent cyst walls.
- The cyst fluid is commonly clear and colorless but can occasionally be hemorrhagic or proteinaceous [2].
- Arachnoid cysts can be congenital or acquired, usually beginning in infancy although often not showing symptoms until adolescence or adulthood.
- Microscopically the cyst wall has a vascular collagenous membrane lined by arachnoid cells [8] appearing histologically indistinguishable from the normal arachnoid membrane [7].
- Progressive enlargement of arachnoid cysts prompts theories of:
  - Active cyst wall fluid secretion
  - Fluid diffusing into cyst by osmotic gradient and "ball-valve" mechanism

Treatment

- Most patients require no treatment but exhibit excellent prognosis when treatment is required.
- Surgical therapy is reserved for cases where symptoms are clearly linked to location of the arachnoid cyst.
- Surgical options include fenestration, shunting, needle aspiration, and marsupialization [2].

Differential Diagnosis

- The differential of a cystic CPA mass lesion (in addition to arachnoid cyst) includes the following:

A. Epidermoid

- Epidermoids typically show scalloped margins. Arachnoid cysts also show sharp margins.
- *Epidermoids show restricted diffusion* and are bright on DWI with corresponding dark signal on ADC map. Not a feature of arachnoid cysts which follow CSF on all imaging sequences.
- Epidermoids are relatively rare in children [8].
- See Chap. 9, CPA Epidermoid Cyst.

B. Neurenteric (NE) Cyst

- Rare benign endodermal lesions which may be mistaken for other more common non-neoplastic cysts or cystic neoplasms.
- Synonyms: enterogenous cyst, enteric cyst, endodermal cyst, etc.
- 3:1 = spine/brain; posterior fossa > supratentorial locations
- T1: Variable – iso- to hyperintense depending on proteinaceous fluid content [which ↑ T1 signal] [1].
- T2 signal is variable.
- T1 Gd: Non-enhancing for bulk of cyst; ± partial rim enhancement.
- Neurenteric cysts have been reported to *rarely* cause *partial* diffusion restriction. This suggests we should place this in our differential as a "long shot" when restriction of diffusion is *partial* in a CPA cyst [1].

C. Cystic Neoplasms

- Astrocytomas
  - Astrocytomas comprise 1% of CPA masses.
  - Astrocytomas are exophytic with moderate postcontrast enhancement.
  - Astrocytomas can appear cystic.
    - Astrocytomas are usually not perfectly smooth with a thin wall like an arachnoid cyst.
    - Cystic astrocytomas usually show enhancement of cyst rim [2].
- Ependymoma
  - Ependymomas can appear cystic.
  - Ependymomas usually do not have a perfectly smooth, thin wall like an arachnoid cyst.
  - Ependymomas usually show rim enhancement [2].
  - Ependymomas pedunculate from the brainstem showing some focus of enhancement.

D. Parasitic Cysts

- Parasitic cyst walls usually enhance [2].
- Parasitic cysts are usually <1 cm.
- Parasitic cysts are usually seen in the ventricles and subarachnoid spaces.
- Includes:
  - Neurocysticercosis (NCC)
    - Calcifications are common.
    - Radiologists must look for the scolex.
    - Ependymitis or basilar meningitis is commonly associated.
    - Usually find multiple lesions within the cisterns and parenchyma.
    - Most of these cysts are <1 cm.
    - NCC doesn't typically crop up in clusters.
    - NCC often displays enhancing cyst walls.
    - Imaging findings follow disease stages: vesicular, colloidal vesicular, granular nodular, nodular calcified.
  - Hydatid cysts
    - AKA: echinococcosis, hydatid disease, hydatidosis, or echinococcal disease.
    - Uni- or multilocular.
    - Almost all are in children.
    - Daughter cysts are common.
    - Calcifications are rare occurring in <1%.
    - Typically, *no* enhancement on CECT.

T1 cyst is isointense to CSF.

T2 cyst is isointense to CSF with ***hypointense rim*** and ***no*** peri-lesional edema.

T1 Gd typically shows *no enhancement in* bulk of lesion, ± fine peripheral enhancement.

A Closer Look

I. Fast Facts

- Arachnoid cysts cause ≤2.6% of intracranial space-occupying lesions [6, 12].
- PFACs probably arise from incomplete separation of the endomenix during early embryogenesis [9].

II. Historic Highlights

- 1831 Richard Bright first described arachnoid cysts [10]. Yes, this is the same Bright we remember for "albuminuric nephritis" as Bright's disease. The brilliance of Bright's pioneering descriptions appear even more amazing when you consider that he didn't have the help of a microscope or formaldehyde to preserve tissue.
- 1958 Starkman reported ACs lie between two membranes of normal arachnoid and described them as "intra-arachnoid" cysts.
- 1907 Placzek and Krause successfully surgically treated an arachnoid cyst.
- 1981 Stein advocated shunting for primary treatment of AC.
- 2000 German Air Force began head and spine MRI screening for ACs. Kriebel and Maxon (2002) suggested ACs are "time bombs" in pilot's head which should render them "unfit to fly" [11].
- Many may debate whether ACs are problematic for pilots or passengers, but most nations do not pre-screen their pilots with MRI and those pilots presumably have the same 2% prevalence of intracranial arachnoid cysts as the general population. So, add that to your lists of concerns when you fly commercially.

III. Genetics and Associations

- The current consensus continues to counsel that arachnoid cysts arise from "unexplained tearing" of arachnoid membranes.
- The precise primary elemental etiology enigmatically endures. Acknowledged associations include agenesis of the corpus callosum, arachnoiditis, mucopolysaccharidosis, and, of course, the Chudley-McCollough and Marfan's syndromes.
- Reports of intracranial arachnoid cysts in siblings suggest some familial cases where inheritance is influenced by an autosomal recessive or polygenic pattern [13–16].

Selected References

1. Preece MT, Osborn AG, Chin SS, Smirniotopoulos JG. Intracranial neurenteric cysts: imaging and pathologic Spectrum. Am J Neuroradiol. 2006;27:1211–6.
2. Fischbein NJ, Dillon WP, Barkovich AJ. Teaching atlas of brain imaging. New York: Thieme; 2000. p. 78–81.
3. Osborne AG. Diagnostic neuroradiology, Mosby-Year Book, St. Louis, MO; 1994. p. 63–8; 639–42.
4. Rengacharry SS, Watanabe I, Brackett CE. Pathogenesis of intracranial arachnoid cysts. Surg Neurol. 1978;9:139–44.
5. Robertson SJ, Wolpert SM, Runge VM. MR imaging of middle cranial fossa arachnoid cysts: temporal lobe agenesis syndrome revisited. AJNR. 1989:1007–10.
6. Al-Holou WN, Terman S, Kilburg C. Prevalence and natural history of arachnoid cysts in adults. J Neurosurg. 2013;118(2):222–31.
7. Miyagami M. Tsunokawa: histological and ultrastructural findings of benign intracranial cysts. Noshuyo Byori. 1993;10:151–60.
8. Fischbein NJ, Dillon WP, Barkovich AJ. Teaching atlas of brain imaging. New York: Thieme; 2000. p. 78–81.
9. Baskin DS, Wilson CB. Transsphenoidal treatment of non-neoplastic intrasellar cysts. A report of 38 cases. J Neurosurg. 1984;60:8–13.
10. Bright R. Serous cysts in the arachnoid. In Rees O, Brown G, editors. Diseases of the brain and nervous system. Part I. London: Longman Group Ltd; 1831. p 437–439.
11. Lueling F, Zschommler Y. Intracranial arachnoid cysts in German military aircraft pilots. Flugmedizinisches Institut der Luftwaffe. German Air Force Institute of Aviation Medicine.
12. Al-Holou WN, Yew AY, Boomsaad ZE, et al. Prevalence and natural history of arachnoid cysts in children clinical article. J Neurosurg Pediatr. 2010;5(6):578–85.
13. Handa J, Okamoto K, Sato M. Arachnoid cyst of the middle cranial fossa: report of bilateral cysts in siblings. Surg Neurol. 1981;16:127–30. [PubMed: 7280984, related citations] [Full Text].
14. Helland CA, Wester K. Monozygotic twins with mirror image cysts: indication of a genetic mechanism in arachnoid cysts? Neurology. 2007;69:110–1. [PubMed: 17606888, related citations] [Full Text].
15. Pomeranz S, Constantini S, Lubetzki-Korn I, Amir N. Familial intracranial arachnoid cysts. Childs Nerv Syst. 1991;7:100–2. [PubMed: 1863926, related citations] [Full Text].
16. Wilson WG, Deponte KA, McIlhenny J, Dreifuss FE. Arachnoid cysts in a brother and sister. J Med Genet. 1988;25:714–5s. [PubMed: 3225827, related citations] [Full Text].

Part III

Anterior Cranial Fossa/Anterior Skull Base

13 Anterior Fossa Meningioma

Pertinent Points

- Definition: Meningiomas are nonglial tumors which arise from arachnoidal cap cells in the arachnoidal membrane. AFMs (anterior fossa meningiomas) comprise a particularly problematic group of up to 20% of intracranial meningiomas originating along the floor of the anterior cranial fossa [26, 28].
- Anterior fossa meningiomas regularly reach striking sizes while showing only superficial symptoms.
- Classified according to attachment site, the most common ACF meningiomas are olfactory groove, planum sphenoidale, and tuberculum sellae meningiomas [28].
- While each tumor site may exhibit distinct clinical features, in practice they often constitute a continuum and can be considered together [28].
- Most frequent locations are olfactory groove and tuberculum sellae [26].
- *Classic Clue*: Middle-aged female patient presenting with headache, seizures, and personality change found to have visual loss with extra-axial solid anterior fossa mass with broad base abutting dural surface.
- Enhancing "dural tail" is classic but not pathognomonic.
- Approximately 75% of these slow-growing AFMs become large >4 cm. before showing symptoms [26].
- Usually seen in middle-aged to elderly patients but can be seen in children.
- Meningioma incidence: F:M = 2:1 [9]
- Meningiomas are the most common nonglial primary brain tumors constituting 20% of all intracranial tumors [1–3, 12].
- Meningiomas are the most common intracranial extra-axial neoplasms in adults.

Imaging

General Imaging Features

- Sharply circumscribed round or smoothly lobulated extra-axial mass, broad-based against the dura.

CT Features

- See General Imaging Features.
- Three fourths are hyperdense with most of the rest isodense to adjacent brain. However, a few can be hypodense to brain with the occasional lipoblastic or xanthomatous tumor having negative attenuation numbers.
- 25% show diffuse or focal calcification rim-like, sandlike (psammomatous), sunburst, or globular patterns.
- CT shows osseous reaction at tumor attachment in >50% of cases [6].
- CT when positive depicts localized hyperostosis and spur formation [6].
- CT is often better than MRI at demonstrating tumor's attachment to skull, a finding important to neurosurgeons [6].
- Typically iso- or hyperdense precontrast with avid post-contrast enhancement.

MRI Features

- T1: Most show heterogeneous low T1 signal (60%). (See Fig. 13.1a Coronal T1.)
- T2: Most show high signal on T2 (68%).
- T1 Gd:
  - 100% show enhancement with 80% avid and 20% moderate. (See Fig. 13.1b–c.)
  - > 50% show "dural tail" sign. (See Fig. 13.1b–d.)

F. A. Midyett, S. K. Mukherji, *Skull Base Imaging*, https://doi.org/10.1007/978-3-030-46447-9_13

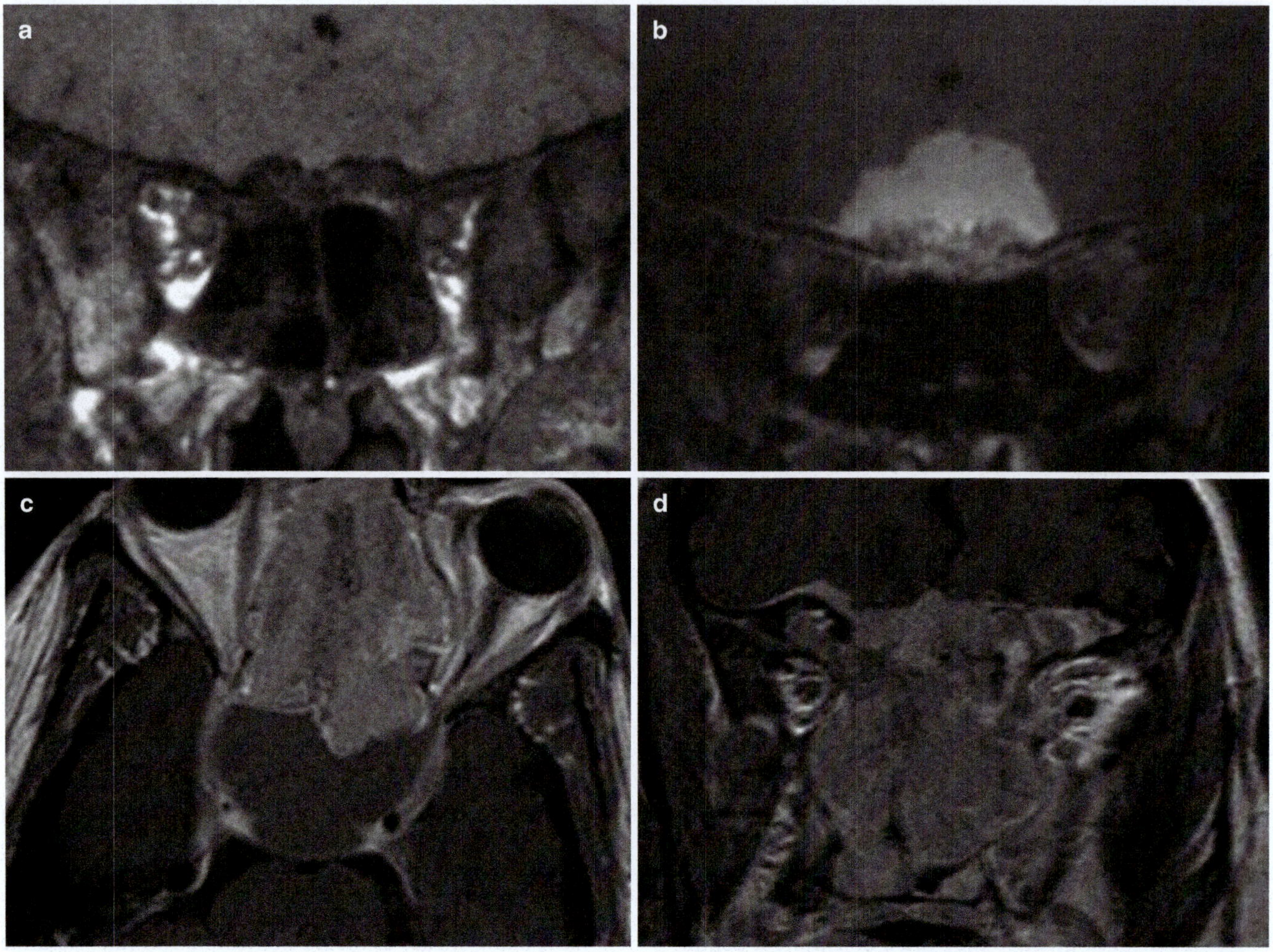

Fig. 13.1 (**a**) Coronal T1 shows abnormal thickening of sphenoid sinus roof with extension into anterior cranial fossa. Low signal suggests the cranial margin is calcified. Asymmetric loss of marrow on right. Abnormal heterogeneity of overlying frontal lobe with focal areas of hypo-attenuation. Abnormal heterogeneous signal involves sphenoid sinuses. (**b**) Coronal T1 Gd shows large avidly enhancing well-circumscribed mass, broad-based against anterior skull base. Conspicuous loss of normal cortex caudal to lesion with irregular expansion into tumor probably represents bony response to tumor. Tumor breaches the skull base extending into sphenoid sinus from above. Bilateral enhancing "dural tails" more conspicuous on right. (**c**) Axial T1 Gd shows huge heterogeneously enhancing mass, involving the anterior skull base, breeching the orbital lamina papyracea displacing the orbital contents laterally. Margins are quite indistinct. (**d**) Coronal T1 Gd shows huge heterogeneously enhancing mass, breaching the skull base to extend caudally to the level of the hard palate. Tumor margins are quite indistinct. Prominent enhancing "dural tail" extends over cranial aspect of right cranial fossa. The floor of left anterior cranial fossa appears largely destroyed

  - "Dural tail" sign is frequent but nonspecific as it may be seen with any tumor which invades the dura or provokes a dural reaction. Dural tails usually represent hypervascular dural reaction rather than tangible tumor involvement [21].
- FLAIR: ~ 70% show high signal on FLAIR.
- DWI:
  - DWI signal is variable and appears to correlate with histologic subtypes.
  - Atypical and malignant meningiomas have less extracellular space for water, reducing ADC values.
  - DWI appears to be a useful tool for separating atypical and malignant meningiomas from more common benign meningiomas.
  - Most meningiomas are benign and typically isointense/slightly hyperintense with ADC isointense/slightly hyperintense.
  - Restricted diffusion with markedly hyperintense (light bulb bright) DWI images which correspond to hypointense (black hole) on ADC map suggests atypical or malignant meningioma [20].

- Most frequent associated findings: *dural tail sign and bone infiltration* [20].
- See General Imaging Features.

Angiographic Features

- Most are dural-based, vascular tumors.
- May demonstrate a radial or "sunburst" pattern of vascular supply.
- Prominent, homogeneous prolonged vascular blush in late arterial and capillary phases.
- Shows Smirniotopoulos' "mother-in-law" sign. The blush "comes early and stays late."
- It occasionally displays early draining veins.

Clinical Issues

1. Presentation
   - Visual impairment is a primary presenting symptom, especially when tumor arises from tuberculum sellae [28, 30].
   - Olfactory groove meningiomas commonly cause headache, seizures, and/or personality disorders.
2. Natural History
   - Location, resectability, and histology are major determinants of clinical outcome.
   - Anterior fossa meningiomas are generally slow-growing and easily compress adjacent structures.
   - Meningioma incidence: F:M = 2:1 [9]
   - More often found in middle-aged patients but can be seen in children.
   - One third of intracranial meningiomas do not show symptoms.
   - There are significant differences in recurrence rates depending on histologic types.
   - Using the WHO criteria, the 5-year recurrence rate ranges from 3% for "benign" meningiomas, increasing by more than tenfold to 38% for "atypical" tumors and more than 75% for "anaplastic" or malignant meningiomas [11, 18, 19].
3. Epidemiology and Pathology
   - Approximately one half of all primary brain tumors are gliomas.
   - The most common nonglial primary brain tumors are meningiomas [11].
   - Meningiomas are usually spherical or lobulated but occasionally are flat and carpet-like when the "en plaque" lesion infiltrates the dura occasionally invading underlying bone.
   - They are sharply circumscribed with well-defined tumor brain interfaces.
   - Often observe distinct arachnoid "clefts" containing trapped CSF and surrounding vessels.
   - They contain hemorrhagic and necrotic foci but usually lack gross hemorrhage.

Treatment

- At time of diagnosis, large lesions coupled with close contact to crucial neurovascular structures regularly make their resection at best "challenging" [28].
- Up to 25% of meningiomas cannot be completely removed because tumor encases a carotid artery, cavernous sinus, or optic nerve [1, 26].
- This should come as no surprise since Harvey Cushing originally used Dr. Bovie's "new" electrocautery device to remove meningiomas from the inside. This was an improvement over using a sharp spoon which he had used previously [28, 33].
- Facing an almost 10% post-surgical mortality, surgeons still stress the importance of early diagnosis to improve patient outcomes [26].
- Today, a wide variety of surgical strategies includes endoscopic and radiosurgery [4, 5, 7, 8, 13–17, 23, 28, 29].

Differential Diagnosis

- While the imaging appearance of an anterior cranial fossa meningioma is usually characteristic, some meningiomas "mimic" other entities, and other entities may masquerade as meningiomas [11].
- The differential diagnosis for an atypical meningioma may include the following.

A. Esthesioneuroblastoma (ENB) [34]

- Rare neuroendocrine malignancy of neural crest origin arising from olfactory epithelium.
- AKA: Olfactory neuroblastoma.
- Classically show avidly enhancing dumbbell-shaped mass with "waist" at cribriform plate.
- May involve anterior cranial fossa, skull base, and orbit.
- Intermediate signal on T1 and T2.
- Cystic areas (with foci of ↑T2) at tumor/brain interface are diagnostic and may be pathognomonic.
- Avid enhancement on T1 Gd.
- Can be confused with meningioma when ENB sometimes shows a "dural tail."
- DWI shows moderate restricted diffusion.
- ENB exhibits an epicenter near the cribriform plate.
- ENB displays no gender preference.
- [See Chap. 28, ENB, Esthesioneuroblastoma.]

B. Inverted Papilloma (IP) [34]
- Exhibits an epicenter near the middle meatus.
- IP shows benign-appearing expansile bone changes.
- IPs occur predominately in males with M: F = 10:1 incidence.
- There is ***no*** signature MRI signal appearance for intracranial IP.
- A distinctive CCP (convoluted cerebriform pattern) of enhancement may be seen when tumor involves maxillary sinus.
- *[See Chap. 14, Inverted Papilloma.]

C. Juvenile Nasal Angiofibroma (JNA)
- AKA: Juvenile angiofibroma (JAF).
- Since the tumor typically begins in the nose (not the nasopharynx), some consider juvenile angiofibroma the more correct terminology.
- Non-encapsulated vascular mass found exclusively in adolescent males.
- While it may occasionally involve the anterior skull base, its origin and usual epicenter is near the posterior wall of the nasal cavity near the near the margin of the sphenopalatine foramen.
- T1 and T2 show heterogeneous signal with conspicuous vascular flow voids.
- T1 Gd exhibits avid enhancement.
- [See Chap. 15, Juvenile Nasal Angiofibroma.]

D. Allergic Fungal Sinusitis (AFS)
- Young immunocompetent patient from the Southwestern United States presents with therapy-resistant chronic sinusitis.
- Hypo-attenuation on T2 MRI corresponds to *characteristically* hyperdense sinus with *characteristic serpiginous* pattern.
- While AFS starts in the sinus, it may have already invaded the skull base before it comes to imaging.
- [See Chap. 32, Allergic Fungal Sinusitis for unabridged description.]

E. Fibrous Dysplasia [35]
- Pre-adolescent patient presenting with painless proptosis and diplopia.
- Expanding enhancing sphenoid wing mass showing intact bony cortex.
- FD shows three basic varieties: sclerotic (35%), lytic (25%), and mixed (40%).
- Plain films classically show "ground-glass" appearance with lesions commonly crossing sutures.
- CT shows bony expansion keeps its original shape but spares the cortex.
- T1 is heterogeneous low to intermediate signal.
- T2 is heterogeneous, usually low but may have regions of higher signal.
- T1 Gd shows avid enhancement.
- [See Chap. 13, Fibrous Dysplasia.]

A Closer Look

I. Fast Facts
- The olfactory grooves (AKA olfactory sulci) are sagittal grooves on the inferior (or orbital) surface of the frontal lobes which demarcate the straight gyri from the orbital gyri [27].
- The tuberculum sella (tubercle of sella turcica) is a small sphenoid bony protuberance which forms the posterior boundary of the chiasmatic groove and the anterior boundary of the hypophyseal fossa.

II. Historic Highlights
- 1614: Felix Plater, Professor of Medicine, University of Basel, first reported at autopsy, a lesion most compatible with meningioma describing a "noble knight" intracranial tumor.
- 1774: French surgeon Antoine Louis called the tumor "fungus dura matris."
- 1847: Virchow recognized meningiomas as "sandlike" calling them "psammomas."
- 1879: Scottish surgeon Sir William Macewen resected a frontal meningioma in a 14-year-old girl publishing the procedure in 1881 [28, 31].
- 1884: Italian politician and surgeon Francesco Durante performed a left frontal craniotomy for a more typical cribriform plate meningioma publishing his findings in 1887 [28, 32].
- 1922: Harvey Cushing coined the term "meningioma," although this tumor has been known under various names since the seventeenth century [9, 10]. Other prior iterations of names include epitheliomas, endotheliomas, and relatives to sarcomas. Thanks to Dr. Cushing for bringing order to this colossal confusion [9]!
- 1927: Harvey Cushing dedicated his Macewen Memorial Lecture illustrating two cases of olfactory groove meningiomas citing the value of Dr. Bovie's new electrocautery device, not previously available to earlier pioneering neurosurgeons Macewen and *Durante* [28, 33].

III. Genetics and Environment
- Ionizing radiation exposure is the environmental risk factor most frequently found with meningiomas although <1% of irradiated individuals develop meningiomas [22].

- Endogenous and exogenous hormones have been implicated in meningioma development, although their precise role requires further study [22].
- The code for tumor suppressor Merlin resides in the NF2 gene and is disrupted in one half of all patients with meningiomas [24].
- Mutation of the NF2 gene with resultant neurofibromatosis type II (NF2) is a dominantly inherited disorder where patients commonly present with bilateral vestibular schwannomas, multiple meningiomas, as well as other CNS tumors [23–25].
- There is hereditary susceptibility for meningioma involving mutations involving multiple other genes in addition to the more commonly recognized NF2 gene.
- Currently impugned genes and locations associated with meningiomas read like an alphabet soup and include chromosomes 1, 9, 10, 14, 17, 18, and 22 and SWI/SNF with subunits SMARCB1 and SMARCE1, and the list grows daily.
- The sonic hedgehog (SHH)-GLI1 signaling pathway gene, SUFU, is clearly the causal culprit for hereditary multiple meningiomas in a Finnish family.

Selected References

1. Velho V, Argarwal V, Mallay R, Palande DA. Posterior Fossa Meningioma "our experience" in 64 cases. Asian J Neurosurg. 2012;7(3):116–24.
2. Castellano F, Ruggiero G. Meningiomas of the posterior fossa. Acta Radiol Suppl. 1953;104:1–177.
3. Laird FJ, Harmer SG, Laws ER, Reese DF. Meningiomas of the cerebellopontine angle. Otolaryngol Head Neck Surg. 1985;93:163–7.
4. Saleh EA, Taibah AK, Achilli V, Aristegui M, Mazzoni A, Sanna M. Posterior Fossa meningioma surgical strategy. Skull Base Surg. 1994;4:202–12.
5. Lobato RD, Gonzaáez P, Alday R, Ramos A, Lagares A, Alen JF, et al. Meningiomas of the basal posterior fossa. Surgical experience in 80 cases. Neurocirugia. 2004;15:525–42.
6. Helie O, Soulie D, Sarrazin JL, Dewrosier C, Cordoliani YS, Cosnard G. Magnetic resonance imaging and meningioma of posterior cerebral fossa, 31 cases. J Neuroradiol. 1995;22:252–70.
7. Hakuba A, Nishimura S, Tanaka K, Kishi H, Nakamura T. Clivus meningioma,: six cases of total removal. Neurol Med Chir. 1977;17:63–77.
8. Mayberg MR, Symon L. Meningiomas of the clivus and apicalpetrous bone: report of 35 cases. J Neurosurg. 1986;65:160–7.
9. Dumitrescu GF, Imndrei A, Husseini ME, et al. Posterior fossa meningiomas: Correlation between site of origin and pathology. Romanian Neurosurg. 2010;XVII 3:327–38.
10. Kaye H. Posterior fossa meningiomas. In: Sindou M, editor. Practical handbook of neurosurgery: from leading neurosurgeons, vol 2. Germany: Springer; 2009. p. 181.
11. Osborne AG. Diagnostic neuroradiology. St Louis, Mo, USA: Mosby, Elsevier; 1994. p. 579–625.
12. Javalkar V, Banerjee AD, Nanda A. Posterior cranial fossa meningioma. J Neurol Surg B Skull Base. 2012;73(1):1–10.
13. Sekhar LN, Wright DC, Richardson R, Monacci W. Petroclival and foramen magnum meningiomas: surgical approaches and pitfalls. J Neuro-Oncol. 1996;29(3):249–59.
14. Williams SJ, Faye-Peterson O, Aronin P, Faith S. Capillary hemangioma of the meninges. AJNR. 1993;14:529–36.
15. Cosentino CM, Poulton TB, Esquerra JV, Sanss SF. Giant cranial hemangiopericytoma: MR and angiographic findings. AJNR. 1993;14:253–6.
16. Gumbs RV, Higginbotham-Ford EA, Teal JS, et al. Thoracic extramedullary hematopoiesis in sickle-cell disease. AJR Am J Roentgenol. 1987;149(5):889–93.
17. Singer A, Quencer R. Intracranial extramedullalry hematopoiesis: a rare cause of headaches. J Neuroimaging. 2014;24(5):524–7.
18. Jaaskelainen J, Haltia M, Servo A. Atypical and anaplastic meningiomas: radiology, surgery, radiotherapy, and outcome. Surg Neurol. 1986;25(3):233–42.
19. Maier H, Öfner D, Hittmair A, et al. Classic, atypical, and anaplastic meningioma: three histopathological subtypes of clinical relevance. J Neurosurg. 1992;77:616–23.
20. Filippi CG, Edgar MA, Ulug AM, et al. Appearance of Meningiomas on diffusion-weighted images: correlating diffusion constants with histopathologic findings. AJNR. 2001;22:65–72.
21. Gasparetto EL, Leite Cda C, Lucato LT, et al. Intracranial meningiomas: magnetic resonance imaging findings in 78 cases. Arq Neurosiquiatr. 2007;65(3A):610–4.
22. Claus EB, Calvocoressi L, Bondy ML, et al. Clinical article. Family and personal medical history and risk of meningioma. J Neurosurg. 2011. https://doi.org/10.3171/2011.JNS11129. Accessed 1/9/2016.
23. Smith MJ. Germline and somatic mutations in meningiomas. Cancer Genetics. 2015;208(4): 107–14. https://doi.org/10.1016/cancergen.2015.02.003. Accessed 1/9/2016.
24. Choy W, et al. The molecular genetics and tumor pathogenesis of meningiomas and the future directions of meningioma treatments. Neurosurg Focus. 2011;30:E6.
25. Liu Y, Pang JC, Dong S, Mao B, Poon WS, Ng HK. Aberrant CpG island hypermethylation profile is associated with atypical and anaplastic meningiomas. Hum Pathol. 2005;36:416–25.
26. Rubin G, David UB, Gornish M, Rappaport ZH. Meningiomas of the anterior cranial fossa floor. Acta Neurochir. 1994;129(1):26–30.
27. Olfactory groove. Dictionary.com. The American Heritage® Science Dictionary. Houghton Mifflin Company. http://dictionary.reference.com/browse/olfactory groove. Aaccessed; January 16, 2016.
28. Morales-Valero SF, Van Gompel JJ, Loumiotis I, et al. Craniotomy for anterior cranial fossa meningiomas: historical overview. Neurosurg Focus. 2014;36(4):E14.
29. Rachinger W, Grau S, Tonn JC. Different microsurgical approaches to meningiomas of the anterior cranial base. Acta Neurochir. 2010;152:931–9.
30. Mahmoud M, Nader R, Al-Mefty O. Optic canal involvement in tuberculum sellae meningiomas: influence on approach, recurrence, and visual recovery. Neurosurgery. 2010;67(3):119.
31. Macewen W. Intra-cranial lesions: illustrating some points in connexion with the localization of cerebral affections and the advantages of antiseptic trephining. Lancet. 1881;2:581–3.
32. Durante F. Contribution to endocranial surgery. Lancet. 1886;130:654–5.
33. Cushing H. The Meningiomas arising from the olfactory groove and their removal by the aid of electro-surgery. Jackson, Wylie & Co: Glasgow; 1927.
34. Midyett FA, Mukherji SK. Chapter 22, Esthesioneuroblastoma. Orbital imaging. Elsevier/Saunders. 2015. pp. 91–5. ISBN : 978-0-323-34037-3.
35. Midyett FA, Mukherji SK. Chapter 50, Fibrous dysplasia. Orbital imaging. Elsevier/Saunders. 2015. pp. 241–6. ISBN : 978-0-323-34037-3.

14 Inverted Papilloma

Pertinent Points

- Definition: Uncommon tumor originating from nasal cavity and paranasal sinus mucosa, possessing distinctive pathologic and imaging features. Papilloma portends neoplasia with epithelial growth [1].
- *Classic Clue*: Adult male presents with unilateral nasal obstruction, postnasal drip, epistaxis, and headache with unilateral mass arising in nasal cavity exhibiting CCP ("convoluted cerebriform pattern") on T2 images.
- *AKA*: Inverting Papilloma, endophytic papilloma, sinonasal inverted papilloma, cylindrical epithelioma, Schneiderian papilloma, etc.
- Inverted papillomas are characterized by frequent recurrences and a prominent potential for malignancy [2].
- Inverted papillomas are most frequently found in adult males 40–60 years of age [3, 4].
- Caucasians are more commonly affected than persons of other races [1].
- Inverted papillomas frequently present with findings of unilateral nasal mass. *Bilaterality is rare.*
- Approximately 75% of patients with inverted papillomas show some form of bony changes including thinning, remodeling, erosion, and sclerosis [1, 5].
- Although many inverted papillomas show benign-appearing expansile bone changes, others display destructive bony alteration and possess a notorious propensity for malignant modification [4].
- Inverted papillomas are often mistaken for inflammatory sinus disease [4].
- Inverted papillomas can contain bony trabecular rests [4].
- Inverted papillomas often exhibit an epicenter near the middle meatus.
- Inverted papillomas occur predominately in males with M > F = 3:1 incidence [1, 6].
- Biopsy is often an important tool when inverted papillomas are suspected. Considering potential intracranial involvement, both medical and legal protocols dictate that imaging studies should precede biopsy.
- A distinctive CCP ("convoluted cerebriform pattern") of enhancement may be seen when the tumor involves the maxillary sinus [7].

Imaging

General Imaging Features

- Moderately advanced tumors commonly show unilateral nasal fossa mass with opacification of the contiguous maxillary sinus [8].
- Other radiologic patterns are encountered making it impossible to cite any one pattern specific for IP [8].
- Inverted papillomas commonly occur on the lateral wall of the nasal cavity, more frequently found near the middle turbinate and maxillary ostium [8].
- Enlargement of the mass results in bony remodeling and resorption as it extends into the maxillary antrum [8].
- Inverted papillomas commonly obstruct maxillary antral drainage, but oddly enough, concomitant mucocoeles are rare [8].
- CT and MRI are complimentary when evaluating this complex entity [2].

CT Features

- *See General Imaging Features.*
- Relatively nonspecific soft tissue density mass showing some enhancement.

F. A. Midyett, S. K. Mukherji, *Skull Base Imaging*, https://doi.org/10.1007/978-3-030-46447-9_14

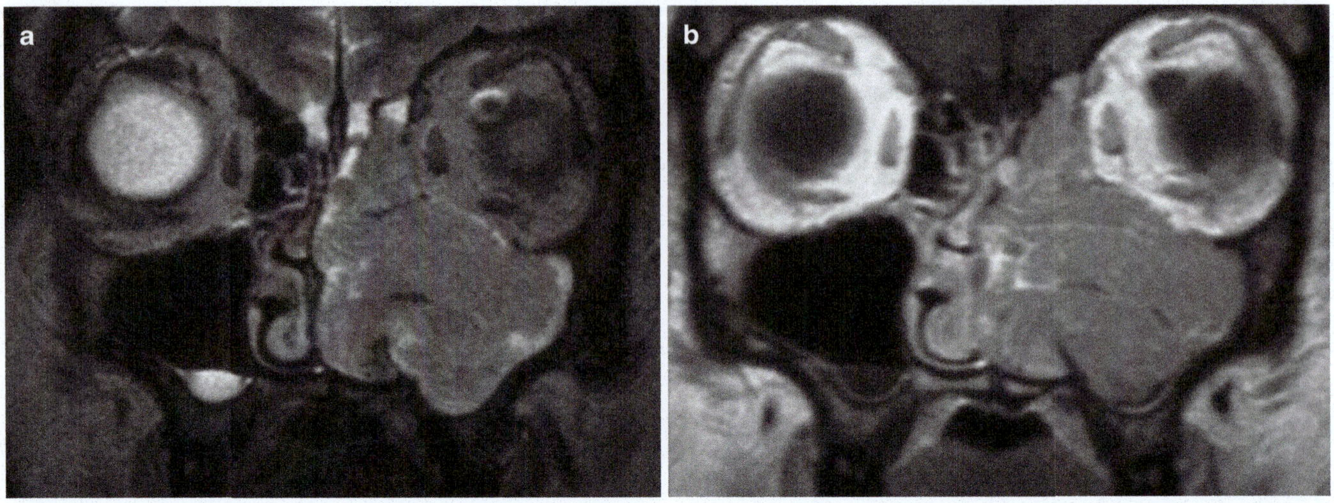

Fig. 14.1 (**a**) Coronal T2 shows large abnormal mass occupying the left maxillary and ethmoid sinuses which is relatively heterogeneous, relatively isointense to brain with high signal around its periphery, probably fluid. The mass extends into the left nasal cavity abutting the nasal septum. The medial wall of the maxillary sinus has been destroyed along with the nasal turbinates. The left inferior orbital wall is contiguous with the mass and probably has been compromised. Tumor abuts the floor of the left anterior cranial fossa medially. The mass is hyperintense to EOMs. (**b**) Coronal T1 Gd again demonstrates the large mass described on the prior T2 image. The bulk of the mass is mildly hyperintense to brain with multiple slow flow contrast-filled vessels coursing through the tumor. The mass is isointense to EOMs

- Like real estate, mass *location* is probably the *best clue* for the correct diagnosis.
- Intratumoral calcifications and focal hyperostosis, while helpful in making the diagnosis, are probably more important in surgical planning [2].
- *Hyperostosis* is *highly predictive* of tumor origin [2].
- CT is superior to MRI in evaluating bone erosion, destruction, and hyperostosis [2].
- Combined bony sclerosis and deformity with an antromeatal mass suggests a slow-growing tumor such as inverted papillomas [9].
- The nasal septum is often bowed to the contralateral side.

MRI Features

- *See General Imaging Features.*
- T1: Iso- to slightly hyperintense to muscle [3].
- T2: Iso- to hyperintense to muscle often showing alternating hypointense lines constituting CCP (*convoluted cerebriform pattern*) [10]. (See Fig. 14.1a.)
- T1 Gd:
  - Heterogeneous enhancement [3]. (See Fig. 14.1b, where the mass is isointense to EOMs.)
  - Often show alternating hypointense lines constituting a *convoluted cerebriform* pattern [10].
- MRI is superior to CT in defining the lesion's extent by distinguishing between tumor and inflammation [2, 3, 9].
- But alas, there is *no* signature signal MRI appearance for inverted papillomas [1, 3]. Although the CCP is present in most inverted papillomas, CCP can be seen in several malignant sinonasal tumors as well [1].

Angiographic Features

- Angiography has no significant role to play in diagnosis or assessment.
- When angiography is performed, most appear to be avascular [8].

Clinical Issues

1. Presentation
   - Common start-up symptoms include unilateral nasal obstruction, rhinorrhea, epistaxis, sinusitis, facial pain, anosmia, and frontal headache [1].
   - Subsequent symptoms may include proptosis or diplopia as the lesion extends from the lateral wall of the nasal cavity to the maxillary sinus and orbit.
2. Epidemiology and Pathology
   - Grossly, inverted papillomas look like polyps with narrow or broad-based stalks.
   - They vary from red to pale pink. They are irregular friable polypoid masses of variable consistency, possessing a propensity for hemorrhage [1, 8].
   - Inverted papilloma's high recurrence rate and association with SCC (squamous cell carcinoma) make them clinically aggressive despite their seemingly benign pathologic personality.

- Histologically, their epithelial cells customarily extend into the underlying supportive stromal structures.

Treatment

- Surgery:
  - Inverted papillomas may be treated by internal or external surgical approaches.
  - The specific surgical approach is determined by tumor stage with endoscopic endonasal resection suggested for early-stage tumors.
  - As the tumor stage increases, endoscopic endonasal resection is used in conjunction with other approaches including the Caldwell-Luc procedure, lateral rhinotomy with medial maxillectomy, or lateral rhinotomy with endoscopic-assisted medial maxillectomy [11].

Differential Diagnosis

A. Allergic Fungal Sinusitis (AFS)

- Young immunocompetent patient from the Southwestern United States presents with therapy-resistant chronic sinusitis.
- Hypo-attenuation on T2 MRI corresponds to *distinctive hyperdense sinus* with *characteristic serpiginous* pattern.
- While AFS starts in the sinus, it may have already invaded the skull base before the patient comes to imaging.
- [See Chap. 32, *Allergic Fungal Sinusitis*, for unabridged description.]

B. Esthesioneuroblastoma (ENB) [7]

- ENB is a rare neuroendocrine malignancy of neural crest origin arising from olfactory epithelium.
- AKA: Olfactory neuroblastoma.
- Classically shows avidly enhancing dumbbell-shaped mass with "waist" at the cribriform plate.
- May involve the anterior cranial fossa, skull base, and orbit.
- Intermediate signal on T1 and T2.
- Cystic areas (with foci of ↑T2) at tumor/brain interface are diagnostic and may be pathognomonic.
- Exhibits avid enhancement on T1 Gd.
- DWI shows moderate restricted diffusion.
- ENB exhibits an epicenter near the cribriform plate.
- ENB displays no gender preference.
- [See Chap. 28, Esthesioneuroblastoma.]

C. Juvenile Nasal Angiofibroma (JNA)

- AKA: Juvenile angiofibroma.
- Non-encapsulated vascular mass found exclusively in adolescent males.
- Although JNAs may occasionally involve the anterior skull base, their origin and usual epicenter is near the posterior wall of the nasal cavity near the margin of the sphenopalatine foramen.
- T1 and T2 show heterogeneous signal with conspicuous vascular flow voids.
- T1 Gd exhibits avid enhancement.
- [See Chap. 15, JNA, Juvenile Nasal Angiofibroma.]

D. Antrochoanal Polyp (AP) [7]

- An antrochoanal polyp is a "dumbbell"-shaped mass involving the nasal cavity and maxillary sinus.
- An antrochoanal polyp is a *non-enhancing* mass with benign-appearing bone changes. Inverted papillomas exhibit *heterogeneous enhancement.*
- Antrochoanal polyps sometimes show cystic changes. Not a feature of inverted papillomas.

E. Primary Paranasal Sinus Tumors

- Paranasal sinus SCCAs are usually found in older males 50–70 years old. Inverted papilloma is most frequently found in patients 40–60 years of age [3].
- Paranasal sinus SCCAs show gross bony destruction. IP's bony changes are more suggestive of slow-growing tumors, with intratumoral calcifications, and focal hyperostosis. Although bony destruction does occur with inverted papilloma, the changes are relatively less severe.

A Closer Look

I. Fast Facts

- While CCP is a reliable imaging feature of sinonasal IPs, it is sometimes seen in malignant sinonasal tumors as well [10].
- Focal loss of the CCP may be a harbinger that an IP contains a concomitant malignancy [1, 10].

II. Historic Highlights

- 1854: Ward first described Schneiderian sinonasal papillomas [12].
- 1935: Kramer and Som classified IPs as true nasal neoplasms, thus distinguishing them from inflammatory nasal polyps [13].
- 1938: Ringertz touted the tumor's tendency to invert into the underlying connective tissue stroma, thus distinguishing them from the plethora of more pedestrian papillomas [14].

III. Genetics and Associations

- *Etiology:* The etiology of inverted papilloma is currently considered "unknown."
- *EBV*: An association with the Epstein-Barr virus (EBV) appears inconclusive.
- *HPV*: Following three decades under suspicion, the human papillomavirus (HPV), seems indisputably involved somewhere in the etiology of inverted papilloma, although present published pronouncements provide no resource to reliably reveal its role [15, 16].

Selected References

1. Wassef SN, Batra PS, Barnett S. Skull base inverted papilloma: a comprehensive review. ISRN Surg. 2012; 2012:Article ID 175903, 34 pages. https://doi.org/10.5402/2012/175903
2. Lee DK, Chung SK, Dhong HJ, et al. Focal hyperostosis on CT of sinonasal inverted papilloma as a predictor of tumor origin. AJNR Am J Neuroradiol. 2007;28(4):618–21.
3. Yousem DM, Fellows DW, Kennedy DW, et al. Inverted papillomas: evaluation with MR imaging. Radiology. 1992;185(2):501–5.
4. Lufkin R, Borges A, Villablanca P. Teaching atlas of head and neck imaging. New York: Thieme; 2000. p. 319–23.
5. Som PM, Lawson W, Lidov W. Simulated aggressive skull base erosion in response to benign sinonasal disease. Radiology. 1991;180(3):755–9.
6. Saha SN, et al. Inverted papilloma: a Clinico-pathological dilemma with special reference to recurrence and malignant transformation. Indian J Otolaryngol Head Neck Surg. 2010;62(4):354–9.
7. Midyett FA, Mukherji SK. Chapter 22, Esthesioneuroblastoma. Orbital imaging. Elsevier/Saunders. 2015. pp. 91–5. ISBN: 978-0-323-34037-3.
8. Momose KJ, Weber AL, Goodman M, et al. Radiological aspects of inverted papilloma. Radiology. 1980;134(1):73–9.
9. Savy L, Lloyd G, Lund VJ, et al. Optimum imaging for inverted papilloma. J Laryngol Otol. 2000;114:891–3.
10. Jeon TY, Kim HJ, Chung SK, et al. Sinonasal inverted papilloma: value of convoluted cerebriform pattern on MR imaging. AJNR Am J Neuroradiol. 2008;29(8):1556–60.
11. Durucu C, Baglam T, Karatas E, et al. Surgical treatment of inverted papilloma. J Craniofac Surg. 2009;20(6):1985–8.
12. Ward N. A mirror of the practice of medicine and surgery in the hospitals of London. London Hosp Lancet. 1854;2:480–2.
13. Kramer R, Som ML. True papilloma of the nasal cavity. Arch Otolaryngol. 1935:22–43.
14. Ringertz N. Pathology of malignant tumors arising in the nasal and paranasal cavities and maxilla. Acta Otolaryngol (Stockh). 1938;27(Suppl):31–42.
15. Lisan Q, Laccourreye O, Bonfils P. Sinonasal inverted papilloma: from diagnosis to treatment. Eur Ann Otorhinolaryngol Head Neck Dis. 2016;133:337–41.
16. Lawson W, Schlecht NF, Brandwein-Gensler M. The role of the human papillomavirus in the pathogenesis of Schneiderian inverted Papillomas: an analytic overview of the evidence. Head Neck Pathol. 2008;2(2):49–59.

Juvenile Nasopharyngeal Angiofibroma 15

Pertinent Points

- *Definition*: Rare, highly vascular, locally invasive benign nasopharyngeal neoplasm occurring almost entirely in adolescent and young adult males displaying a distinct tendency for recurrence.
- *AKA*: Juvenile angiofibroma (JAF), fibromatous or angiofibromatous hamartoma.
- The preferred name for this tumor continues to be contested based on the site of origin. New research strongly supports evidence that the tumor arises from the concha or nasopharynx [1]. This would favor JNA over JAF.
- While comprising only 0.5% of all head and neck tumors, JNA is, surprisingly, still the most common benign tumor arising from the nasopharynx [2, 3].
- *Classic Clue*: Adolescent male presenting with epistaxis has avidly enhancing, heterogeneous posterior nasal mass with MRI showing *characteristic salt and pepper appearance* from the presence of prominent flow voids [4, 5]
- Informed clinicians absolutely avoid preoperative biopsy fearing collossal catastrophic hemorrhage [6]. This could be calamitous for the clinician, not to mention feasibly fatal for the ill-fated patient.
- Age:
  - Most commonly seen in young adult males between 14 and 25 with the mean age at diagnosis being 14 years.
  - JNA may regress in late teens or persist into adulthood.
  - Cases involving men >25 or women of any age, while reported, are *extremely rare* [7, 8].
- JNAs have a general incidence of 1: 1,500,000 [1].
- T1 and T2 have heterogeneous signal with conspicuous vascular flow voids.
- T1 Gd exhibits excessive enhancement.
- Most sequences show *characteristic salt and pepper appearance* from the presence of prominent flow voids [4, 5].

Imaging

General Imaging Features

- Young male with posterior nasal mass which classically first involves the choana and nasopharynx routinely extends into the PPF (pterygopalatine fossa), sphenopalatine foramen, and Vidian canal [1]. See Chap. 51, Vidian Canal.
- JNAs exhibit characteristic anterior bowing of the posterior wall of the maxillary sinus.
- JNA's characteristic imaging appearance should ban biopsy as being notoriously hazardous.

CT Features

- *See General Imaging Features.*
- Typically has the Holman-Miller sign with archetypical anterior bowing of the posterior maxillary sinus wall. See Fig. 15.1a, b

F. A. Midyett, S. K. Mukherji, *Skull Base Imaging*, https://doi.org/10.1007/978-3-030-46447-9_15

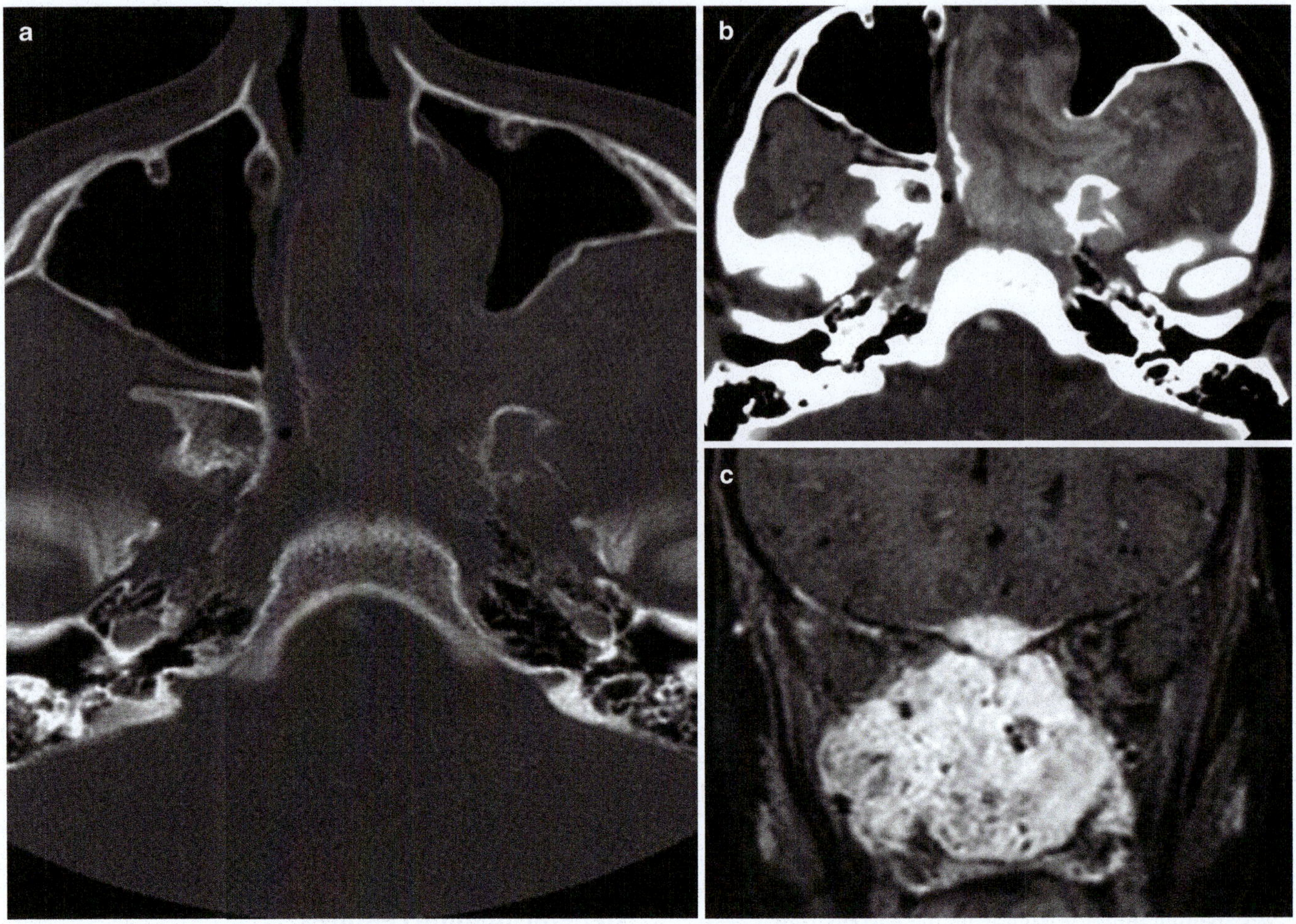

Fig. 15.1 (a) Axial NECT shows a huge mass filling and expanding the nasopharynx and extending into the masticator space through a grossly enlarged sphenopalatine fissure. The medial wall of the left maxillary sinus has been breached admitting tumor into the antrum. The posterior wall of the left maxillary antrum is bowed anteriorly creating the classic Holman-Miller sign. The medial wall of the left nasal cavity and the nasal septum has been totally destroyed along with the posterior wall of the canal for the nasolacrimal duct. The left pterygoid is partially destroyed. (b) Axial CECT shows heterogeneous tumor enhancement with zebra-like pattern of enhancing tissue separated by lower attenuation bands. The mass destroys the septum and left nasal cavity wall. The tumor shows multiple internal contrast-filled vessels. The posterior wall of the left maxillary antrum is dramatically bowed anteriorly creating the classic Holman-Miller sign. (c) Coronal T1 Gd shows avidly enhancing mass which has breached the floor of the ACF with intracranial extension causing bilateral "dural tails." The epicenter of the mass is in the nasopharynx and shows striking heterogeneity clearly related to innumerable tortuous vascular "flow voids"

- Depicts expansion of ipsilateral nasal cavity and pterygopalatine fossa (PPF). See Chap. 51, PPF.
- With growth, JNAs often enlarge the Vidian canal and the foramen rotundum as they extend to the pterygoid plate and middle cranial fossae.
- Other common changes include widened superior orbital fissure, distorted pterygoid plates, nasal septal displacement, and erosion of medial maxillary sinus and hard palate.
- A recent study showed involvement of the choana and nasopharynx in 100% of patients with expansion of the choana in 97% of cases [1].

Angiographic Features

- Catheter angiography illustrates a plethora of dilated tortuous vessels and depicts an intense characteristic capillary blush. See Fig. 15.2a.

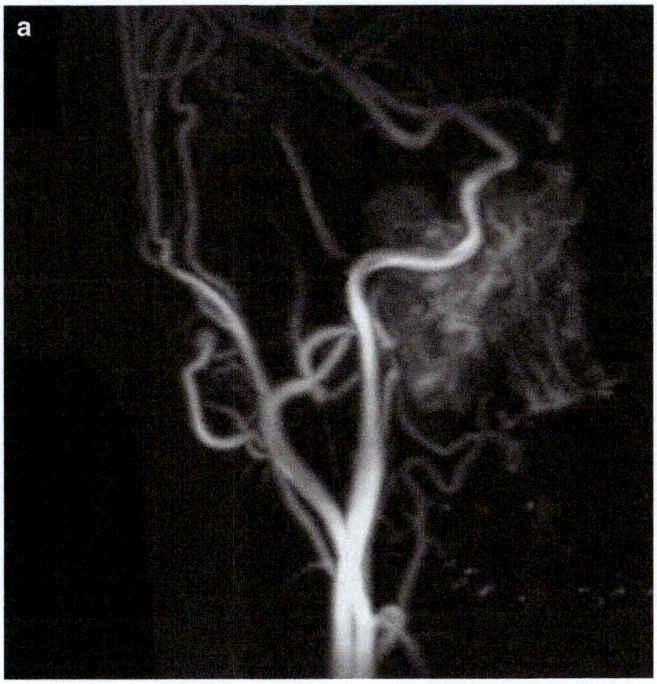

Fig. 15.2 (**a**) AP view of right common carotid catheter angiogram shows huge vascular nasopharyngeal mass filled with abnormal-appearing serpiginous vessels of varying size. This (is a different case than the prior images which) shows a huge tumor component extending into the middle cranial fossa. Intense vascular blush is just beginning and peaked on subsequent images. Selective ICA and ECA injections were necessary to sort out the multiple feeder connections

- JNAs feed from enlarged ECA branches, most frequently from ascending pharyngeal branches of the internal maxillary artery.
- Occasionally the tumor takes vascular contributions from the contralateral ECA.
- When the tumor extends into the skull base or cavernous sinus, it commonly enlists feeders from the ICA.
- Catheter angiography of the ICA and ECA is usually performed for surgical planning during preoperative embolism to reduce intraoperative hemorrhage.

MRI Features

- *See General Imaging Features.*
- T1: Habitually has heterogeneous intermediate signal.
- T2: Habitually has heterogeneous signal with dark flow voids. See Fig. 15.3b.
- T1 Gd: Exhibits avid enhancement. Axial and coronal fat saturation images are essential to define involvement of skull base, sphenoid, and cavernous sinuses. See Figs. 15.1c and 15.3a, c, d.
- Most sequences show *characteristic salt and pepper appearance* from presence of prominent flow voids [4, 5].

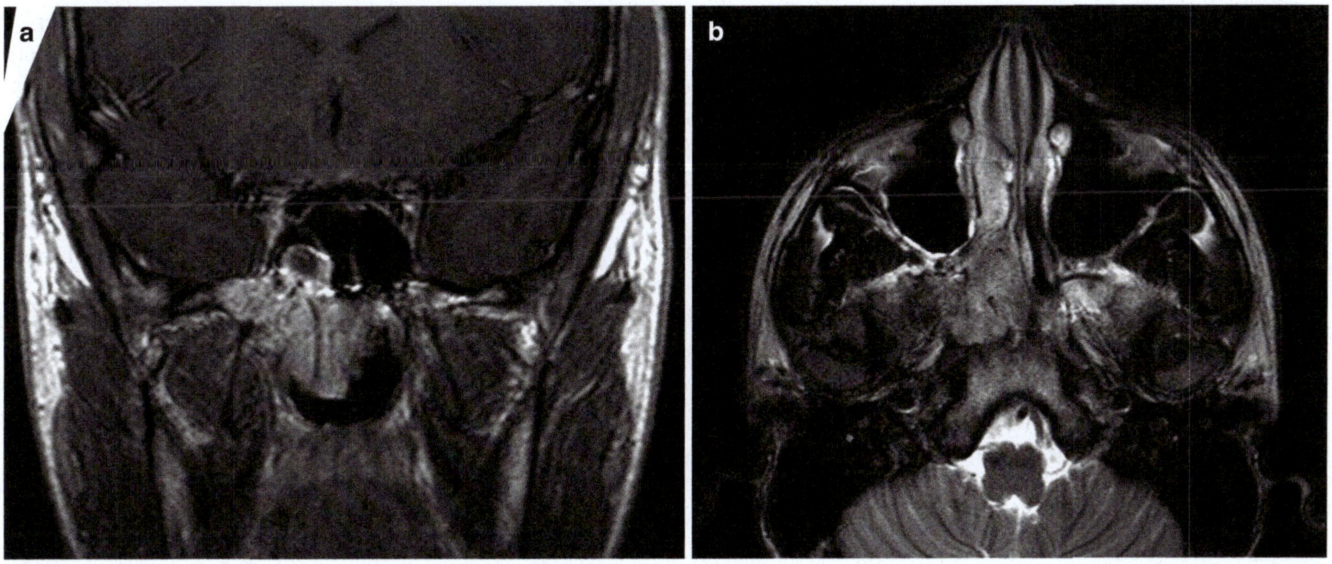

Fig. 15.3 (**a**) Coronal T1 Gd exhibits an avidly enhancing nasopharyngeal mass breaching the floor of the right sphenoid sinus and invading the adjacent right skull base. (**b**) Axial T2 shows a large heterogeneous nasopharyngeal mass expanding and obstructing the right choana. Shows somewhat "salt and pepper" appearance

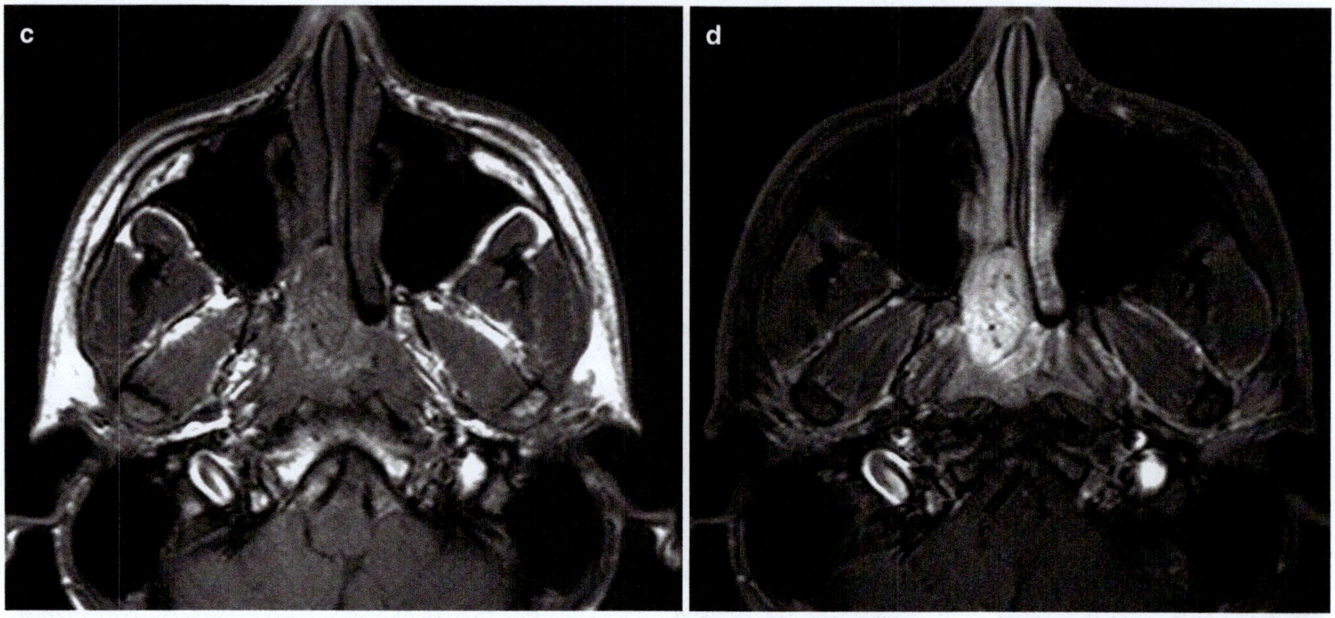

Fig. 15.3 (continued) Axial T1 Gd images performed without (**c**) and with (**d**) fat suppression clearly better define margins of the mass expanding and obstructing the right choana

Plain Films

- Alas, plain films are not relied on much anymore, but those familiar findings can be appreciated on CT.
- Historically these classic findings were heralded when the lateral sinus view depicted anterior displacement of the posterior wall of the maxillary antrum accompanying sinus opacification in a teenage boy exhibiting exigent epistaxis.
- First described by Mayo radiologists Colin Holman and W. Eugene Miller, this is known as the Holman-Miller (or antral) sign. Once considered pathognomonic of JNA, all admit the Holman-Miller sign could be produced by any slowly growing mass. But, really, how many slowly growing nasopharyngeal masses do we see in this characteristic clinical setting of an adolescent male with epistaxis?
- Continuing to search for the holy grail, more sophisticated H&N imagers now suggest erosion of the pterygoid lamina or an intranasal mass causing enlargement of the choana as the real "pathognomonic" sign for JNA.
- The ordinarily obvious Holman-Miller sign is best shown on CT.

Clinical Issues

1. Presentation
   - Common presenting symptoms include unilateral nasal obstruction, rhinorrhea, epistaxis, sinusitis, facial pain, anosmia, and frontal headache [9].
   - Later, the lesion can produce proptosis or diplopia as the tumor travels from the nasal cavity into the maxillary sinus and orbit.
2. Epidemiology and Pathology
   - Gross Examination
     - Red-pink to tan-grey, sessile, lobulated, rubbery solid mass.
     - Rarely polypoid or pedunculated.
     - Usually non-encapsulated and composed of vascular tissue with fibrous stroma and collagen fibers.
     - Late-stage tumors invade the cavernous sinus, optic chiasmatic region, and/or pituitary fossa.
   - The classification system according to Sessions is most commonly used [10].
   - Stage I:
     - 1a: Limited to the nasal cavity/nasopharynx
     - 1b: Extension into one or more paranasal sinuses
   - Stage II:
     - 2a: Minimal extension through sphenopalatine foramen into pterygomaxillary fossa.
     - 2b: Fills the pterygomaxillary fossa bowing the posterior wall of the maxillary antrum anteriorly or extending into the orbit via the inferior orbital fissure.
     - 1c: Extends beyond the pterygomaxillary fossa into infratemporal fossa.
   - Stage III: Intracranial extension

Treatment

A. Embolism

- Selective preoperative embolism of arterial feeding vessels has significantly decreased intraoperative hemorrhage facilitating resection of larger tumors.

- Embolism is typically performed 24–72 hours prior to resection.
- Gelfoam and PVA (polyvinyl alcohol) are frequent embolic agents.

B. Surgery

- Surgical resection after embolism is the treatment of choice and may be performed using and open or endoscopic approaches.

C. Radiation Therapy

- Radiation therapy may be an option when surgery is impossible or incomplete.
- With skull base involvement, ≤50% recur after surgery [2, 11].

Differential Diagnosis

A. Allergic Fungal Sinusitis (AFS)

- Young immunocompetent patient from the Southwestern United States presents with therapy-resistant chronic sinusitis.
- Hypo-attenuation on T2 MRI corresponds to *distinctive hyperdense sinus* with *characteristic serpiginous* pattern.
- Although AFS starts in the sinus, it may have already invaded the skull base before it comes to imaging.
- [See Chap. 32, *Allergic Fungal Sinusitis*.]

B. Esthesioneuroblastoma (ENB) [5]

- Rare neuroendocrine malignancy of neural crest origin arising from olfactory epithelium.
- AKA: Olfactory neuroblastoma.
- ENB classically shows avidly enhancing dumbbell-shaped mass with "waist" at cribriform plate.
- May involve anterior cranial fossa, skull base, and orbit.
- Shows intermediate signal on T1 and T2.
- Cystic areas (with foci of ↑T2) at the tumor/brain interface are diagnostic and may be pathognomonic.
- Exhibits avid enhancement on T1 Gd.
- DWI shows moderate restricted diffusion.
- [See Chap. 28, Esthesioneuroblastoma.]

C. Rhabdomyosarcoma (RMS) [12]

- RMS has a predilection for the head and neck.
- While relatively rare, RMS is the most common childhood soft tissue sarcoma.
- RMS is frequently found in children age 1–5 causing ~3% of childhood cancers.
- Typically has a homogeneous soft tissue mass isodense to normal muscle [but may rarely resemble a cystic lesion with areas of hemorrhage].
- Commonly appears as well-circumscribed mass with irregular margins.
- The tumor is *not calcified* and *almost never has hyperostosis* of adjacent bones.
- T1 is isointense to EOMs but hypointense to orbital fat.
- T2 is usually hyperintense to both orbital fat and EOMs.
- T1 Gd exhibits enthusiastic enhancement.
- Demonstrates *restricted diffusion* with bright DWI images.
- CT and FDG PET/CT play major roles in detection of metastasis. DWI and whole-body MRI may be helpful for staging.
- While RMS and JNAs are both pediatric problems, 90% of RMS are <16 years of age (with a mean onset of 5–7 years). JNA is classically associated with adolescent males.
- Curious cases of RMS have been documented in elderly and newborns.
- [See Chap. 49, Rhabdomyosarcoma.]

D. Antrochoanal Polyp (AP) [13]

- Antrochoanal Polyp portrays a "dumbbell"-shaped mass involving the nasal cavity and maxillary sinus.
- Antrochoanal polyp exhibits a non-enhancing (or occasionally peripheral-enhancing) mass with benign-appearing bone changes. JNA exhibits enthusiastic enhancement.
- Antrochoanal polyps sometimes show cystic changes. Not a feature of JNA.
- Antrochoanal polyps frequently fill the nasal antrum but do *not* extend into the PPF. JNA exhibits early extension into the PPF.
- Antrochoanal polyps herniate into the anterior nasal cavity before involving the nasopharynx. By contrast, JNA begins in the choana or nasopharynx [14].

E. Primary Paranasal Sinus Tumors

- Paranasal sinus SCCAs are frequently found in older males 50–70 years old. This is *not* the age group for JNA.
- Paranasal sinus SCCAs classically cause gross bony destruction.

A Closer Look

I. Genetics

- While some subscribe to theories that JNAs replicate vascular malformations or stem from remnant embryologic vascular components, substantial progress has been made to unravel genetic and molecular mechanisms involved in JNAs [1].

- The androgen receptor (AR) offers a potential explanation for this tumor's predilection for males [1].
- The 25-fold increased prevalence of JNA in the male familial adenomatous polyposis (FAP) population has highlighted the role of the adenomatous polyposis coli (APC) gene mutation and abnormal regulation of the Wnt/beta-catenin pathway in JNAAR receptor with a "double-hit" mechanism [1].

II. Fast Facts

- Definition: Choana, choanae (plural), represent the paired openings between the nasal cavity and the nasopharynx.
- In contrast to commonly held assertions that JNAs arise from the pterygopalatine fossa or sphenopalatine foramen, new research suggests JNAs arise in the region of the choana and nasopharynx [1, 14].

III. Historic Highlights

- Hippocrates described the tumor in the fifth century BC [6, 9].
- 1940: Friedberg first used the term angiofibroma [6, 10].
- 1981: Maurice and Milad noted JNAs showed striking similarity to genital erectile tissue and the time course for development of male erectile tissue closely parallels that of JNAs [15].
- Maurice and Milad proposed that JNA could arise from midline genital erectile tissue sequestered during fetal development [15].

Selected References

1. Bryan RN, Sessions RB, Horowitz BL. Radiographic management of juvenile angiofibromas. AJNR Am J Neuroradiol. 1981;2(2):157–66.
2. Momeni AK, Roberts CC, Chew FS. Imaging of chronic and exotic sinonasal disease: review. AJR Am J Roentgenol. 2007;189(6):S35–45.
3. Davis KR. Embolization of epistaxis and juvenile nasopharyngeal angiofibromas. AJR. 1987;148:209–18.
4. Seo CS, Han MH, Chang KH, et al. Angiofibroma confined to the pterygoid muscle region: CT and MR demonstration. AJNR Am J Neuroradiol. 1996;17(2):374–6.
5. Hurst RW, Rosenwasser RH. Interventional neuroradiology. Informa HealthCare. 2007. ISBN:0849395623.
6. Moorthy PNS, Reddy BR, Qaiyum HA, et al. Management of Juvenile Nasopharyngeal Angiofibroma: a five year retrospective study. Indian J Otolaryngol Head Neck Surg. 2010;62(4):390–4.
7. Finerman WB. Juvenile nasopharyngeal angiofibroma in the female. AMA Arch Otolaryngol. 1951;54(6):620–3. PubMed PMID: 14877367
8. Maurice M, Milad M. Pathogenesis of juvenile nasopharyngeal fibroma. (A new concept). J Laryngol Otol. 1981;95(11):1121–6. PubMed PMID: 72299258
9. Harma RA. Nasopharyngeal angiofibroma. Acta Otolaryngol. 1958;146(Supp l):1–74.
10. Friedberg SA. Vascular fibroma of the nasopharynx (nasopharyngeal fibroma). Arch Otolaryngol. 1940;31:313–26.
11. Kania RE, Sauvaget E, Guichard JP, et al. Early postoperative CT scanning for juvenile nasopharyngeal angiofibroma: detection of residual disease. AJNR Am J Neuroradiol. 2005;26(1):82–8.
12. Midyett FA, Mukherji SK. Chapter 23, Rhabdomyosarcoma. Orbital imaging. Philadelphia: Elsevier/Saunders; 2015. p. 99–102. ISBN: 978-0-323-34037-3.
13. Midyett FA, Mukherji SK. Chapter 22, Esthesioneuroblastoma. Orbital imaging. Philadelphia: Elsevier/Saunders; 2015. p. 91–5. ISBN : 978-0-323-34037-3.
14. Mcknight CD, Palmar HA, Watcharotone K, Mukherji SK. Reassessing the Anatomic Origin of the Juvenile Nasopharyngeal Angiofibroma. J Comput Assit Tomogr. 2017;41(4):559–564. https://doi.org/10.1097/RCT000000000000566.
15. Antonelli AR, Cappiello J, Di Lorenzo D, et al. Diagnosis, staging, and treatment of juvenile nasopharyngeal angiofibroma (JNA). Laryngoscope. 1987;97(11):1319–25. https://doi.org/10.1288/00005537-198711000-00014. PubMed PMID: 2823033

Neuroendocrine Tumors

16

Pertinent Points

- *Definition*: Neuroendocrine tumors comprise a vast variety of tumors which may have either epithelial or neural origins [15–17, 24].
- *Classic Clue*: Destructive paranasal sinus mass shown in a setting where the panel seems to be soliciting a differential diagnosis other than sinonasal carcinoma and the other "usual suspects."
- Classification Controversy:
  - There is no doubt that we got off to a bad start with these tumors in 1897 when Russian anatomist and histologist Nikolai Kulchitsky said they looked like cancers but were not [1].
  - This confusion was perpetuated by pathologist Siegfried Oberndorfer who ostensibly created the term "carcinoid" to mean carcinoma-like [24].
  - To be fair, it was only in 1938 when publications first confirmed some of these tumors were malignant.

    And the controversy continued to the millennial turn in 2000 when WHO finally put its foot down and eliminated carcinoid from its histopathologic classifications conclusively making this a politically incorrect term [12].
  - So, we are left with an entity which causes 2% of cancers and affects 200,000 people in the United States which has previously been called "carcinoma-like."
  - And clearly many in this group of tumors are not "carcinoma-like"; they *are* cancer. So, it is easy to agree "carcinoid" does not apply. The case we present is clearly the "real deal," manifestly malignant, destroying the skull base, and it deserves to be at least called a neuroendocrine carcinoma (NEC).
  - Lumpers vs. splitters: In the terminology arena, there are lumpers and splitters. Currently the lumpers are winning with NETs comprising a disparate group of cancer subtypes supposedly ranging from NENs and pPNETs to small cell lung and large cell NECs [24].
  - Clearly, when these don't even look alike under the microscope, we can all predict that it is only a matter of time before the splitters surface to give some of them yet another name.
  - Already some suggest the term "neuroendocrine" is not helpful as it implies a biologically benign behavior [24].
  - What people currently agree on is that these tumors, because of their low incidence and prevalence, are currently "orphans," with many clinicians going so far as to calling them "zebras." Certainly, in the skull base, they fit into that category.
  - Whatever we call them, we cannot simply ignore 2% of cancers with NETs involving 200,000 people in the United States.

- *Incidence and Prevalence*:
  - *Incidence*: The annual incidence of neuroendocrine tumors is approximately 5 per 100,000 [3].
  - *Prevalence*:

    Estimated at 35 per 100,0000 but probably is higher if clinically silent tumors are included [3].

    Current prevalence for NETs for the entire United States is <200,000[24].

    NETs comprise ~2% of all malignancies.
- The incidence of brain metastasis from extracranial NETs is ~5%, usually from lung. Primary intracranial NETs are very rare but have been reported [12].
- Head and neck NETs are rare with limited information available regarding frequency, prognosis, and site significance. Virtually every variant of NET can occur in the head and neck region [13].

F. A. Midyett, S. K. Mukherji, *Skull Base Imaging*, https://doi.org/10.1007/978-3-030-46447-9_16

- Head and neck paragangliomas are well-recognized and are not considered in this chapter which is confined to nonlaryngeal NECs.
- Nonlaryngeal NETs of the head and neck are rare tumors, most frequently found in the proximity of paranasal sinuses [15].
- Although NETs can arise in many different areas of the body, they are most frequently found in the intestine, pancreas, or lungs [9]. Neuroradiologists are more familiar with NETs in the pituitary, thyroid, and parathyroid regions.
- Age, Sex, and Incidence for NECs:
  - The median age of presentation is 56 years, with equal sex distribution [19, 20].
  - NECs account for 5% of sinonasal malignancies [19, 21].
  - The most common site of origin is ethmoid sinus (64%), nasal cavity (32%), and maxillary sinus (14%) [19, 20].

Imaging

General Imaging Features

- They commonly expand and erode sinus walls.
- Most conclude there are *no characteristic* CT or MRI features for this entity [15].

MRI Features

- *See General Imaging Features.*
- T1: *Relatively iso- or slightly hyperintense to brain.* Heterogeneous with scattered areas of additional hyperintensity. (See Fig. 16.1a, c)
- T2: *Relatively iso- or slightly hyperintense to brain.* Heterogeneous with scattered areas more hyperintensity. (See Fig. 16.1e.)
- T1 Gd: Mild heterogeneous enhancement. (See Fig. 16.1b, d.)
- DWI: Moderate diffusion restriction. (See Fig. 16.1f.)

CT Features

- *See General Imaging Features.*
- Typically shows a soft tissue mass which expands and erodes the involved sinus.
- The mass may extend into the nasal cavity and nasopharynx.
- Skull base involvement is a frequent finding.
- (See Fig. 16.2a, b for normal coronal CT anatomy of this region.)

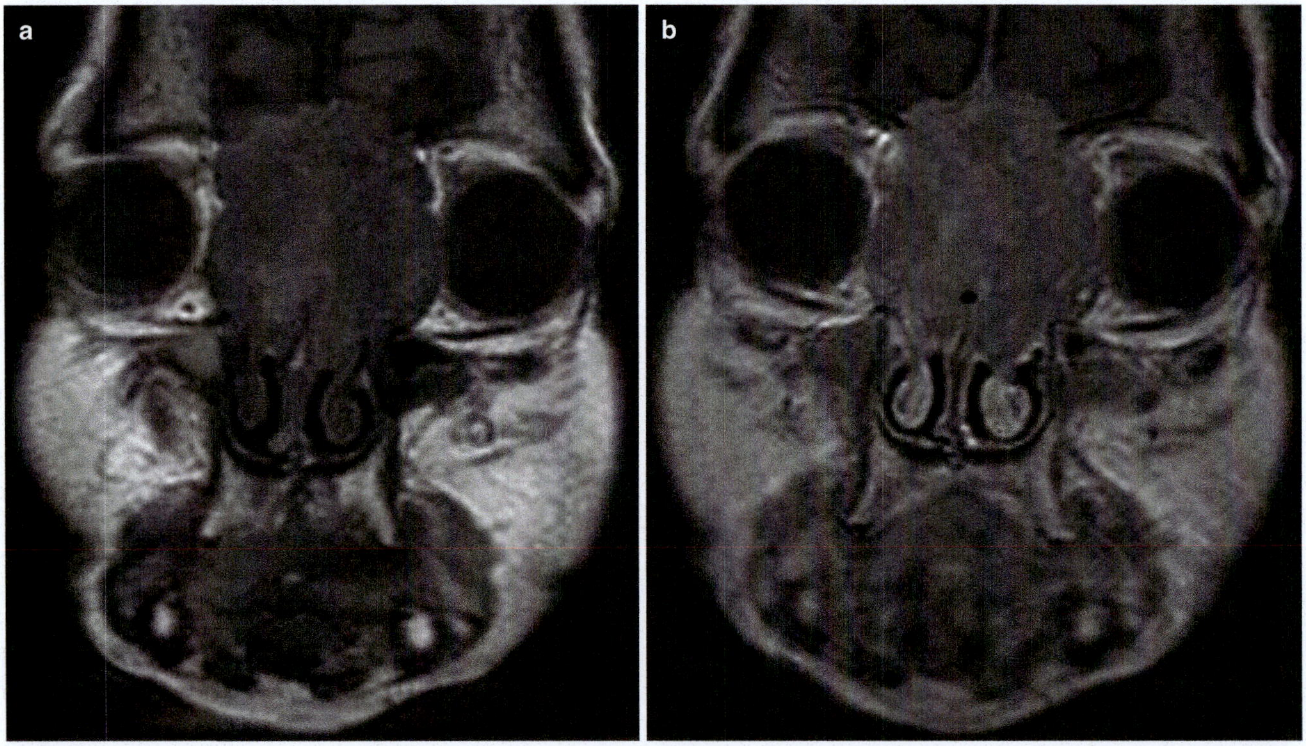

Fig. 16.1 (**a**) Coronal T1 shows huge mass filling and expanding the nasopharynx. Its cephalic extension takes it through the ethmoid and the floor of the anterior cranial fossa where it abuts the frontal lobes. Its epicenter is, however, much more caudal, and caudally it reaches and destroys the middle nasal turbinate. It extends laterally into the orbits, L > R flattening of the medial aspect of the left globe. Its signal is relatively *iso- or slightly hyperintense to brain* and moderately heterogeneous. (**b**) Coronal T1 Gd at the same level of the prior image shows *mild heterogeneous enhancement* with enhancing tumor contiguous with the falx. This image clearly depicts the abrupt loss of anterior cranial fossa floor and brutal breaching of the medial orbital walls with extensive intraorbital extension

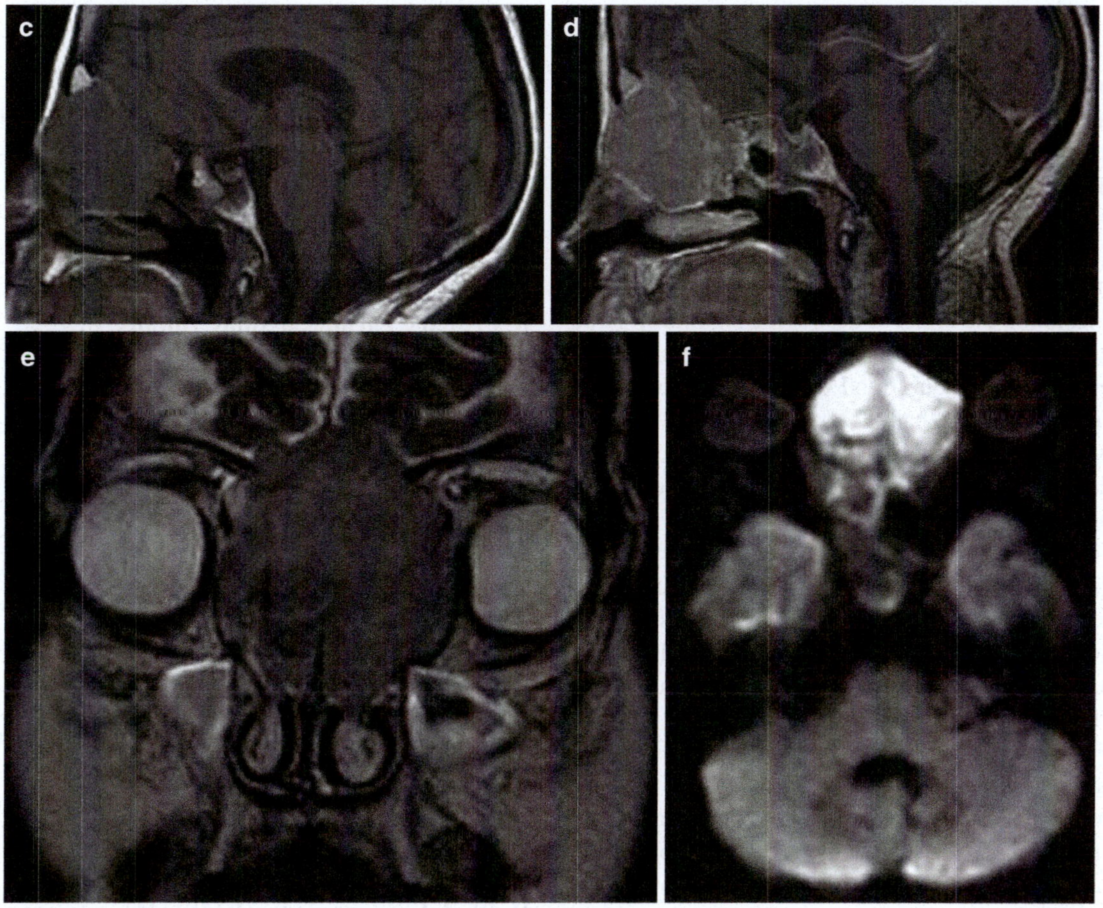

Fig. 16.1 (continued) (**c**, **d**) Sagittal T1 without (**c**) and with (**d**) Gd again sepict flagrant destruction of the ethmoid sinus and anterior cranial fossa floor. Moderate heterogeneous enhancement shows the mass to be hyperintense to brain extending cranially to abut and displace the frontal lobes. It extends caudally to narrow the nasal airway. It completely destroys the ethmoid and frontal sinuses and extends into the sphenoid sinus. Tumor abuts the inferior and posterior aspects of the crista galli depicted by bright T1 signal at the tumor's anterior superior aspect. The remainder of the cribriform plate has been destroyed. (**e**) Coronal T2 depicts a huge heterogeneous mass filling, expanding, and obliterating the nasal cavity and ethmoid sinuses with deliberate destruction of the anterior cranial fossa floor causing abrupt absence of its dark signal. Signal is *relatively iso- or slightly hyperintense to the brain* and moderately heterogeneous. Intraorbital extension L > R with flagrant flattening of the left globe. (**f**) Axial DWI reveals remarkable restricted diffusion corresponding to the large mass near the floor of the anterior cranial fossa. Coupled with the other images from this case, this finding suggests a histologically menacing malignancy

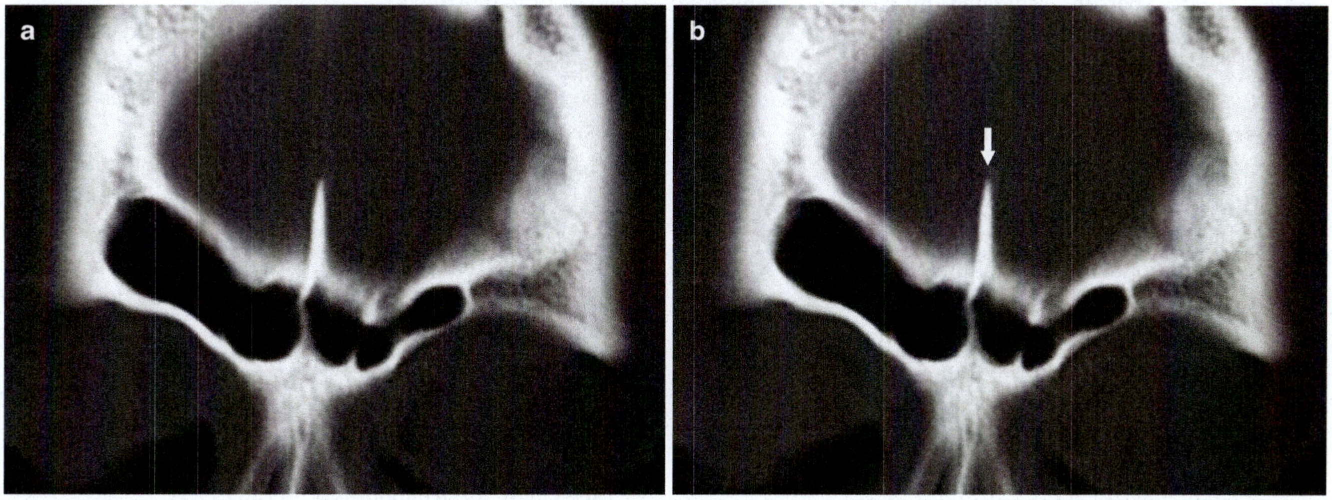

Fig. 16.2 (**a**, **b**) Coronal CT showing crista galli in a normal patient without (**a**) and with arrow (**b**). Crista galli comes from Latin meaning the crest of the rooster

Clinical Issues

1. Presentation
   - Neuroendocrine carcinomas originate in various locations including the lung, brain, GI tract, and head and neck.
   - Although some hormone-producing varieties proclaim their presence through hormonal responses, others just wait to publicize their presence in the old fashion way like invading the orbits or destroying significant structures like the skull base and olfactory bulbs.
   - The myriad symptoms of NECs can include headache, anxiety, persistent pain, hyperglycemia, hypoglycemia, diarrhea, unexpected weight gain or loss, night sweats, changes concerning bowel or bladder, cough or hoarseness, etc.
   - So, it is no wonder that radiologists are eventually enlisted to explain these complex clinical situations.
   - Much like ENB's presenting symptoms for skull base region, NECs most frequently include nasal obstruction, drainage, and epistaxis. Variations of visual acuity are found in about 1/5. Facial pain, swelling, diplopia, and V_2 numbness are uncommonly found [19, 20].
2. Epidemiology and Pathology
   - Gross: NETs are typically tan or yellow masses frequently found in the submucosa and when more deeply intramural exhibit firming from desmoplastic reaction.
   - Microscopic [23]:
     - Histologically, NEC remains relegated to a category (containing conspicuous neuroendocrine appearances) which otherwise portrays poor histologic delineation [23].
     - NEC displays defectively differentiated nests of tumor cells showing scant cytoplasm, finely granular nuclear chromatin, and benign glandular epithelium, sparsely separated by cellular connective tissue branches [23].

Differential Diagnosis (DDx)

A. Esthesioneuroblastoma (ENB) [4, 10]

- Rare neuroendocrine malignancy of neural crest origin arising from olfactory epithelium.
- Newer genetic information suggests that ENB is a distinct entity and does not belong to primitive peripheral neuroectodermal tumor-Ewing's tumor (pPNETs-ETs) [22]. This suggests that ENB is not a NEC.
- AKA: Olfactory neuroblastoma.
- Classically shows avidly enhancing dumbbell-shaped mass with "waist" at the cribriform plate.
- May involve anterior cranial fossa, skull base, and orbit.
- Intermediate signal on T1 and T2.
- Cystic areas (with foci of ↑T2) at the tumor/brain interface are diagnostic and may be pathognomonic.
- Exhibits avid enhancement on T1 Gd.
- DWI shows moderate restricted diffusion.
- [See Chap. 28, Esthesioneuroblastoma.]

B. Primary Paranasal Sinus Tumors

- Paranasal sinus SCCs often occur in older males 50–70 years old.
- Paranasal sinus SCCs show gross bony destruction.
- [See Chap. 22, Paranasal Sinus Cancer.]

C. Allergic Fungal Sinusitis (AFS)

- Young immunocompetent patient from the Southwestern United States presents with therapy-resistant chronic sinusitis.
- Hypo-attenuation on T2 MRI corresponds to *distinctive hyperdense sinus* with *characteristic serpiginous* pattern.
- Although AFS starts in the sinus, it may have already invaded the skull base before it comes to imaging.
- *See* Chap. 32, *Allergic Fungal Sinusitis*, for unabridged description.

D. Rhabdomyosarcoma (RMS) [11]

- Rhabdomyosarcoma reveals a predilection for the head and neck.
- While relatively rare, RMS is the most common childhood soft tissue sarcoma.
- Rhabdomyosarcoma is frequently found in children age 1–5 causing ~3% of childhood cancers.
- Typically homogeneous soft tissue mass isodense to normal muscle [but may rarely resemble a cystic lesion with areas of hemorrhage].
- Commonly appears as a well-circumscribed mass with irregular margins.
- The tumor is *not* calcified and almost never has hyperostosis of adjacent bones.
- T1 is isointense to the EOMs but hypointense to orbital fat.
- T2 is usually hyperintense to the EOMs and orbital fat.
- T1 Gd shows substantial enhancement.
- Reveals restricted diffusion with bright DWI images.
- CT and FDG PET/CT play major roles in detection of metastasis. DWI and whole-body MRI may be helpful for staging.
- 90% of RMS occur <16 years of age (with a mean onset of 5–7 years). However, cases of RMS have been documented in elderly and newborn patients.
- [See Chap. 49, Rhabdomyosarcoma.]

Treatment

- Difficulty in diagnosis coupled with the paucity of published cases, along with treatment heterogeneity, hampers creation of ideal treatment strategies [8, 19].
- Some suggest neoadjuvant chemotherapy followed by either chemoradiation or surgery and postoperative radiation [19].
- Others suggest high-dose proton-photon radiotherapy with neoadjuvant chemotherapy reserving radical surgery for non-responders [14].
- These issues are clearly suited for tumor boards and treatment trials

A Closer Look

I. Genetics [5]

- Most NETs are sporadic but can be seen in several inherited familial syndromes, including [4]:
  - MEN 1 (multiple endocrine neoplasia type I) [7]
  - MEN 2 (multiple endocrine neoplasia type II)
  - VHL (Von Hippel-Lindau disease) [4]
  - NF 1 (neurofibromatosis type I) [5]
  - TS (tuberous sclerosis) [6, 7]
  - Carney complex

II. Fast Facts

- The root cell for neuroendocrine carcinoma has not been sufficiently settled. Some suspect they originate from the endocrine cell of the dispersed neuroendocrine system, while others opine they come from pluripotential stem cells adept at epithelial and endocrine differentiation [15, 18].

III. Historic Highlights

- 1897: Russian anatomist and histologist Nikolai Kulchitsky suggested serotonin-secreting enterochromaffin cells created "carcinoids" [1].
- 1907: Carcinoids were first distinguished from other tumors and so named because their slow growth was considered "cancer-like" rather than truly malignant [1, 2].
- 1938: Some "carcinoids" were recognized to be malignant, forming the first authentic evidence that their name was actually a misnomer [1, 2].
- 1953: Serotonin's role in the "flushing effect" was first recognized [1].
- 2000: The WHO finally eliminated "carcinoid" from its histopathologic classification repertoire [12].
- This was almost a century after this misnomer's inception. How long will it take to conclusively clear this popular term from our medical lexicon?

Selected References

1. Modlin IM, Shapiro MD, Kidd M. Siegfried oberndorfer: origins and perspectives of carcinoid tumors. Hum Pathol. 2004;35(12):1440–51. https://doi.org/10.1016/j.humpath.2004.09.018.
2. Arnold R, Göke R, Wied M, Behr T. Chapter 15 neuroendocrine Gastro-Entero-Pancreatic (GEP) tumors. In: Scheppach W, Bresalier RS, Tytgat GNJ, editors. Gastrointestinal and liver tumors. Berlin: Springer; 2003. p. 195–233. isbn:3-540-43462-3.
3. Öberg K, Castellano D. Current knowledge on diagnosis and staging of neuroendocrine tumors. Cancer Metastasis Rev. 2011;30:3–7. https://doi.org/10.1007/s10555-011-9292-1.
4. Jensen RT, Berna MJ, Bingham DB, Norton JA. Inherited pancreatic endocrine tumor syndromes: advances in molecular pathogenesis, diagnosis, management, and controversies. Cancer. 2008;113(7 Suppl):1807–43. https://doi.org/10.1002/cncr.23648. PMC 2574000
5. Hirsch NP, Murphy A, Radcliffe J. Neurofibromatosis: clinical presentations and anaesthetic implications. Br J Anaesth. 2001;86(4):555–64. https://doi.org/10.1093/bja/86.4.555. PMID
6. Lodish MB, Stratakis CA. Endocrine tumours in neurofibromatosis type 1, tuberous sclerosis and related syndromes. Best Pract Res Clin Endocrinol Metab. 2010;24(3):439–49. https://doi.org/10.1016/j.beem.2010.02.00.
7. Dworakowska D, Grossman AB. Are neuroendocrine tumours a feature of tuberous sclerosis? A systematic review. Endocrine Related Cancer. 2008;16(1):45–58. https://doi.org/10.1677/ERC-08-0142. PMID 18978035
8. Ramage JK, Davies AH, Ardill J, et al. Guidelines for the management of gastroenteropancreatic neuroendocrine (including carcinoid) tumours. Gut. 2005;54(Suppl 4):iv1–16. https://doi.org/10.1136/gut.2004.053314. PMC 1867801
9. Liu Y, Sturgis CD, Grzybicki DM, et al. Microtubule-associated protein 2: a new sensitive and specific marker for pulmonary carcinoid tumor and small cell carcinoma. Mod Pathol. 2001;14(9):880–5. https://doi.org/10.1038/modpathol.3880406. Retrieved 1/21/2016
10. Midyett FA, Mukherji SK. Chapter 22, Esthesioneuroblastoma. Orbital imaging. Elsevier/Saunders. 2015. pp. 91–5. ISBN: 978-0-323-34037-3.
11. Midyett FA, Mukherji SK. Chapter 23, Rhabdomyosarcoma. Orbital imaging. Elsevier/Saunders. 2015. pp. 99–102. ISBN : 978-0-323-34037-3.
12. Tamura R, Kuroshima Y, Nakamura Y. Primary neuroendocrine tumor in brain. Case Reports in Neurological Medicine, vol. 2014, Article ID 295253, 6 pages, 2014. https://doi.org/10.1155/2014/295253.
13. Mills SE. Neuroendocrine tumors of head and neck: a selected review with emphasis on terminology. Endocr Pathol. 1996;7(4):329–43.
14. Fitek MM, Thornton AF, Varvares M, et al. Neuroendocrine tumors of the sinonasal tract. Results of a prospective study incorporating chemotherapy, surgery, and combined proton-photon radiotherapy. Cancer. 2002;94(10):2623–34.

15. Kanamalla US, Kesava PP, McGuff HS. Imaging of nonlaryngeal neuroendocrine carcinoma. AJNR. 2000;21:775–8.
16. Batsakis JG, El-Naggar AK, Luna MA. Neuroendocrine tumors of the larynx. Ann Otol Rhinol Laryngol. 1992;101:710–4.
17. Erlandson RA, Nesland JM. Tumors of the endocrine/neuroendocrine system. Ultrastruct Pathol. 1994;18:149–70.
18. Wenig BM, Gnepp DR. The spectrum of neuroendocrine carcinomas of the larynx. Semin Diag Pathol. 1989;6:329–50.
19. Su SY, Bell D, Hanna EY. Esthesioneuroblastoma, neuroendocrine carcinoma, and sinonasal undifferentiated carcinoma: differentiation in diagnosis and treatment. Int Arch Otorhinolaryngol. 2014;18(Supl. 2): Sao Paulo 2014, On-line version ISSN 1809-4864. Accessed 1/24/2016.
20. Mitchell EH, Diaz A, Yilmaz T, et al. Multimodality treatment for sinonasal neuroendocrine carcinoma. Head Neck. 2012;34(10):1372–6.
21. Renner G. Small cell carcinoma of the head and neck: a review. Semin Oncol. 2007;34(1):3–14.
22. Mezzelani A, Tornielli S, Minoletti F, et al. Esthesioneuroblastoma is not a member of the primitive neuroectodermal tumor-Ewing's group. Br J Cancer. 1999;81(4):586–91.
23. Austin JR, Cebrun H, Kershisnik MM, et al. Olfactory neuroblastoma and neuroendocrine carcinoma of the anterior skull base: treatment results at the M.D. Anderson Cancer Center. Skull Base Surg. 1996;6(1):1–8.
24. Oronsky B, Ma PC, Morgensztern D, Caarter CA. Nothing but NET: a review of neuroendocrine tumors and carcinomas. Neoplasia. 2017;19(12):991–1002.

17 Nasofrontal Encephalocele

Pertinent Points

- *Definition*: Characteristic sac-like protrusion of brain and meninges through an osseous cranial defect resulting from incomplete neural tube closure during fetal development.
- *AKA*: (Latin) cranium bifidum, nasal encephalocele [1], meningocele, meningoencephalocele, transsphenoidal encephalocele, basal encephalocele [3].
- *Scope:* Because this text is on skull base imaging, this chapter concentrates on the nasofrontal encephalocele (NFE) while attempting to shine some light on the entire spectrum of encephaloceles.
- *Classic Clue*: Asian child presents to pediatrician showing symptoms of nasal obstruction, with nasal mass isointense to CSF on all imaging sequences and *no* restriction of diffusion on DWI.
- *Terminology:* An encephalocele consists of brain herniated through cranial bone. Meningocele means herniated dura. When brain *and* dura are herniated, the proper term is meningoencephalocele. But, alas, too many syllables for some, so we commonly call them all encephaloceles.

Imaging

General Imaging Features

- Encephaloceles can protrude in the midline frontal, occipital, or paramedian parietal regions.
- Some separate basal encephaloceles into transethmoidal, sphenoethmoidal, transsphenoidal, and frontosphenoidal subtypes [4].
- Transsphenoidal encephaloceles traverse a sellar floor defect into the nasal cavity. They may also project into the oral cavity and are associated with cleft palates [4].
- Transethmoidal encephaloceles project through a midline or cribriform plate defect into the nasal cavity [4].
- Located anterior to the dorsum sella, the transsphenoidal encephalocele splays the sphenoid displacing the cavernous sinus laterally.

MRI Features

See General Imaging Features.

T1 and T2 sometimes show a fluid-filled midline abnormality outside the calvarium which is isointense to CSF [See Fig. 17.1a,b].

T1 Gd: Follows signal of intracranial CSF and brain. [See Fig. 17.2b, e.]

- This can contain component of the brain which is isointense to intracranial brain. [See Fig. 17.3a–d.]
- DWI: Shows *no* restricted diffusion.

CT Features

- *See General Imaging Features.*
- Typically shows CSF attenuation midline soft tissue mass and depicts bony changes as outlined in *General Imaging Features.*

F. A. Midyett, S. K. Mukherji, *Skull Base Imaging*, https://doi.org/10.1007/978-3-030-46447-9_17

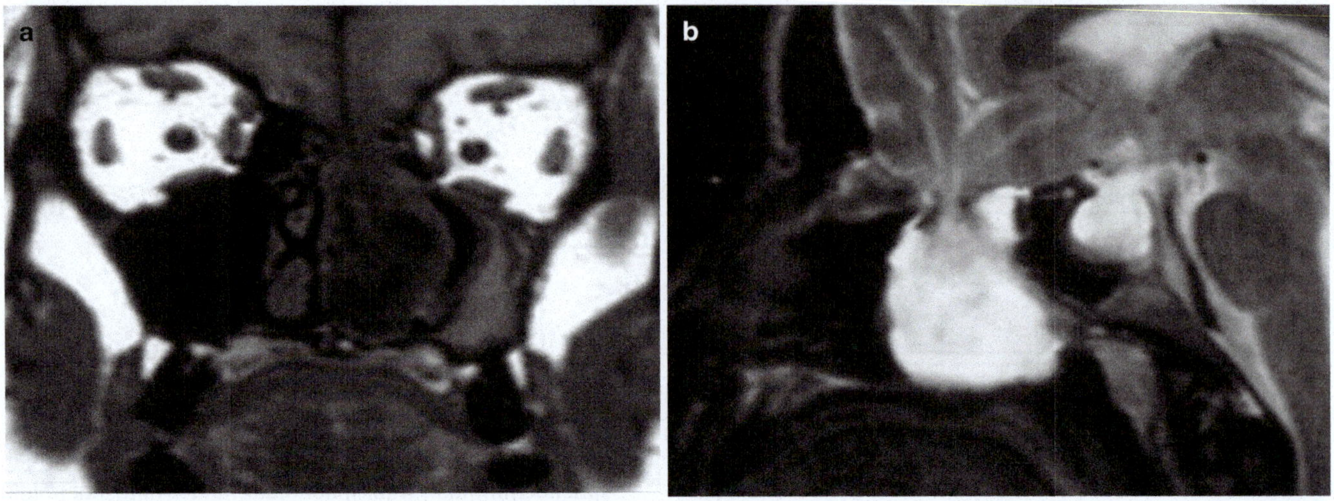

Fig. 17.1 (**a**) Coronal T1 shows large mass filling and expanding the medial aspect of the left nasal cavity. It is moderately heterogeneous containing components isointense to intracranial brain. (**b**) Sagittal midline T2 shows the large mass to be predominately filled with CSF. It clearly contains a component which has an intracranial connection. Intracranial components sag caudally through a bony defect which breaches the skull base. Perusal of the plethora of associated images will tell "the rest of the story"

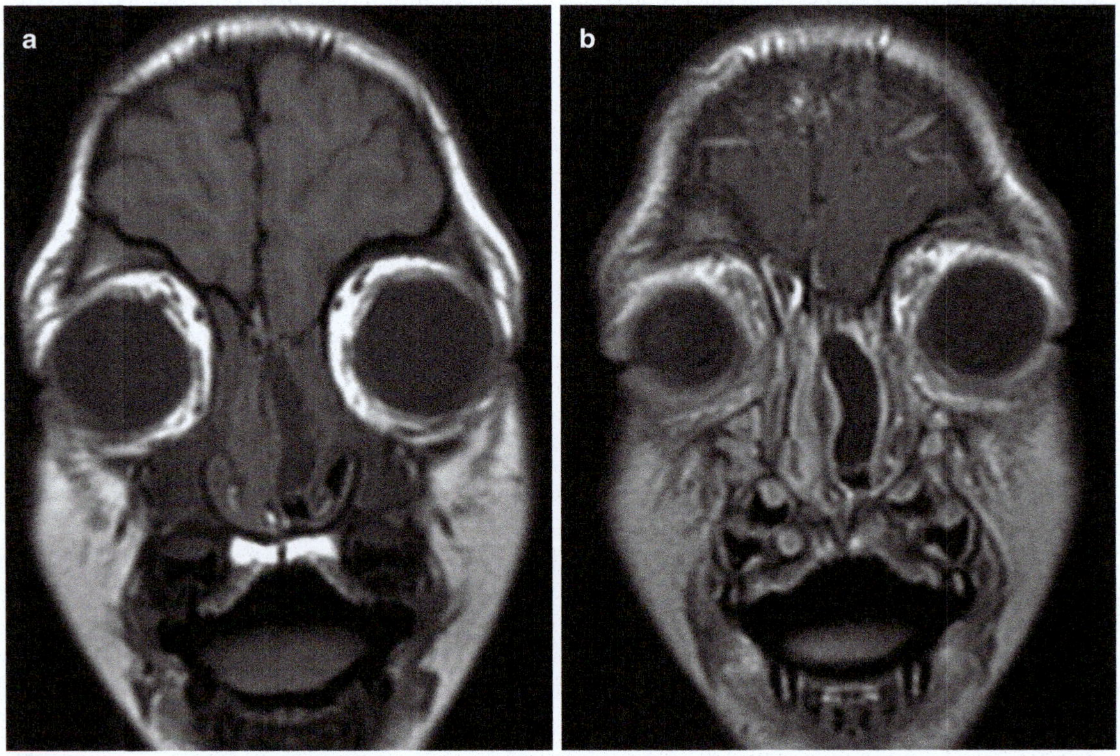

Fig. 17.2 (A and B) Coronal T1 without (**a**) and with Gd (**b**) show low signal mass in the left nasal cavity. Note prominent ptosis of the left anterior cranial fossa contents. The demonstrable defect in hard palate high signal marrow corresponds to the anterior palatine canal on (**a**). Post-Gd T1 (**b**) shows thick enhancing rind around the intranasal mass

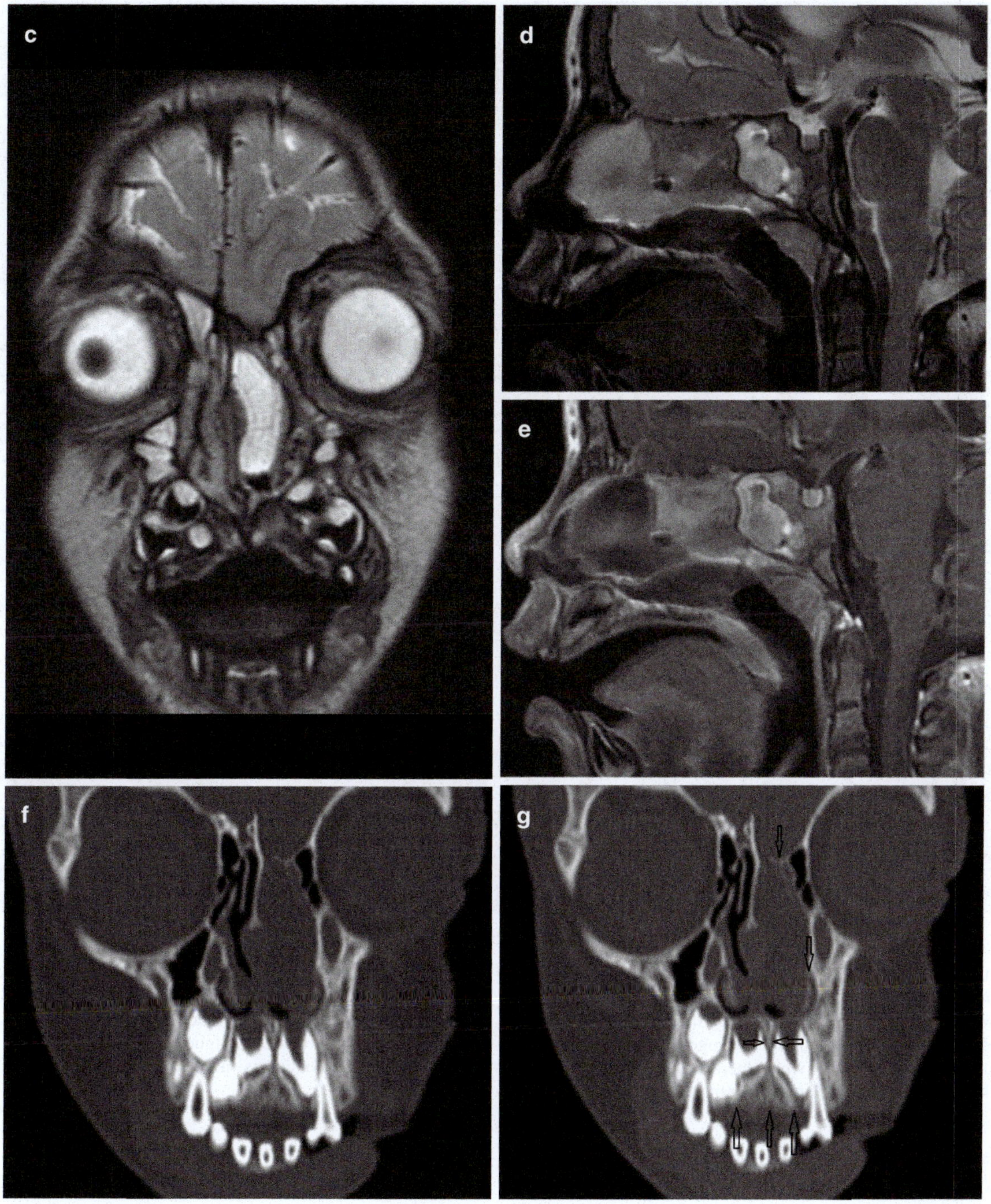

Fig. 17.2 (continued) (**c**, **d**) Coronal (**c**) and sagittal (**d**) T2 images show large anterior nasal mass with signal isointense to CSF. The mass extends cranially to the level of the anterior cranial fossa and caudally almost to the maxilla. Caudal to the mass is a prominent anterior palatine canal. (**e**) Sagittal T1 Gd shows a large anterior nasal mass with signal isointense to CSF. It extends cranially almost to the level of the frontal lobe suggesting the anterior cranial fossa is breached. The mass has a mildly enhancing rim. Caudal to the mass is a prominent anterior palatine canal. (**f**, **g**) Coronal CT contrast cisternogram shows a large left nasal mass enlarging the left nasal cavity and destroying the caudal aspect of the nasal septum. The floor of the left anterior cranial fossa is clearly breached with contrast extending caudally along the left side of the mass through the anterior palatine canal to puddle in the oral cavity. (**f**) Without and (**g**) with arrows. (↑ = contrast in mouth); (→← contrast just cranial to prominent patent anterior palatine canal); (↓ contrast in encephalocele)

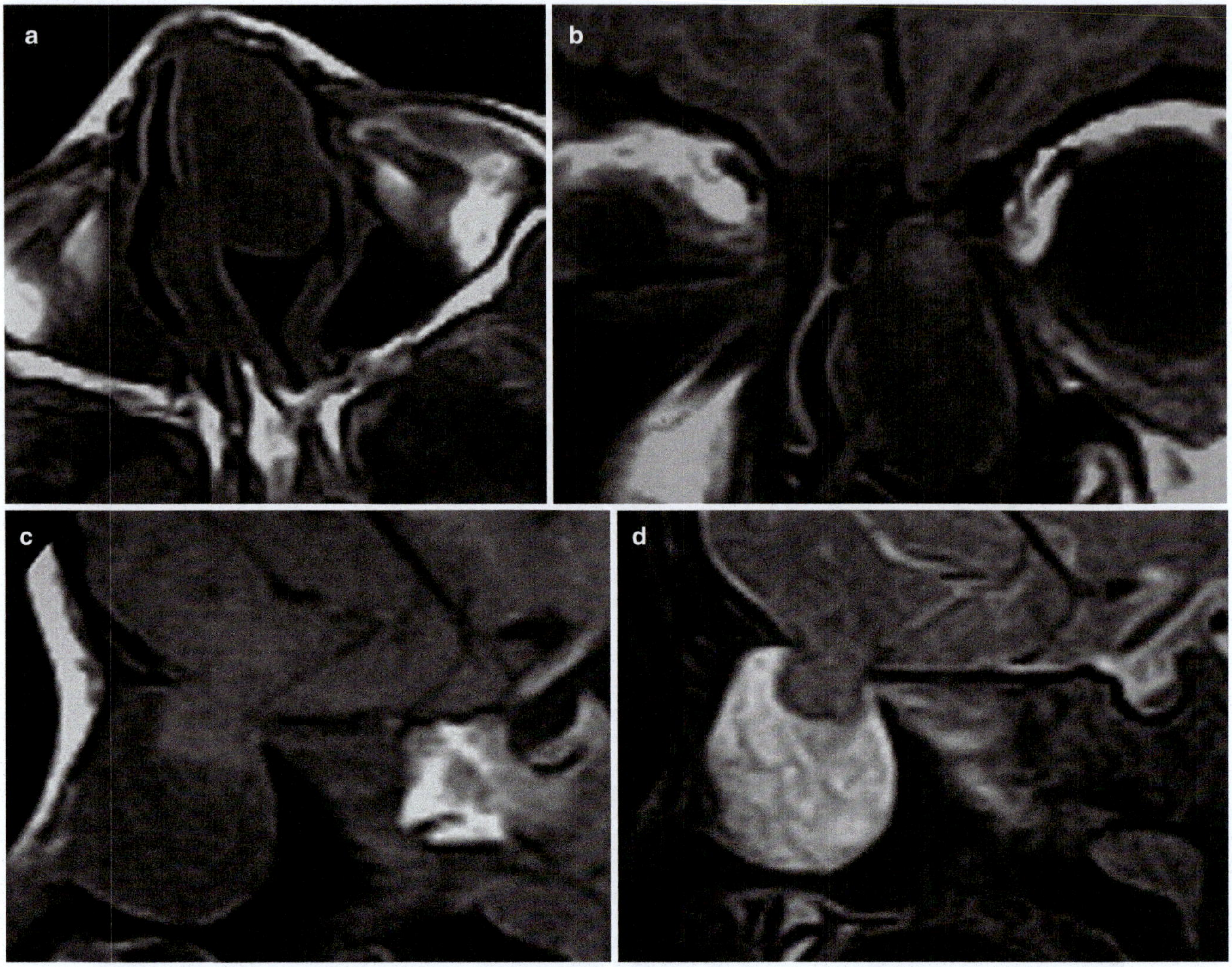

Fig. 17.3 (**a**) Axial and (**b**) coronal T1 images depict a large egg-sized anterior nasal mass, filling and expanding the left nasal cavity deviating the septum to the right. Moderately heterogeneous signal with vague area cranially which is isointense to brain. (**c**) Sagittal T1 again displays large ovoid anterior nasal mass, mildly heterogeneous with signal similar to brain, particularly cranially where there is conspicuous absence of the dark linear signal from the anterior cranial fossa. (**d**) Sagittal T2. Truly one picture is worth a thousand words (and a thousand other imaging sequences! Indeed, this is "money shot.") The large anterior nasal mass is filled with bright CSF. The floor of the anterior cranial fossa is absent and has been breached by this NFE which contains a small component of tissue contiguous with and isointense to the adjacent frontal lobe. Diagnosis: nasofrontal meningoencephalocele containing brain!

- Frequently find a midline hypo-attenuating mass with a thin wall which scallops adjacent intact bony cortex.
- CTC (CT cisternography) [10]:
  - CTC is frequently useful for evaluation of CSF leaks.
  - CTC is usually reserved for patients where high-resolution CT does not identify a bony defect, or those unfortunate patients where there are multiple defects and it is not clear which one is leaking.

Ultrasound Features

- Herniation through a calvarial or skull base defect by a spherical, fluid-filled structure which can contain brain parenchyma.
- 90% occur in the midline.

Embryology

- The neural tube is embryonic tissue which develops into the brain, spinal cord, and surrounding bone. This narrow structure folds and closes during the third and fourth weeks of fetal development during brain and spinal cord construction. Rare neural tube defects (NTDs) develop when this process goes awry with the tube failing to close completely. Of late, this fourth week faux pas is currently regarded as a "late" neurulation defect [1, 11].
- See Fig. 17.4a–f.
- Encephaloceles are frequently found in frontal, occipital, or paramedian parietal regions.
- Transsphenoidal encephaloceles sometimes surface as a nasopharyngeal masses. Hopefully the endoscopist will

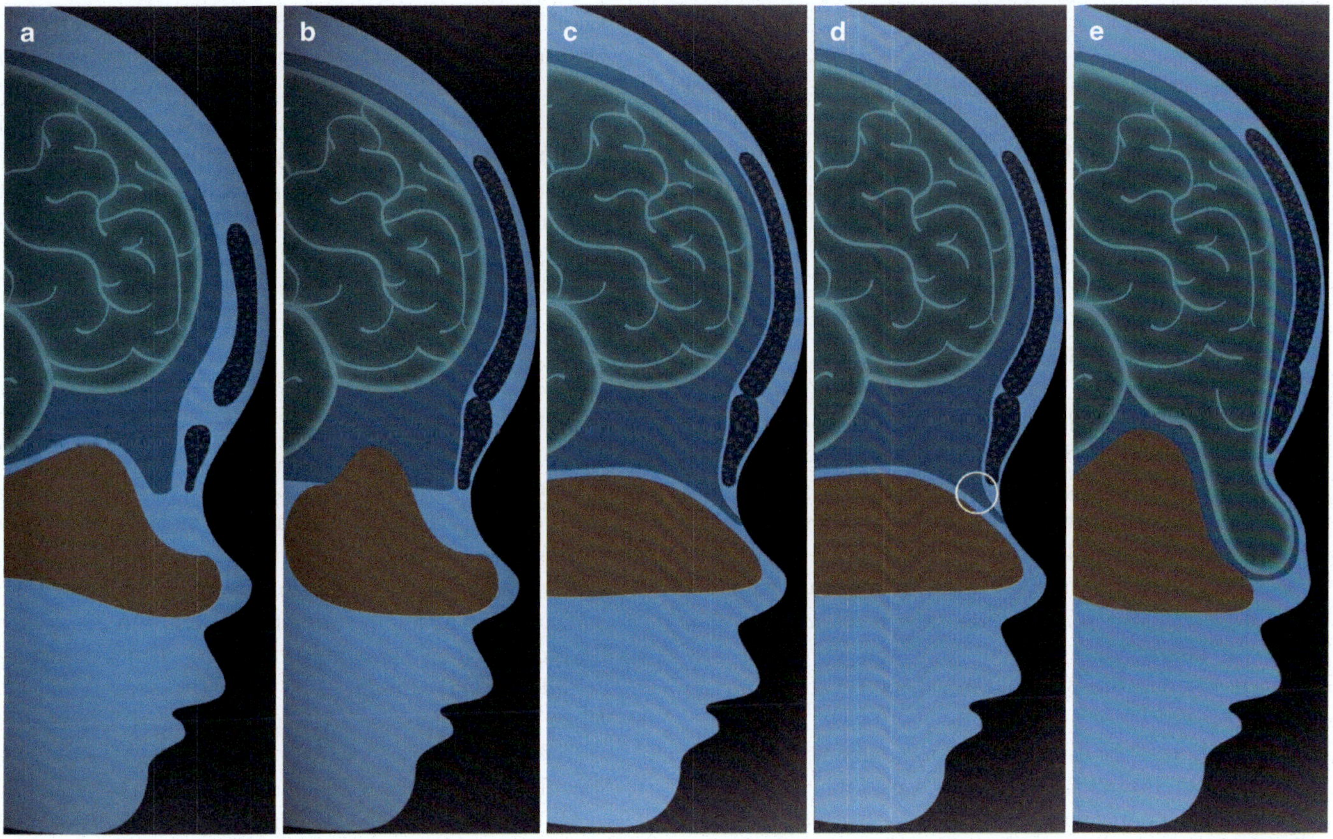

Fig. 17.4 Sagittal view of embryologic brain and frontal skull base development depicts normal nasal development at 6 weeks (**a**) and 8 weeks' (**b**) gestation. Nasal cartilage is portrayed in brown with overlying neural crest cells shown in teal. Anteriorly, developing frontal and anterior nasal bones (speckled slate) are separated at 6 weeks (**a**) but generally adjoin by 8 weeks (**b**). This separation presents a potential site for frontal encephaloceles. (**c**) Portrays path for frontonasal encephalocele protruding through the potential space seen caudal to the frontal bone on figure (**a**) normally present at 6 weeks' fetal development. (**d**) Neural crest cells (teal) migrate anteriorly until contacting ectodermal elements (skin). When the primitive prenasal space diverticulum (teal) touches nasal tip ectoderm, it normally recedes intracranially through the defect depicted by the circle. (**e**) Depicts development of a nasoethmoidal encephalocele with (green) neural tissue protruding through the migration path previously taken by primitive neural crest cells. (Reprinted with permission from Elsevier: Castillo and Mukherji [11])

distinguish dura, dural blood vessels, or pulsating brain and abort an ill-fated biopsy.

- Nasofrontal and sphenoethmoidal meningoencephaloceles are most frequently found in Vietnamese and Southeast Asian women.
- Associated abnormalities include agenesis of the corpus callosum, colobomas, and cleft lips.
- *Incidence*: Reports range from 1 in 40,000 to 1 in 5000 live births, with the higher incidence in Southeast Asia [2].
- *Location:*
  - Girls are more prone to present with occipital encephaloceles.
  - Boys are more frequently found with frontal encephaloceles.
  - In North America, encephaloceles are more common in the occipital region.
  - In Southeast Asia frontoethmoidal encephaloceles predominate [1].
  - Encephaloceles and meningoceles may occasionally involve the mastoids.
  - Encephaloceles' favored anatomic areas include [4]:
    Occipital 75%
    Frontoethmoidal 15%
    Basal 10%

Clinical Issues

Presentation

- Encephaloceles are frequently found during fetal ultrasound with most of the others encountered soon after birth.
- At birth, sphenoidal encephaloceles are classically clinically occult usually revealing their presence during the first year of life.
- Children with transsphenoidal encephaloceles may present with nasal obstruction [4] and are frequently occult until found by the clinician using a nasoscope.

Treatment

- Therapy involves resection, closure of the dural defect, and reconstruction of any associated bony defect [1].
- Since frontoethmoidal encephaloceles are not typically related to anomalies which control prognosis, their outcome tends to be better than occipital and parietal encephaloceles [1, 2].

Differential Diagnosis [1]

A. Nasal Glioma [4, 5]

- Congenital heterotopic non-neoplastic mass occurring near the nasal root which is composed of dysplastic glial tissue.
- 15% connect to the brain by a stalk but *do not* communicate with the CSF-filled subarachnoid space.
- Nasal gliomas are distinctly different from an encephalocele which *does connect with subarachnoid space* and *does contain CSF.*
- Nasal gliomas are 30% intranasal, 60% extranasal, and 10% mixed.
- Nasal gliomas are usually isointense to the brain on MRI.
- High-resolution surface coil MRI is useful in demonstrating an intracranial stalk.
- *[See Chap. 20, Nasal Glioma.]

B. Dermoid and Epidermoid Cysts

- Found in various locations around the skull and midface.
- Dermoids contain ectoderm and skin elements. Epidermoids contain ectoderm with *no* skin elements.
- CT attenuation varies depending on fat content *showing fat with dermoids* and *fluid with epidermoids.*
- MRI signal varies with fluid content ranging from pure fluid isointense to CSF on T1 and T2 in epidermoids to a more complex intensity for dermoids (T1 hyperintense, T2 hypointense).
- A key factor here is that epidermoid cysts typically show restricted diffusion and are bright on DWI with a dark area on corresponding ADC map. This is *not* a feature for encephaloceles.
- [See Chap. 9, Epidermoid.]

C. Antrochoanal Polyp (AP) [6]

- Antrochoanal polyps demonstrate a "dumbbell"-shaped mass involving the nasal cavity and maxillary sinus.
- Antrochoanal polyps exhibit non-enhancing (or occasionally peripheral-enhancing) mass with benign-appearing bone changes.
- Antrochoanal polyps can contain cystic changes.
- Antrochoanal polyps frequently fill the nasal antrum but *do NOT* extend into the PPF.
- Antrochoanal polyps habitually herniate into the anterior nasal cavity before involving the nasopharynx.

D. Nasal Teratomas [7, 8]

- Teratomas are neoplasms *containing all three germ layers.*
- In general, head and neck teratomas tend to be benign in children, whereas in adults they are mostly malignant.
- Most head and neck teratomas *contain calcifications.* Not a feature for encephaloceles.

E. Intra-oral salivary gland cyst

- May occasionally mimic a basal encephalocele.

A Closer Look

I. Genetics

- The worldwide general population's chance of having a child with spina bifida is less than 0.2%.
- If a woman already has a child with spina bifida, the chance of having another affected child is 1 in 20.
- A woman who has spina bifida has a 5% chance of having a child with spina bifida.
- When both parents have spina bifida, the risk increases to 15%.
- Specific genes currently linked to spina bifida include:
  - MTHFR and SHMT1 which are involved in folic acid metabolism.
  - VANGL1 gene which encodes for glucose metabolism.

II. Fast Facts

- And, if you thought you really understood the embryology, there is more.
- Transsphenoidal encephaloceles are theorized to be related to skull base formation during migration of cephalic neural crest cells.

III. Historic Highlights [2, 9]

- Nasofrontal encephaloceles have been recorded since the 16th century [2].
- 1755: Corvinus described draining CSF and resecting the surrounding membrane in a patient with a NFE.
- 1774: Freeand published an article on "'hernia of brain'" and advocated supporting the surgical repair with boiled leather to facilitate firm scar formation. Apparently not too many product liability suits back then.
- 1830: Grossheim encouraged excising extruding brain during repair.
- 1813: Richter first documented NFEs (nasofrontal encephaloceles).
- 1895: Fenger first described a successful treatment of NFEs.
- 1947: First Anderson and then in 1959 Davis and Alexander advocated modern-day treatment using bifrontal craniotomies for NFE.

Selected References

1. Hoving EW. Nasal encephaloceles. Childs Nerv Syst. 2000;16: 702–6.
2. Tirumandas M, Gbenimacho SA, Shoja MM, et al. Nasal encephaloceles: a review of etiology, pathophysiology, clinical presentations, diagnosis, treatment, and complications. Childs Nerv Syst. 2013;29(5):739–44.
3. Koral K1, Geffner ME, Curran JG.Trans-sphenoidal and spheno-ethmoidal encephalocele: report of two cases and review of the literature. Australas Radiol. 2000;44(2):220–4.
4. Moron FE, Morriss MC, Jones JJ, Hunter JJ. Lumps and bumps on the head in children: use of CT and MR imaging in Solvint the clinical diagnostic dilemma. Radiographics. 2004;24(6) https://doi.org/10.1148/rg.246045034.
5. Lowe LH, Booth TN, Joglar JM, Rollins NK. Midface anomalies in children. Radiographics. 2000;20:907–22.
6. Midyett FA, Mukherji SK. Chapter 22, Esthesioneuroblastoma. Orbital imaging. Elsevier/Saunders. 2015. pp. 91–5. ISBN: 978-0-323-34037-3.
7. Cukurova I, Gumusssoy M, Yaz A, et al. A benign teratoma presenting as an obstruction of the nasal cavity: a case report. J Med Case Rep. 2012;6:147. Accessed on line 1/25/2016. https://doi.org/10.1186/1752-1947-6-147
8. Barnes L, Eveson J, Reichart P, Sidransky D. Germ cell tumours. 3. In: Cardesa A, Luna M, editors. Pathology and genetics of head and neck tumors. France: IARC Press; 2005. p. 76–9.
9. McGee, Jimenez DF. The history of Nasofrontal Encephaloceles. American Association of Neurological Surgeons. May 2004.
10. Stone JA, Castillo M, Neelon B, Mukherji SK. Evaluation of CSF leaks: high-resolution CT compared with contrast-enhanced CT and radionuclide cisternography. AJNR Am J Neuroradiol. 1999;20(4):706–12.
11. Castillo M, Mukherji SK. Imaging of facial anomalies. Curr Problems Diagnostic Imaging. 1996;15:169–88.

Sinonasal Melanoma

18

Pertinent Points

- *Definition*: Sinonasal melanoma (SNM) is a very rare and unique subtype of malignant melanoma which is noted for its poor prognosis and unique staging systems.
- *AKA*: Sinonasal mucosal melanoma.
- *Classic Clue*: Older patient presenting for nasal congestion or epistaxis exhibits on MRI a nasal cavity mass having high T1 and *low T2 signal compared to gray matter.*
- *Location*: Sinonasal melanoma is found in the nasal cavity more commonly than in the paranasal sinuses showing the anterior nasal septum, lateral nasal wall, and inferior turbinates to be the preferred sites [10, 12].
- *Melanosis:* Sinonasal melanomas sometimes show melanosis with melanin deposits along the mucosal surface of the sinonasal cavity.
- Multiple Foci: Multiple lesional foci suggest melanoma.
- Melanomas may contain melanin with paramagnetic effects demonstrating T1 and T2 shortening causing characteristic high signal on T1 and low signal on T2.
- However, amelanotic melanomas may show low T1 and bright T2. And, if this is not enough to confuse things, bleeding is common and can show about any signal combination depending on the hemorrhage's hemoglobin transitional stage.
- *Spread:* Melanoma readily spreads using hematogenous and perineural routes.
- *Rare:* Sinonasal melanomas are rare accounting for <1% of head and neck cancers, 1% of malignant melanomas, and < 4% of sinonasal neoplasms [2, 3, 10, 11].
- *Older Patients*: Sinonasal melanomas are frequently found in older patients (60–90 years of age) [3].
- *Incidence:* In North America, SNM accounts for 2% of malignant melanomas, 4% of H&N melanomas [5, 6], and 3.5% of sinonasal malignancies [5, 7]. SNM has a higher incidence in Asian populations where more complete studies have been published [4, 8].

Imaging

General Imaging Features

- Sinonasal melanoma may be multifocal.
- 2/3 are melanotic, 1/3 is amelanotic [10, 12].
- CT and MRI share complimentary roles in tumor mapping.
- CT is crucial in defining bony structure, while MRI is superior in separating secretions from tumor.

CT Features

- *See General Imaging Features.*
- Shows sessile or polypoid mass flaunting flagrant post-contrast enhancement.
- Frequently find bony remodeling and erosion [4]. [See Fig. 18.1a.]

MRI Features [10]

- *See General Imaging Features.*
- *Gray matter* is probably the *best internal standard* for comparing MRI signal [10].

F. A. Midyett, S. K. Mukherji, *Skull Base Imaging*, https://doi.org/10.1007/978-3-030-46447-9_18

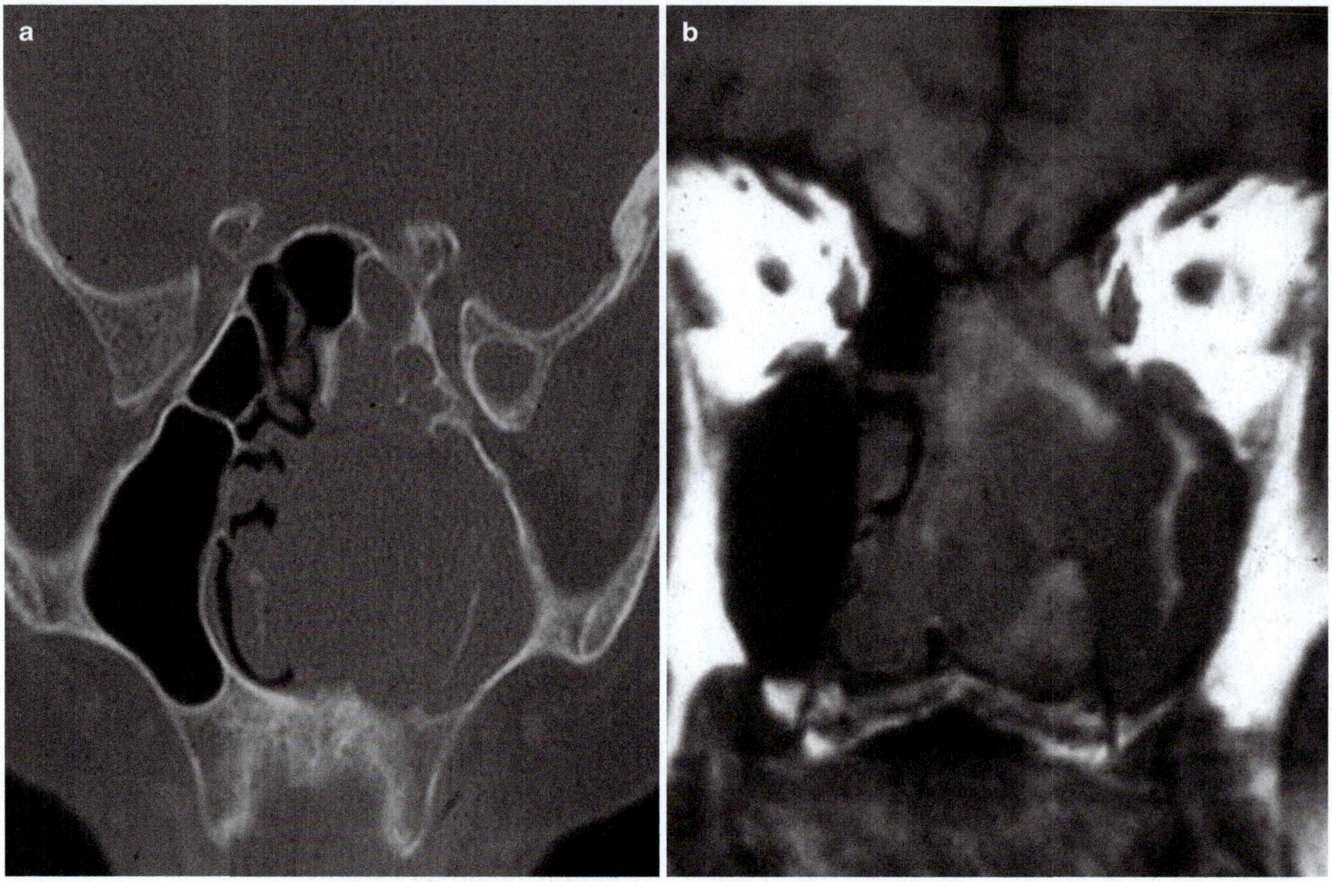

Fig. 18.1 (**a**) Coronal NECT shows large sinonasal mass filling and expanding the left nasal cavity extending into the maxillary and ethmoid sinuses. It has destroyed the nasal septum extending into the contralateral nasal cavity. (**b**) Coronal T1 confirms a large tumor fills the left nasal cavity, and maxillary sinus extending caudally to the hard palate, and cranially through the ethmoid sinuses to the skull base. The tumor is relatively isointense to gray matter. Scattered hyperintense foci indicate intratumoral hemorrhage, often seen with SNM. [See DDx, E. Hemorrhagic Neoplasms]

- The *most common pattern* for these *uncommon lesions* encountered at conferences and board examinations is *high signal on T1* and *low signal on T2*. But, alas, things are not always so simple. Here are some general guiding principles.
- T1 homogeneous signal:
  – Sometimes see ↑ T1 secondary to melanin or hemorrhage [4, 10]. [See Fig. 18.1b.]
  – Amelanotic melanomas show intermediate T1 signal compared to gray matter [10]. [See Fig. 18.2a.]
  – Melanotic melanomas have ↑ T1 compared to gray matter [10]. [See Fig. 18.3a.]
- T2 *exhibits erratic* intermediate signal compared to gray matter.
- T1 Gd: Mild to moderate heterogeneous enhancement. The specific signal varies with histology [10].
- DWI: Shows significant restricted diffusion with bright DWI and dark ADC map. [See Fig. 18.4a, b.]

Nuclear Radiology

- ^{18}F-FDG-PET/CT imaging helps stage SNM [18].

Clinical Issues

1. Presentation
   - Nasal congestion and epistaxis are common complaints.
   - Pain and polyps are less frequent presentations.
   - *Melanorrhea*: A characteristic "coal-flecked" brown nasal discharge (*melanorrhea*) sometimes suggests the diagnosis to a clever clinician.
2. Epidemiology
   - May be related to smoking or chemical exposure like formaldehyde.

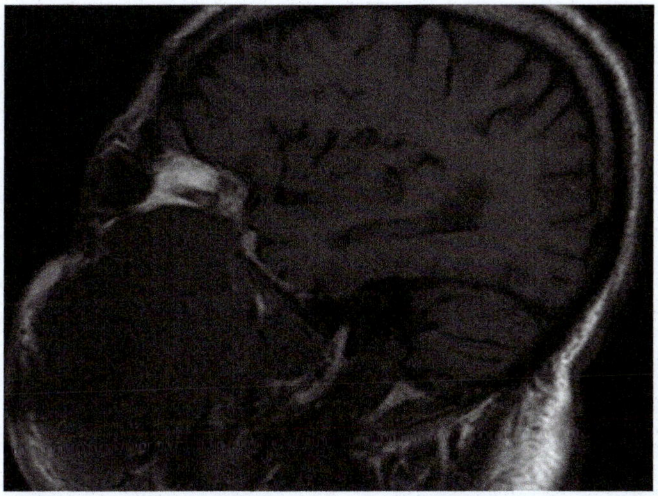

Fig. 18.2 Sagittal T1 Gd shows a mammoth mass occupying the left face extending cranially to the orbital floor and skull base. At one point the tumor appears almost adjacent to the anterior temporal lobe. The tumor is relatively isointense to gray matter, a pattern frequently found with amelanotic melanomas

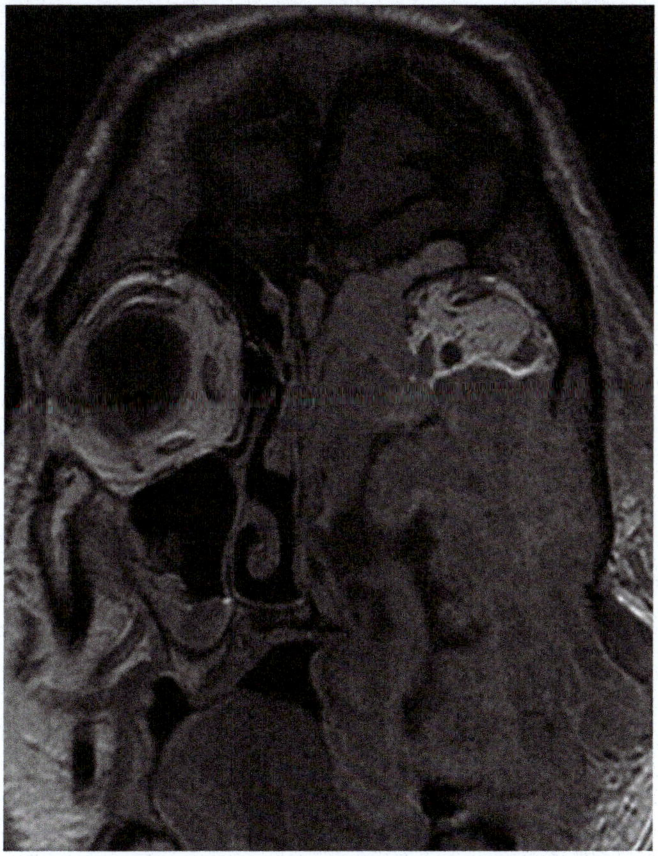

Fig. 18.3 Coronal T1 shows an enormous tumor hyperintense to gray matter involving the left nasal cavity, maxillary, and ethmoid sinuses. This mammoth mass extends cranially into the frontal sinuses, L > R. It invades the orbit displacing orbital contents. It extends caudally through the hard palate into the oral cavity abutting and displacing the tongue

- Sinonasal melanoma is locally invasive and spreads through lymphatics to the nodes, brain, bone, lung, and liver.

3. Pathology
   - *Gross*: Usually ulcerated, polypoid, and pigmented (brown or black) [17].
   - *Microscopic*: Cell shapes vary but usually contain melanin pigment within the cytoplasm. If melanin granules are *not present*, pathologists regularly stain for vimentin, S100, and melan-A.
4. Staging
   A. Freedman Classification System [10, 14]:
   - Stage T_1: Tumor limited to one side of the nasal cavity.
   - Stage T_2: Tumor spread into other nasal structures or the palate.
   - Stage T_3: Tumor spreads beyond the ipsilateral nasal cavity into the maxillary or ethmoid sinus, contralateral nasal cavity, or skin.
   - Stage T_4: Tumor extends to the orbit, pterygopalatine fossa, brain, or sphenoid sinus.

   B. TNM [15]:
   - This variant of the TNM staging system reflects SNM's poor prognosis.
   - T_1 and T_2 do *not exist* for SNM in this system.
   - T_3: Confined to the mucosa.
   - T_{4a}: Invades the deep soft tissue, cartilage, bone, or skin.
   - T_{4b}: Invades the brain, dura, cranial nerves, carotid artery, paravertebral space, or the mediastinum.
   - N Stage: N_0, no regional lymph node metastasis; N_1, regional lymph node metastasis.
   - M Stage: M_0, no distant metastasis; M_1, distant metastasis.
   - Final Stage.

Stage	T	N	M
III	T_3	N_0	M_0
IVA	T_{4a}	N_0	M_0
	T_{3-4a}	N_1	
IVB	T_{4b}	N_{any}	M_0
IVB	T_{any}	N_{any}	M_1

Treatment

- Sinonasal melanoma continues to elude effective treatment innovations.
- Recurrences are habitually high and survival is abysmally low [5].
- Surgery:
  - Surgical resection with clear margins is the primary goal.

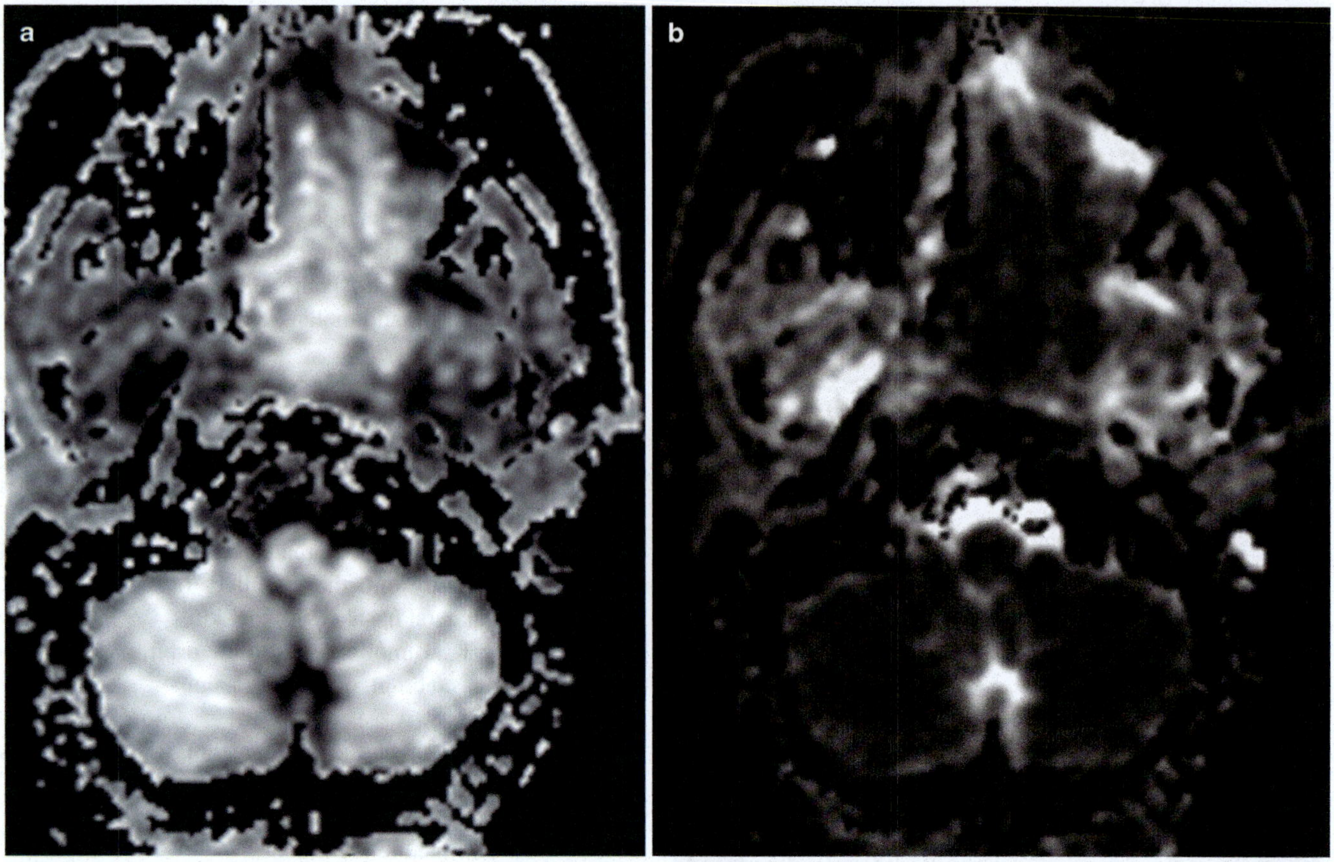

Fig. 18.4 (**a**) Axial DWI shows a large area of *bright signal* corresponding to the large left sinonasal mass demonstrated on prior images. (**b**) Axial ADC map shows large area of *dark signal* corresponding to the large left sinonasal mass. The dark area on this ADC map corresponds to the bright area on the (prior 4A) DWI image. Taken together (images 4**a** and 4**b**) demonstrate remarkable restricted diffusion denoting dismal disease

- Radiation therapy:
  - While some studies show complete clinical response to radiation therapy alone, most advocate radiation therapy for recurrent or inoperable tumors.
- Chemotherapy:
  - Targeted chemotherapy probably holds the best hope for these patients in the foreseeable future.
  - Currently the B-Raf and KIT genes have been identified in mucosal melanoma patients, and therapy has added additional survival time.

Prognosis [1]

- Sinonasal malignant melanoma has a worse prognosis than other nasal cavity neoplasms, and local recurrence represents aggressive disease with short survival.
- Infiltration into the skull base, orbit, or facial soft tissues portents a particularly poor prognosis with a 5-year survival of ~30% [9].
- Recently reported median disease-free interval was 18 months, and the median survival was 23 months [1].
- At the time of diagnosis, approximately 10% have hematogenous, and nearly 20% have lymphatic spread. During treatment, lymphatic spread sometimes increases to involve one third of patients.

Differential Diagnosis [1]

A. Sinonasal Undifferentiated Carcinoma (SNUC) [19]

- Rare and highly aggressive paranasal sinus neoplasm first recognized as a distinct pathologic entity in 1987.
- Its rapid growth, local and regional recurrence, and distant metastasis portent a particularly poor prognosis.
- CT shows aggressive bone destruction often extending from the sinonasal region into orbit, anterior cranial fossa, and occasionally the cavernous sinus.
- SNUCs are typically large (>4 cm) *non-calcified* masses, presenting poorly defined margins more often than not

emerging from the ethmoid sinuses or superior nasal cavity. They regularly result in sinus obstruction.
- T1 signal is isointense to muscle, while T2 is iso-hyperintense to muscle.
- Some say SNUCs cannot be distinguished from other tumors of this region on the basis of imaging alone *except for SNM* [20]. [See imaging features for SNM in this chapter.]
- [See Chap. 26, Sinonasal Undifferentiated Carcinoma.]

B. Inverted Papilloma (IP)
- These moderately advanced tumors commonly show a *unilateral nasal fossa mass* with opacification of the contiguous maxillary sinus.
- Inverted papillomas most commonly occur on the lateral wall of the nasal cavity, more frequently found near the middle turbinate and maxillary ostium.
- Enlargement of the mass results in bony remodeling and resorption as it extends into the maxillary antrum.
- While they commonly obstruct the maxillary antrum drainage, oddly enough, concomitant *mucoceles Sp are rare.*
- CT: *Hyperostosis* is *highly predictive* of tumor origin.
- Combined bony sclerosis and deformity with an antro-meatal mass suggests a slow-growing tumor such as IP.
- MRI:
  - T1: Iso- to slightly hyperintense to muscle
  - T2: Iso- to hyperintense to muscle often showing alternating hypointense lines constituting CCP (*convoluted cerebriform pattern*)
  - T1 Gd: Heterogeneous enhancement often showing alternating hypointense lines constituting CCP (*convoluted cerebriform pattern*)
- [See Chap. 14, Inverted Papilloma.]

C. Esthesioneuroblastoma (ENB)
- Rare neuroendocrine malignancy of neural crest origin arising from olfactory epithelium. AKA: Olfactory neuroblastoma.
- Classically exhibits avidly enhancing dumbbell-shaped mass with "waist" at the cribriform plate on T1 Gd.
- May involve the anterior cranial fossa, skull base, and orbit.
- Shows intermediate signal on T1 and T2.
- Cystic areas (with foci of ↑T2) at tumor/brain interface are diagnostic and may be pathognomonic.
- DWI demonstrates moderate restricted diffusion.
- ENB exhibits an epicenter near the cribriform plate.
- ENB gives no gender preference.
- [See Chap. 28, Esthesioneuroblastoma.]

D. Allergic Fungal Sinusitis (AFS)
- NECT usually shows hyperdense sinus opacification surrounded by a thin rim of hypodense mucosa.
- T1 is variable with hypointensity most common.
- T2 shows *hypointense* signal from ↑ metals, ↑ protein, and ↓free water in mucin.
- [See Chap. 32, Allergic Fungal Sinusitis.]

E. Hemorrhagic Neoplasms
- Certain neoplasms can contain intratumoral hemorrhage and blood products with methemoglobin which ↑ T1 signal. [See Fig. 18.1b.]
- Habitually hemorrhagic primary neoplasms include hemangioma, lymphangioma, and JNA (juvenile nasal angiofibroma).
- May have hemorrhagic metastasis from the thyroid, lung, breast, or kidney.
- [See Chap. 15, Juvenile Nasal Angiofibroma.]

A Closer Look

I. Genetics
- Genetic mutations were found for NRAS (14%) as well as KIT and BRAF (4%) in a review of 56 SNM cases [3, 13].

II. Fast Facts
- Multiple mucosal melanomas may be seen in close proximity, typically in the same site.
- SNM has been reported to simultaneously involve oral and the nearby but noncontiguous nasal cavity.
- Hematogenous metastases occur in up to 50% of cases [10].
- An association between SNM and occupational formalin exposure has been suggested [16].

Selected References

1. Roth TN, Gengler C, Huber GF, et al. Outcome of sinonasal melanoma: clinical experience and review of the literature. Head Heck. 2010;32(10):1385–92. https://doi.org/10.1002/hed.21340.
2. Narasimhan K, Kucuk O, Lin HS, et al. Sinonasal mucosal melanoma: a 13-year experience at a single institution. Skull Base. 2009;19(04):255–62. https://doi.org/10.1055/s-0028-1115321.
3. Batra K, Chhabra A, Rampure J, et al. CT and MRI appearances of primary sphenoid melanoma: a rare case. AJNR Am J Neuroradiol. 2006;26(10):2642–4.
4. Eggesbø HB. Imaging of sinonasal tumours. Cancer Imaging. 2012;12(1):136–52. https://doi.org/10.1102/1470-7330.2012.0015.
5. Narasimhan K, Kucuk O, Lin H-S, et al. Sinonasal Mucosal Melanoma: a 13-year experience at a single institution. Skull Base. 2009;19(4):255–62. https://doi.org/10.1055/s-0028-1115321

6. Thompson AC, Morgan DA, Bradley PJ. Malignant melanoma of the nasal cavity and paranasal sinuses. Clin Otolaryngol. 1993;18:34–6.
7. Conley JJ, Ackerman AB. Melanoma of the head and neck. 1st ed. New York: Georg Thieme Verlag; 1990. p. 154–78.
8. Cheng YF, Lai CC, Ho CY, Shu CH, Lin CZ. Toward a better understanding of sinonasal mucosal melanoma: clinical review of 23 cases. J Chin Med Assoc. 2007;70(1):24–9.
9. Nguyen B. Sinonasal malignant melanoma with diffuse metastasis: F-18 FDG PET/CT imaging. Radiol Case Rep. 03;3(1): https://doi.org/10.2484/rcr.v3i1.118
10. Yousem DM, Li C, Montone KT, et al. Primary malignant melanoma of the Sinonasal cavity: MR imaging evaluation. Radiographics. 1996;16:1101–10.
11. Lund VJ. Malignant melanoma of the nasal cavity and paranasal sinuses. Ear Nose Throat J. 1993;72:285–90.
12. Barnes L, Peel RL. Head and neck pathology: a text/atlas of differential diagnosis. New York: Igaku-Shoin; 1990. p. 122–3.
13. Zebary A, Jangard M, Omholt K, et al. KIT, NRAS and BRAF mutations in sinonasal mucosal melanoma: a study of 56 cases. Br J Cancer. 2013;109:559–64. https://doi.org/10.1038/bjc.2013.373.
14. Freedman HM, DeSanto LW, Devine KD, Weiland LH. Malgnant melanoma of the nasal cavity and paranasal sinuses. Arch Otolaryngol. 1973;97:322–5.
15. National Comprehensive Cancer Network. NCCN Clinical Practice Guidelines in Oncology: Head and Neck Cancers. V 1.2015. Available at http://www.nccn.org/professionals/physician_gls/pdf/head-and-neck.pdf. Accessed: December 31, 2015.
16. Holmstrom M, Lund VJ. Malignant melanomas of the nasal cavity after occupational exposure to formaldehyde. Br J Ind Med. 1991;48(1):9–11.
17. Thompson LD, Wieneke JA, et al. Sinonasal tract and nasopharyngeal melanomas: a clinicopathologic study of 115 cases with a proposed staging system. Am J Surg Pathol. 2003;27(5):594–611.
18. Haerle SK, Soyka MB, Fisher DR, et al. The value of 18F-FDG-PET/CT imaging for sinonasal malignant melanoma. Eur Arch Otorhinolaryngol. 2012;269(1):127–33/Springer-Verlag, 2011. https://doi.org/10.1007/s00405-011-1664-1.
19. Pitman KT, Costantino PD, Lassen LF. Sinonasal undifferentiated carcinoma: current trends in treatment. Skull Base Surg. 2011;5(4):269–72.
20. Phillips CD, Futter SF, Lipper MH, Levine PA. Sinonasal undifferentiated carcinoma: CT and MR imaging of an uncommon neoplasm of the nasal cavity. Radiology. 1997;202(2). https://doi.org/10.1148/radiology.202.2.9015077

19 Nasal Dermoid

Pertinent Points

- *Definition*: Most common midline nasal mass appearing as congenital abnormality in which a subcutaneous sac-like structure develops near the nose sometimes showing external ostia or hair tufts.
- *Embryology:* Incomplete regression of the embryonic frontonasal diverticula traps nonglial tissue developing dermoids, epidermoids, and teratomas. (See Fig. 19.1c, d.) Congenital dermoids are developmental anomalies and not true neoplasms [2, 3].
- *AKA*: Dermoid, dermoid cyst, dermal cyst, nasal dermal sinus cyst, nasal dermoid sinus cyst.
- *Classic Clue*: Imaging studies show hair arising from cyst or sinus tract near the base of the nose with an associated fatty mass.
- *Location:* Can occur anywhere along the course of the primitive prenasal space diverticulum from the nasal septum to the foramen cecum in the anterior cranial fossa.
- *Incidence*:
  - 1 in 30,000; M > F [1]; 7% of dermoids occur in H&N region.
  - Nasal dermoids comprise up to 3% of all dermoids and 7% of head and neck dermoids.

Imaging

General Imaging Features

- Unlike intracranial dermoids which characteristically contain fat, extracranial dermoids exhibit an erratic alterable appearance and may appear as fat or fluid.
- *Infection:*
  - If infected (or previously infected), they may enhance.
  - Infection may progress to a nasal septal abscess.
- Dermoids may truncate the tip of the nasal septum. [See Fig. 19.2b.]
- MRI should probably not be the primary tool for working up developmental nasal midline masses.
- *CNS Involvement*: Nasal dermoids connecting to the CNS are variably reported as <50%.

CT Features [4]

- *See General Imaging Features.*
- Typically see a midline centrally hypodense lesion with a thin wall overlying the nasofrontal junction.
- Usually a well-defined hypodense mass approximately −20 HU (Hounsfield units), consistent with fatty components. [See Fig. 19.2a–c]

F. A. Midyett, S. K. Mukherji, *Skull Base Imaging*, https://doi.org/10.1007/978-3-030-46447-9_19

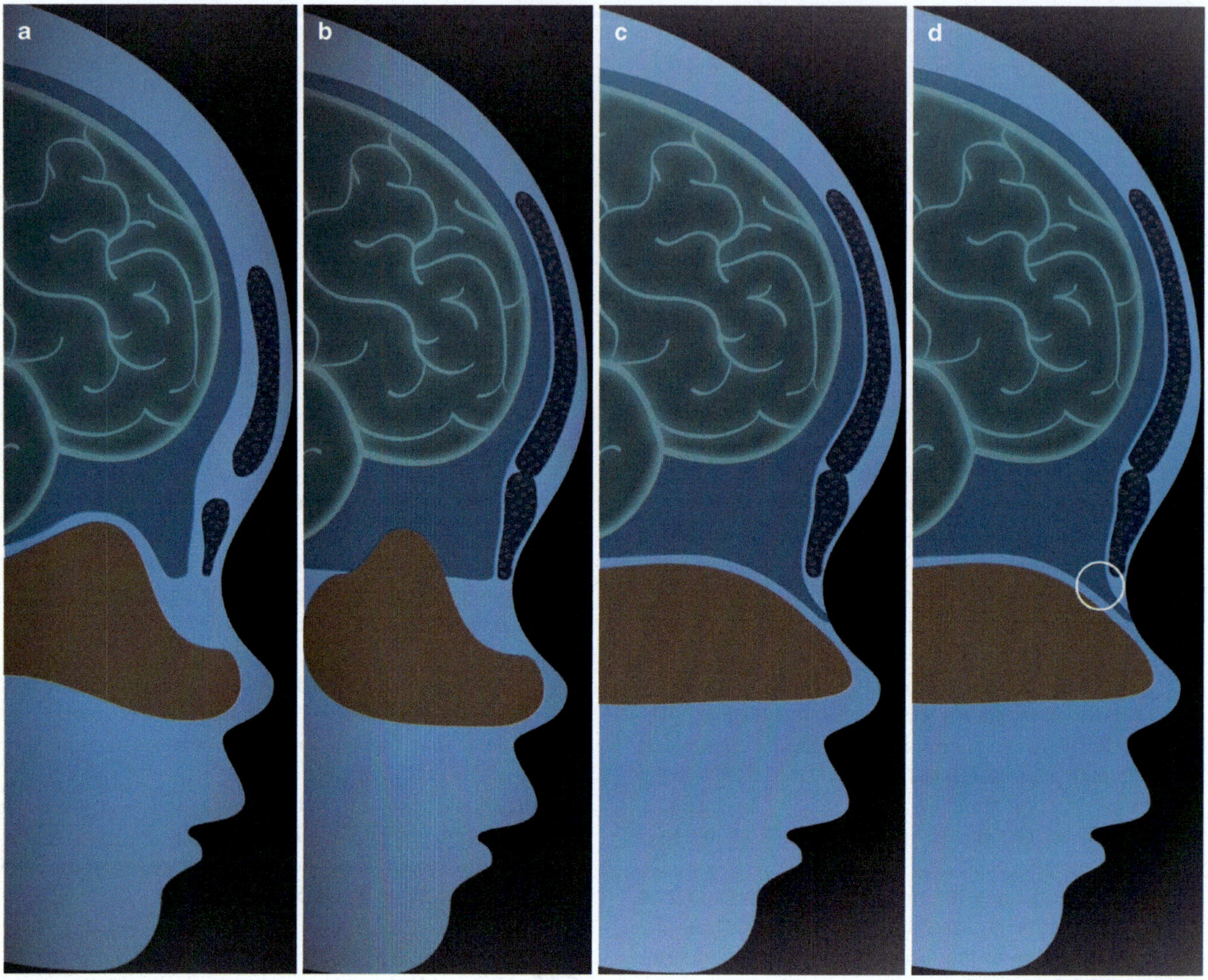

Fig. 19.1 (**a**, **b**) Color drawing depicts sagittal view of normal nasal development at 6 weeks' (**a**) and 8 weeks' (**b**) gestation. Nasal cartilage is portrayed in brown and neural crest cells are rendered in teal. Anteriorly, the developing frontal and nasal bones are separated by a few millimeters at 6 weeks (**a**) but are juxtaposed by 8 weeks (**b**). This is a potential location for frontonasal encephaloceles. [See Chap. 17, Encephalocele.] (**c**, **d**) Color drawing depicts sagittal view of nasal development. Neural crest cells (depicted in teal) have migrated anteriorly to contact ectodermal elements (skin). When the (teal) primitive prenasal space diverticulum reaches the nasal tip ectoderm, it normally recedes intracranially. During this process, if it takes ectodermal elements along with it, a tract may form between the septum and the nasal bone. Trapped ectodermal element cells can potentially proliferate producing a dermoid, an epidermoid, or a teratoma anywhere along this tract. Circle on image (**d**) depicts a common location for a dermoid caudal to the nasion and cranial to the (brown) nasal cartilage. (Reprinted with permission from Elsevier: Castillo and Mukherji [1])

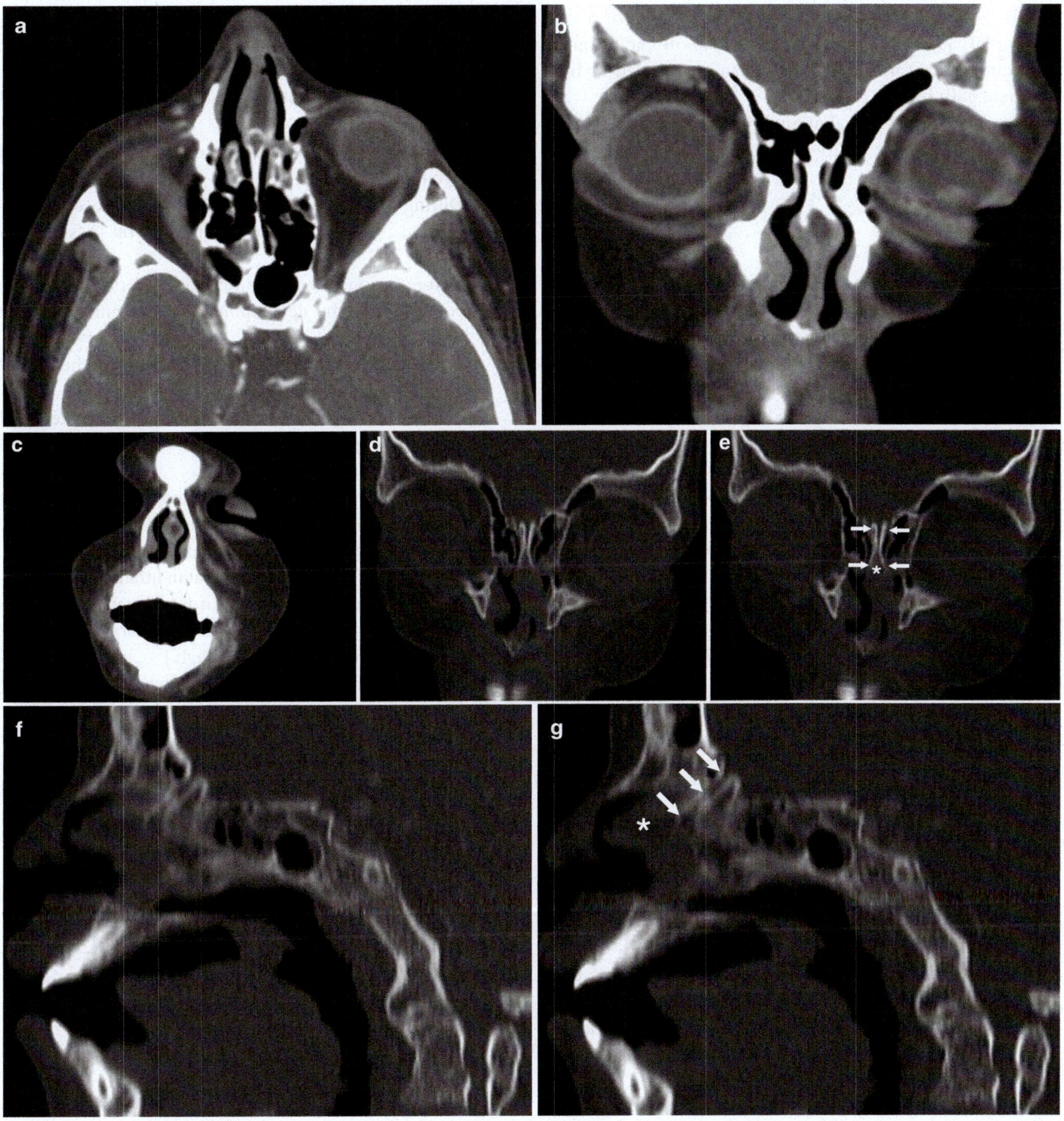

Fig. 19.2 Axial (**a**) and coronal (**b**, **c**) CECT soft tissue algorithms show low attenuation mass expanding the nasal septum. It is isodense with subcutaneous and intraorbital fat. The bony septum is truncated and bifid with the fatty mass residing in its "fork." Coronal bone algorithm CECT (**d**) without and with arrows (**e**) demonstrate an abnormal bony canal *(arrows)* crossing through the anterior skull base. This has formed along the path of the primitive prenasal space diverticulum [depicted in Fig. 19.1a]. Its caudal aspect extends to the demonstrated nasal dermoid (∗*star*) and its cranial orifice extends intracranially into the anterior fossa. (**f**, **g**) sagittal bone show prominent well-defined, well-corticated foramen cecum without (**f**) and with (**g**) arrows

- Bony skull base findings comprise scalloping or alteration of adjacent bone with widening of the foramen cecum, cribriform plate defects, and an eroded or bifid crista galli [5, 6].
- Sometimes shows an abnormal bony canal with sclerotic margins. [See Fig. 19.2d–g]

MRI Features [1]

- *See General Imaging Features.*
- *Pitfall*: Don't mistake high T1 signal from the crista galli or nasal septum for a dermoid.
- T1: Unlike intracranial dermoids which have brightly ↑ T1 signal, extracranial dermoids have a variable, often nonspecific appearance depending on their fat content [2]. [See Figs. 19.3a and 19.4c, d.]
- T2: Variable depending on content. They are often heterogeneous with ↑ signal. [See Figs. 19.3b and 19.4a, b.]
- T1 Gd: Enhancement varies from slight enhancement of a thin cyst wall if uninfected to more avid internal enhancement when infected or previously infected. [See Fig. 19.3c.]
- *DWI*: Restricted diffusion is a variably positive feature for dermoids (and therefore cannot reliably be used to distinguish from epidermoids) [4].
- Sometimes see chemical shift artifact with dermoids, lipomas, and teratomas.

Clinical Issues

1. Presentation
   - Dermoids periodically proclaim their presence with a crater, fistula, or squishy swelling anywhere from the nasal tip to the gabella [2, 7].
   - Hair protruding from a cyst or sinus tract, while typical, is seen in <50% [2, 5].
   - Patients with a patent pore or sinus ostium have a significantly higher risk of an intracranial connection [2, 5].
   - Failure to promptly diagnose and treat dermoids (and epidermoids) allows time for the lesions to enlarge. This risks recurrent infection, meningitis, brain abscess, cavernous or superior orbital venous thrombosis, periorbital cellulitis, and/or orbital abscess [2, 7].
2. More Embryology [1]
   - The neural tube develops between the third and fourth gestational weeks.
   - Neural tube closure begins at its midportion extending caudally and cranially.
   - With neural tube closure, neural crest cells migrate anteriorly and laterally around eyes to the frontonasal prominence.
   - The nose develops from the frontonasal processes and two nasal placodes.
   - During formation of the skull base and nose, mesenchymal structures form from several ossification centers.
   - Before fusion of these ossification centers, three spaces contribute to the development of congenital midline nasal masses:
     1. Fonticulus Frontalis: The space between the frontal and nasal bones.
     2. Prenasal Space: Between the nasal bones and nasal capsule (precursor of nasal septum and cartilages).
     3. Foramen Cecum. This is located in the anterior cranial fossa, anterior to the ethmoid cribriform plate, and the crista galli, posterior to the frontal bone. Frequently found to be patent in infants and uncommonly patent in children, it is only open in <1.5% of adults. It rarely transmits emissary veins to the nasal cavity. [See Fig. 19.5a, b.]
        – See Chap. 51, Sect. A3, Foramen Cecum.
3. Pathology
   - *Gross*: Dermoids are covered by a thick dermis-like wall and contain epidermis and subcutaneous tissue with hair follicles as well as sebaceous and sweat glands [2, 8].
   - *Microscopic*: Dermoids are classically cysts lined by keratinizing squamous epithelium with hallmark intramural pilosebaceous structures.

Treatment

- Surgery
  – Surgery is the archetypal standard treatment, but remember the caveat, don't biopsy before imaging. Preoperative imaging evaluation is essential to exclude intracranial extension.
  – Surgical strategies depend on location and lesion extent ranging from local excision to a combined intracranial-extracranial approach.
  – While recurrences are uncommon and easily managed, it is essential to excise the entire tract to prevent a recurrence [6].

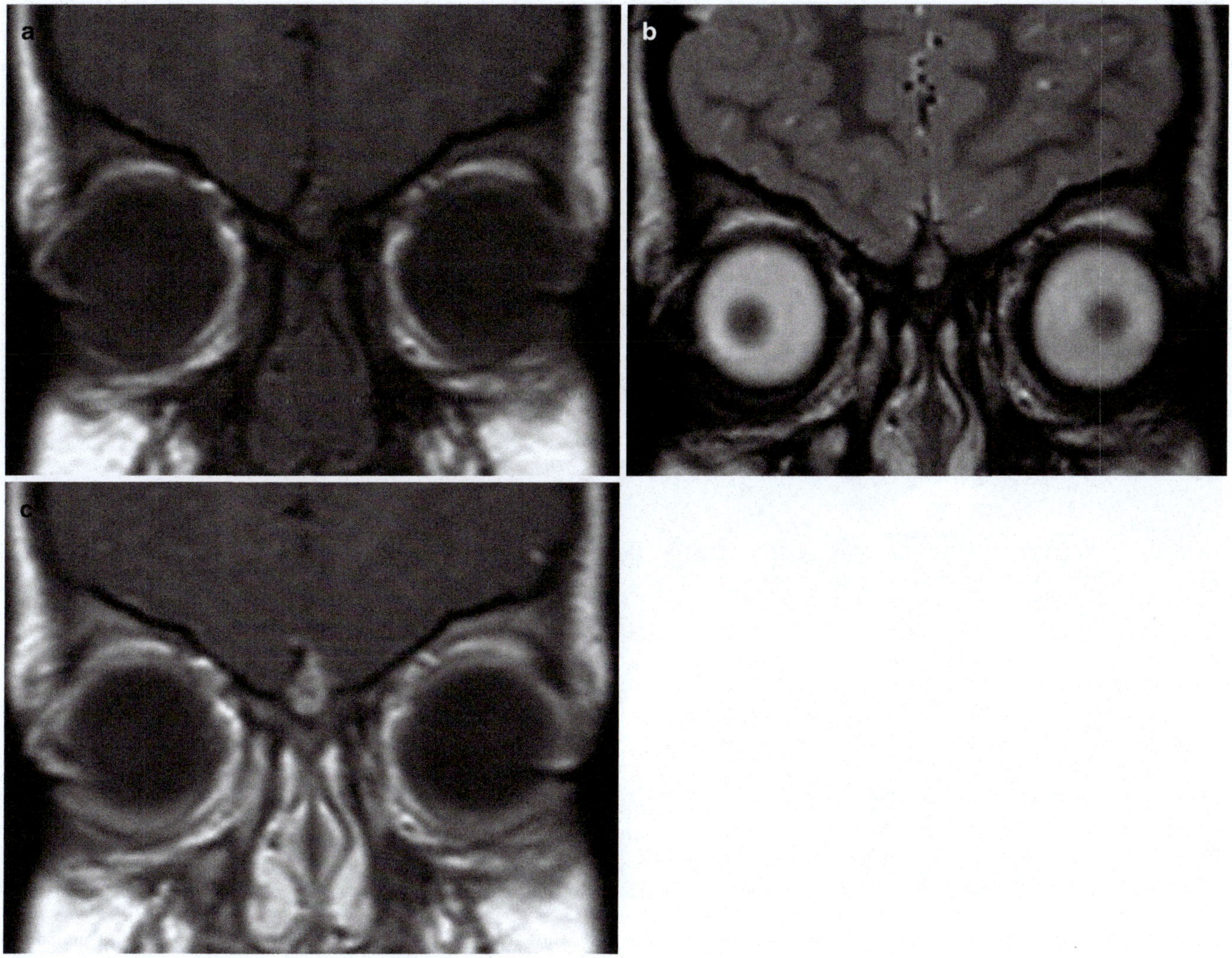

Fig. 19.3 (**a**) Coronal T1 shows small midline mass adjacent to the skull base. This should not be confused with the normal crista galli. (**b**) Coronal T2 shows small midline mass adjacent to the skull base. This is moderately heterogeneous with some higher signal foci. (**c**) Coronal T1 Gd shows small midline mass adjacent to the skull base. This is moderately heterogeneous, mostly high signal, with multiple low signal foci. The mass, in general, appears isointense to other fatty structures

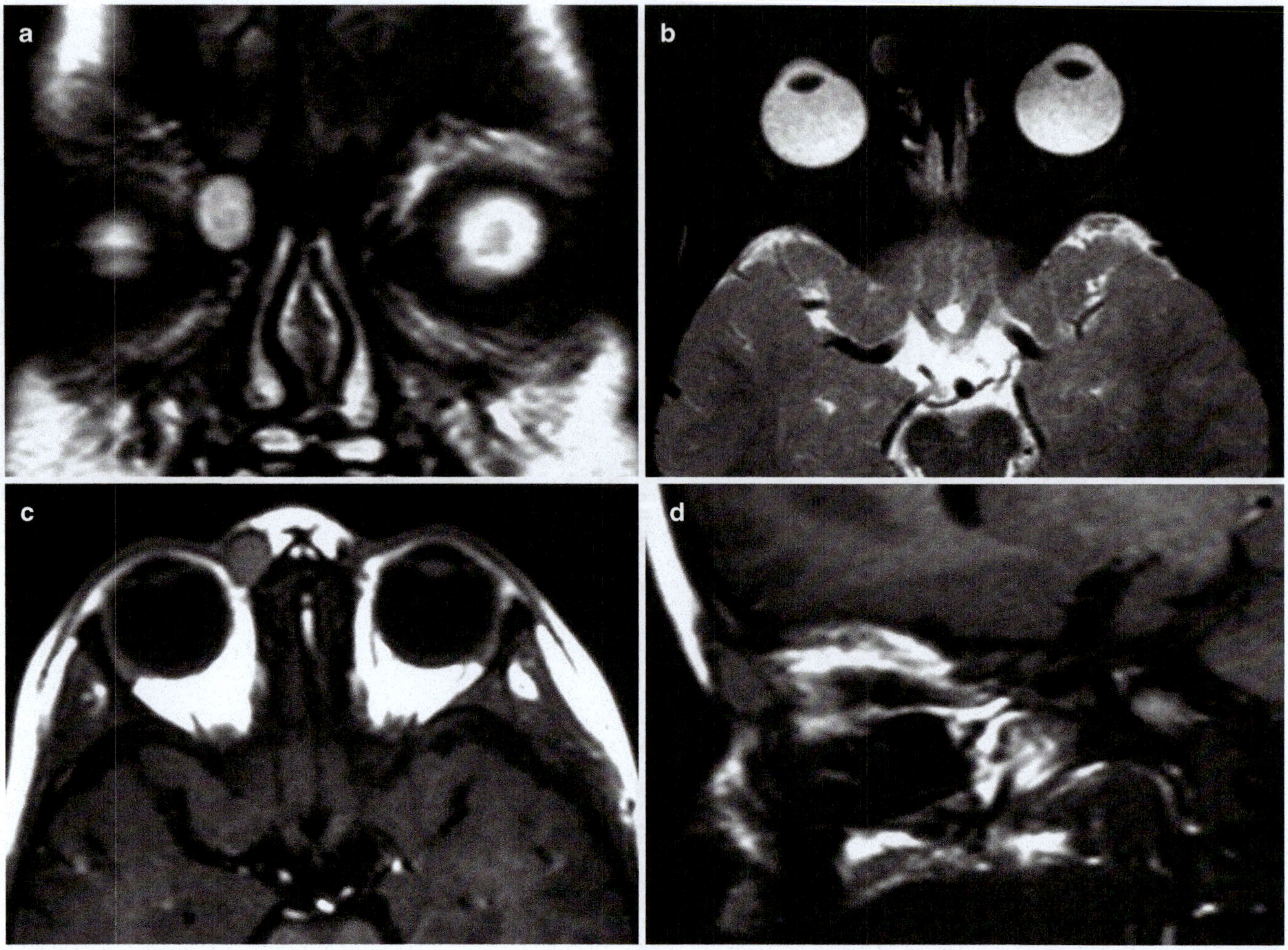

Fig. 19.4 (**a**) Coronal and (**b**) axial T2 images show ~1.5 × 2 cm abnormality with its epicenter ~2 cm lateral to the midline. Its peripheral signal follows CSF and the globes suggesting fluid surrounding a lower signal component. The lesion extends cranially to abut the skull base and laterally protruding into the right orbit. The asymmetric bright margin along the orbital aspect of the mass probably is related to chemical shift artifact and is better seen on the axial image. (**c**) Coronal and (**d**) sagittal T1 again demonstrate the paranasal mass. It is sharply circumscribed with a low signal capsule around its periphery clearly separating its internal contents from adjacent fat. Its T1 signal is mildly heterogeneous and its capsule is relatively isointense to bony cortex. This is a small nasal dermoid

Differential Diagnosis [2]

A. Teratomas

- Teratomas are tumors which contain all three germ layers: ectoderm, mesoderm, and endoderm. Dermoids (and epidermoids) exhibit exclusively ectoderm.
- In general, head and neck teratomas tend to be benign in children, whereas in adults they are mostly malignant.
- Most head and neck teratomas contain calcifications.
- Teratomas typically present as large complex masses.
- More mature teratomas contain fat and bone, while immature teratomas tend to have a more ambiguous appearance.
- Although rare, oronasal teratomas are more common than orbital teratomas following in frequency teratomas found near the thyroid.

B. Epidermoids

- They are frequently found around the skull and midface.
- On imaging, epidermoids and dermoids may be indistinguishable. More commonly *dermoids are midline*,

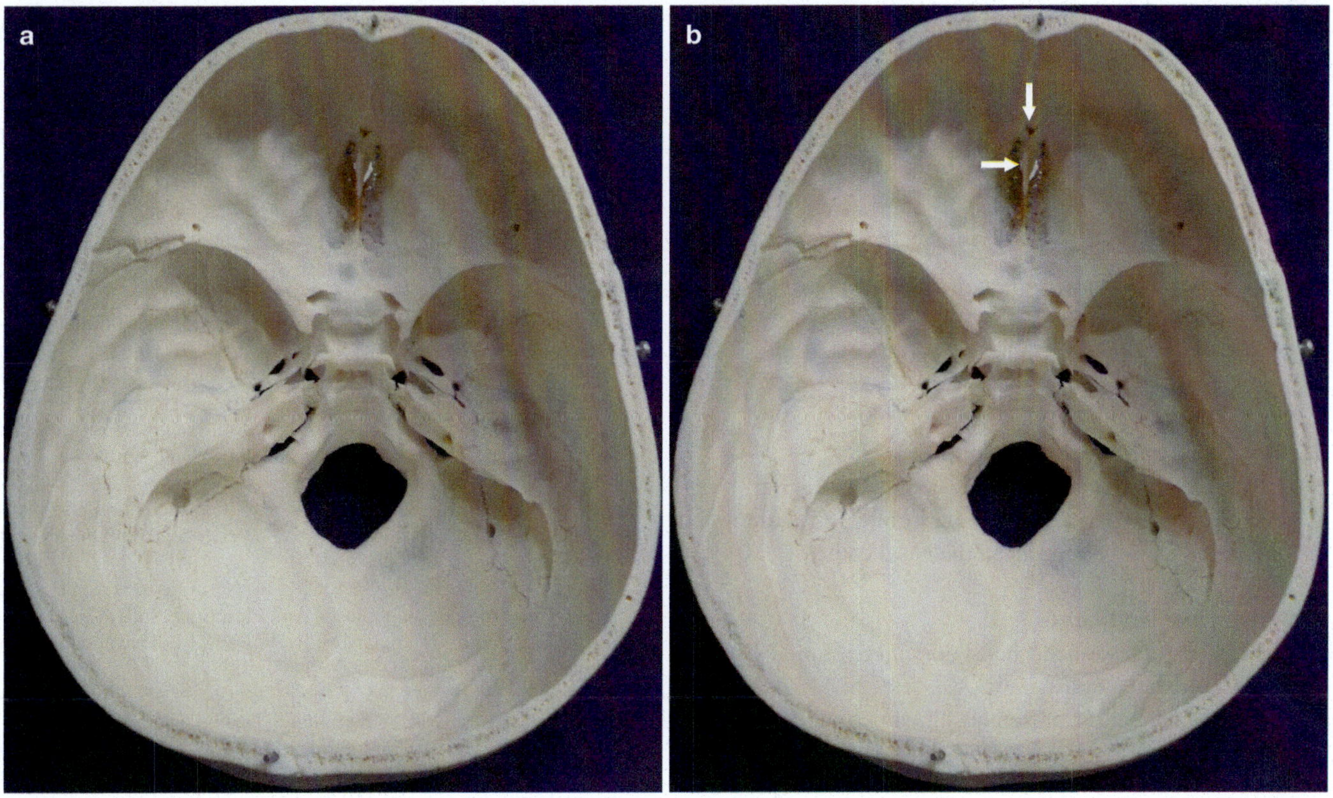

Fig. 19.5 Endocranial skull base (**a**) without and (**b**) with arrows (↓ = foramen cecum), → = crista galli)

whereas epidermoids are paramidline or involve the soft tissue portion of the nasal septum (columella nasi) [4].

- Epidermoids contain ectoderm with *NO* skin elements. [Dermoids contain ectoderm with skin elements.]
- CT attenuation varies depending on fat content commonly *showing fat with dermoids* and *fluid with epidermoids*.
- MRI signal varies with fluid content ranging from pure fluid isointense to CSF on T1 and T2 with epidermoids to a more complex intensity for dermoids (T1 hyperintense, T2 hypointense).
- A *key factor* here is that epidermoid cysts typically show *restricted diffusion* and are bright on DWI with a dark area on corresponding ADC map. By contrast, this feature is variably positive for dermoids [4].
- [See Chap. 9, CPA Epidermoids.]

C. Nasofrontal Encephalocele (NFE)

- Most encephaloceles are found soon after birth or even during fetal ultrasound.
- Children with transsphenoidal encephaloceles may present with nasal obstruction and are frequently occult until confronted by a nasoscope-carrying clinician.
- Frequently find midline CSF attenuation hypo-attenuating soft tissue mass with a thin wall which steadily scallops the adjacent intact bony cortex.
- T1 and T2 show fluid-filled midline abnormality outside the calvarium which is isointense to CSF. This can contain a component of brain which is isointense to intracranial brain.
- T1 Gd: Follows signal of the intracranial CSF and brain.
- DWI: Shows *no* restricted diffusion.
- [See Chap. 17, Nasofrontal Encephalocele.]

D. Nasal Glioma

- Congenital heterotopic non-neoplastic mass occurring near nasal root composed of dysplastic glial tissue.
- 15% connect to the brain by a stalk but *do not* communicate with CSF-filled subarachnoid space.
- Nasal gliomas are distinctly different from encephaloceles which do connect with the subarachnoid space and do contain CSF.
- Nasal gliomas are 30% intranasal, 60% extranasal, and 10% mixed.
- Nasal gliomas are usually isointense to brain on MRI.

- High-resolution surface coil MRI imaging is useful in demonstrating an intracranial stalk.
- [See Chap. 20, Nasal Glioma.]

A Closer Look

I. Genetics

- Patients with nasal dermoids often (41%) have craniofacial malformations [2, 9].
- Nasal dermoids are not normally associated with syndromes.

II. Fast Facts and Statistical Soup

- 7% of dermoids occur in the head and neck region.
- In the head and neck, 50% are periorbital, 25% are in the oral cavity, and 13% occur in the nasal cavity [2, 10].

III. Historical Highlights

- 1891: Cuvier described a nasal dorsum dermoid cyst with a hair-containing sinus.
- 1893: Bland-Sutton presented his superficial sequestration theory.
- 1910: Grunwald proposed the commonly accepted current theory which eventually evolved into the *prenasal theory of Pratt* and the *cranial theory by Bradley* [6].

Selected References

1. Castillo M, Mukherji SK. Imaging of facial anomalies. Curr Problems Diagnostic Imaging. 1996;15:169–88.
2. Valencia MP, Castillo M. Congenital and acquired lesions of the nasal septum: a practical guide for differential diagnosis. Radiographics. 2008;28(1):205–24. https://doi.org/10.1148/rg.281075049
3. Bilkay U, Gundogan H, Ozek C, et al. Nasal dermoid sinus cysts and the role of open rhinoplasty. Ann Plast Surg. 2001;47(1):8–14.
4. Kadom N, Sze RW. Radiological reasoning: pediatric midline nasofrontal mass. AJR 2010:194. https://doi.org/10.2214/AJR.07.7126; Downloaded from www.ajronline.org by 72.221.61.114 on 2/2/2016.
5. Paller AS, Pensler JM, Tomita T. Nasal midline masses in infants and children: dermoids, encephaloceles and gliomas. Arch Dermatol. 1991;127:362–6.
6. Rahbar R, Shah P, Mulliken JB, et al. The presentation and management of nasal dermoid, a 30 year experience. Arch Otolaryngol Head Neck Surg. 2003;120:464–71.
7. Bilkay U, Gundogan H, Ozek C, et al. Nasal dermoid sinus cysts and the role of open rhinoplasty. Ann Plast Surg. 2001;47(1):8–14.
8. Lowe LH, Booth TN, Joglar JM, Rollins NK. Midface anomalies in children. Radiographics. 2000;20:907–22.
9. Wardinsky TD, Pagon RA, Kropp RJ, et al. Nasal dermoid sinus cysts: association with intracranial extension and multiple malformations. Cleft Palate Craniofac J. 1991;28:87–95.
10. Kollias SS, Ball WS, Prenger EC, Myers CM. Dermoids of the eustachian tube: CT and MR findings with histologic correlation. AJNR Am J Neuroradiol. 1995;16:663–8.

Nasal Glioma

20

Pertinent Points

- *Definition:* Nasal gliomas (NGs) are congenital heterotopic non-neoplastic masses found near the nasal root in infants and children. Nasal gliomas are composed of dysplastic glial tissue.
- *AKA:* Intranasal glioma, nasal glial heterotopia, glial heterotopia, nasal cerebral heterotopia, and benign congenital nasal neuroectodermal tumor.
- *Classic Clue*: An infant presents with a nasal cavity mass, often arising medial to the middle turbinate, causing airway obstruction and occasionally tearing. The mass is isodense to brain on CT, bright on T2, with a *bifid crista galli* and a *prominent foramen cecum*. Unlike the encephalocele no CSF surrounds the lesion. (See Chap. 17, Fig. 17.3d.)
- *Incidence*: Rare with approximately 250 cases reported in the literature as of 2008 [7, 9]. They are more frequently found on board examinations or at high-level conferences.
- *Imaging Lite*: Nasal gliomas are usually isointense to brain on T1 and ↑ on T2.
- *Development*:
  - Nasal gliomas are composed of dysplastic glial cells which have habitually lost their intracranial connections and present as nasal masses.
  - We can compare nasal gliomas to nasoethmoidal encephaloceles as during development incomplete regression of the frontonasal diverticulum traps detached glial remnants in the prenasal space [1]. (See Chap. 17, Figs. 17.3d and 17.4e.)
  - A nasal glioma is like an encephalocele which contains brain tissue from extracranial entrapment, except nasal gliomas usually have no connection to intracranial brain and the trapped brain is habitually hamartomatous [1].
  - Nasal gliomas are distinctly different from encephaloceles which do connect with the subarachnoid space and do contain CSF [3].
- *Location*:
  - Nasal gliomas often occur near the nasal root with intranasal lesions manifesting medial to the middle turbinate. Extranasal gliomas are frequently found external to the airway in a paramedian position near the nasal arch [3].
  - 15% of NGs connect to the brain by a stalk but do NOT communicate with a CSF-filled subarachnoid space [3].
  - Nasal gliomas are 30% intranasal, 60% extranasal, and 10% mixed [3].

Imaging

General Imaging Features

- The foramen cecum may be deeper than normal.
- The crista galli may be small or bifid.
- The anterior border of the nasal septum may be truncated or deformed by larger lesions.
- May appear intranasal (30%), extranasal (60%), or mixed (10%).
- Extranasal gliomas form from failed fusion of the fonticulus frontalis [1].
- Most nasal gliomas do not show significant growth. However, some 15% continue to be connected to the brain via a thin trunk and exhibit growth equivalent to the brain [3].

CT Features [5]

- *See General Imaging Features.*
- The nasal septum is usually intact but has a tendency to be truncated by large lesions [1].

F. A. Midyett, S. K. Mukherji, *Skull Base Imaging*, https://doi.org/10.1007/978-3-030-46447-9_20

- Although the anterior cranial fossa floor may appear intact, subtle signs sometimes suggest otherwise.
- A *bifid crista galli*, as well as widening of the foramen cecum or crista galli suggests an occult intracranial connection.
- Nasal gliomas are usually isodense to brain.
- Calcifications are *rarely reported* with nasal gliomas.
- Nasal gliomas sometimes show cystic changes.
- CT cisternography may be required to demonstrate the extent of the CSF space.
- Nasal gliomas are typically medial to the middle turbinate.

MRI Features [1]

- *See General Imaging Features.*
- MRIs superior soft tissue enhancement makes it the imaging modality of choice for assessing nasal gliomas [2, 3].
- T1: Shows intermediate signal intensity [1]. See Fig. 20.1c, d which also shows high signal from focal fat.
- T2: Shows ↑ signal secondary to gliosis [1]. See Fig. 20.1e.
- T1 Gd:
  - Non-enhancing to slightly enhancing [9]. See Fig. 20.1f, g.
- Sometimes shows a tract extending from a nasal glioma to the anterior skull base [1].
- High-resolution surface coil imaging is important to illustrate an intracranial stalk [3].
- MRI can currently be performed in the prenatal period for diagnosis and pre-surgical planning [9].

Ultrasound

- Nasal gliomas are sometimes seen during incidental prenatal US.
- US may be helpful in determining whether the mass is cystic or solid [2].
- Doppler shows characteristic low arterial flow velocity during end diastole [2].

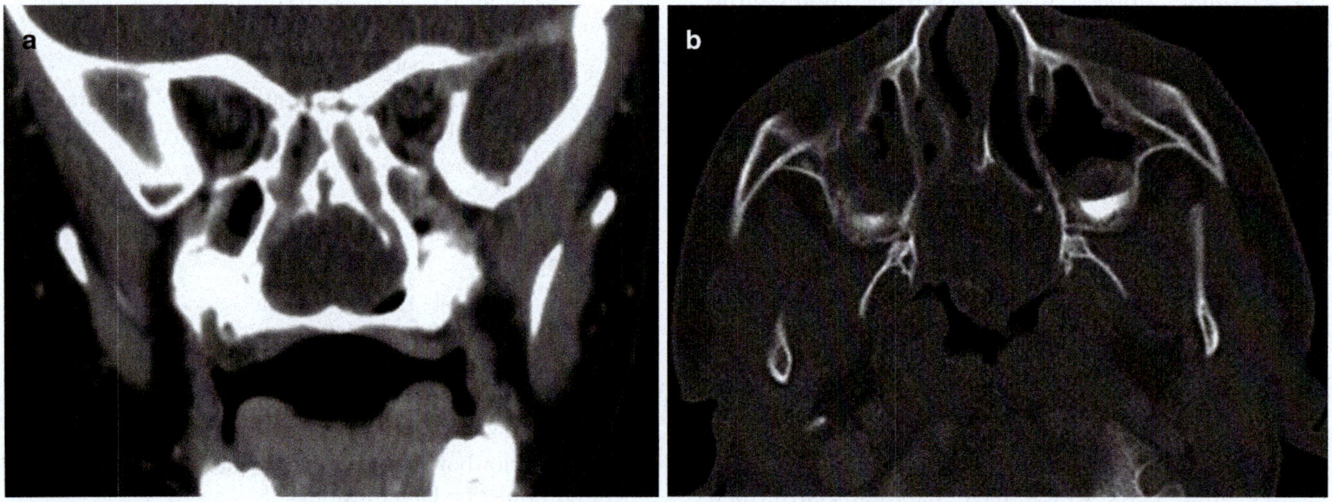

Fig. 20.1 (**a**) Coronal CECT soft tissue algorithm shows large (~ 3 × 4 cm) mass splaying the lower nasal septum extending caudally to abut the hard palate. Attenuation is relatively isodense to brain. (**b**) Axial bone algorithm CECT again shows large mass which has enlarged the nasopharynx causing bowing and sclerosis of adjacent bone. There is a remnant of a small bony "fork" at the remaining septum anteriorly. The mass clearly compromises the airway. The posterior margins of the nasolacrimal canals appear dehiscent. Nasal gliomas are known to block the nasolacrimal ducts causing tearing

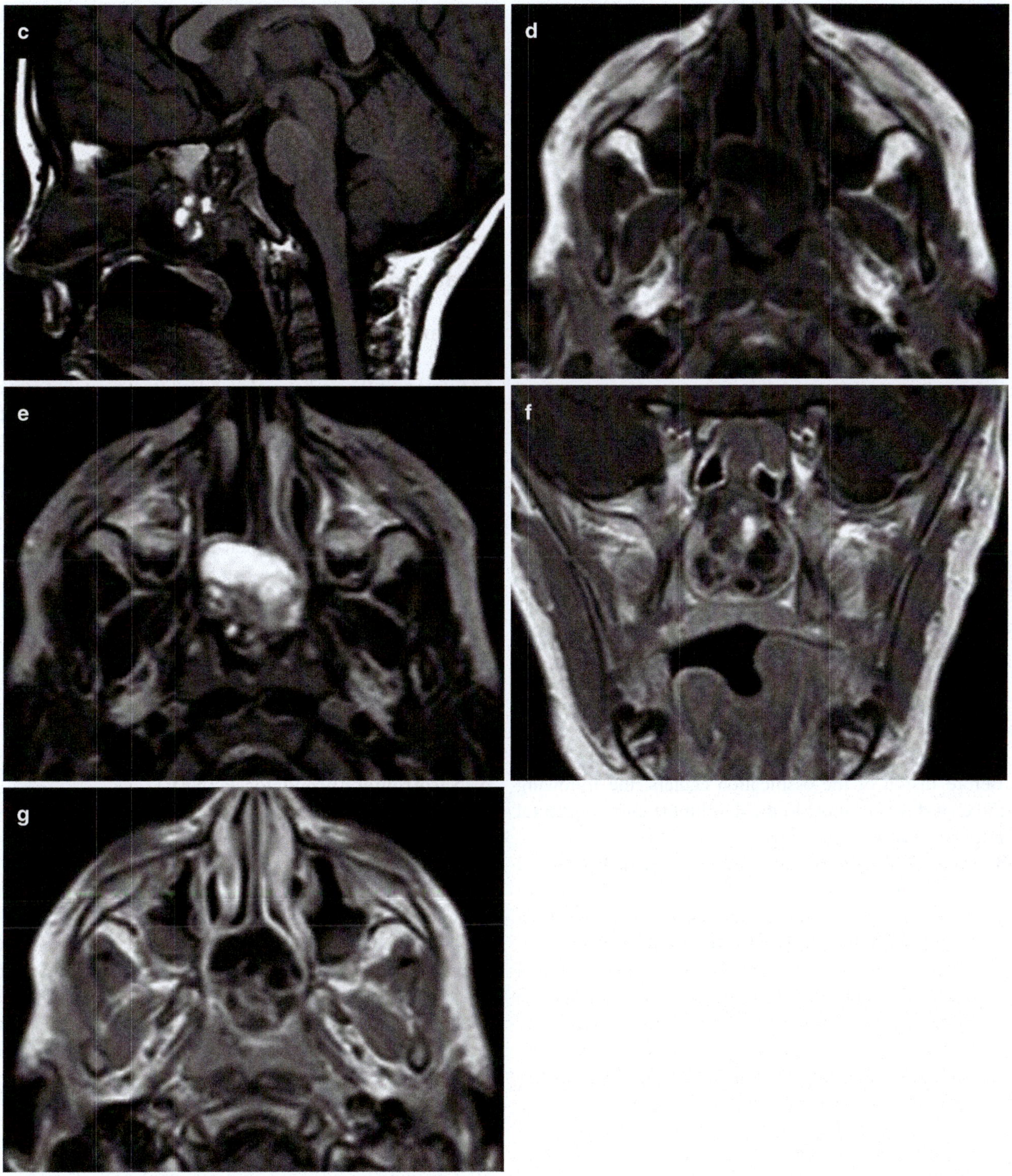

Fig. 20.1 (continued) (**c**) Sagittal T1 depicts a huge heterogeneous nasopharyngeal mass. The core components are homogeneous with brain. There are, however, multiple foci of bright signal which appear isointense to fat specifically when compared to the crista galli marrow. The mass extends cranially to abut the (dark) cortex of the anterior cranial fossa, which appears intact on this image. The mass extends caudally to abut the hard and soft palates. The large area of low signal fluid anteriorly and inferiorly is isointense to CSF and is shown on the next image axial imaging set. It extends posteriorly into the basosphenoid portion of the clivus. No clear cortex is demonstrated in the basosphenoid clivus anteriorly and superiorly as is clearly seen in the more posterior and caudal basiocciput below the spheno-occipital synchondrosis. Axial T1 (**d**) and T2 (**e**) show a huge nasopharyngeal mass that contains loculated fluid components which are predominantly low on T1 and high on T2 consistent with fluid. Solid components are isointense to brain. One small hyperintense area on the T1 (**d**) probably represents proteinaceous fluid. (**f**) Coronal T1 Gd shows huge heterogeneous mass extending cranially into the sphenoid sinuses, to abut the floor of the anterior cranial fossa which appears on this image to be intact. It extends caudally to abut the hard palate. It shows multiple enhancing septa but, in general, remains relatively isointense to brain except for a central area of high intensity which probably represents proteinaceous fluid. (**g**) Axial T1 Gd shows a huge heterogeneous mass extending anteriorly to the nasal septum and posteriorly into the clivus. The anterior 1/3 of the mass contains a low signal fluid collection. The posterior 2/3 contains multiple enhancing septa which separate low signal fluid collections

Clinical Issues

Presentation

- Nasal gliomas present during infancy or childhood as large, firm, red to bluish submucosal masses extending toward the nostril.
- Nasal gliomas don't demonstrate pulsation or enlargement with a Valsalva maneuver [9].
- Typically, nasal gliomas don't grow much unless they have an intracranial connection.
- They can cause airway obstruction, respiratory compromise, epiphora (from obstruction of the nasolacrimal duct), CSF rhinorrhea, epistaxis, and meningitis.

Embryology

- The neural tube develops during the third and fourth gestational weeks.
- Neural tube closure begins at its midportion extending caudally and cranially.
- With neural tube closure, neural crest cells migrate anteriorly and laterally around the eyes to the frontonasal prominence.
- The nose develops from the frontonasal processes and two nasal placodes.
- During formation of the skull base and nose, mesenchymal structures form from several ossification centers.
- Before fusion of the ossification centers, the following three spaces contribute to the development of congenital midline nasal masses.
  1. *Fonticulus frontalis*: The space between the frontal and nasal bones.
  2. *Prenasal space:* Between the nasal bones and nasal capsule (precursor of nasal septum and cartilages).
  3. *Foramen cecum*. This is located in the anterior cranial fossa, anterior to the ethmoid cribriform plate and the crista galli, posterior to the frontal bone. Frequently found to be patent in infants and uncommonly patent in children, it is only open in <1.5% of adults. It rarely transmits emissary veins to the nasal cavity (see Fig. 19.4a, b). See Chap. 51, Sect. A3/Foramen Cecum.

Pathology

- Gross: Firm, noncompressible, reddish blue to purple lesion occurring near the nasal root or bridge.
- Microscopic:
  - Integration with immunohistologic studies provides definitive documentation of NG [2].
  - Shows unencapsulated rests of astrocytes and neuroglial fibers embedded in fibrovascular connective tissue stroma [4].
  - Sometimes see multinucleated giant cells but mitotic figures are rare or absent.
  - Occasionally find focal calcifications [9].
  - Immunohistochemical demonstration of S100 protein and GFAP show a high specificity for neuroglial cells.

Treatment

Surgery

- Surgery is the archetypal standard treatment, but remember the caveat – don't biopsy before imaging. Preoperative imaging evaluation is essential to exclude intracranial extension.
- Surgical strategies depend on location and lesion extent.
- Surgeons require radiologists to separate nasal gliomas from encephaloceles which require an altered approach [4].
- Surgical risks include meningitis, recurrence, and CSF leaks.
- See Chap. 27, Skull Base CSF Leaks

Differential Diagnosis [1]

A. Nasofrontal Encephalocele (NFE)

- Most encephaloceles are found soon after birth or even during prenatal fetal ultrasound.
- Children with transsphenoidal encephaloceles may present with nasal obstruction and are frequently occult until first found by a clinician carrying a nasoscope.
- Often see midline hypo-attenuating soft tissue mass with a thin wall which often scallops an adjacent intact bony cortex.
- T1 and T2 show a fluid-filled midline abnormality outside the calvarium which is isointense to CSF. This can contain a component of brain which is isointense to intracranial brain.
- T1 Gd: Follows signal of intracranial CSF and brain.
- DWI: Shows *no* restricted diffusion.
- A pedicle is almost always present with encephaloceles but is uncommon with nasal gliomas [6].
- Furstenberg Sign: The size of encephaloceles frequently fluctuate from changes in intracranial pressure. By contrast, nasal gliomas should not change size during a Valsalva maneuver. This relates to absence of a patent connection to the CNS [9].
- See Chap. 17, Nasofrontal Encephalocele

B. Teratomas

- Teratomas are tumors which contain all three germ layers: ectoderm, mesoderm, and endoderm. Dermoids (and epidermoids) exhibit exclusively ectoderm.
- In general, H&N teratomas tend to be benign in children whereas in adults are mostly malignant.
- Most head and neck teratomas contain calcifications.
- Teratomas typically present as large complex masses.
- More mature teratomas contain fat and bone, while immature teratomas tend to conceal themselves with more ambiguous appearances.
- Although rare, oronasal teratomas are more common than orbital teratomas following in frequency teratomas found near the thyroid.

C. Epidermoids and Dermoids

- Frequently found in various locations around skull and midface.
- On imaging, epidermoids and dermoids may be indistinguishable. More commonly *dermoids are midline, whereas epidermoids are paramidline* or involve the soft tissue portion of the nasal septum (columella nasi) [5].
- Epidermoids contain ectoderm with *no* skin elements. Dermoids contain ectoderm with skin elements.
- CT attenuation varies depending on fat content commonly *showing fat with dermoids* and *fluid with epidermoids*.
- MRI signal varies with fluid content ranging from pure fluid isointense to CSF on T1 and T2 with epidermoids to a more complex intensity for dermoids (T1 hyperintense, T2 hypointense).
- A *key factor* here is that epidermoid cysts typically show *restricted diffusion* and are bright on DWI with a dark area on corresponding ADC map. By contrast, this feature is variably positive for dermoids [5].
- See Chap. 19, Nasal Dermoid

A Closer Look

I. Genetics

- The PAX3 gene which is involved in neural tube closure has ↑ susceptibility to neural tube defects with folate restriction [8].

II. Fast Facts and Statistical Soup

- Congenital midline nasal masses occur in one in 30,000 live births.
- Nasal gliomas account for 5% of all congenital nasal masses.
- The term "nasal glioma" is actually a muddling misnomer for a benign congenital abnormality which is not really a "brain tumor."
- Current developmental theories include:
  - A. Sequestration of glial tissue trapped by the olfactory bulb during cribriform plate fusion.
  - B. Ectopic neural tissue cells.
  - C. Encephalocele which lost its intracranial and meningeal connections.
  - D. Inappropriate closure of the anterior neuropore (fonticulus frontalis).
- Whichever of these theses turns out to be the "true theory" will probably be just fine with the average radiologist who didn't really have a dog in this fight anyway.

III. Historical Highlights.

- 1900 Schmidt first described the nasal glioma.

Selected References

1. Valencia MP, Castillo M. Congenital and acquired lesions of the nasal septum: a practical guide for differential diagnosis. Radiographics. 2008;28(1):205–23. https://doi.org/10.1148/rg.281075049.
2. Dasgupta NR, Bentz ML. Nasal gliomas: identification and differentiation from hemangiomas. J Craniofac Surg. 2003;14(5):736–8.
3. Moron FE, Morriss MC, Jones JJ, Hunter JJ. Lumps and Bumps on the head in children: use of CT and MR imaging in solving the clinical diagnostic dilemma. Radiographics. 2004;24(6):1655–74. https://doi.org/10.1148/rg.246045034.
4. Penner CR, Thompson L. Nasal glial heterotopia: a clinicopathologic and immunophenotypic analysis of 10 cases with a review of the literature. Ann Diagn Pathol. 2003;7(6):354–9.
5. Kadom N, Sze RW. Radiological reasoning: pediatric midline nasofrontal mass. AJR. 2010;194. https://doi.org/10.2214/AJR.07.7126; Downloaded from www.ajronline.org by 72.221.61.114 on 2/2/2016.
6. Shah J, Patkar D, Patankar T, Krishnan A, Prasad S, Limdi J. Pedunculated nasal glioma: MRI features and review of the literature. J Postgrad Med. 1999;45:15.
7. Niedzielska G, Niedzielska A, Kotowski M. Nasal ganglioma-difficulties in radiological imaging. Int J Pediatr Otorhinolaryngol. 2008;72(2):285–7.
8. Burren KA, Savery D, Massa V, et al. Gene-environment interactions in the causation of neural tube defects: folate deficiency increases susceptibility conferred by loss of PAX3 function. Hum Mol Genet. 2008;17(23):3675–85.
9. Olubunmi Ajose-Popoola BA, Lin HW, Silvera VM, et al. Nasal glioma: prenatal diagnosis and multidisciplinary surgical approach. Skull Base Rep. 2011;1(2):83–8. https://doi.org/10.1055/s-0031-1284210. Accessed 2/3/2016.

Paranasal Sinus Mucoceles

21

Pertinent Points

- *Definition:* Mucoceles are space-occupying masses filled with secretions stemming from blockage of a sinus drainage passageway. They are surrounded by mucus secreting epithelium.
- *Classic Clue*: Large mass whose epicenter is usually co-located with a paranasal sinus, showing signs of slow growth with expansion, remodeling, and thinning of sinus walls. MRI signal is frequently bright on T1 and T2 parading *peripheral* T1 Gd *rim enhancement*.
- *Location:* 90% occur in frontal or ethmoid sinuses. Less frequently found in sphenoid and maxillary sinuses.
- *AKA:* Mucoceles, paranasal sinus mucocele, mucocele of paranasal sinus.
- Mucoceles develop when the ostium draining a sinus (or septated sinus) is obstructed.
- *Contributing Causes:* Risk factors for mucoceles include sinusitis, allergies, and trauma including instrumentation.
- *Incidence*: There are no reliable incidence figures. Japan reports an elevated incidence of maxillary sinus mucoceles following radical sinus surgery for sinusitis.
- *Pitfall*: While MRI signal varies with concentration of water and protein, signal is *often bright on both T1 and T2. When signal is dark on both T1 and T2, this may present a pitfall* particularly when MRI is the only imaging study as dark signal may be confused with a normal air-containing sinus.
- Associations: Cystic fibrosis, particularly when found in children [2]. Aside from children with cystic fibrosis, the median age for mucoceles is approximately 53 years [4].

Imaging

General Imaging Features

- Typically expansile, slow-growing lesions related to the paranasal sinuses.
- Sometimes show signs of recurrent sinusitis with sinus wall thickening.
- The affected sinus is completely filled.
- CT and MRI are complimentary for this entity:
  - CT findings which best demonstrate sinus wall changes include:
    - Expansion
    - Remodeling
    - Thinning
    - Dehiscence (more often seen with large mucoceles)
  - MRI
    - Best detects mucocele's interface with intracranial and intraorbital structures.
    - T1 Gd is very useful in showing *peripheral rim enhancement* of *mucocele* (as contrasted to *solid enhancement of neoplasm*).
    - See Fig. 21.1f.

CT Features [5]

- *See General Imaging Features.*
- Mucocele contents vary from water-like to hyperdense dehydrated tenacious secretions (See Fig. 21.2a, b).
- The material within these expansile lesions is frequently hyperdense on soft tissue algorithms of NECT because of its mucoid material.
- Peripheral calcifications are *sometimes seen* [1].

F. A. Midyett, S. K. Mukherji, *Skull Base Imaging*, https://doi.org/10.1007/978-3-030-46447-9_21

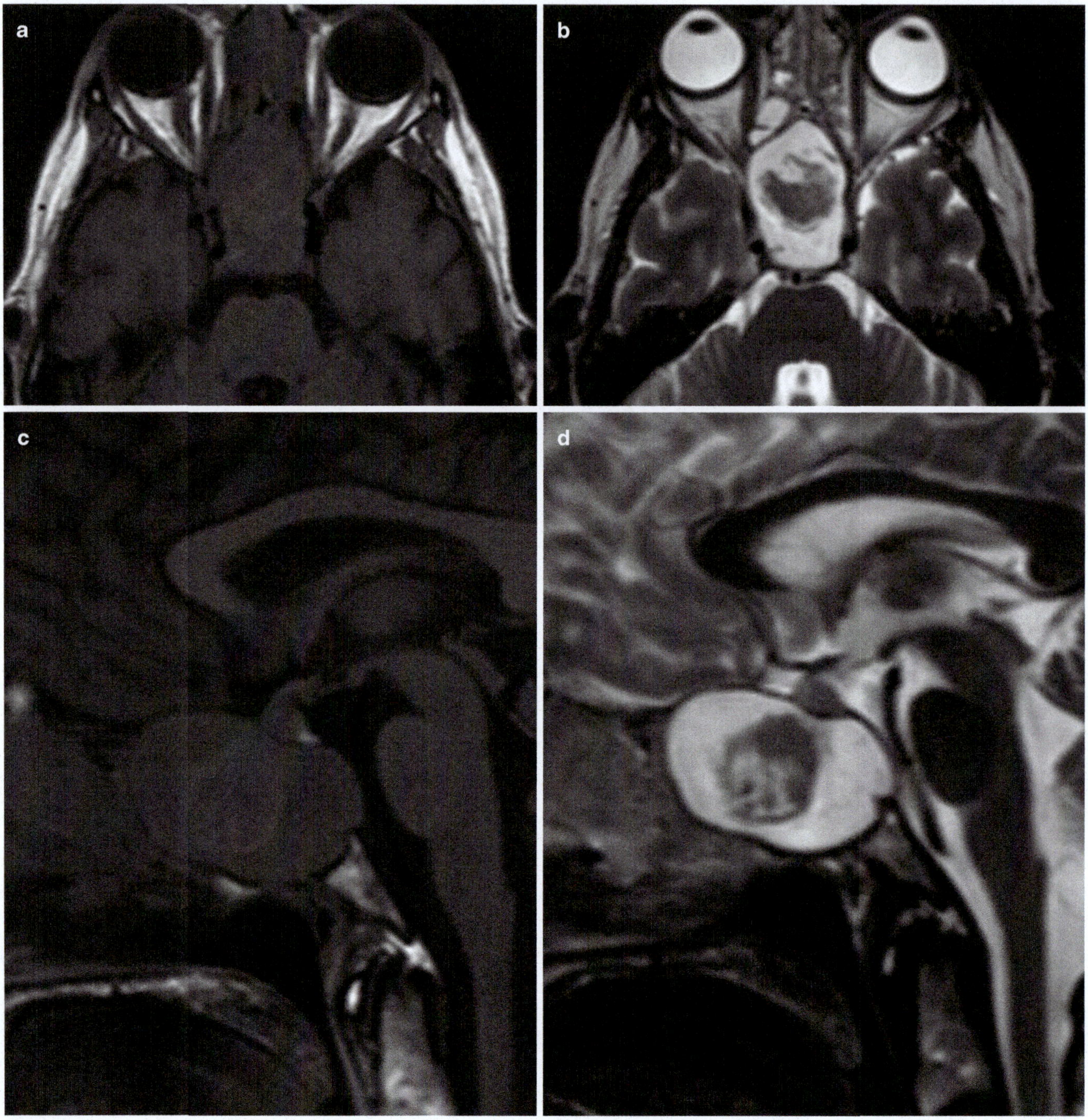

Fig. 21.1 (**a**) Axial T1 shows a large (~ *2.5 × 4 cm)* mass involving the central and anterior skull base. It is mildly heterogeneous and relatively isointense to brain. It protrudes laterally to the carotid siphons and posteriorly almost touching the basilar artery (black flow void). It expands anteriorly encroaching on the orbital apices along the planum sphenoidale. (**b**) Axial T2 confirms the position of the mass described on T1 (**a**). The mass is filled with fluid which has ↑ T2 signal roughly isointense to CSF and globes. Centrally, it contains debris with ↓T2 signal. There is similar fluid in adjacent ethmoid sinuses. (**c**) Sagittal T1 depicts a huge mass which has almost obliterated the basisphenoid down to the spheno-occipital synchondrosis which appears to have survived the devastation inflicted on its northern neighbor. The mass appears to be wearing the pituitary like a crown, displacing it cranially with the sellar floor partially dehiscent. Again, shown within the mass center is higher signal from internal debris courtesy of an occupying fungal colony. (**d**) Sagittal T2 depicts the huge mass occupying the basisphenoid clivus, with an epicenter suggesting the sphenoid sinus is its home. It wears the pituitary like a crown and contains the heterogeneous debris from the "friendly" fungal colony. It is surrounded by a distinct low signal layer of mucus-secreting epithelium

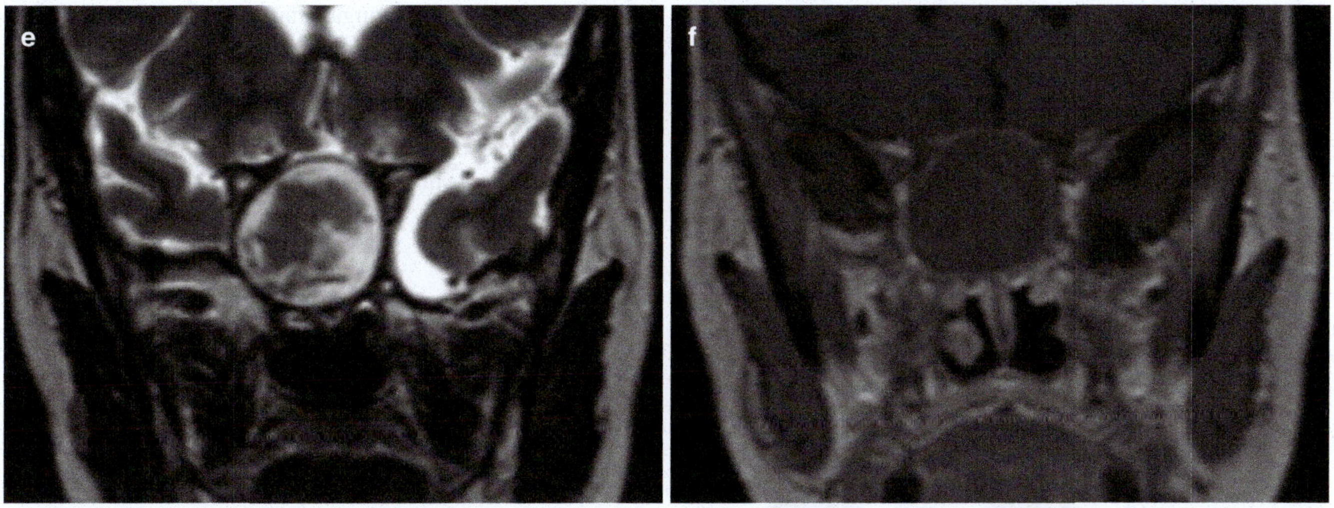

Fig. 21.1 (continued) (**e**) Coronal T2 depicts a well-circumscribed central mass surrounded by a low signal layer of mucus-secreting epithelium. Lateral enlargement contacts the temporal fossa contents. Cephalic extension elevates intracranial structures while caudal expansion encroaches on the adjacent airway below. T2 signal fluid is high like CSF but includes central low signal debris from the fungal colony. (**f**) Coronal T1 Gd depicts moderate *rim enhancement* of the wall surrounding the mass corresponding to low signal seen on other sequences, particularly on the previous coronal T2 (**e**). The internal signal is predominately isointense to brain with scattered ↑ T1 signal related to internal fungal debris

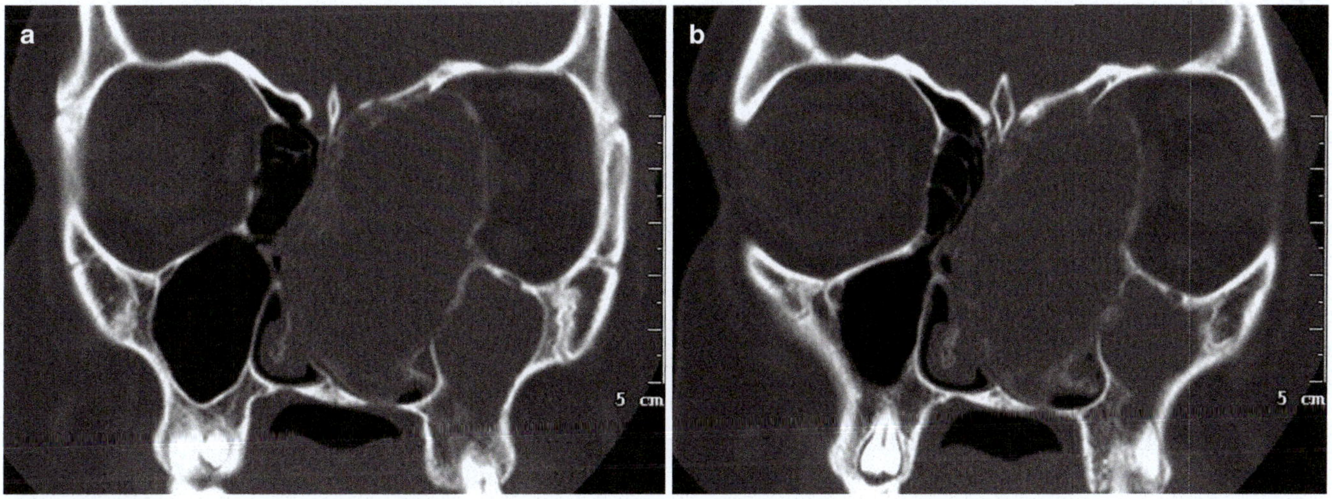

Fig. 21.2 (**a**, **b**) Coronal NECT (from a different case) shows a huge mucocele which has grown from its humble ethmoidal beginnings to fill the left nasal cavity displacing the nasal septum. It has taken territory from the left orbit as well as left maxillary and frontal sinuses. And, it did all this using basic nonmalignant techniques which most mucoceles have definitely mastered: expansion, remodeling, thinning, and dehiscence

- Paranasal sinus hyperdensity suggests inspissated secretions, fungal disease, or hemorrhage. By contrast *tumor is not hyperdense* on NECT.

MRI Features

- *See General Imaging Features.*
- T1 signal varies depending on content:
  - Water-rich content: ↓ T1 signal (most frequent)
  - Protein-rich content: ↑ T1 signal
- T2 signal varies depending on content:
  - Water-rich content: ↑ T2 signal (most frequent)
  - Protein-rich content: ↓ T1 signal
- T1 Gd: Shows moderate *peripheral enhancement* of mucus secreting epithelial mass wall (See Fig. 21.1f).
- DWI: Variable, so not particularly helpful.
- Although the *MRI signal varies with concentration of water and protein*, internal material observed as hyperdense on CT is often heterogeneously hyperintense on T1 and T2 MRI.
- Frequently found fungal components have heterogeneous amorphous shape showing ↑ CECT attenuation and ↑ T1 and ↓ T2 signal (See Fig. 21.1b–e).
- Protein content causing diversely different MR signals is depicted by the following table.

MRI of sinus secretions [8]		
Protein content	T1 signal	T2 signal
<10%	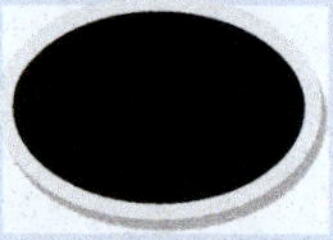	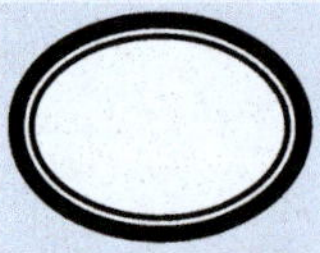
20–25%	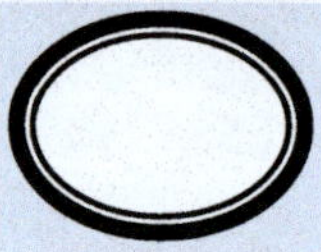	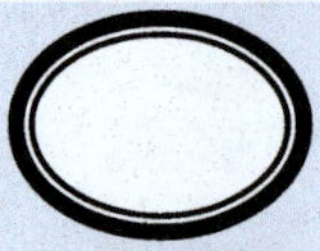
>25%	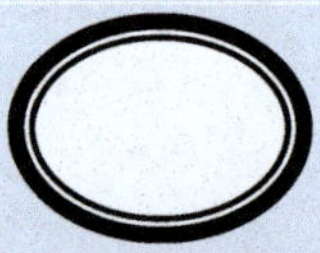	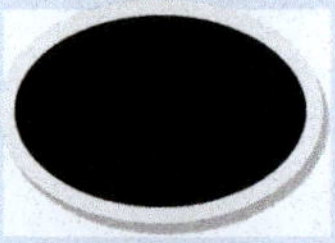
>28%	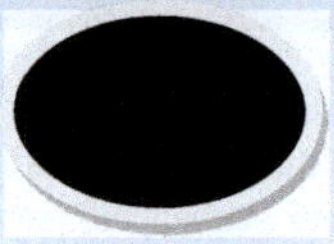	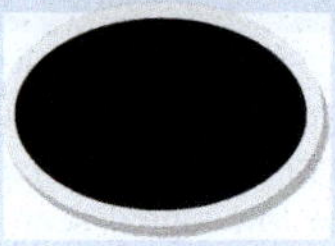

Clinical Issues

Presentation

- Symptoms, when present, mirror the mass location:
  - Orbital involvement can cause pain, diplopia, proptosis, or visual impairment.
  - Encroachment on the pituitary and brainstem can cause confusion, headache, syncope, vertigo, visual symptoms, and cranial nerve symptoms.
  - Frontal sinus involvement with osteomyelitis and Pott's puffy tumor can cause recurrent fever, headache, periorbital swelling, photophobia, eye movement discomfort, scalp pain, nuchal rigidity, and purulent eye discharge [3].
  - Complications include mucopyocele as well as intraorbital or intracranial involvement more frequently follow prior sinus wall fractures.

Embryology

- Associations: Cystic fibrosis, particularly when found in children [2].

Pathology

- Usually result from obstructed sinus ostium from inflammation, trauma, or mass causing mucus accumulation which expands the sinus.
- Chronic noninvasive fungal sinusitis has also been associated with mucocele formation (See Chap. 32, Allergic Fungal Sinusitis).
- Gross: While content is variable, most simple mucoceles contain clear thick mucus. With prior infection, the contents can seem similar to pus.

Treatment

Surgery

- Most mucoceles are currently treated by an endonasal endoscopic or a combined transfacial/endonasal approach.
- Endoscopic surgery sometimes supplies seemingly simple solutions for multifaceted mucoceles.
- However, there remains an almost 25% post-surgical mucocele recurrence rate in patients who have had multiple surgical procedures with chronic sinusitis [4].

Differential Diagnosis [1]

A. Pituitary Adenoma

- Typically see sellar expansion, erosion, and remodeling.
- Usually see combined sellar and suprasellar mass with "waist" at the sellar diaphragm.
- Characteristic "figure of eight" or "Biker on Harley" appearance on coronal or sagittal imaging.
- Usually homogeneously isointense on both T1 and T2 (except with hemorrhage).
- Habitually have a solid mass with moderate homogeneous enhancement on T1 Gd.
- When pituitary adenomas are cystic or have both cystic and solid components, they can be confusing.
- *A cystic pituitary adenoma with rim enhancement can be very similar to a mucocele.*
- See Chap. 2, Pituitary Adenoma, Fig. 2.4a–f.

B. Craniopharyngioma

- Like liquids in your automobile, the varying viscosity of craniopharyngioma's cystic fluid fluctuates from yellowish proteinaceous fluid to classic 'crank-case oil' containing cholesterol and blood by-products.
- Craniopharyngiomas often have mixed cystic and enhancing solid components. Except for *peripheral rim enhancement*, mucoceles are non-enhancing with *no* solid components. Mucoceles are cystic but can contain internal amorphous debris, particularly when harboring a fungus colony.

- Craniopharyngiomas are often calcified. Mucoceles may occasionally present peripheral calcifications [1].
- Craniopharyngiomas often infiltrate adjacent structures on MRI. Not a feature for mucoceles.
- Craniopharyngiomas can occasionally enlarge and/or erode the sella. Craniopharyngiomas commonly emanate from above, while mucoceles habitually hail from below.
- See Chap. 3, Craniopharyngioma.

C. Rathke's Cleft Cyst (RCC)
- RCC usually does not erode the sella. Sphenoid mucoceles sometimes destroy the sella from below (See Fig. 21.1c, d).
- Cystic pituitary adenoma may be difficult to distinguish from RCC (See Fig. 2.4a–f).
- See Chap. 1, Rathke's Cleft Cyst.

D. Intrasellar Arachnoid Cyst
- Characteristic arachnoid-like, thin transparent, cyst walls are barely seen on imaging. By contrast, the mucocele's epithelial wall is well defined (See Fig. 21.1d–f).
- CT attenuation in Hounsfield units is identical to CSF for intrasellar arachnoid cysts. CT attenuation of mucoceles is frequently hyperdense.
- Intrasellar arachnoid cysts often show suprasellar extension.
- Intrasellar arachnoid cysts show no hemorrhage or calcification. Mucoceles sometimes show peripheral calcifications.
- Intrasellar arachnoid cysts are usually isointense to CSF on T1, T2, and T1 Gd with *no enhancement*. Mucoceles characteristically demonstrate peripheral rim enhancement on T1 Gd (See Fig. 21.1f).
- Intrasellar arachnoid cysts typically arise in the sella sparing the sphenoid sinus below. By contrast, mucoceles arise within the sinus sometimes extending superiorly into the sella (See Fig. 21.1c, d).
- See Chap. 7, Intrasellar Arachnoid Cyst.

E. Inverted Papilloma (IP)
- Moderately advanced tumors commonly show a unilateral nasal fossa mass with opacification of the contiguous maxillary sinus.
- Inverted papillomas most commonly occur on the lateral nasal cavity wall, more frequently found near the middle turbinate and maxillary ostium.
- Enlargement of the mass results in bony remodeling and resorption as it extends into the maxillary antrum.
- Commonly obstructs the maxillary antrum drainage, but oddly enough, concomitant *mucoceles are rare.*
- CT: *Hyperostosis* is *highly predictive* of tumor origin site.
- Combined bony sclerosis and deformity with an antromeatal mass suggests a slow growing tumor such as IP.
- MRI:
  - T1: Iso- to slightly hyperintense to muscle.
  - T2: Iso- to hyperintense to muscle often showing alternating hypointense lines constituting CCP (*convoluted cerebriform pattern*)
  - T1 Gd: Heterogeneous enhancement often showing alternating hypointense lines constituting CCP (*convoluted cerebriform pattern*)
  - See Chap. 14, Inverted Papilloma.

F. Esthesioneuroblastoma (ENB)
- AKA: Olfactory neuroblastoma.
- Rare neuroendocrine malignancy of neural crest origin arising from olfactory epithelium.
- Newer genetic information suggests that ENB is a distinct entity not belonging to primitive peripheral neuroectodermal tumor-Ewing's tumor (pPNETs-ETs). This suggests that ENB is *not* a NEC.
- Classically shows avidly enhancing dumbbell-shaped mass with "waist" at the cribriform plate.
- May involve the anterior cranial fossa, skull base, and orbit.
- ENBs show intermediate signal on T1 and T2.
- Cystic areas (with foci of ↑T2) at tumor/brain interface are diagnostic and may be pathognomonic. By contrast, mucoceles *are* completely cystic although they may contain internal debris.
- ENBs exhibit avid enhancement on T1 Gd. (Mucoceles show *only* peripheral rim enhancement.)
- *ENB exhibits moderate restricted diffusion on DWI.* By contrast, DWI is variable with mucoceles.
- See Chap. 28, Esthesioneuroblastoma.

G. Allergic Fungal Sinusitis (AFS)
- Young immunocompetent patient from the Southwestern United States presents with therapy-resistant chronic sinusitis.
- Hypo-attenuation on T2 MRI corresponds to *distinctive hyperdense sinus* with *characteristic serpiginous* pattern.
- While AFS starts in the sinus, it may have already invaded the skull base before it presents for imaging.
- See Chap. 32, Allergic Fungal Sinusitis.

A Closer Look

I. Associations
- Cystic fibrosis, particularly when found in children [2].

II. Fast Facts

- Paranasal sinus mucoceles *usually* develop following obstruction of the sinus ostium.
- *Rarely*, they develop when a distended mucous gland (submucosal retention cyst) fills the entire sinus.
- For imaging purposes, *submucosal retention cysts fill only a part of the sinus* while paranasal sinus mucoceles *fill the entire sinus* [7].

III. Historical Highlights

- 1820 Langeback was first to describe paranasal sinus mucoceles.
- 1900s Rollet and Gerber named and popularized them publishing 178 cases of PNS mucoceles.
- 1995 Lambert credited mucoceles for being the most common condition causing proptosis [5, 6].

Selected References

1. Mafee MF, Valvassori GE, Becker M. Imaging of the head and neck. New York, NY: George Thieme Verlag; 2004. ISBN:1588900096.
2. Guttenplan MD, Wetmore RF. Paranasal sinus mucocele in cystic fibrosis. Clin Pediatr Philadelphia. 1989;28(9):429–30.
3. Midyett FA, Mukherji SK. Chapter 46: Pott's puffy tumor. In: Orbital imaging. Philadelpshia: Elsevier/Saunders; 2015. p. 215–9. ISBN : 978-0-323-34037-3.
4. Devars du Mayne M, Moya-Plana A, Malinvaud D, et al. Sinus mucocele: natural history and long-term recurrence rate. Eur Ann Otorhinolaryngol Head Neck Dis. 2012;129(3):125–30. https://doi.org/10.1016/j.anorl.2011.10,002. Epub 2012 Jan 5.
5. Gendeh BS. Chapter 23. Paranasal sinus mucoceles-opthalmic manifestations, radiological imaging, endoscopic endonasal marsupilization and outcome. In: Opthalmology- current clinical and research updates. p. 567–93. https://doi.org/10.5772/58331.
6. Alberti PW, Marshall HF, Black JI. Fronto-ethmoidalmucocele as a cause of unilateral proptosis. Br J Ophthalmol. 1968;52:833–8.
7. Van Tassel P, Lee YY, Jing BS, De Pena CA. Mucoceles of the paranasal sinuses: MR imaging with CT correlation. AJR Am J Roentgenol. 1989;153(2):407–12.
8. Loevner L, Bradshaw J, Paranasal sinuses – MRI, head neck, radiology assistant. 2009. https://radiologyassistant.nl/en/p191710c96a36d/paranasal-sinuses-mri.html. Accessed 02/12/2016.

Paranasal Sinus Cancer

22

Pertinent Points

- *Definition*: Tumors arising from paranasal sinus epithelium comprise the most common group of anterior skull base malignancies.
- *AKA*: Squamous cell carcinoma, epidermoid carcinoma, transitional carcinoma, and adenocarcinoma.
- *Classic Clue*: Older male woodworker with moderately enhancing mass destroying the skull base and adjacent paranasal sinus habitually having its epicenter near a paranasal sinus.
- *Incidence*: Approximately 1 per 1,000,000.
- *Distributions*: Age, 50–70; gender prevalence, M > F probably related to occupational exposure.
- *Diagnostic Delay*:
  - As the early symptoms are often ignored by both patients and doctors, patients perpetually present for imaging at advanced stages [3].
  - Even patients presenting for imaging at early stages may have their studies interpreted by less experienced radiologists who fail to fathom the early tumor signs [3].

Imaging

General Imaging Features

- CT is the gold standard for imaging recurrent and chronic sinusitis [3].
- MRI compliments CT with superior soft tissue characterization, more easily evaluating the extent of tumor invasion.
- Often see a solid mass affecting aggressive osseous obliteration.

CT Features

- *See General Imaging Features.*
- CT superbly portrays osseous involvement including cortical thickening, sclerosis, erosion, remodeling, and destruction [3].
- It is important to reconstruct images using both bone and soft tissue algorithms [3].
- NECT shows a solid mass with aggressive bone destruction. CECT depicts moderate enhancement.

MRI Features:

- *See General Imaging Features.*
- Although MRI is acknowledged to be the preferred modality for complete assessment of skull base paranasal sinus cancer, experts remind us that it is *only superior* when optimal pulse sequences and imaging planes are performed [6].
- T1:
  - Heterogeneous, intermediate signal mass (see Fig. 22.1a).
  - T1 is superb at evaluating tumor extending into cortical bone or fatty marrow causing loss of dark (cortical bone) or bright (marrow) signal, respectively.
- T2: Intermediate signal mass. Useful in separating tumor from obstructed sinus secretions which have higher signal. (See Fig. 22.1c. Please compare to T1 (Fig. 22.1a, b) with attention to signal from the frontal sinus.)
- T1 Gd (see Fig. 22.1e–g):
  - Moderate tumor enhancement.
  - T1 Gd fat saturation images are beneficial in defining the degree of invasion and are particularly practical for depicting perineural tumor spread.

F. A. Midyett, S. K. Mukherji, *Skull Base Imaging*, https://doi.org/10.1007/978-3-030-46447-9_22

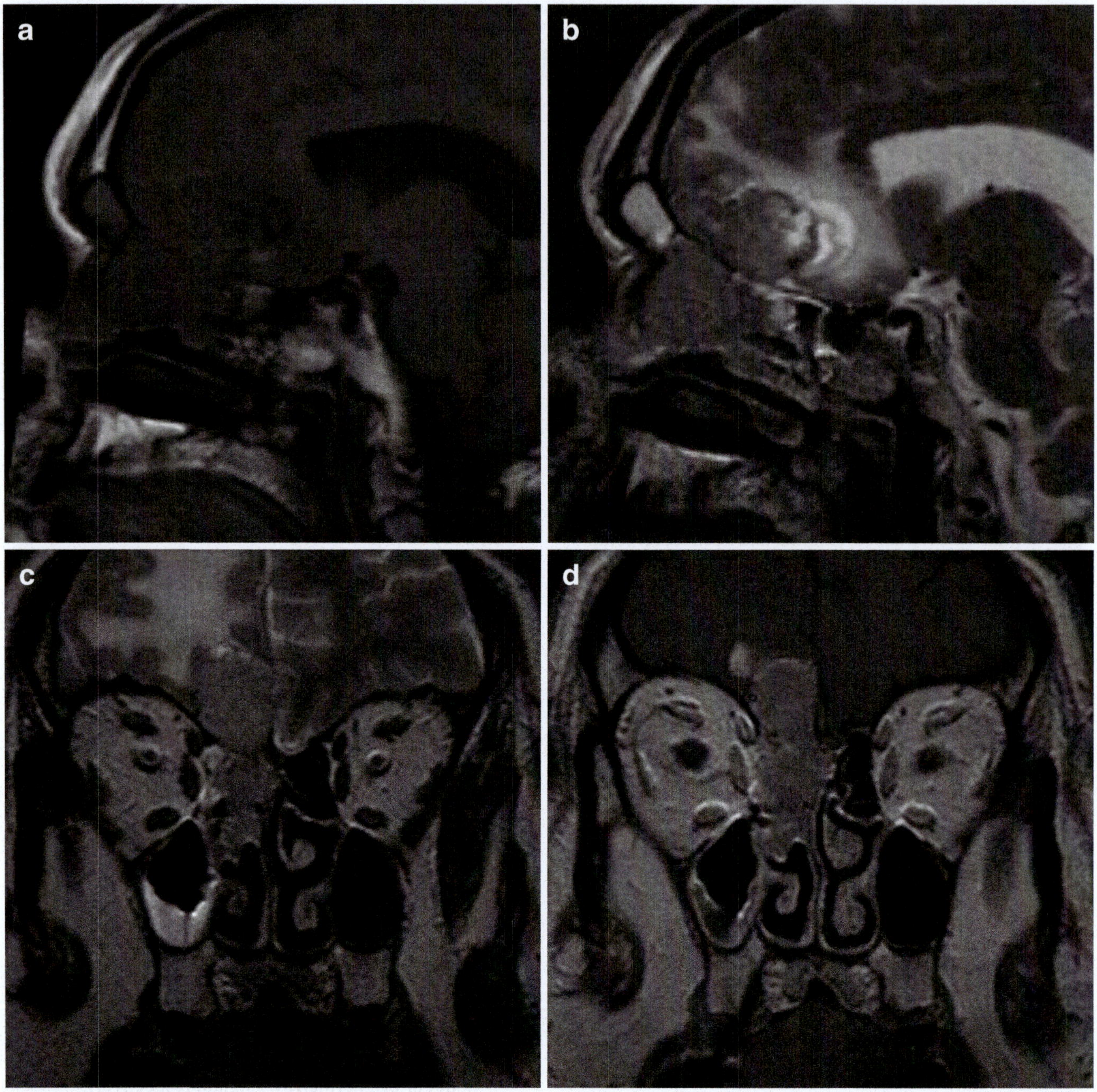

Fig. 22.1 Sagittal T1 (**a**) and T2 (**b**) show a huge anterior skull base mass extending caudally into the nasal cavity and cranially into the frontal lobes. The floor of the anterior cranial fossa is clearly compromised with the tumor "waist" near the breached floor. MR signal is relatively isointense to brain on both T1 and T2, except that the T2 images show foci of fluid within the tumor superiorly. The tumor provokes significant edema in the adjacent brain. High T2 signal anteriorly represents fluid trapped in the right frontal sinus and corresponds to relatively hyperintense fluid on T1 which contains proteinaceous material. Note significant deformity of the anterior horn of the right lateral ventricle by this aggressive mass invading the frontal lobe. Coronal T2 (**c**) and T1 Gd (**d**) show the huge anterior skull base mass portrayed on prior images. It seems solid and is relatively homogeneous showing moderate post-contrast enhancement. It extends laterally to abut and probably involves the right orbit but does not appear to have arisen from the orbit. Its epicenter suggests it arose near the skull base or ethmoid sinus

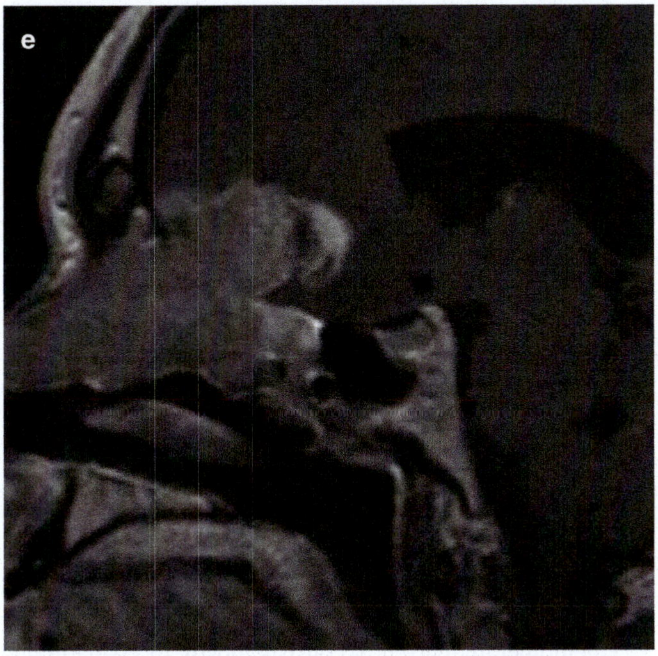

Fig. 22.1 (continued) (**e**) Sagittal T1 Gd shows the huge anterior skull base mass demonstrated on prior images. It appears solid with relatively moderate homogeneous enhancement. It extends anteriorly into the nasal cavity. The floor of the anterior cranial fossa (black line) has been deliberately destroyed by this aggressive tumor which has extended not only through the skull base but also through the dura into the frontal lobe. This is clearly a bad, bad tumor portending a poor prognosis

  - Linear dural enhancement is not sufficient to diagnose dural invasion. That diagnosis should be reserved for cases demonstrating dural thickening >5 mm, focal dural nodules, or concurrent pial enhancement [3, 6].
- ADC (apparent diffusion coefficient) mapping:
  - ADC mapping shows significant promise for separating benign inflammatory lesions from malignant paranasal sinus tumors [5].
  - ADCs of malignant tumors are consistently lower than benign tumors or inflammatory lesions [5].
- STIR (short tau inversion recovery).
  - Useful in detecting lymph node involvement and marrow edema [3].

Nuclear Medicine Features

- ^{18}F FDG PET/CT has high sensitivity and moderate specificity and seems superior to conventional CT and MR imaging for finding residual/recurrent tumor. It, however, is not routinely recommended for diagnosis and staging.
- Because therapy-generated inflammation creates false-positive uptake, it is recommended that FDG imaging be performed >3 months following completion of treatment [3].
- Most malignant tumors have high metabolic activity with increased FDG uptake. However, exceptions are evident. Benign tumors like pleomorphic adenomas and Warthin tumors also have high FDG uptake, while highly malignant tumors like adenoid cystic carcinoma can have low metabolic activity and low FDG uptake!

Plain Films

- Patients should have annual chest radiographs beginning at initial diagnosis to exclude pulmonary metastasis.
- These should supplement more sophisticated imaging procedures provided for diagnosis and follow up.

Angiography

- Angiography tends to be typically reserved for surgical candidates whose tumors surround the carotid artery when vessel sacrifice is contemplated to obtain tolerable tumor margins.

Clinical Issues

Presentation

- Symptoms of local tumor involvement inform imagers where to look:
  - I. Extension into the Nasal Cavity:
    - Patients are typically treated for symptoms of chronic sinusitis, often delaying their diagnosis until late disease stages.
    - As the tumor enlarges, patients develop additional symptoms including:
      1. Unilateral nasal obstruction
      2. Nasal discharge
      3. Anosmia
      4. Facial numbness
      5. Epistaxis
  - II. Extension into the Orbit:
    - Ocular dysfunction, proptosis, diplopia, and pain
  - III. Extension into the Oral Cavity:
    - Toothache
    - Loosening of upper teeth
    - New complaint that "dentures don't fit anymore"
  - IV. Extension into the Inferior Pterygoid Muscle:
    - Trismus

Epidemiology and Risk Factors

- Surprisingly, there is no known link to smoking.
- Observed occupational exposures affect people who work with wood dust, leather, textiles, isopropyl alcohol, formaldehyde, and welding fumes [3],
- Frequently found in miners of minerals like arsenic, chromium, cadmium, and nickel [3].

- Woodworkers report an increased risk of sinonasal adenocarcinoma 500 times that of an average male and 900 times that found in the general population [3, 4].
- Occupational exposure probably accounts for the male predominance.

Pathology

- Paranasal sinus cancers comprise three predominant histologic types: [2]
  I. SCC (Squamous Cell Carcinomas)
    - SCC is most common, accounting for 50% paranasal sinus malignancies.
    - SCC is most frequently found in maxillary (85%), followed by ethmoid (10%) and frontal/sphenoid (5%) sinuses.
    - These tumors are more common in Asia.

  II. Adenocarcinomas
    - Comprise ~35% of paranasal sinus cancer.
    - Primarily arise in the ethmoid sinuses or upper nasal cavity.

  III. Adenoid Cystic Carcinomas
    - Comprise ~11% of tumors and arise from minor salivary glands.
    - Characterized by their diffuse infiltration and a propensity for perineural propagation.
    - See Chap. 37, Adenoid Cystic Carcinoma.

  IV. Other Rare Tumor Types
    - Other rare types of cancers occurring in the sinonasal region include NEC, SNM, SNUC, and ENB and are not specifically covered in this chapter but are discussed in other chapters.
    - See following chapters:
      - See Chap. 16, Neuroendocrine Tumor.
      - See Chap. 18, Sinonasal Melanoma.
      - See Chap. 26, Sinonasal Undifferentiated Carcinoma.
      - See Chap. 28, Esthesioneuroblastoma.
- <1% of paranasal sinus cancer arise from the frontal and sphenoid sinuses.
- Gross Features: Friable fungating polypoid tan/white or red/pink mass.
- Microscopic features
  - Depends on types outlined earlier
  - Two typical subtypes of SCC include keratinizing (80%) and nonkeratinizing (20%)

Treatment and Prognosis

- Today's typical treatment regimens favor surgery and irradiation.
- Sometimes see concurrent dissection or irradiation of ipsilateral neck nodes.

Surgery

- Tumors invading the skull base present some of the most complex and technically difficult surgical problems, commonly compromising complete excision.
- Image-guided needle biopsy is often obtained to confirm cytology.
- Relatively recent advancements in skull base surgery have improved the prognosis for these unfortunate patients.
- Potential complications comprise CSF leakage, meningitis, pneumocephalus, and abscess formation [2].
- Persistent pneumocephalus is *pathognomonic* for the presence of a CSF leak [2].

Chemotherapy

- Some studies suggest radiation and chemotherapy should precede surgery [2].
- Chemotherapy currently consists mostly of cisplatin and 5-fluorouracil.

Radiotherapy

- Typically deliver doses of 6000 to 8000 cGy over 6 weeks.
- Newer delivery methods (including intensity modulation) attempt to decrease morbidity from dry eyes, radionecrosis, and optic nerve damage [2].

Prognosis

- Tumor stage provides a powerful predictor of outcome:
  - For all tumor types and stages, the 5-year survival rate is 75%.
  - Stage T1 tumors show a 100% survival when treated aggressively.
  - Stage T4 survival rates currently hover at 60%.
- Factors predicting a preferred prognosis include low tumor stage, prior history of inverted papilloma, origination in an ethmoid sinus, and a treatment regimen which combines surgery and radiation therapy.

Differential Diagnosis

A. Acute Invasive Fungal Sinusitis

- Typically exhibit acute onset fever, cough, nasal mucosal ulceration, epistaxis, and headache.
- Usually involves immunocompromised individuals.
- Associated conditions include diabetes mellitus, malignancy, neutropenia, and severe malnutrition.

- Imaging shows hyperdense sinus on CT corresponding to hypointense sinus on MRI with rapid development of adjacent progressive bony destruction.
- Periodically progress to ICA invasion causing thrombosis.
- See Chap. 32, Allergic Fungal Sinusitis and Chap. 45, Invasive Fungal Sinusitis.

B. Wegener's Granulomatosis (WG) [1]

- WG is a systemic vasculitis causing necrosis and granulomatous inflammation.
- German pathologist Friedrich Wegener described the disease entity in 1936.
- Two-third of affected patients show signs of concurrent sinus and orbital disease with associated bony erosions.
- Relative to orbital fat typically see ↑ T1 and ↓ T2 signal. The ↓ *T2 signal suggests this diagnosis*.

C. Chondrosarcoma (CS)

- Chondrosarcomas are chondroid malignancies which commonly chose a synchondrosis when selecting the skull base.
- *Classic Clue*: Skull-based mass exhibiting an affinity for the POF (petro-occipital fissure) sometimes showing chondroid matrix, characterized by low T1 and high T2 signals.
- Chondrosarcomas appear as well circumscribed, often scalloped, or lobulated lytic lesions exhibiting chondroid calcifications. In contrast, skull base paranasal sinus cancer usually does *not* show calcifications.
- Age: 10–79 years (mean 39).
- Low attenuation may make them subtle on brain soft tissue algorithms (See Chap. 46, Fig. 46.1i).
- T2: Very high T2 signal (See Fig. 46.1b, d).
- See Chap. 46, Skull Base Chondrosarcoma.

D. Juvenile Nasopharyngeal Angiofibroma (JNA)

- Rare, highly vascular, locally invasive benign nasopharyngeal neoplasm occurring almost entirely in adolescent and young adult males displaying a distinct tendency for recurrence.
- *Classic Clue*: Adolescent male presenting with epistaxis has an avidly enhancing, heterogeneous posterior nasal mass with MRI showing *characteristic salt and pepper appearance* from the presence of prominent flow voids.
- Typically have Holman-Miller sign with archetypical anterior bowing of posterior maxillary sinus wall.
  - T1: Heterogeneous intermediate signal.
  - T2: Heterogeneous signal with dark flow voids.
  - T1 Gd: Exhibits avid enhancement. Axial and coronal fat saturation images are essential to define involvement of skull base, sphenoid, and cavernous sinuses.
- Most sequences show *characteristic salt and pepper appearance* from the presence of prominent flow voids.
- Catheter angiography illustrates a plethora of dilated, tortuous vessels and depicts an intense characteristic capillary blush.
- See Chap. 15, Juvenile Nasopharyngeal Angiofibroma.

E. Ewing's Sarcoma (ES)

- Ewing's sarcoma is an aggressive malignant tumor of *childhood and adolescence* containing small blue round cells which usually presents in the second decade.
- *Classic Clue*: *Caucasian child or adolescent* presenting with pain, fever, and ↑ ESR found on imaging to have an extra-axial mass extending cranially and caudally from its skull base epicenter. On examination, patients often demonstrate orbital or cranial nerve symptoms.
- Ewing's sarcoma accounts for 10–15% of childhood malignant bone tumors and is *second* only to osteosarcoma.
- Ewing's sarcoma is *rare* among Asians and African-Americans.
- Usually demonstrates destructive, permeative bone destruction with soft tissue components showing *no* soft tissue calcifications.
- Depending on tumor stage, Ewing's sarcoma can cause cortical erosion with rarefaction and "moth-eaten" permeative destruction.
- T1: Low to intermediate signal, isointense with the brain and muscle (See Chap. 47, Fig. 47.1a).
- T2: Heterogeneous signal, relatively isointense to the brain with focal fluid collections which show high T2 signal (See Chap. 47, Fig. 47.1c). Low signal striations sometimes suggest "hair on end" appearance.
- T1 Gd:
  - *Mild heterogeneous enhancement* (See Chap. 47, Fig. 47.1b, d).
  - *Fat saturation* techniques are very helpful.
  - Bony involvement by Ewing's sarcoma may be more conspicuous on DWI than other MRI sequences particularly when small and metastatic.
- See Chap. 47, Ewing's Sarcoma.

F. Esthesioneuroblastoma (ENB)

- Rare neuroendocrine malignancy of neural crest origin arising from olfactory epithelium.
- AKA: Olfactory neuroblastoma.
- ENB is more often found in middle-aged patients but is sometimes seen in children.
- ENB classically shows avidly enhancing dumbbell-shaped mass with "waist" at cribriform plate.
- May involve anterior cranial fossa, skull base, and orbit.
- ENBs exhibit intermediate signal on T1 and T2 with avid enhancement on T1 Gd.
- Cystic areas (with foci of ↑ T2) at tumor/brain interface are diagnostic and may be pathognomonic.
- DWI displays moderate restricted diffusion.

- ENBs exhibit an epicenter near the cribriform plate.
- ENB exhibits no gender preference.
- See Chap. 28, Esthesioneuroblastoma.

G. Metastatic Neoplasm

- A metastatic neoplasm can cause a destructive mass anywhere along the skull base.
- Frequently find *multiple metastases* in patients having recognized primary neoplasms.
- In children, metastatic neuroblastoma should be considered in the differential.

A Closer Look

I. Genetics and Associations

- Currently, there are no known inherited tendencies for paranasal sinus cancer.
- However, scientists are finding changes in genes which have occurred during the patient's lifetime.
- For example, researchers report mutations involving TP53, the tumor suppressor gene, in many head and neck cancers.

II. Statistical Soup

- Sinonasal tumors are rare, comprising 3% of head and neck cancers and 1% of all malignancies.

Selected References

1. Midyett FA, Mukherji SK. Wegener's granulomatosis. In: Orbital imaging. Philadelphia: Elsevier/Saunders; 2015. p. 227–9. ISBN : 978-0-323-34037-3.
2. Vrionis FD, Kienstra MA, Rivera M, Padhya TA. Malignant tumors of the anterior skull base. Cancer Control. 2004;11(3): 144–51.
3. Eggesbo HB. Imaging of sinonasal tumors. Cancer Imaging. 2012:136–52. https://doi.org/10.1102/1470-7330.2012.0015.
4. Acheson ED, Cowdell RH, Hadfield E, Macbeth RG. Nasal cancer in woodworkers in the furniture industry. BMJ. 1968;2:587–96. https://doi.org/10.1136/bmj.2.5605.587.
5. Sasaki M, Eida S, Sumi M, Nakamura T. Apparent diffusion coefficient mapping for sinonasal diseases: differentiation of benign and malignant lesions. AJNR Am J Neuroradiol. 2011;32(6): 1100–6.
6. Casselman JW. The skull base: tumoral lesions. Eur Radiol. 2005;15:534–42. https://doi.org/10.1007/s00330-004-2532-9.

Skull Base Osteoma

23

Pertinent Points

- *Definition*: Osteomas are mature, slow-growing, benign bone tumors composed of dense cortical bone comprising the most common primary bone tumor involving the calvarium; however, skull base involvement remains relatively rare [1].
- *Classic Clue:* 50-year-old male comes for CT because of severe frontal pain when flying, particularly after takeoff during initial climb out. This has been so severe that he avoids flying whenever possible. He has learned to travel with a nasal decongestant spray, and this has helped somewhat. A prior cranial MRI was unremarkable, but his newly acquired ENT physician specifically requested a sinus CT. This seems at first glance unremarkable except for a small benign appearing focus of increased attenuation near the caudal aspect of one of the frontal sinuses.
- *AKA*: Homoplastic osteoma.
- *Age*: Fourth to fifth decade, mean age is 50 years; Sex: M > F = 1.5:1 [4].
- *Locations*:
  - Osteomas commonly occur in the calvarium and mandible. Calvarial osteomas arise more frequently from the frontal bone near the frontal sinuses, but they can occur anywhere within the cranial vault.
  - Occurrence: Frontal > ethmoid > maxillary > sphenoid
- Osteomas are slow growing and usually asymptomatic but can cause sinus symptoms or become large enough to compress the brain.
- *Prevalence*: The prevalence of paranasal sinus osteomas is 3% [3, 4].
- *Gardner's:* When osteomas are multiple, Gardner's syndrome should surely be considered. (If it is really big or in your head, you probably would consider Gardener's with just one!)

Imaging

General Imaging Features

- Imaging features reflect the underlying pathology with ivory osteomas demonstrating no marrow and mature osteomas showing central marrow [1, 2].
- Most osteomas vary between 2 and 30 mm [3] but exceptionally they may be much larger (See Figs. 23.1a, b and 23.2a–d).
- More than one third are accompanied by abnormal sinonasal findings [3].
- Sometimes see an associated mucocele when an osteoma blocks a sinus drainage passageway.
- May produce pneumocephalus when an osteoma breaches the sinus wall through the inner table.

CT Features

- *See General Imaging Features.*
- Although osteomas sometime seem stealthy on MRI, they are usually unashamedly conspicuous on CT.
- They frequently flaunt themselves as a conspicuous markedly hyperdense mass poking into a sinus or protruding out from a calvarial table.
- CT findings correlate well (but not perfectly) with histologic subtypes, because of overlapping findings (which may relate to specimen sampling) [11].
- CT findings show three general types:
  - I. Ivory Osteomas
    - Predominately very dense bone
    - Often small foci of more lucent areas
  - II. Mature Osteomas
    - More equal distribution of very dense and less dense bone
  - III. Osteomas with Osteoblastoma-Like Features
    - Contain larger areas of less dense bone with peripheral rim of dense bone [11]

F. A. Midyett, S. K. Mukherji, *Skull Base Imaging*, https://doi.org/10.1007/978-3-030-46447-9_23

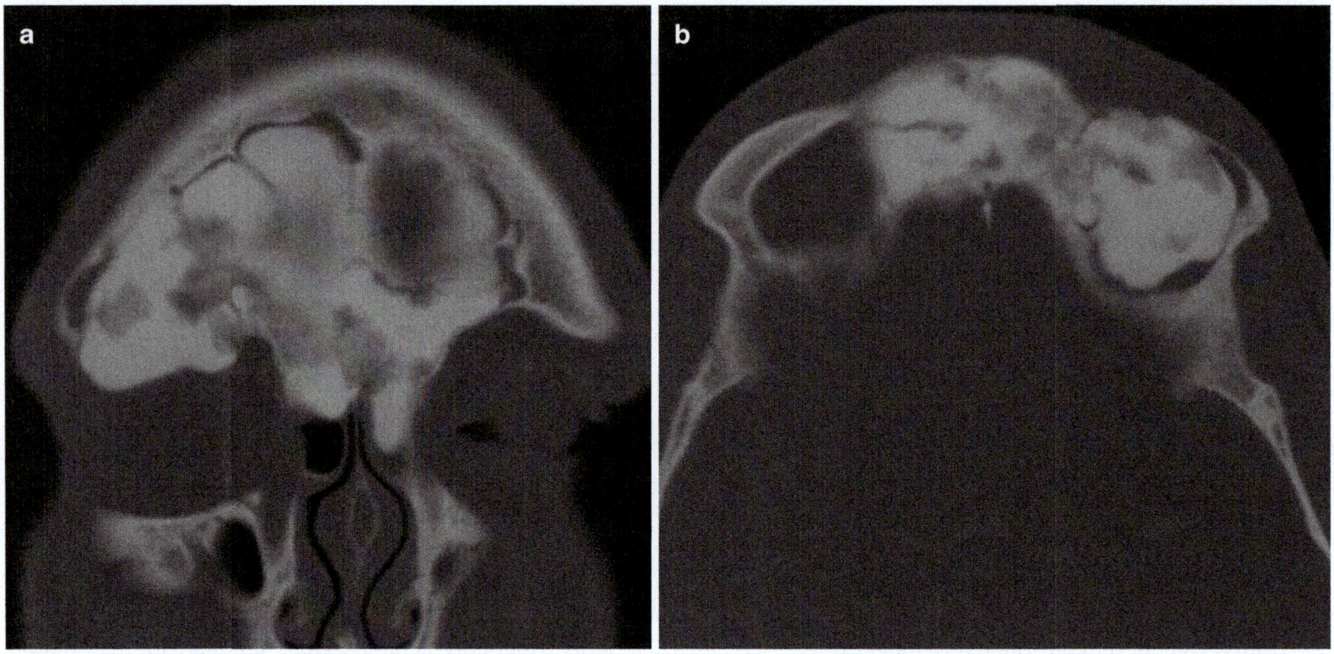

Fig. 23.1 (**a**) Coronal and (**b**) Axial NECT exhibit an extensive mass filling the frontal sinuses and extending caudally into the right orbit and upper nasal cavity. The tumor is a very dense, high attenuation mass, appearing as white as cortical bone suggesting the diagnosis of a "giant osteoma." Some of the tumor margins merely abut the adjacent cortical sinus margins where others have been clearly breached by this slow-growing although tenacious tumor

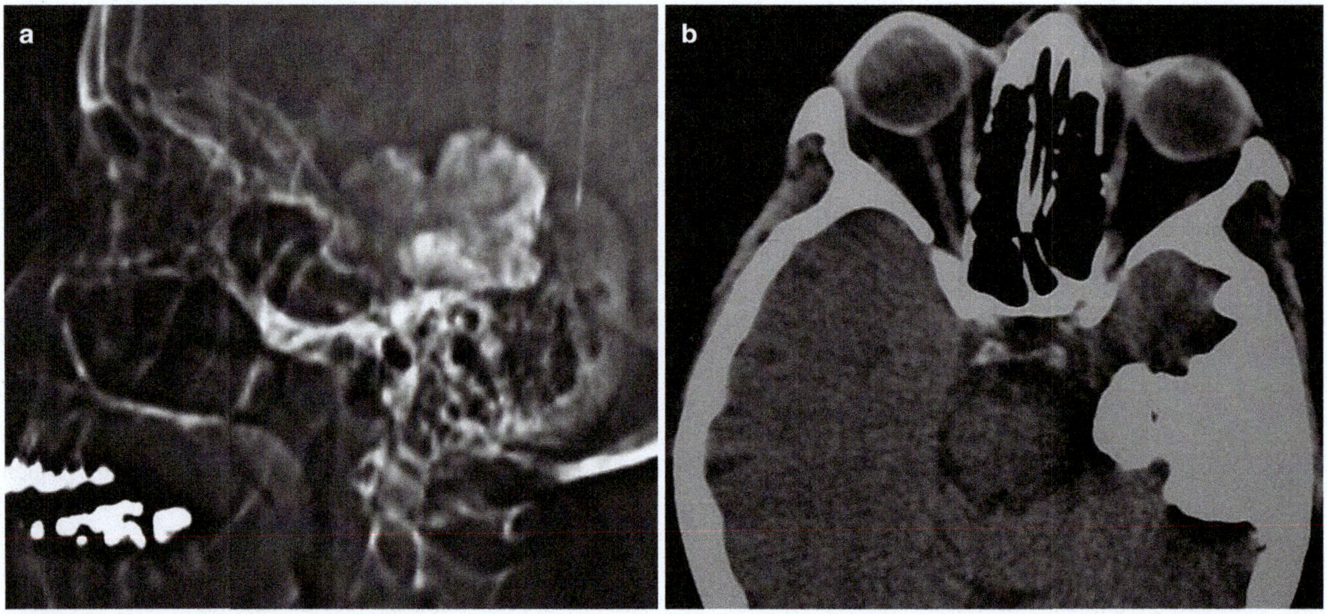

Fig. 23.2 (**a**) Lateral skull shows a large cauliflower-like mass occupying much of the left middle cranial fossa. While moderately heterogeneous, much of its density approximates cortical bone in this giant skull base osteoma. (**b**) Axial NECT with brain algorithm demonstrates a huge left middle fossa mass extending medially to the ambient cistern claiming space previously occupied by the contralateral temporal lobe. Is it any wonder that the patient "can't really remember" when his headaches began?

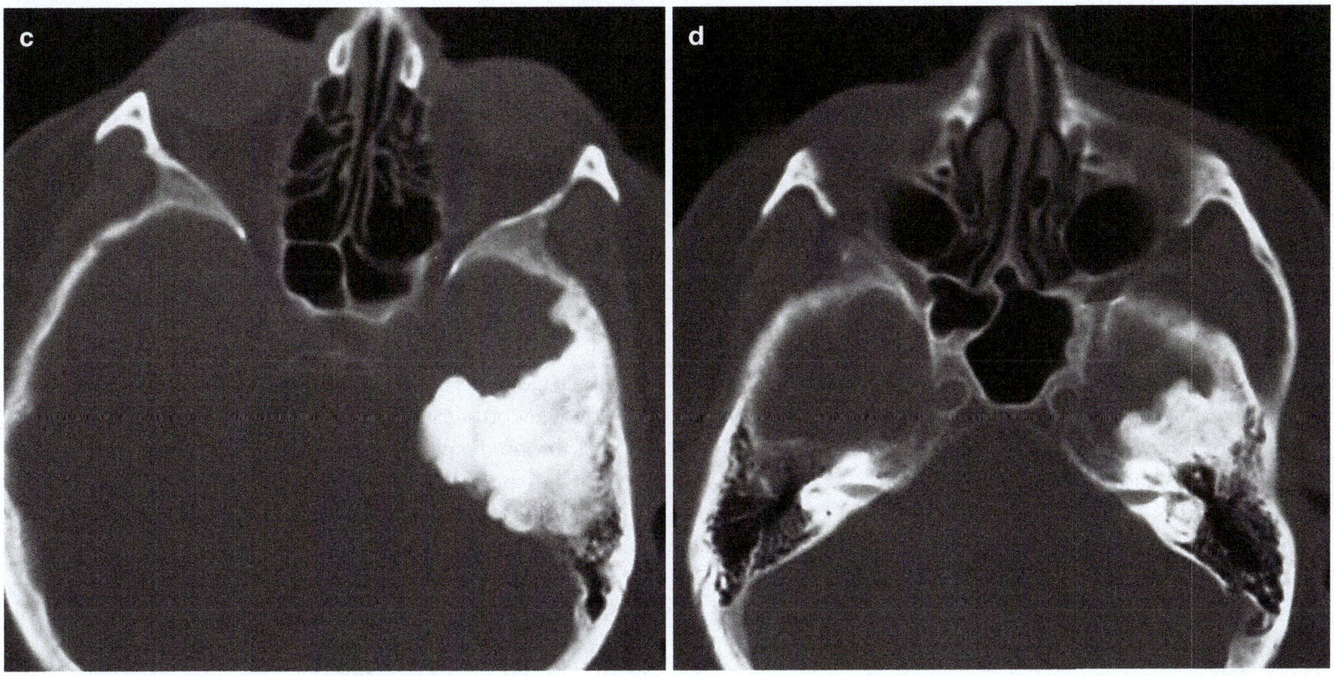

Fig. 23.2 (continued) (**c**, **d**) Axial NECT with bone algorithm again depicts a huge space-occupying left middle fossa mass. The more caudal image (**d**) clearly confirms the attachment of this giant skull base osteoma

MRI Features

- *See General Imaging Features.*
- MRI sometimes seems insensitive to cortical bone and calcifications. Because osteomas are composed of dense cortical bone, they are truly stealth to MRI and sometimes seem to be completely "invisible". Remember, even the impressive "invisible man" left tracks in the snow.
- MRI, however, may be beneficial in accessing adjacent dural or soft tissue tumor incursion [8].
- T1 and T2: Low signal simulating aeration. Osteomas are seemingly stealth when surrounded by low signal air in sinuses. They sometimes show less contrast than when photographing a black cat in front of a black fence.
- T1 Gd: Some show moderate heterogeneous enhancement [8]. Enhancement, however, varies according to the histologic subtype with the extent of enhancement varying inversely proportional to the degree of dense cortical bone.

Clinical Issues

Presentation

- Most calvarial osteomas are usually asymptomatic and are frequently found and incidentally identified on routine imaging.
- They may be confirmed as the underlying cause of the patient's sinusitis or mucocele.
- Occasionally osteomas can cause mass effect on adjacent brain (See Fig. 23.2a, b).
- Ethmoid osteomas tend to present earlier with mass effect leading to symptoms.
- Orbital involvement can cause headache, diplopia, exophthalmos, and proptosis [6].
- Other clinical presentations include orbital invasion and deformity, dural erosion causing CSF leak with pneumocephalus resulting in rhinorrhea, or intracranial infection including meningitis and cerebral abscess [7, 8, 10].

Pathophysiology

- Osteomas are benign, slow growing, and usually asymptomatic.
- Osteomas arising from bone are dubbed homoplastic osteomas, while those forming from soft tissue can be called heteroplastic osteomas.
- Histologic features which tend to correlate with CT include [11]:
  - I. Ivory osteomas are typically composed of very dense bone containing a very few small lucent areas [11].
  - II. Mature osteomas demonstrate very dense bone of variable thickness adjacent to less dense areas sometimes similar to fibrous dysplasia [11].

III. Osteoblastoma-like osteomas can be characterized by a central area of less dense fibrous matrix surrounded by a thinner periphery of very dense bone [11].

Treatment

Surgery

- Cranial osteomas are benign and usually asymptomatic, not requiring surgical resection [7]. Some advocate surgical excision only when they create cosmetic or mass effect problems.
- Osteomas with mass effect can cause:
  I. Sinusitis
  II. Mucocele
  III. Mass effect on brain (see Fig. 23.2a, b)
- It is generally agreed that sino-orbital osteomas should be removed when [9, 11]:
  I. Symptomatic
  II. Enlarging
  III. Extending beyond paranasal sinus
- However, some suggest that because they possess the potential to progressively compress visual pathways resulting in blindness, surgery should be considered for orbital and sphenoid osteomas despite their lack of specific signs and symptoms [5].
- While traditionally removed via external surgical approaches, endoscopy is increasingly being used in some selected cases [4].
- Fortunately for everyone, sphenoid sinus osteomas are extremely rare [8, 9].

Differential Diagnosis (DDx) [12]

A. Fibrous Dysplasia (FD) [12]
- Fibrous dysplasia is a benign slowly progressing tumor-like process in which normal cancellous bone is replaced by fibrous tissue and immature woven bone.
- Fibrous dysplasia favors frontal, sphenoid, ethmoid, and maxillary bones.
- Fibrous dysplasia comes in three typical types: sclerotic, lytic, and mixed with skull base lesions *mostly sclerotic* and *least likely lytic*.
- Fibrous dysplasia classically causes medullary cavity expansion sparing its cortex and preserving its original shape. Severe expansion can cause cortical crevices or even "vanishing cortex."
- Reaction of the periosteum should suggest either malignant modification or an incipient pathologic fracture.
- Lytic lesions imply malignant transformation, particularly when progressing on imaging.
- Classically exhibits ground-glass appearance, commonly crossing sutures, and may be sclerotic or show bubbly cystic foci.
- Fibrous dysplasia's fondness for the calvarium and orbit can cause crucial eye problems.
- T1 shows heterogeneous low to intermediate signal.
- T2 has heterogeneous, predominately low T2 signal (but may find foci of higher signal).
- T1 Gd demonstrates avid enhancement.
- Heterogeneous signal caused by cysts and hemorrhage varies according to the age of blood and protein content.
  – Fibrous dysplasia widens the diploic space primarily by displacing the outer table while at the same time sparing the inner table.
  – Facial bone involvement is common with fibrous dysplasia.
- See Chap. 25, Fibrous Dysplasia.

B. Paget's Disease [12] **(PD)**
- Sir James Paget first described this disease in 1877.
- Paget's disease typically involves *both* the inner and outer bony tables.
- Facial bone involvement is uncommon with Paget's disease.
- Paget's disease typically starts initially in the frontal or occipital regions sparing the skull vertex.
- Paget's disease demonstrates well-defined lytic lesions lacking sclerotic margins.
- Paget's tendency toward bone softening promotes basilar invagination.
- Paget's healing phase causes its classic "cotton-wool" appearance.
- See Chap. 41, Paget's Disease.

C. Hyperparathyroidism (HPT) [12, 13]
- Some show mottled demineralization with "ground-glass" appearance.
- While rare, hyperparathyroidism's brown tumor can cause focal destruction and usually involves multiple calvarial foci.
- Look for indistinct cortical margins of vascular grooves, subperiosteal absorption in hand radiographs, and loss of lamina dura in dental radiographs.

D. Intraosseous Meningioma [12]
- Except for the very rare intraosseous variety, meningiomas are extradiploic causing cortical thickening without showing an intraosseous epicenter.
- Intraosseous meningiomas are rare, accounting for $<1\%$ of bone tumors.
- T1 is isointense to grey matter.

- T2 is variable mostly isointense to grey matter (some are, however, hyperintense).
- T1 Gd exhibits avid uniform enhancement.
- Intraosseous meningiomas can cause proptosis.
- 65% are sclerotic while 35% appear lytic.

E. Sclerotic Metastasis [12]

- Sclerotic or blastic bony metastasis may occasionally resemble osteomas.
- Sclerotic metastasis can come from prostate, breast, transitional cell carcinoma, carcinoid, medulloblastoma, neuroblastoma, mucinous adenocarcinoma, and lymphoma.

F. Langerhans Cell Histiocytosis (LCH)

- LCH is the modern moniker bestowed on a rare, ill understood but significant, pathologic process related to proliferation of macrophages and dendrites (formerly dubbed histiocytes).
- *Classic Clue*: Pediatrics refer for MRI a child with a history of diabetes insipidus who is found to have an avidly enhancing infundibular stalk enlargement and an absent posterior pituitary bright spot.
- LCH predominately involves the pediatric population age 1–5, typically appearing during the first decade.
- May see lytic lesions involving the calvarium and/or temporal bones.
- CNS manifestations of LCH occur in ≤50% and are more frequent in patients with multisystem disease. Patients *rarely* present with isolated CNS involvement.
- See Chap. 8, Langerhans Cell Histiocytosis.

A Closer Look

I. Genetics

- Osteomas are linked to Gardner's syndrome, an autosomal-dominant variation of familial adenomatous polyposis.
- Gardner's syndrome involves multiple cranial osteomas, colonic polyposis, and soft tissue tumors. These colonic polyps possess a 100% chance for malignant transformation if left untreated. This is a good reason for radiologists to at least mention Gardner's when encountering osteomas.

II. Fast Facts

- Osteomas are the most common paranasal sinus tumors [11].
- Osteomas are uncommon tumors which comprise 1% of all bone tumors and 11% of benign bone tumors.
- Osteomas >3 cm in diameter and weighing >110 g are considered *giant* tumors.
- Cranial osteomas can be comprehensively classified as follows [7]:
  - I. Intraparenchymal
  - II. Dural
  - III. Skull base
  - IV. Skull vault
    - – Exostotic
    - – Enostotic

Selected References

1. Greenberg M. Handbook of neurosurgery. 7th ed. New York: Thieme; 2010.
2. Maroldi R, Nicolai P, Antonelli AR. Imaging in treatment planning for sinonasal diseases. Berlin: Springer; 2005. ISBN: 3540423834.
3. Erdogan N, Demir U, Songu M, et al. A prospective study of paranasal sinus osteomas in 1,889 cases: changing patterns of localization. Laryngoscope. 2009;119(12):2355–9. https://doi.org/10.1002/lary.20646.
4. Georgalas C, Goudakos J, Fokkens WJ. Osteoma of the skull base and sinuses. Otolaryngol Clin N Am. 2011;44(4):875–90. https://doi.org/10.1016/j.otc.2011.06.008.
5. Muderris T, Bercin S, Sevil E, et al. Endoscopic removal of a giant ethmoid osteoma with orbital extension. Acta Inform Med. 2012;20(4):266–8.
6. Yiotakis I, Eleftheriadou A, Giotakis E, et al. Resection of giant ethmoid osteoma with orbital and skull base extension followed by duraplasty. World J Surg Oncol. 2008;6:110. https://doi.org/10.1186/1477-7819-6-110.
7. Haddad FS, Haddad GF, Zaatri G. Cranial osteomas: their classification and management-report on a giant osteoma and review of the literature. Surg Neurol. 1997;48(2):143–7.
8. Chen CY, Ying SH, Yao MS, et al. Sphenoid sinus osteoma at the sella turcica associated with empty sella: CT and MR imaging findings. AJNR Am J Neuroradiol. 2008;29:550–1. https://doi.org/10.3174/ajnr.A0935.
9. Strek P, Zagoliski O, Wywial A, et al. Osteoma or the sphenoid sinus. B-ENT. 2005;1:39–41.
10. Hsu CC, Kwan GN, Bhuta SS. Non-traumatic cerebrospinal fluid rhinorrhea caused by ethmoid sinus osteoma. J Clin Neurosci. 2010;17(9):1185–6. https://doi.org/10.1016/j.jocn.2009.11.028.
11. McHugh JB, Mukherji SK, Lucas DR. Sino-orbital osteoma: a clinicopathologic study of 45 surgically treated cases with emphasis on tumors with osteoblastoma-like features. Arch Pathol Lab Med. 2009;133:1587–93.
12. Midyett FA, Mukherji SK. Chapter 50. Fibrous dysplasia. In: Orbital imaging. Philadelphia: Elsevier/Saunders; 2015. p. 241–6. ISBN: 978-0-323-34037-3.
13. Midyett FA, Mukherji SK. Chapter 49. Orbital plasmacytoma and myeloma. In: Orbital imaging. Philadelphia: Elsevier/Saunders; 2015. p. 233–40. ISBN: 978-0-323-34037-3.

24 Giant Cell Tumor

Pertinent Points

- *Definition:* Giant cell tumors (GCTs) are "common" lytic, locally aggressive expansile tumors which are characterized by regular recurrence and sporadic metastasis [1]. Although generally benign, 5–10% are malignant [2].
- *Classic Clue:* Young adult female presenting with headache and cranial nerve deficits is found to have an aggressive appearing, destructive, lytic skull base lesion exhibiting avid enhancement with fluid-fluid levels. (Fig. 24.1b.)
- *AKA:* Osteoclastomas, osteoblastoclastoma, myeloid sarcoma, tumor of myeloplaxus, and benign metastasizing GCT [2].
- *Incidence*:
  - Only in medicine would we call "common" a bone tumor which involves one person in a million [3].
  - While 2% of giant cell tumors involve the head and neck [1], only 1% involve the skull [4].
  - Giant cell tumors represent ~5% of all primary bone tumors and 20% of all benign bone tumors [5, 6, 2].
  - Cranial GCTs prefer the skull base over the calvarium [7, 5].
  - Giant cell tumors have a higher incidence in China and Southern India [2].
- *Age:* GCTs are frequently found in the third and fourth decades [1]. Patients with skull base GCTs tend to be older than those with long bone GCTs [8].
- *Gender Preference*: F > M. When 5–10% undergo malignant transformation, the sex preference shifts to males with M: F = 3:1 [2].
- *Locations*:
  - While we expect to encounter GCTs in long bones, we should not be so surprised when we happen upon them in the head and neck where they show a preference for the sphenoid and temporal bones and occasionally the mandible and maxilla [1, 9].
  - Although controversial, when involving long bones, GCTs typically arise eccentrically from the metaphysis often extending through the epiphysis to within 1 cm of the subarticular surface [2].
  - While usually solitary, they are occasionally multiple [10].
- Metastatic Issues:
  - GCTs typically tend to be histologically benign but locally aggressive. However, 5–10% undergo malignant transformation [6, 10, 11, 12, 13].
  - They may metastasize when both the primary and secondary lesions are "histologically benign" [10, 12, 13].
  - Somewhat suggestive of the "Strange Case of Dr. Jekyll and Mr. Hyde," GCTs present pathologists with "histologically benign" patterns while simultaneously parading malevolent manifestations before radiologists. GCTs regularly appear radiographically indistinguishable from malignant tumors [3]. And, they may metastasize while the pathologist is still signing them off as being benign!
- Tumor Classification:
  - Some say GCT is a tumor which is predominantly benign but portrays potential for malignant transformation.
  - Some separate these into benign and malignant GCT.
  - However pathologists eventually classify these lesions; they are clearly problematic for patients, pathologists, and radiologists.

F. A. Midyett, S. K. Mukherji, *Skull Base Imaging*, https://doi.org/10.1007/978-3-030-46447-9_24

Imaging

General Imaging Features

- Cranial GCTs often omit their characteristic "soap bubble" appearance seen in the long bones [1, 4].
- Radiographic findings for skull base GCTs may not be suggestive of a specific tumor diagnosis, although features clearly advocate an aggressive lesion [8].
- Adjacent soft tissues (including cerebral parenchyma) typically *do not exhibit edema* (See Fig. 24.1a).

CT Features

- *See General Imaging Features.*
- As a rule, GCTs appear as nonspecific expansile lytic lesions lacking a sclerotic margin with their contiguous cortex thinned, expanded, or breached.
- Periosteal reaction is present in about one fourth.
- Giant cell tumors exhibit no bony matrix mineralization or calcification.
- Most show narrow (normal to lesion) transition zones although these zones are broader with more aggressive GCTs.
- CECT shows slightly hyperdense homogeneous post-contrast enhancement.
- Frequently find a soft tissue mass with nearly half exhibiting extraosseous involvement [14].
- Frequently find fluid-fluid levels on CT.

MRI Features

- *See General Imaging Features.*
- T1 and T2 typically are isointense to gray matter, but signal may be ↓ by hemosiderin and/or fibrous components.
- T1:
  - Solid components show heterogeneous signal similar to the cortical brain.
  - Frequently find multiple cystic components with fluid-fluid levels (See Fig. 24.1c).
- T2:
  - Solid components are isointense to the cortical brain (See Fig. 24.1a).
  - Cystic components can show high signal (similar to vitreous) which may layer on top of lower signal fluid.
  - *Typically do not exhibit edema in the adjacent brain.*
  - See Fig. 24.1b.
- T1 Gd:
  - Enhancement varies but often exhibits avid enhancement of solid components. Heterogeneity varies proportional to the cystic component content.
  - See Fig. 24.1d, e.
- DWI:
  - Demonstrates restricted diffusion appearing bright on DWI images.
- *Fat Sat:* Fat saturation techniques often improve imaging of bony lesions, particularly when abnormalities abut orbital fat (See Fig. 24.1e).
- *MRA*:
  - Shows findings similar to angiography [2]

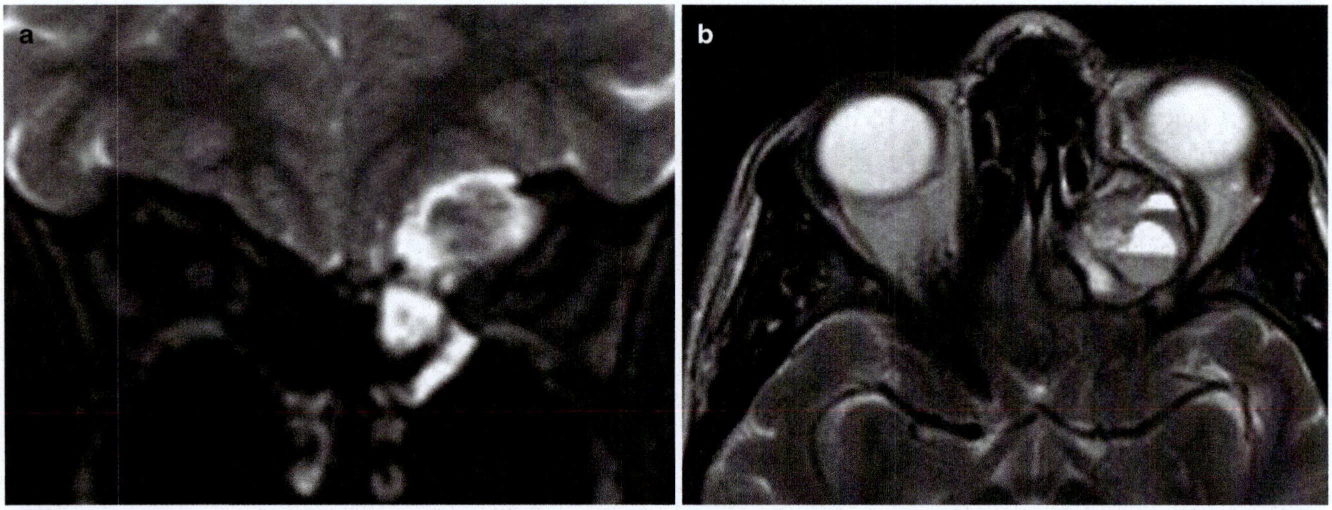

Fig. 24.1 (**a**) Coronal T2 shows large left orbital mass extending through the demolished (dark signal) skull base to abut the frontal lobe. The mass extends caudally and medially into the nasal cavity. NB (L. nota bene), the adjacent a frontal lobe shows *no* edema. (**b**) Axial T2 demonstrates large left orbital mass displacing adjacent orbital contents laterally and extending medially into the nasal cavity. Conspicuous fluid-fluid levels with less viscous, higher signal material resembles ocular vitreous

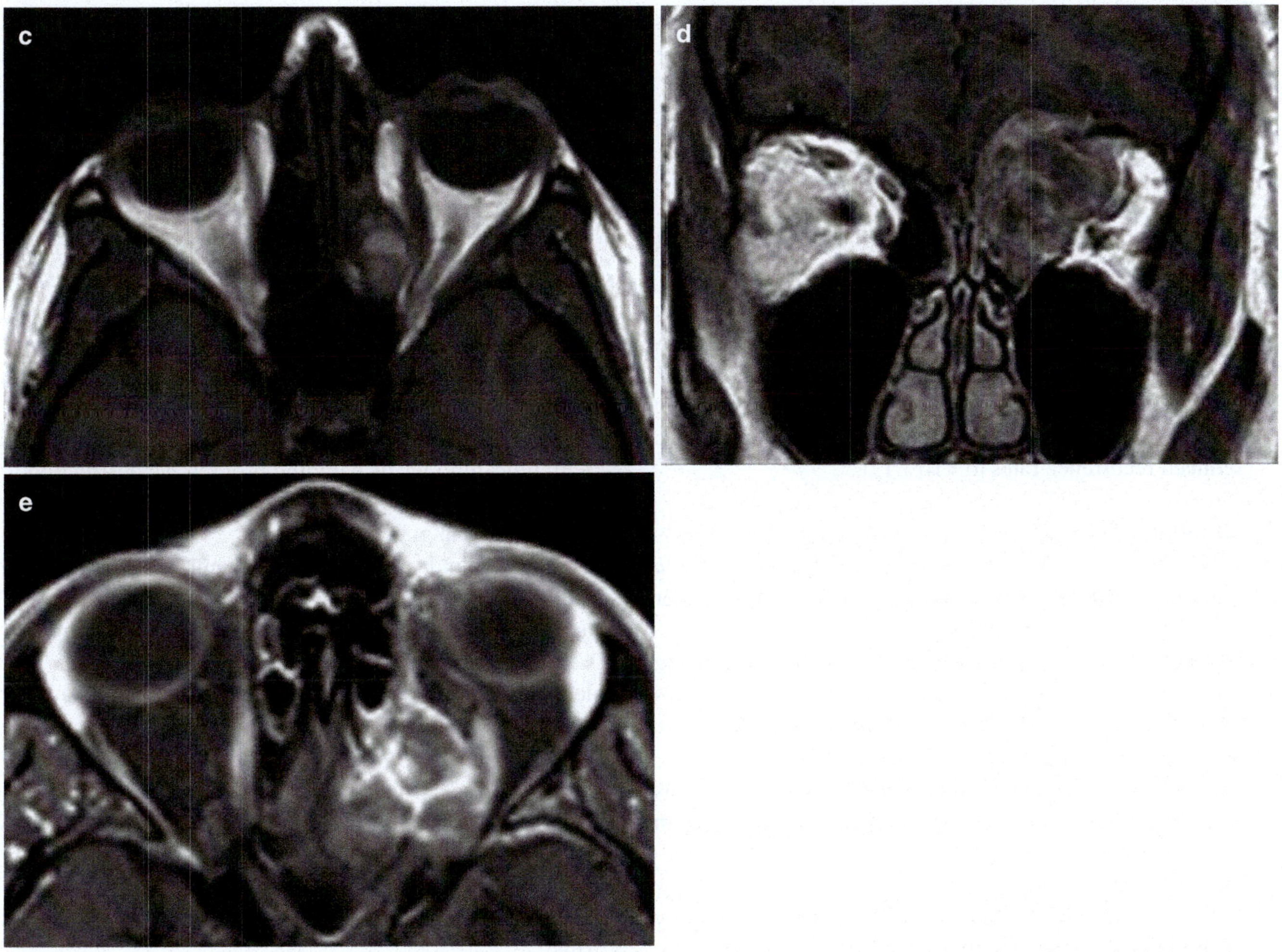

Fig. 24.1 (continued) (**c**) T1 depicts large left orbital mass displacing orbital contents. Fluid-fluid level depicts less viscous, higher signal material layered superiorly showing signal similar or slightly > ocular lens. (**d**) Coronal T1 Gd. Large left orbital mass exhibits moderate heterogeneous enhancement of solid components but clearly contains significant non-enhancing components consistent with cysts seen on other sequences. Tumor has breached the left orbital roof/skull base with absence of a large segment of skull base. By comparison, the skull base (black line) is clearly demonstrated on the contralateral right. Tumor clearly abuts and displaces the adjacent orbital fat and the left frontal lobe. (**e**) Axial T1 Gd with fat saturation. Large left orbital mass destroys the left medial orbital wall and extends into the nasal cavity. It displaces orbital contents medially. Enhancement of solid tumor components has been accentuated and confirms the multicystic structure seen on prior imaging sequences

Angiography

- Although not normally performed for primary diagnosis, angiography acquired during preoperative embolization usually portrays:
  - 2/3 have hypervascular and 1/3 have hypo- or avascular lesions [2].

Nuclear Imaging

- Most GCTs demonstrate ↑ uptake on delayed images.
- Uptake characteristically involves the lesion's periphery and contains central photopenia demonstrating a "doughnut sign."
- Blood pool images illustrate increased activity in the lesion as well as adjacent bone secondary to regional hyperemia.

Clinical Issues

Presentation

- Presentation and physical findings depend on the exact site of origin and typically include pain, swelling, and neurologic deficits. Frequently find diplopia, proptosis, and visual disturbances with sphenoid involvement [5].
- Skull base GCTs possess the possibility of presenting with myriad maladies depending on involvement site and include [1]:
  - Headache
  - Ophthalmoparesis
  - Trigeminal hypesthesia
  - Visual deficits
  - Ear pain
  - ↓ Hearing
  - Facial weakness

- Diagnostic delay: Pain is often present for several months before a correct diagnosis is made [2].

Treatment and Prognosis

I. Surgery

- While wide local excision reduces recurrence rates, it is also associated with increased morbidity.
- Typical treatment consisting of curettage and packing [with bone chips or PMMA (polymethylmethacrylate)] is coupled with a 50% recurrence rate [1, 15].
- Newer intraoperative improvements including treating surgical margins (using thermal or chemical means) have reduced recurrence rates to <10% [2].

II. Radiation Therapy

- IMRT (intensity modulated radiotherapy) is a viable option for patients where complete resection is either impossible or impractical [6].
- The issue of malignant transformation of GCT following radiation therapy sounded significant when initial rates ranged up to 24%. However, more modern megavoltage techniques confer current rates <1% [6, 16].
- The average latent period between initial GCT diagnosis and detection of a secondary malignancy was 9 years in patients treated with radiation and 19 years for "spontaneous" transformation [17].
- While some GCTs treated with radiation therapy undoubtedly undergo malignant transformation, it should be remembered that Dahlin and Cupps reported sarcomatous development in 4% of GCTs *not* treated by radiation [6, 18].

III. Chemotherapy

- While adjuvant chemotherapy has revealed respectable results, no prevailing protocol has emerged [4].

IV. Other Adjuvant Therapies

- Monoclonal antibodies show striking results, causing considerable tumor necrosis [18].

Pathology

A. *Gross:* Giant cell tumors vary in appearance related to the degree of hemorrhage, fibrosis, and whether there is an associated ABC. Some studies show nearly half of GCTs have concurrent ABCs [14].

B. *Histology:* Giant cell tumors characteristically contain prominent, diffuse osteoclastic histiocyte-like mononuclear and giant cells. Frequently find many mitotic figures, particularly in pregnant patients and those on oral contraceptives [2].

Differential Diagnosis

A. Aneurysmal Bone Cysts (ABC)

- Aneurysmal bone cysts are benign, osteolytic, expansile, occasionally locally destructive bone lesions more frequently found involving long bone metaphyses, flat bones, and posterior vertebral elements. However, 2–6% of ABCs involve the skull with involvement of the calvarium more often than the skull base.
- Typically rapidly growing enhancing multi-cystic mass with fluid-fluid levels parading progressive destruction.
- Aneurysmal bone cysts are frequently found in a younger age group than giant cell tumor.
- Frequently find an expanding eccentric mass "blowing out" bony contours causing a characteristic "aneurysmal" appearance.
- CT typically shows an expansile, multiloculated lytic lesion bordered by a thin low-attenuation rim.
- CT bone algorithms typically show a lytic, expansile mass surrounded by a thin bony shell, frequently focally eroded or appearing almost invisible.
- CT soft tissue algorithms sometimes show a "Swiss cheese" pattern of multiloculated higher-attenuation septae filled with lower-attenuation fluid.
- Habitually shows a smooth, sharp, curving peripheral rim.
- CT often exhibits expansion of bone with widened diploic spaces, narrowed neural and vascular foramina, "ground-glass" opacity, and post contrast enhancement.
- MRI findings include:
  - T1:
    - Solid components show heterogeneous signal similar to the cortical brain.
    - Multiple septations separate cystic components.
    - Multiple internal cystic components contain blood depicting diverse signals which vary according to differing ages of their degradation products.
    - May have a hypointense demarcating rim separating the lesion from surrounding structures.
  - T2:
    - Solid components are isointense to the cortical brain.
    - Cystic components have high signal isointense to ocular vitreous.
    - Frequently find fluid-fluid levels.
    - Sometimes shows a hypointense surrounding rim demarcating the lesion from surrounding structures.

– T1 Gd:
  Exhibits avid heterogeneous enhancement of solid components including septa surrounding non-enhancing cysts. Sometimes shows a “soap bubble” appearance.
– See Chap. 38, Aneurysmal Bone Cysts.

B. Giant Cell Granuloma (GCG) [19]

- Jaffe coined the term “giant cell reparative granuloma” in 1953 [20].
- As most giant cell granulomas have a history of prior trauma, Jaffe portrayed their pathology as a reparative reaction to injury induced intraosseous hemorrhage [20, 19]
- Giant cell tumors were subsequently shown to occur without antecedent trauma, and pathologists removed the term “reparative” [19].
- Giant cell granulomas are infrequent benign masses seen in a small segment of H&N tumors [19].
- Giant cell granuloma is typically a slow-growing mass commonly showing significant diagnostic delay [19].
- CT usually shows expansion, remodeling, and lytic destruction of adjacent bone with intralesional mineralization.
- Giant cell granulomas sometimes show fluid-fluid levels [21].
- T1 Gd demonstrates discernible homogeneous enhancement [19].
- T1 and T2 sometimes show ↓ signal secondary to hemosiderin and/or high collagen content [20, 22–23].
- Giant cell granuloma is radiologically indistinguishable from and frequently misdiagnosed as giant cell tumor [21].
- Giant cell granuloma undergoes neither malignant transformation nor metastasis [21]. By contrast, giant cell tumors demonstrate both.

C. Fibrous Dysplasia (FD)

- While fibrous dysplasia gives no gender preference, giant cell tumor favors females. Malignant transformation of FD, however, is more prevalent in males. M:F = 3:1 [2].
- More frequently find expansile fibrous dysplasia in the ethmoid sinuses where it classically cavalcades its characteristic “ground-glass” appearance [24]. This is not a feature for GCT.
- FDs cortical margins are intact with minimal thinning [24]. GCTs have overlying cortex which is thinned, expanded, or incomplete.
- FD sometimes shows bubbly blistering cysts with hemorrhage, but we find few fluid-fluid levels to cause confusion with GCTs [5].
- FD is more prevalent in children and young adults [24]. GCTs are frequently found in the third and fourth decades [1], and patients with skull base GCTs tend to be older than those with long bone GCTs [8].
- FD displays three basic varieties: sclerotic, lytic, and mixed with sclerotic lesions leading in the skull base [24].
- Fibrous dysplasia demonstrates *avid enhancement* on T1 Gd [24].
- See Chap. 25, Fibrous Dysplasia.

D. Metastasis

- Most cases of metastasis show more than one lesion.
- Approximately half of patients with metastasis from breast cancer are aware that they have cancer [25]. However, most patients presenting with metastatic lung cancer do not even know they have cancer. A chest radiograph is recommended for workup [25].
- T1:
  – T1 is the “go to” sequence for excluding bone marrow metastasis.
  – Metastatic carcinoma is graphically hypointense when compared to normal “bright” marrow signal.
  – A high homogeneous fatty signal excludes metastasis. Problematic areas may be further evaluated with T2 fat saturation or fast STIR sequences.
- T2: Usually has hyperintense signal.
- T1 Gd: Most metastatic lesions exhibit avid enhancement of bone and soft tissue components [26].

E. Brown Tumor of Hyperparathyroidism (HPT)

- Von Recklinghausen first described HPT as osteitis fibrosa cystica in 1891.
- Although rare, “brown tumors” of the skull base have been reported [27].
- HPT may show “ground-glass” appearance with mottled demineralization. This is *not* a feature of GCT [28].
- HPT shows subperiosteal resorption of bone which classically involves the radial aspects of the proximal and middle phalanges of the second and third fingers. Originally described in 1951 by bone radiologist David Pugh, this is virtually pathognomonic for HPT. This is *not* a feature of GCT [28].
- HPT also shows *subperiosteal resorption of the lamina dura* which may progress to cause *floating teeth* [28].
- HPT usually causes multiple skull defects with diffuse trabecular resorption giving a granular *salt and pepper* appearance [28].
- HPT can cause indistinctness involving the inner and outer tables as well as cortical margins of vascular grooves. This is *not* a feature of GCT [28].

- HPT's "brown tumor" is rare but can cause focal bony destruction which could be problematic in the differential of GCT [28].

F. Plasmacytoma [8]

- CT shows focal lytic lesions which expand bone with soft tissue components which can cause bone remodeling or erosion.
- Solitary bone plasmacytomas arising in marrow cause characteristic bony destruction.
- T1 and T2 show a homogeneous appearance of pure soft tissue components while having a markedly heterogeneous appearance in calcified/ossified portions of the tumor.
- T1 is isointense to the muscle and brain but hypointense to orbital fat.
- T2 is isointense to muscle and brain. May be quite heterogeneous, depending on content of calcification/bone formation.
- T1 Gd is variable. Often shows significant contrast enhancement with central heterogeneity. This heterogeneity correlates with calcification/ossification (often shown on CT).
- Sometimes shows "grapefruit-like" septations.
- Unlike other lesions in the differential like FD which stops at sutures, a plasmacytoma can cross almost anything in its path.
- Plasmacytomas may progress to erosion, expansion, and destruction of bony cortex with thick peripheral ridging causing a characteristic "soap bubble" appearance. This "soap bubble" appearance which is shared with ABCs can clearly create confusion for the clinician and radiologist, particularly since a significant percentage of GCTs contain coexisting ABCs.

A Closer Look

I. Genetics

- The precise ontogeny of GCT is currently confusing.
- The short answer is GCTs are currently considered to be the consequence of an overachieving RANK/RANKL signaling pathway producing extraordinarily exuberant osteoclastic proliferation [11].
- The long answer is a subject for yet another treatise.

II. Potpourri

- ~5% of patients with benign GCTs have "benign" pulmonary metastasis [6, 10, 14].
- GCTs usually appear "histologically benign" while at the same time being indistinguishable on imaging from many malignant lesions. Moreover, some GCTs are definitely malignant and some metastasize while appearing "histologically benign" [10, 29]. Is there any wonder that a world class pathologist like Dahlin often routinely reviewed the imaging studies with bone radiologists before signing out his final pathologic diagnosis?
- So, we again ponder Jaffe's assertion. The final diagnosis "has a lot to do with the pathologist's state of mind" when signing out the case.
- And most of us will not be too surprised when bone pathologists once again assess their "state of mind" and reassess the remarkable riddle regarding this truly thorny tumor.

III. Historic Highlights

- In 1818, Sir Astley Cooper first described giant cell tumor of the bone [30, 31, 15].

Selected References

1. Silvers AR, Som PM, Brandwein M, et al. The role of imaging in the diagnosis of giant cell tumor of the skull base. AJNR Am J Neuroradiol. 1996;18:1392–5.
2. Murphey MD, Nomikos GC, Flemming DJ, et al. Imaging of giant cell tumor and giant cell reparative granuloma of bone: radiologic-pathologic correlation. Radiographics. 2001;21(5):1283–309.
3. Tsai YF, Chen LK, Su CT, et al. Giant cell tumor of the skull base: a case report. Chin J Radiol. 2000;25:223–7.
4. Mondal S, Mallik S, Goswami J, et al. Base of the skull giant cell tumor: rare presenting features of a rare tumor. Clin Cancer Investig J. 2014;3:444–6.
5. Zorlu F, Selek U, Soylemezoglu F, Oge K. Malignant giant cell tumor of the skull base originating from clivus and sphenoid bone. J Neuro-Oncol. 2006;76:149–52. https://doi.org/10.1007/s11060-005-4343-5.
6. Roeder F, Timke C, Zwicker F, et al. Intensity modulated radiotherapy (IMRT) in benign giant cell tumors – a single institution case series and a short review of the literature. Radiat Oncol. 2010;5(1):18. https://doi.org/10.1186/1748-717X-5-18.
7. Rock JP, Mahmood A, Cramer HB. Giant cell tumor of the skull base. Am J Otol. 1994;15(2):268–72.
8. Bertoni F, Unni KK, Beabout JW, Ebersold MJ. Giant cell tumor of skull. Cancer. 1992;70:1124–32.
9. Lee HJ, Lum C. Giant-cell tumor of the skull base. Neuroradiology. 1999;41(4):305–7.
10. Kay RM, Eckardt JJ, Seeger LL, et al. Pulmonary metastasis of benign giant cell tumor of bone: six histologically confirmed cases, including one of spontaneous regression. Clin Orthop. 1994;302:219–30.
11. Abbas AK, Kumar V, Fausto N, et al. Robbins and Cotran pathologic basis of disease, professional edition e-book: expert consult – online and print. Philadelphia: W.B. Saunders Company; 2010. ISBN: 1437721826.
12. Chen CC, Liau CT, Chang CH, et al. Giant cell tumors of the bone with pulmonary metastasis. Orthopedics. 2016;39(1):e68–73. https://doi.org/10.3928/01477447-20151228-04. Accessed 4/23/2016.
13. Bertoni F, Present D, Enneking WF. Giant-cell tumor of bone with pulmonary metastases. J Bone Joint Surg Am. 1985;67:890–900.
14. Pereira HM, Marchiori E, Severo A. Magnetic resonance imaging aspects of giant-cell tumours of bone. J Med Imaging Radiat Oncol. 2014;58(6):674–8. https://doi.org/10.1111/1754-9485.12249.

15. Cooper AS, Travers B. Surgical essays. London: Cox Longman & Co; 1818. p. 178–9.
16. McGrath PJ. Giant-cell tumor of bone: an analysis of fifty-two cases. J Bone Joint Surg. 1972;54:216–24.
17. Bertoni F, Bacchini P, Staals EL. Malignancy in giant cell tumor of bone. Cancer. 2003;97(10):2520–9.
18. Dahlin DC, Cupps RE, Johnson EW. Giant-cell tumors: a study of 195 cases. Cancer. 1970;25:1061–70. https://doi.org/10.1002/1097-0142(197005)25:5<1061::AID-CNCR2820250509>3.0.CO;2-E.
19. Nackos JS, Wiggins RH III, Harnsberger HR. CT and MR imaging of giant cell granuloma of the craniofacial bones. AJNR Am J Neuroradiol. 2006;27:1651–3.
20. Sinha NR, Szmigielski W, Khanna M. Aneurysmal bone cyst of the ethmoid sinus: a case report. Pol J Radiol. 2010;75(3):65–7.
21. Aralasmak A, Aygun N, Westra WH, Yousem DM. Giant cell reparative granuloma of the sphenoid bone. AJNR Am J Neuroradiol. 2006;27:1675–7.
22. Hrishikesh KA, Narlawar RS, Deasi SB, et al. Aneurysmal bone cyst of the ethmoid bone. Br J Radiol. 2002;75:916–8.
23. Aoki J, Tanikawa H, Ishii K, et al. MR findings indicative of hemosiderin in giant-cell tumor of bone: frequency, cause, and diagnostic significance. AJR Am J Roentgenol. 1996;166:145–8.
24. Midyett FA, Mukherji SK. Fibrous dysplasia. In: Orbital imaging. Philadelphia: Elsevier/Saunders; 2015. p. 241–6. ISBN: 978-0-323-34037-3.
25. Midyett FA, Mukherji SK. Optic nerve metastasis. In: Orbital imaging. Philadelphia: Elsevier/Saunders; 2015. p. 87–90. ISBN: 978-0-323-34037-3.
26. Vanel D. MRI of bone metastasis: the choice of the sequence. Cancer Imaging. 2004;4(1):30–4. https://doi.org/10.1102/1470-7330.2003.0029.
27. Al-Gahtany M, Cusimano M, Singer W, et al. Brown tumors of the skull base. Case report and review of the literature. J. Neurosurgery. 2003;98(2):417–20.
28. Midyett FA, Mukherji SK. Orbital plasmacytoma and myeloma. In: Orbital imaging. Philadelphia: Elsevier/Saunders; 2015. p. 233–40. ISBN: 978-0-323-34037-3.
29. Finch EF, Gleave HH. A case of osteoclastoma (myeloid sarcoma, benign giant cell tumour) with pulmonary metastasis. J Pathol Bacteriol. 1926;29:399–406. https://doi.org/10.1002/path.1700290408.
30. Cooper A, Travers B. Surgical essays. 3rd ed. London: Cox & Son; 1818.
31. Chakarun C, Forrester D, Gottsegen C, et al. Giant cell tumor of bone: review, mimics, and new developments in treatment. Radiographics. 2013;33(1):197–211. https://doi.org/10.1148/rg.331125089.

25 Fibrous Dysplasia Involving the Skull Base

Pertinent Points

- *Definition*: Fibrous dysplasia (FD) is a slowly progressive tumor-like process where normal cancellous bone is replaced by immature woven bone and fibrous tissue. This is often associated with endocrine dysfunction, abnormal pigmentation, and, in girls, precocious puberty [10]. With its fondness for the skull base and orbit, fibrous dysplasia can cause serious neurologic problems.
- *Classic Clue*: Young adolescent patient presents with painless proptosis and diplopia with an expanding enhancing sphenoid wing mass showing a "ground-glass" appearance with an intact bony cortex.
- *Presentation*: Fibrous dysplasia involving the skull base may present in myriad manners [28].
- *AKA*: Lichtenstein-Jaffe disease, leontiasis ossea.
- *Sex*: M = F. There is no known gender preference [1].
- *Age*: 75% present ≤30 year old with peak incidence 3–15 years.
- *Prevalence*: Fibrous dysplasia is a nonfamilial bone disorder with prevalence predictions showing their span through: "relatively uncommon," "not uncommon," "relatively rare," and "rare" [6, 7, 11].
- *Locations*: Fibrous dysplasia flaunts a fondness for the frontal, sphenoid, ethmoid, and maxillary bones [7, 12].
- Fibrous dysplasia falls into three basic types: sclerotic, lytic, and mixed.
- Sclerotic lesions dominate the skull base with lytic lesions least likely.
- Fibrous dysplasia's matchless medullary cavity expansion conserves original bone shape while concurrently conserving its cortex.
- Like a referee, the radiologist has been provided with several "red flags" which he should be vigilant in employing early and properly.
- Classically fibrous dysplasia displays a "ground-glass" appearance. Conversely, cystic degeneration is a "red flag" which when near the orbit has a high propensity for visual impairment.
- Periosteal reaction also raises a second "red flag" for a pathological fracture or underlying malignant metamorphosis.
- While fibrous dysplasia's cortex is classically preserved, severe expansion may cause the cortex to virtually "vanish."
- A third "red flag" is readied for progressive lytic lesions which suggest malignant degeneration.

Imaging

General Imaging Features

- Fibrous dysplasia's bony expansion retains its original shape while sparing the cortex.
- Relatively radiolucent expansile medullary lesions with lucency vary depending on the degree of osteoid.
- Fibrous dysplasia displays well-defined sclerotic margins with endosteal scalloping.
- Skull base fibrous dysplasia is typically *sclerotic*.
- Frequently find frontal bossing and facial asymmetry.
- Fibrous dysplasia may "mimic" a variety of bone lesions.

CT Findings

- *See General Imaging Features.*
- The "ground-glass" appearance is "classic" for fibrous dysplasia. However, when not choosing to conform to the classic "ground-glass" craze, avant-garde lesions may appear astoundingly heterogeneous.

F. A. Midyett, S. K. Mukherji, *Skull Base Imaging*, https://doi.org/10.1007/978-3-030-46447-9_25

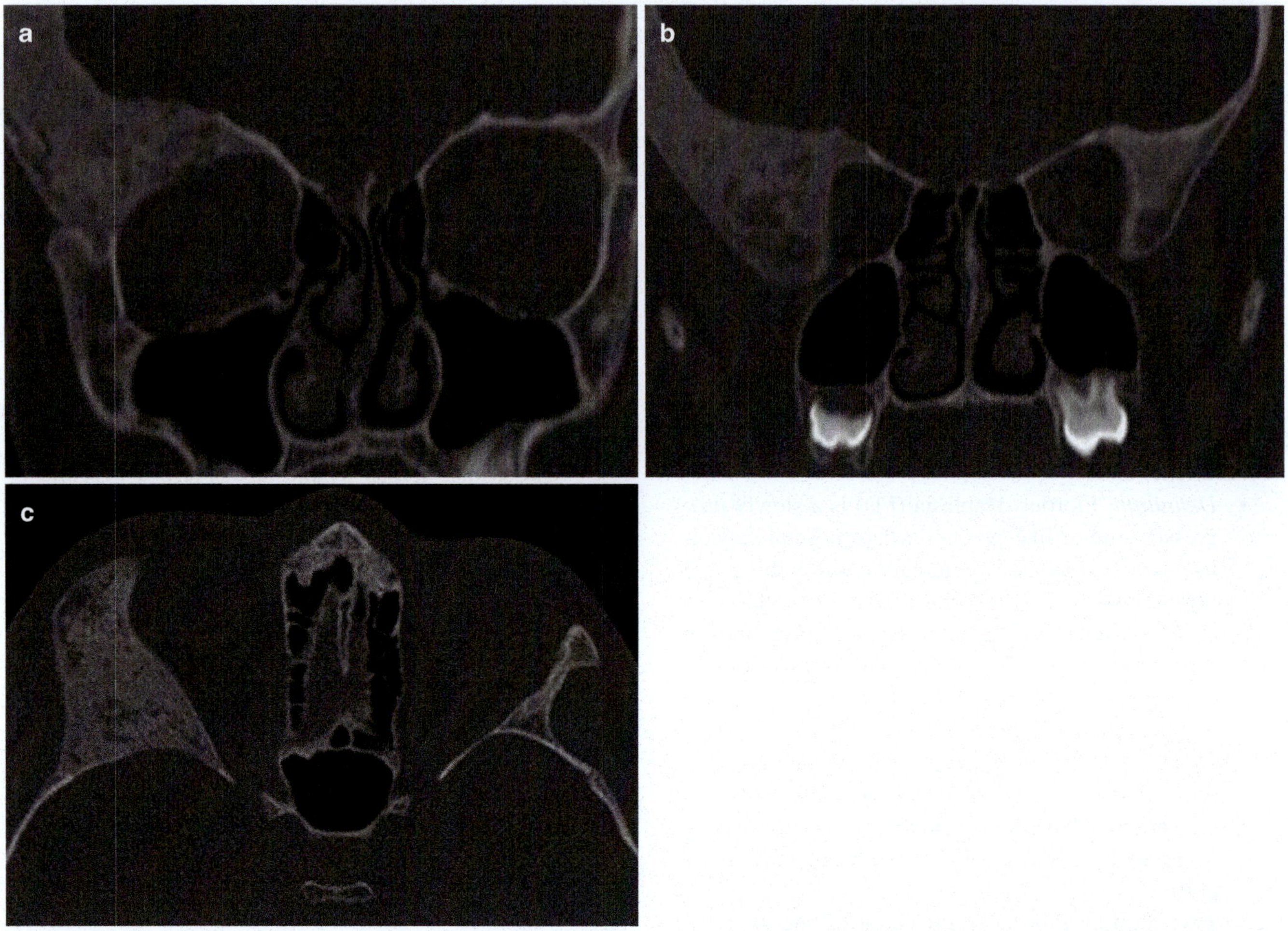

Fig. 25.1 (**a**, **b**) Coronal and axial (**c**) NECT shows a diffuse intradiploic abnormality, depicting uniform diploic thickening involving the right orbit, particularly the greater sphenoid wing. The general bony shape has been preserved with a "ground-glass" appearance. While some of the cortex has been preserved, much of it has virtually "vanished." [NECTs are from different patient than MRs]

- Fibrous dysplasia classically expands bone while keeping its original shape and simultaneously sparing the cortex.
- Clinicians frequently find 3D CT reconstructions to be useful pre-surgical planning roadmaps.
- While fibrous dysplasia's cortex is classically preserved, severe expansion can cause the cortex to virtually "vanish."
- See Fig. 25.1a–c.

MRI

- *See General Imaging Features.*
- Regrettably, fibrous dysplasia's MRI findings do not share those unique features frequently found on CT/radiography. Alas, fibrous dysplasia's MRI facades regularly resemble tumor [24].
- When fibrous dysplasia preserves the original bony shape, the diagnosis is relatively easy. Exceptionally, extraosseous localized involvement presents a potential pitfall [24].
- T1: Heterogeneous usually low to intermediate signal is often isointense to brain [24].
- T2: Often variable. Heterogeneous, usually low, often isointense to brain but may reveal regions of higher signal [24] (See Fig. 25.2c).
- T1 Gd:
  - Usually exhibits enthusiastic enhancement. However, please note where there is no significant enhancement.

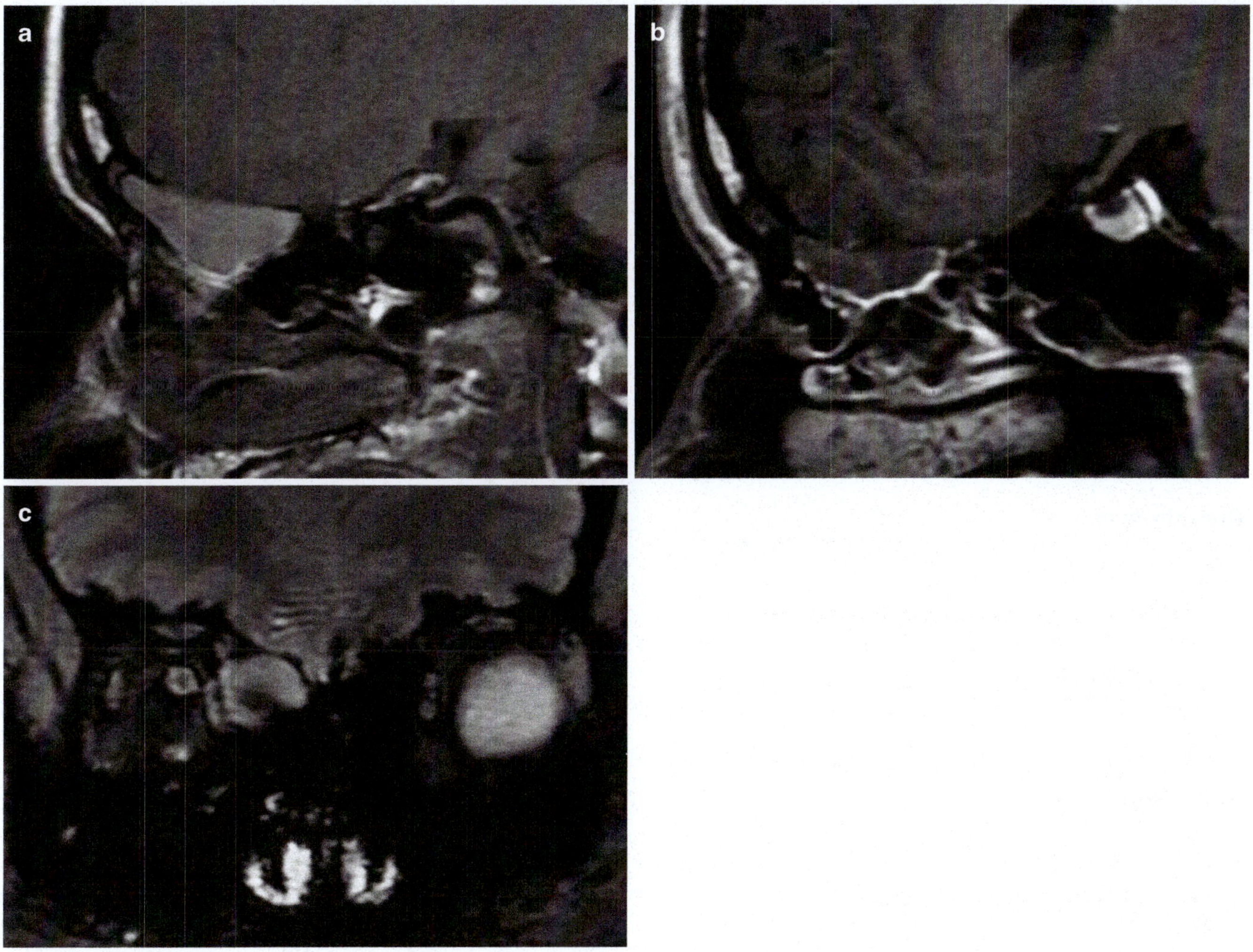

Fig. 25.2 (**a**) Sagittal T1 shows relatively homogeneous focus of abnormal marrow involving the right anterior skull base. This is clearly an intradiploic process which has expanded bone preserving its original shape and much of its cortex. There is however, moderate indistinctness of the cortex composing the anterior skull base (with loss of the normal black line). The lesion's signal intensity is hyperintense to brain but hypointense to nearby normal frontal fatty marrow. (**b**) Sagittal T1 Gd shows a relatively homogeneous focus of abnormal marrow involving the right anterior skull base. This intradiploic process has expanded bone while preserving its original shape and much of its cortex. There is however moderate indistinctness of the cortex composing the floor of the anterior cranial fossa. The lesion's signal intensity is isointense to the brain but hypointense to nearby normal frontal fatty marrow. No significant intralesional enhancement. (**c**) Coronal T2 shows heterogeneous high signal mass adjacent the inferior aspect of the right anterior cranial fossa along the right orbit's medial margin

  - Cysts and hemorrhage can cause heterogeneous signals which vary depending on protein content and age of blood products.
- *Confidence*: Confidence in MRI can be high with low T1 and T2 signal (despite post-contrast enhancement) [24].
- *Confusion*: Confusion crops up with intermediate T1 and high T2 when the lesions exhibit enthusiastic enhancement. These cases should be resolved by CT [24].

Nuclear Medicine

- *Tc*^{99m} *Hot*: Bone scans show ↑ uptake of Tc^{99m} with "hot" lesions in affected areas.
  - By contrast, plasmacytoma portrays ↓ uptake [29].

Clinical Issues

Signs and Symptoms

- Fibrous dysplasia involving the skull base may present in myriad manners [2].
- When involving the orbit, FD may present with proptosis, diplopia, globe displacement, ↓ extraocular motility, visual impairment, or overlying soft tissue swelling [7, 13, 20].
- Fibrous dysplasia can compromise any cranial nerve causing clinical findings similar to those shown by skull base Paget's disease.
- See Ch-41/Paget's/Complications.

Prevalences

- Age:
  - More prevalent in children and young adults.
  - 75% present <30 year old with peak incidence of 3–15 years.
- Gender: M = F. There is no known gender preference [1].

Pathology

- *Gross:* Involved marrow cavity is filled with fibrous tissue causing a whitish abnormal appearance.
- *Microscopic:*
  - The bony matrix comprises small scantily shaped trabeculae of immature, mistakenly mineralized bone.
  - The seemingly sporadic shapes shown by bony trabeculae have been compared to *Chinese characters* [3].
  - Fibrous dysplasia is not contained by a capsule.
- Cortical bone is typically spared by fibrous dysplasia, although the cortex can sometimes be thinned and transgressed by abnormal medullary cavity expansion.
- <1% undergo malignant transformation, most often after radiation therapy and may give rise to osteo-, fibro-, or chondrosarcomas [3].
- Fibrous dysplasia's *secondary cystic degeneration* is often a more frequent cause of optic symptoms than its *primary impingement* on the optic nerve [7, 20].

Treatment and Prognosis

- Treatment for fibrous dysplasia is *principally palliative* focused on fracture and deformity management.
- Fibrous dysplasia is usually managed conservatively with little consideration for intervention unless faced with significant functional impairment or neurologic deficit [3].
- Surgery to correct cosmetic problems is typically postponed pending growth cessation with lesional stabilization [3].
- Craniofacial surgical resections confront significant postoperative complications including recurrence rates of ~25% in the first 3 years [3].

I. Nonsurgical

- *Conservative Management*: Currently preferred unless significant functional impairment or neurologic deficits develop [3, 20].
- *Steroids*: Some support the short-term use of systemic steroids for medical management [7, 20].
- *Radiotherapy*: While used in the past, radiotherapy is *currently considered contraindicated* because of potential sarcomatous degeneration [6, 7, 20].

II. Surgical

- *Vision*:
  - The etiology and treatment for fibrous dysplasia's visual impairment continue to be controversial some 3/4 century after Dandy first challenged its transcranial surgical solution [7, 8, 20].
  - Some suggest saving surgical decompression for when the optic nerve is "markedly" compressed. Nevertheless, post-surgical visual deficits can crop up despite scrupulous surgical skills [20].
  - Orbital fibrous dysplasia is seldom confined to the orbit and regularly requires team tactics with neurosurgical involvement.
- *Hearing*:
  - Interventions to correct stenosis of both EAC and IAC involvement have shown some surgical successes.
- *Cosmetics*:
  - Cosmetic surgery should be postponed until the lesions stabilize [3].

III. Complications

- Fibrous dysplasia can compromise any cranial nerve causing clinical findings similar to those exhibited by Paget's disease (See Chap. 41, Paget's Disease/ Complications).
- Patients with fibrous dysplasia are 400 times more likely to develop a malignant bone tumor compared to the general population.

IV. Prognosis

- Postoperative recurrences occur in approximately 25% within 3 years after surgery [3, 20].
- The most common causes for visual loss in patients with orbital fibrous dysplasia are probably iatrogenic [7].

Differential Diagnosis (DDx)

A. Paget's Disease of the Bone

- 1877 Sir James Paget, English surgeon and pathologist, first described this disorder in a small group of patients who exhibited an "odd overgrowth" on their heads and extremities, resulting in regular occurrence of long bone bowing with recurrent fractures.
- Paget's involves both inner and outer tables. By contrast, fibrous dysplasia widens the diploic space displacing the outer table while sparing the inner table.
- While facial bone involvement is uncommon with Paget's, it is common with fibrous dysplasia [7, 14].
- Paget's typically spares the skull vertex, usually starting in the frontal or occipital regions.
- Paget's well-defined lytic lesions characteristically lack sclerotic margins.
- Paget's bony skull base softening encourages basilar impression.
- Paget's healing phase can cause the classic "cotton-wool" appearance [4].
- See Chap. 41, Paget's Disease.

B. Hyperparathyroidism (HPT) [20]

- Most display "mottled" demineralization confirming a classic "ground-glass" appearance.
- Vascular grooves display indistinct cortical margins.
- HPT's rare "brown tumor" can cause focal destruction.
- Frequently find multiple skull defects with HPT [16].
- Radiologists should search for secondary signs of HPT including subperiosteal absorption of bone in hand radiographs.

C. Sclerotic Metastasis [18, 19, 20]

- Sclerotic or blastic bony metastasis may occasionally fall into the differential diagnosis of skull base fibrous dysplasia.
- Patients frequently are aware of an existing or pre-existing malignancy.
- Sclerotic metastasis can come from the prostate (most common), breast (may be mixed), transitional cell carcinoma (TCC), carcinoid, medulloblastoma, neuroblastoma, mucinous adenocarcinoma, and lymphoma.

D. Intraosseous Meningioma (IM)

- Intraosseous meningiomas are really rare tumors causing <1% of all bone tumors.
- Most meningiomas are extra diploic often causing cortical thickening but most do not involve an intraosseous epicenter.
- A blatant exception is the intraosseous meningiomas which may mimic the intrinsically intradiploic fibrous dysplasia which only occasionally breaches its cortex to extend afar.
- 65% of intraosseous meningiomas are sclerotic and 35% are osteolytic [17, 20].
- MRI features of intraosseous meningiomas include:
  - T1: isointense to grey matter.
  - T2: Most are isointense to grey matter although some show hyperintense signals.
  - T1 Gd: Exhibit enthusiastic enhancement.

A Closer Look

I. Fast Facts

- Fibrous dysplasia's definitive diagnosis is based on clinical, radiological, histological data.
- Visual impairment is the most common, dreaded, and debilitating of FD's neurologic complications [7, 15, 20].

II. Potpourri

- Fibrous dysplasia comprises 2.5% of all bone tumors.
- Fibrous dysplasia comprises 7.5% of all benign bone tumors.

III. Genetics and Molecular Biology

- Fibrous dysplasia's exact cause continues to be unknown but current theories favor developmental over traumatic and neoplastic etiologies [3].

- Fibrous dysplasia is noticeably *not hereditary* with no known parent-to-child transmission.
- Fibrous dysplasia is a diverse disease capable of collating any combination of craniofacial, axillary, or appendicular ossicles [21].
- Abnormal regulation of cyclic adenosine monophosphate or protein kinase A has been proposed as a possible etiologic factor in development of fibrous dysplasia [27].
- Fibrous dysplasia probably results from post-zygotic activating mutations of the GNAS locus at 20q13.2-q13.3 which codes for the alpha subunit of the G_S G-coupled protein receptor [22].
- Increased G_S alpha signaling results bone marrow stromal cell proliferation prompting replacement of normal marrow with fibrous tissue. The resultant irregular, thin bony trabeculae are commonly compared to "Chinese characters" [23].

IV. Historic Highlights

- 1891 von Recklinghausen was the first physician to describe the unique lesions of fibrous dysplasia [25].
- 1938 Lichtenstein recognized this distinctive condition and coined the moniker "fibrous dysplasia" for this exceptional entity [26].
- 1941 Dandy published his classic monograph describing the first transcranial approach for removal of orbital fibrous dysplasia [7, 8].
- 1936 and 1937 McCune and Albright recognized the frequent correlation between fibrous dysplasia and endocrinopathy [7–9].
- The McCune-Albright syndrome came to be recognized by the triad of polyostotic fibrous dysplasia, cutaneous pigmentation (café au lait spots), and precocious puberty [7–9].
- Clearly, fibrous dysplasia has been around a long time, having been found in the seventh century Anglo Saxon skulls and in a skull from 1480 more recently discovered in an ancient Tennessee cavern [4–6].

Selected References

1. Larheim TA, Westesson P. Maxillofacial imaging. Cham: Springer; 2008. p. 406.
2. Dähnert W. Radiology review manual. 3rd ed. Baltimore: Williams & Wilkins; 1996. p. 54–6.
3. Lufkin R, Borges A, Villablanca P. Teaching atlas of head and neck imaging. New York/Stuttgart: Thieme; 2000. p. 13–7.
4. Wells C. Polyostotic fibrous dysplasia in a 7th century Anglo-Saxon. Br J Radiol. 1963;36:925–6.
5. Gregg JB, Reed A. Monostotic fibrous dysplasia in the temporal bone: a late prehistoric occurrence. Am J Phys Anthropol. 1980;52:587–93.
6. Bibby K, McFadzean R. Fibrous dysplasia of the orbit. Br J Ophthalmol. 1994;78:266–70.
7. Dumont AS, Boulos PT, Jane JA, et al. Cranio-orbital fibrous dysplasia: with emphasis on visual impairment and current surgical management. Neurosurg Focus. 2001;10(5):1–8.
8. Dandy WE. Orbital tumors: results following the transcranial operative attack. New York: Piest; 1941. p. 3–7.
9. McCune DJ. Osteitis fibrosa cystic: the case of a nine year old girl who also exhibits precocious puberty, multiple pigmentations of the skin and hyperthyroidism. Am J Dis Child. 1936;52:743.
10. Albright F, Butler MA, Hampton AO, et al. Syndrome characterized by osteitis fibrosa disseminata, areas of pigmentation and endocrine dysfunction with precocious puberty in females. N Engl J Med. 1937;216:727–46.
11. Ricalde P, Horswell BB. Craniofacial fibrous dysplasia of the fronto-orbital region: a case series and literature review. J Oral Maxillofac Surg. 2001;59:157–68.
12. Michael CB, Lee AB, Patrinely JR, et al. Visual loss associated with fibrous dysplasia of the anterior skull base. Case report and review of the literature. J Neurosurg. 2000;92:350–4.
13. Moore AT, Buncic JR, Munro IR. Fibrous dysplasia of the orbit in childhood. Clinical features and management. Ophthalmology. 1985;92:12–20.
14. Doran SE, Gebarski SS, Hoff JT. Tumors of the skull. In: Youmans JR, editor. Neurological surgery, vol. 4. 4th ed. Philadelphia: WB Saunders; 1996. p. 2998–3023.
15. Sassin JF, Rosenberg RN. Neurological complications of fibrous dysplasia of the skull. Arch Neurol. 1968;18:363–9.
16. Zee CS. Neuroradiology: a study guide. New York: McGraw-Hill; 1996. p. 2–3.
17. Tokgoz N, Oner YA, Kaymaz M, et al. Primary intraosseous meningioma: CT and MRI appearance. AJNR Am J Neuroradiol. 2005;26(8):2053–6.
18. Char DH, Miller T, Kroll S. Orbital metastases: diagnosis and course. Br J Ophthalmol. 1997;81(5):386–90.
19. Jacquemin C, Bosley TM, Svedberg H. Orbit deformities in craniofacial neurofibromatosis type 1. AJNR Am J Neuroradiol. 2003;24(8):1678–82.
20. Midyett FA, Mukherji SK. Fibrous dysplasia. In: Orbital imaging. Philadelphia: Elsevier/Saunders; 2015. p. 241–6. ISBN: 978-0-323-34037-3.
21. Kelly MH, Brillante B, Collins MT. Pain in fibrous dysplasia of bone: age-related changes and the anatomical distribution of skeletal lesions. Osteoporos Int. 2008;19(1):57–63. https://doi.org/10.1007/s00198-007-0425-x. ISSN 0937-941X. PMID 17622477.
22. Weinstein LS, Shenker A, Gejman PV, et al. Activating mutations of the stimulatory G protein in the McCune-Albright syndrome. N Engl J Med. 1991;325(24):1688–95. https://doi.org/10.1056/NEJM199112123252403. ISSN 0028-4793. PMID 1944469.
23. Riminucci M, Fisher LW, Shenker A, et al. Fibrous dysplasia of bone in the McCune-Albright syndrome: abnormalities in bone formation. Am J Pathol. 1997;151(6):1587–600. ISSN 0002-9440. PMC 1858361. PMID 9403710.

24. Chong VF, Khoo JB, Fan YF. Fibrous dysplasia involving the base of the skull. AJR Am J Roentgenol. 2002;178(3):717–20.
25. von Recklinghausen F. Die Fibrose oder deformierende Ostitis, die Osteomalacie und die osteoplastische Carcinose in ihren gegenseitigen Beziehungen, vol. 13. Berlin: Germany; 1891.
26. Lichtenstein L. Polyostotic fibrous dysplasia. Arch Surg. 1938;36:874–98.
27. Lee PA, Van Dop C, Migeon CJ. McCune-Albright syndrome: long-term follow-up. JAMA. 1986;256(21):2980–4.
28. Lustig LR, Holliday MJ, McCarthy EF, Nager GT. Fibrous dysplasia involving the skull base and temporal bone. Arch Otolaryngol Head Neck Surg. 2001;127(10):1239–47.
29. Curaudeau GA, Chan L, Hammoud K, et al. Quite a slippery slope: pictorial review of the radiographic appearance of mass lesions and pseudolesions of the clivus. Neurographics. 2019;9(4):293–300.

26 Sinonasal Undifferentiated Carcinoma

Pertinent Points

- *Definition*: Sinonasal undifferentiated carcinoma (SNUC) is a rare, highly aggressive cancer arising from nasal or paranasal sinus epithelium [1]. SNUCs propensity for late stage advanced presentation together with its traditional terrible temperament portends *pathetically poor survival rates.*
- *AKA*: Anaplastic carcinoma [11]
- *Prevalence:*
  - Age: Range is third to ninth decade with median presentation in sixth decade [4].
  - Gender: M > F = ≤3:1 [7, 11].
  - Habits: 85% of SNUC patients are smokers.
- *Classic Clue*: A 60-year-old male smoker patient presents with seemingly insignificant interval including one or more of following symptoms: nasal obstruction, facial pain, diplopia, epistaxis, proptosis, periorbital swelling, and symptoms of cranial nerve involvement. Imaging shows an aggressive mass involving the skull base, superior nasal cavity, and/or ethmoids and may already extend into the orbits or brain.
- *Poor Prognosis:* Its rapid growth, potential for local and regional recurrence, and distant metastasis portent a particularly poor prognosis [13].

Imaging

General Imaging Features

- Tumors tend to be large at presentation with poorly defined margins.
- Most arise from ethmoid sinuses or superior nasal cavity.
- Often see aggressive bone destruction with tumor extending from the sinonasal region into the orbit(s), skull base, or occasionally the cavernous sinuses.
- SNUCs are typically large (>4 cm) *non-calcified* masses, presenting poorly defined margins more often than not emerging from the ethmoids or superior nasal cavity. They commonly cause sinus obstruction.

CT Features

- *See General Imaging Features.*
- Sinonasal mass causing opacification with or without bone erosion.
- *Erratic enhancement*: Exhibits *erratic* post contrast *enhancement.*

MRI Features

- *See Section General Imaging Features.*
  - Often demonstrate bone destruction with tumor completely obliterating the skull base (see Fig. 26.1a, b).
  - May extend through the skull base to involve dura and brain (see Fig. 26.1a, b).
  - May extend into the orbits (see Fig. 26.1c–e).
- T1 Signal
  - Hypo- to Isointense to brain. Generally homogeneous with occasional foci of high signal related to mucus (see Figs. 26.1a, c and 26.2a, c).
- T2 Signal
  - Moderately heterogeneous, mostly iso- to hyperintense to brain. Scattered fluid containing high signal foci isointense to CSF (see Fig. 26.1e).
- T1 Gd:
  - Exhibits *avid* heterogeneous enthusiastic *enhancement*, containing multiple non-enhancing foci (See Figs. 26.1b, d and 26.2b–e).

F. A. Midyett, S. K. Mukherji, *Skull Base Imaging*, https://doi.org/10.1007/978-3-030-46447-9_26

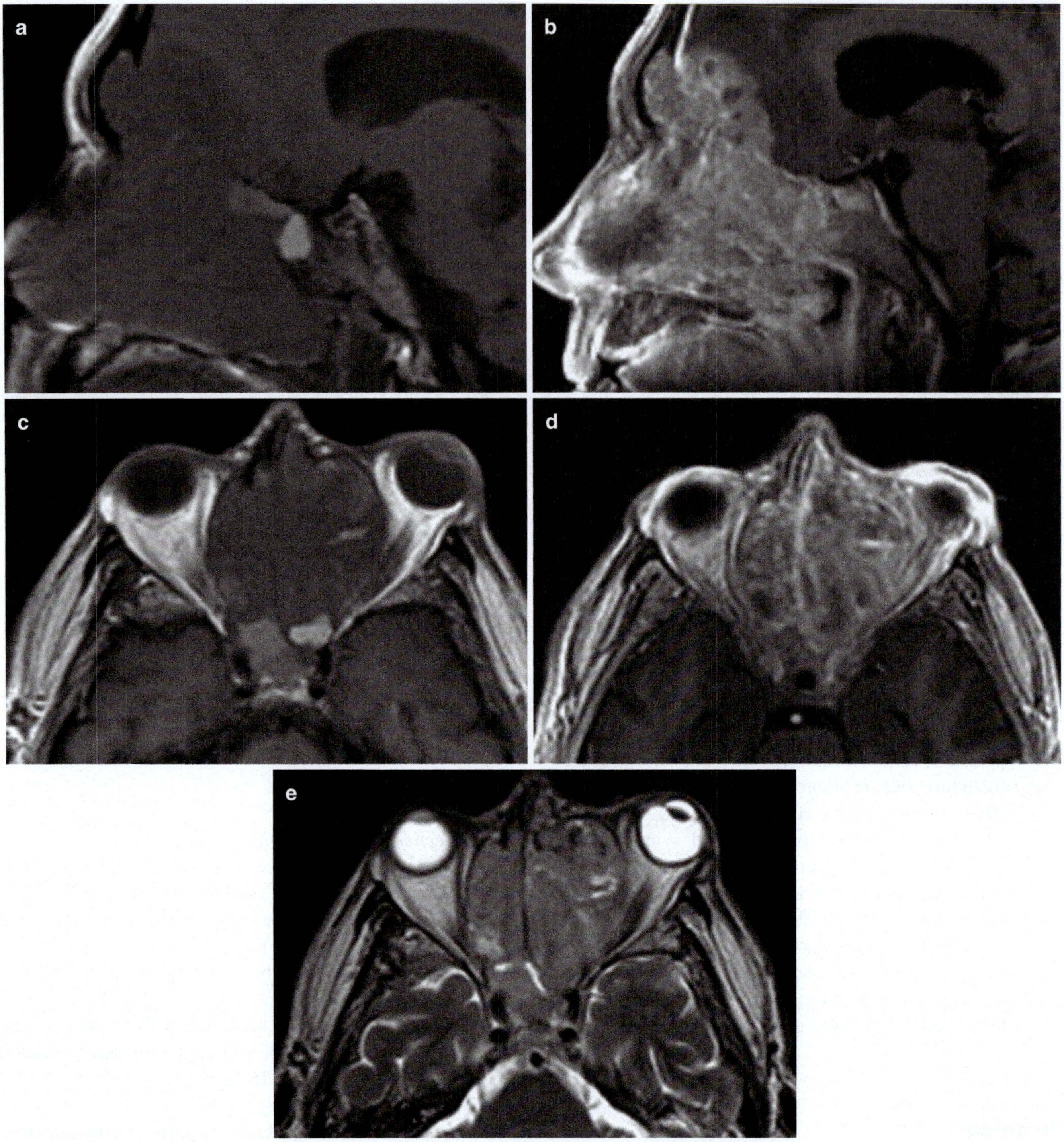

Fig. 26.1 Sagittal T1 without (**a**) and with Gd (**b**) show a huge skull base mass hypo/isointense to brain before Gd exhibits avid enthusiastic heterogeneous postcontrast enhancement. The extensive pathologic process involves the visualized sinuses and nasal cavity extending through the skull base to invade the meninges and brain. There is dural thickening with avid enhancement extending in the frontal region to the top of the image and posteriorly along the skull base to the clival tip. Much of the skull base (denoted by its inherent black line) has been destroyed by this blatantly aggressive tumor. Axial T1 without (**c**) and with Gd (**d**) show a huge skull base mass isointense to brain before Gd exhibits avid enthusiastic heterogeneous postcontrast enhancement. This massive tumor has extended into the orbits displacing their contents laterally, destroying much of the bony structure in its path. Scattered foci of high signal (**c**) are related to fluid with varying mucus components. While there is significant avid tumor enhancement, it is laced with non-enhancing foci (**d**). (**e**) Axial T2 shows huge mass extending into both orbits, displacing orbital contents laterally. The mass is relatively isointense to brain, moderately heterogeneous with some scattered dark and bright foci. The bright foci show signal intensity similar to CSF

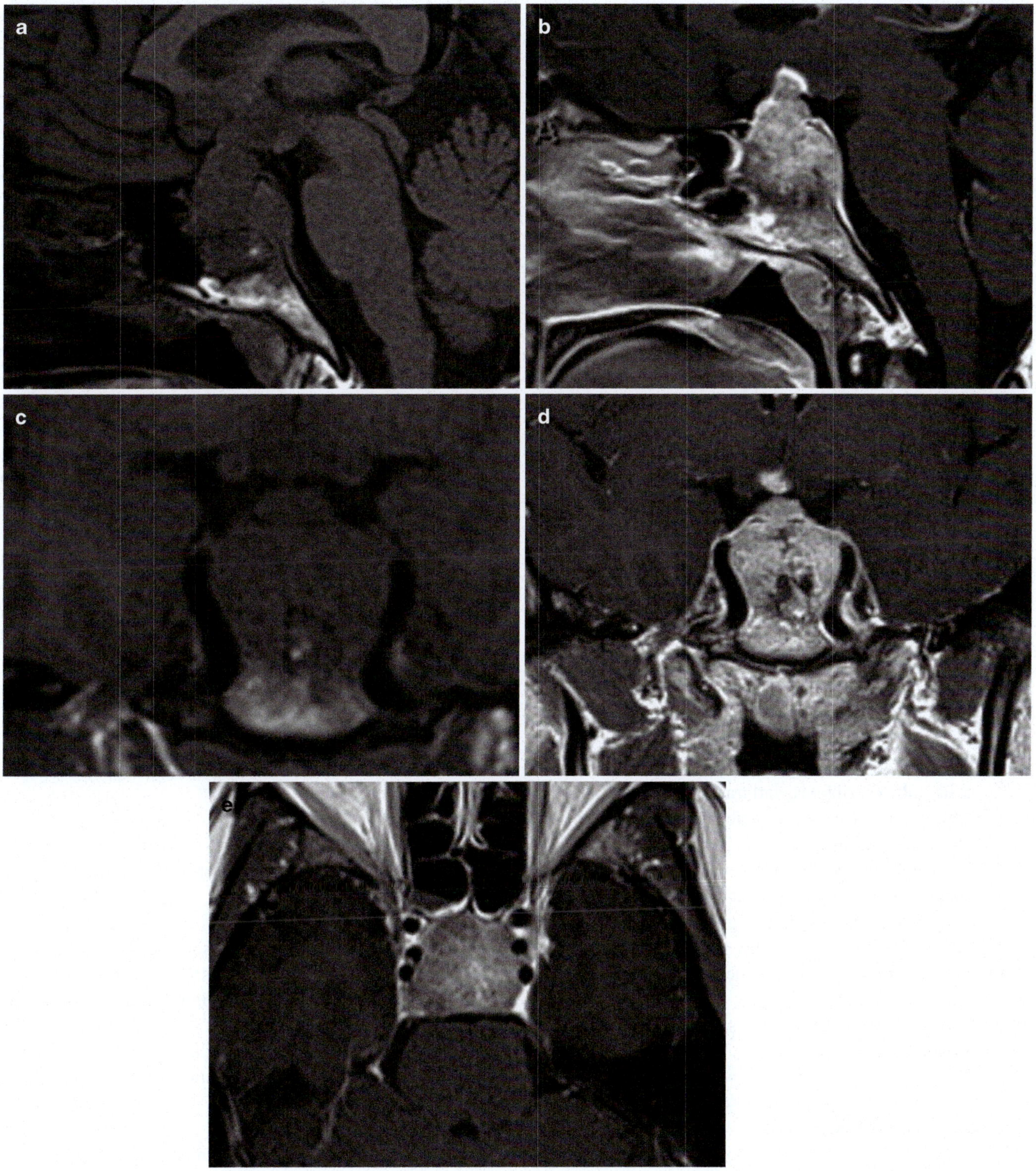

Fig. 26.2 Sagittal T1 without (**a**) and with Gd (**b**) show a sellar mass isointense to brain before Gd which exhibits avid enthusiastic heterogeneous postcontrast enhancement. The pathologic process breaches the sellar floor invading and replacing brighter marrow inferiorly (**a**). Post-Gd (**b**) demonstrates destruction of the posterior clival cortex superiorly with tumor extending posteriorly to abut the dura. Enhancement is avid but highly heterogeneous with areas of lower signal. Tumor extends superiorly into the suprasellar chiasmatic region. The anterior tumor margin is irregular as it extends into the sphenoid sinus. Coronal T1 without (**c**) and with Gd (**d**) show a large sellar and suprasellar mass isointense to brain before Gd (**c**) exhibiting avid enthusiastic heterogeneous post-Gd enhancement (**d**). Tumor extends laterally to the carotid siphons and cephalad above the chiasm. It extends caudally to the sellar floor which appears intact. As the upper sphenoid is clearly breached on sagittal images superiorly, this may be a hint that this is *not* of pituitary origin. Axial T1 Gd (**e**) shows moderately enhancing heterogeneous sellar mass. Nothing on this image suggests anything other than a pituitary adenoma. But, this was a sellar SNUC. Well, another case clearly cautions us to use a DDx! And (oh yes), this is another case when the cranial fossa classification system showed an exception as this is clearly in the MCF/Pituitary Region

Clinical Issues

Signs and Symptoms

- Patients present sometimes showing a seemingly insignificant interval of nasal obstruction, facial pain, diplopia, epistaxis, proptosis, periorbital swelling, and symptoms of cranial nerve involvement [1, 11].
- As is frequently found with other sinonasal tumors, SNUC patients perpetually present with far developed disease [13].

Pathology

- Various carcinoma types involve the paranasal sinuses including [7–9]:

SCC	Squamous cell carcinoma
NKSCC	Nonkeratinizing squamous cell carcinoma
CCC	Cylindrical cell carcinoma
TCC	Transitional cell carcinoma
NPTC	Nasopharyngeal-type undifferentiated Ca
SNUC	Sinonasal undifferentiated carcinoma

- *Gross* (SNUC)
  - Generally greater than 4 cm [11].
  - Usually fungating with ill-defined borders frequently invading into bone as well as contiguous compartments of anatomic anatomy [11].
- *Microscopic* SNUC [1]
  - SNUC is composed of cohesive cells shown in sheets, nests, lobules, ribbons, and trabeculae [11].
  - Cells exhibit hyperchromatic nuclei and ↑ nuclear/cytoplasmic ratios.
  - Prominent features include ↑mitotic rate, tumor necrosis, as well as lymphovascular and perineural invasion.
  - Confirmation of SNUC using light microscopy alone can be challenging and may require correlation with clinical, immunohistochemical, and ultrastructural characteristics [1].
  - Current histochemical studies are considered noncontributory for SNUC [10].

Treatment and Prognosis

- Clinical treatment has proven multimodality therapy to be the most successful of available options offering patients the best chance for survival.
- Carefully customized craniofacial resections are often currently combined with concomitant chemoradiation [11].
- However, currently there is not general agreement even for the best sequence for surgery, radiation therapy, and chemotherapy. Most do agree that optimal treatment has yet to be determined.
- Prognosis.
  - Given the relative rarity of SNUC, definitive prognostic information is absent [13].
  - Prognosis for patients with SNUC is currently considered to be poor with median survival rates of <18 months and 5-year survivals <20% [10, 11].
  - This is, however, considerably better than for the original group reported in 1986 whose grim mean survival was only 4 months [13].
  - SNUC can metastasize to the cervical lymph nodes, liver, lung, bone, and brain [10, 11].

Differential Diagnosis

- Although SNUC comprises <1% of all neoplasms, numerous tumors occurring near the same skull base region tend to present in similar locations with undifferentiated or poorly differentiated morphology [4].
- Some suggest that SNUC cannot be distinguished from other tumors of this region on the basis of imaging alone *except for SNM* [3]. This is *even more reason for radiologists to render* informed differential diagnoses.
- Per cubic centimeter, the sinonasal tract spawns the body's greatest mixture of malignancies [4].
- These uniquely diverse tumors which are frequently problematic for patients, pathologists, and radiologists include the following:

A. Sinonasal Melanoma (SNM)

- Sinonasal melanoma is a very rare and unique subtype of malignant melanoma noted for its poor prognosis and unique staging systems.
- *Classic Clue*: Older patient presenting for nasal congestion or epistaxis exhibits on MRI a nasal cavity mass having high T1 and low T2 signal compared to gray matter.
- Location: SNM is found in the nasal cavity more commonly than in the paranasal sinuses showing anterior nasal septum, lateral nasal wall, and inferior turbinate to be its preferred sites [10, 12].
- SNMs sometimes produce melanosis depositing melanin along the mucosal surface of the sinonasal cavity. Multiple lesional foci suggest melanoma.
- Melanoma may contain melanin with its paramagnetic effect demonstrating T1 and T2 shortening with characteristic high signal on T1 and low signal on T2.
- However, amelanotic melanomas may show low T1 and bright T2. And, if this not enough to confuse things,

bleeding is common and can show about any signal combination depending on the stage of hemoglobin breakdown.

- Melanoma swiftly spreads via hematogenous and perineural routes.
- Found in older patients (60–90) years of age with a higher incidence in Asia.
- May manifest as a multifocal sessile or polypoid mass. Frequently find bony remodeling and erosion.
- *Gray matter* is probably the *best internal standard* for comparing MRI signal.
- The *most common pattern* for these *uncommon lesions* encountered at conferences and board examinations is *high signal on T1* and *low signal on T2*. But alas, things are not always that simple. So, here are some general guiding principles.
- T1: Homogeneous signal.
  - May see ↑ T1 secondary to melanin or hemorrhage.
  - Melanotic melanomas have ↑ T1 compared to gray matter.
  - Amelanotic melanomas show intermediate T1 signal compared to gray matter.
- T2 shows variable intermediate signal compared to gray matter.
- T1 Gd: Mild to moderate heterogeneous enhancement. Signal varies with histology.
- DWI: Shows significant restricted diffusion with bright DWI and dark ADC map.
- See Chap. 18, Sinonasal Melanoma.

B. Rhabdomyosarcoma (RMS)

- RMS is the most common childhood soft tissue sarcoma caused by primitive mesenchymal cells retaining their capacity for skeletal muscle differentiation. RMS is most frequently found in children <age 10 currently comprising 5% of childhood cancers.
- Rhabdomyosarcoma originates from the Greek words *rhabdo* meaning rod shape and *myo* meaning muscle.
- *Classic Clue*: Child presents with headache showing signs of cranial nerve involvement with imaging depicting a large homogeneous well-circumscribed skull base mass without hyperostosis or calcification. It is similar to muscle on NECT and T1 with blatant restricted diffusion.
- Incidence in the United States is 6 cases per 1,000,000 per year in children <15 years.
- Distributions:
  - Age: Peak incidence is 1–5 years old.
  - Gender: Slight M > F = 1.5:1 prevalence.
  - Race: First recognized race predilection for RMS is Maori.
- The embryonal type of RMS is most common and is the most likely to involve the skull base.
- NECT classically appears as a homogeneous well circumscribed non-calcified soft tissue mass with irregular margins isodense to muscle. Rarely resembles a cystic mass with hemorrhagic foci.
- CECT shows the mass to be slightly hyperintense to surrounding muscle.
- RMS classically erodes and destroys adjacent bone but usually does not contain calcifications or provoke hyperostosis from adjacent bone.
- T1: Isointense to muscle but hypointense to orbital fat.
- T2: Heterogeneous hyperintense to muscle with multiple foci of high T2 signal.
- T1 Gd: Demonstrates avid heterogeneous enhancement.
- DWI: Demonstrates *restricted diffusion* with *bright DWI* images and corresponding *dark ADC* images.
- Nuclear Medicine: Shows ↑ uptake on bone scans.
- See Chap. 49, Rhabdomyosarcoma.

C. Ewing's Sarcoma (ES)

- Ewing's sarcoma is an aggressive malignant tumor of *childhood and adolescence* containing small blue round cells which usually presents in the second decade.
- *Classic Clue*: *Caucasian child or adolescent* presenting with pain, fever, and ↑ ESR found on imaging to have an extra-axial mass extending cranially and caudally from its skull base epicenter. On examination, the patient demonstrates orbital or cranial nerve symptoms.
- Ewing's accounts for 10–15% of childhood malignant bone tumors and is second only to osteosarcoma.
- ES is rare among Asians and African-Americans.
- Usually demonstrates destructive, permeative bone destruction with soft tissue components showing *no* soft tissue calcifications.
- Depending on the tumor stage, Ewing's sarcoma can cause cortical erosion with rarefaction and "moth-eaten" permeative destruction.
- T1: Low to intermediate signal, isointense to brain and muscle.
- T2: Heterogeneous signal, relatively isointense to brain with focal fluid collections which show high T2 signal. Low signal striations sometimes suggest a "hair on end" appearance.
- T1 Gd: *Mild heterogeneous enhancement.*
- DWI: Bony involvement may be more conspicuous on DWI.
- See Chap. 47, Ewing's Sarcoma.

D. Esthesioneuroblastoma (ENB)

- Rare neuroendocrine malignancy of neural crest origin arising from olfactory epithelium.
- AKA: Olfactory neuroblastoma.
- While esthesioneuroblastoma is more frequently found in middle aged patients, it is sometimes seen in children.

- Classically show avidly enhancing dumbbell-shaped mass with "waist" at the cribriform plate.
- May involve the anterior cranial fossa, skull base, and orbit.
- ENBs show intermediate signal on T1 and T2 with avid enhancement on T1 Gd.
- Cystic areas (with foci of ↑ T2) at the tumor/brain interface are diagnostic and may be pathognomonic.
- DWI shows moderate restricted diffusion.
- ENB exhibits an epicenter near the cribriform plate.
- ENB gives no gender preference.
- See Chap. 28, Esthesioneuroblastoma.

E. Neuroendocrine Carcinoma (NEC)

- Neuroendocrine tumors (NETs) may have either epithelial or neural origins. NETs arising from neural origin are paragangliomas and those arising from epithelial origin are neuroendocrine carcinomas (NECs).
- Nonlaryngeal NETs of the H&N are rare tumors, most frequently found near the paranasal sinuses with common origin sites including nasal cavity, ethmoid, and maxillary sinuses.
- The median age of presentation is 56 years, showing equal sex distribution.
- Although NECs expand and erode sinus walls most feel, there are *no characteristic* CT or MR features.
- CT typically shows a soft tissue mass which expands and erodes the involved sinus possibly extending into the nasal cavity and/or nasopharynx. Skull base involvement is frequent.
- T1: Relatively iso- or slightly hyperintense to the brain. Heterogeneous with scattered areas of more hyperintensity.
- T2: Relatively iso- or slightly hyperintense to the brain. Heterogeneous with scattered areas of more hyperintensity.
- T1 Gd: Mild heterogeneous enhancement.
- DWI: Moderate diffusion restriction.
- See Chap. 16, Neuroendocrine Carcinoma.

F. Juvenile Nasopharyngeal Angiofibroma (JNA)

- Rare, highly vascular, locally invasive benign nasopharyngeal neoplasm occurring almost entirely in adolescent and young adult males displaying a distinct tendency for recurrence.
- *Classic Clue*: Adolescent male presenting with epistaxis has avidly enhancing, heterogeneous posterior nasal mass with MRI showing *characteristic salt and pepper appearance* from presence of prominent flow voids.
- Typically have the Holman-Miller sign with archetypical anterior bowing of the posterior maxillary sinus wall.
  - T1: Heterogeneous intermediate signal.
  - T2: Heterogeneous signal with dark flow voids.
  - T1 Gd: Exhibits avid enhancement. Axial and coronal fat saturation images are essential to define involvement of the skull base, sphenoid, and cavernous sinuses.
- Most sequences show *characteristic salt and pepper appearance* from the presence of prominent flow voids.
- Catheter angiography illustrates a plethora of dilated tortuous vessels and depicts an intense characteristic capillary blush.
- See Chap. 15, Juvenile Nasopharyngeal Angiofibroma.

A Closer Look

I. Genetics and Molecular Biology

- Although SNUC is currently of uncertain histogenesis, it does possess unique clinicopathologic characteristics [11].
- While not universally found, EBV has been isolated in some SNUC cases and is particularly prominent in EBV endemic areas [7].
- A somatic mutation at the RB-1 locus on chromosome 13 has been described and may be involved in the formation or progression of these tumors. But it is uncertain whether this mutation is spontaneous or radiation-induced [6].

II. Statistical Soup

- ≤90% of patients present with stage T4 disease [4].
- ≤50% of patients present with orbital or skull base and brain involvement [4].
- ~10% have nodal metastasis at presentation [4].
- SNUC causes 3% of all H&N malignancies [14].

III. Historic Highlights

- In 1986 Frierson et al. first recognized SNUC as a rare but distinctly different pathologic entity. SNUC is a highly aggressive paranasal sinus tumor.

Selected References

1. Houston GD, Gilles E. Sinonasal undifferentiated carcinoma: a distinctive cllinicopathologic entity. Adv Anat Pathol. 1999;6(6):317–23.
2. Pitman KT, Costantino PD, Lassen LF. Sinonasal undifferentiated carcinoma: current trends in treatment. Skull Base Surg. 2011;5(4):269–72.
3. Phillips CD, Futter SF, Lipper MH, Levine PA. Sinonasal undifferentiated carcinoma: CT and MR imaging of an uncommon neoplasm of the nasal cavity. Radiology. 1997;202(2):477–80. https://doi.org/10.1148/radiology.202.2.9015077.
4. Su SY, Bell D, Hanna EY. Esthesioneuroblastoma, neuroendocrine carcinoma and sinonasal undifferentiated carcinoma: differentiation in diagnosis and treatment. Int Arch Otorhinolaryngol. 2014;18(2):S149–56.

5. Jones AV, Robinson I, Speight PM. Sinonasal undifferentiated carcinoma: report of a case and review of literature. Oral Oncol Extra. 2005;41(10):299–302.
6. Greger V, Schirmacher P, Bohl J, et al. Possible involvement of the retinoblastoma gene in undifferentiated sinonasal carcinoma. Cancer. 1990;66(9):1954–9.
7. Jeng YM, Sung MT, Fang CL. Sinonasal undifferentiated carcinoma and nasopharyngeal-typ undifferentiated carcinoma: two clinically, biologically, and histopathologically distinct entities. Am J Surg Pathol. 2002;26:371–6.
8. Franchi A, Moroni M, Massi D, et al. Sinonasal undifferentiated carcinoma, nasopharyngeal-type undifferentiated carcinoma, and keratinizing and nonkeratinizing squamous cell carcinoma express different cytokeratin patterns. Am J Surg Pathol. 2002;26:1597–604.
9. Perez-Ordonex B. Special tumors of the head and neck. Curr Diagn Pathol. 2003;9:366–93.
10. Wenig BM. Undifferentiated malignant neoplasms of the sinonasal tract. Arch Pathol Lab Med. 2009;133:699–712.
11. Frierson HF. Sinonasal undifferentiated carcinoma. In: Barnes L, Eveson JW, Reichart P, Sidransky D, editors. World Health Organization classification of tumours. Pathology & genetics of head and neck tumours, vol. 19. Lyon: IARC Press; 2005.
12. Frierson HF, Mills S, Fechner R, et al. Sinonasal undifferentiated carcinoma: an aggressive neoplasm derived from schneiderian epithelium and distinct from olfactory neuroblastoma. Am J Surg Pathol. 1986;10:771–9.
13. Enepekides DJ. Sinonasal undifferentiated carcinoma: an update. Curr Opin Otolaryngol Head Neck Surg. 2005;13:222–5.
14. Goel R, Ramalingam K, Ramani P, et al. Sino nasal undifferentiated carcinoma: a rare entity. J Nat Sci Biol Med. 2012;3(1): 101–4.

Skull Base CSF Leaks

27

Pertinent Points

- *Definition*: Skull base CSF leaks become visible when bony and dural defects directly link subarachnoid and extracranial spaces [14].
- *AKA*: Cerebrospinal fluid fistulas.
- CSF leaks pose particularly unique diagnostic difficulties frequently fostering multiple imaging studies, incurring interrelated expenses, and propagation of pain to these ill-fated individuals [1].
- Although CSF leaks occur predominately post trauma (or surgery), nontraumatic cases can occur and should be considered. While we frequently focus on posttraumatic leaks, the diagnosis, treatment, and complications are surprisingly similar for all etiologies.
- CSF leaks may materialize at various venues with engendering events embracing trauma, surgery, arachnoid granulations, and persistently increased intracranial pressure [14].
- It is imperative to recognize the literal leak site and activate appropriate treatment to avoid complications including low-pressure headaches, meningitis, and intracranial abscess with consequent serious neurologic complications [14].
- CSF leaks can confer considerable challenge to clinicians and radiologists alike [1]. Suspected specimens should be sent to the laboratory for β_2 transferrin to prove the presence of a CSF leak [14].
- *β_2 transferrin:* Found almost exclusively in CSF, the detection of *β_2 transferrin* should immediately initiate imaging to forthwith find its origin.
- *Classic Clue*: A patient presents having headaches and persistent runny nose dating back to an earlier episode of craniofacial trauma. More recent symptoms can comprise one or more of the following: irritability, drowsiness, fever, photophobia, or neck stiffness.
- Precise preoperative evaluation of patients with CSF rhinorrhea or otorrhea demands detection of the culpable anatomic defect [1].
- Skull base defects causing CSF leaks can be complicated by meningitis, encephalitis, or brain abscess. Where possible, these leaks are routinely repaired via endoscopic approaches to prevent their more serious complications.
- Untreated patients with CSF leaks face an annual meningitis risk of 10% translating to 40% long term [3].
- The most common cause of CSF leak is closed head injuries with CSF leak occurring in approximately 2% of cases [3]. Other etiologies include tumor, surgery, and developmental defects [3].
- Spontaneous CSF leaks are prominent in the setting of IIH (idiopathic intracranial hypertension) [3, 16].
- 90% of CSF leaks are posttraumatic with 80% revealed as rhinorrhea and 20% observed as otorrhea [14].
- Methodical analysis should be carefully coordinated by the neuroradiologist to confer clinicians the important information they need to provide patients preferred treatment [14].

F. A. Midyett, S. K. Mukherji, *Skull Base Imaging*, https://doi.org/10.1007/978-3-030-46447-9_27

Imaging

General Imaging Features

- Imaging is traditionally employed for location of the leakage site consequent to confirmation of CSF rhinorrhea.
- Multiple modalities have historically been used for the evaluation of CSF leak. Thin-section MDCT (multidetector CT) with 3D reconstructions can currently provide appropriate evaluation in the majority of cases [14].
- Exceptions include cases where there are multiple suspected sites, and it is desirable to define the legitimate leak site from assorted possibilities or when there is a possibility for paradoxical rhinorrhea.
- Typical techniques used for CSF leaks include:

I. High-Resolution CT (HRCT)

- HRCT with thin collimation and MPR (multiplanar reconstruction) reliably detect the site of most CSF leaks [3].
- Sensitivity for HRCT appears higher than for RNC (radionuclide cisternography) and CTC (CT cisternography).
- HRCTs accuracy is independent of (active vs. inactive) leak status [3].
- Comparing HRCT to MRC for sensitivity, specificity, and accuracy [3, 4]:

Modality	Sensitivity	Specificity	Accuracy
HRCT:	92%	100%	93%
MRC:	87%	100%	89%

- Thin-section MDCT (multidetector CT) allows 3D multiplanar reformations and has replaced direct coronal acquisitions in most institutions [14].
- Using current imaging technology with state-of-the-art equipment, the most common scenario is as follows: when the β_2 transferrin test is positive and MDCT shows a single bony defect, no other imaging is required [14].

II. CT Cisternography (CTC)

- Developed in the 1970s using iodinated contrast media, CTC has, until recently, been considered standard procedure for preoperative evaluation of CSF leaks [3, 14].
  - Approximately 3–10 cc of nonionic low-osmolarity iodinated contrast media is administered via lumbar puncture, and the patient is placed in a Trendelenburg position to opacify the basal cisterns with subsequent CT.
  - CTC sensitivity of 92% during active leaking drops to 40% during intermittent leakage [3].
  - CTC carries a low risk of infection as well as puncture site hemorrhage and CSF leakage.
  - When the leak is *not* active, CTC is *no more useful* than HRCT.
- CTC is often reserved for patients with negative MDCT (multidetector CT) in patients with active leaking or multiple bony defects [14].
- When the β_2 transferrin test is positive and MDCT shows multiple bony defects with sinus opacification, CTC is employed to localize the leaking site [14].
- Very rarely when the β_2 transferrin test is positive and MDCT is *negative*, CTC is employed to localize the leaking site [14].
- May see a conspicuous *decrease in density* (attenuation) of contrast due to washout near an active leak site [14].
- See Fig. 27.1a–h.

III. Radionuclide Cisternography (RNC)

- RNC became popular in the 1970s and 1980s along with "Pet Rocks and Mood Rings."
- RNC uses intrathecal placement of a radioactive tracer [such as Tc99m DTPA (diethylene triamine penta acetic acid)] and is sometimes coupled with CTC as the radiopharmaceutical can be concurrently injected with the contrast media.
- RNC carries similar low risks associated with CTC.
- When used *alone,* RNC is *less sensitive* than CTC [1].
- When used with CTC, the combination is *more sensitive* than when CTC is used alone [1].
- RNC shows a low sensitivity of ~75% and a false-positive rate ≤33% [3].
- Frequently found RNC reports seem satisfied to show the leak located in the left or right subnasal space without precise subsite localization [3].
- RNC requires transnasal endoscopic pledget placement adjacent the anterior cribriform plate, middle meatus, or sphenoethmoidal recess [5].
- Even in patients who tolerate the nasal pledgets, RNC typically fails to adequately localize and characterize the defect well enough to be the solitary diagnostic examination [14].
- RNC is presently performed in only the most complex cases of skull base CSF leaks [14].
- And, along with other items from the 1970s and 1980s, we don't seem to see many "Pet Rocks" sold in stores anymore.

IV. MR Cisternography (MRC)

- MRC is typically performed with multiplanar heavily T2-weighted images.
- Reported to be 85% sensitive and 100% specific for CSF leaks between the subarachnoid space and sinonasal spaces [3].
- MRC tends to be an anatomic study independent of leak activity.
- MRC absolves both the patient and the physician from lumbar puncture problems.

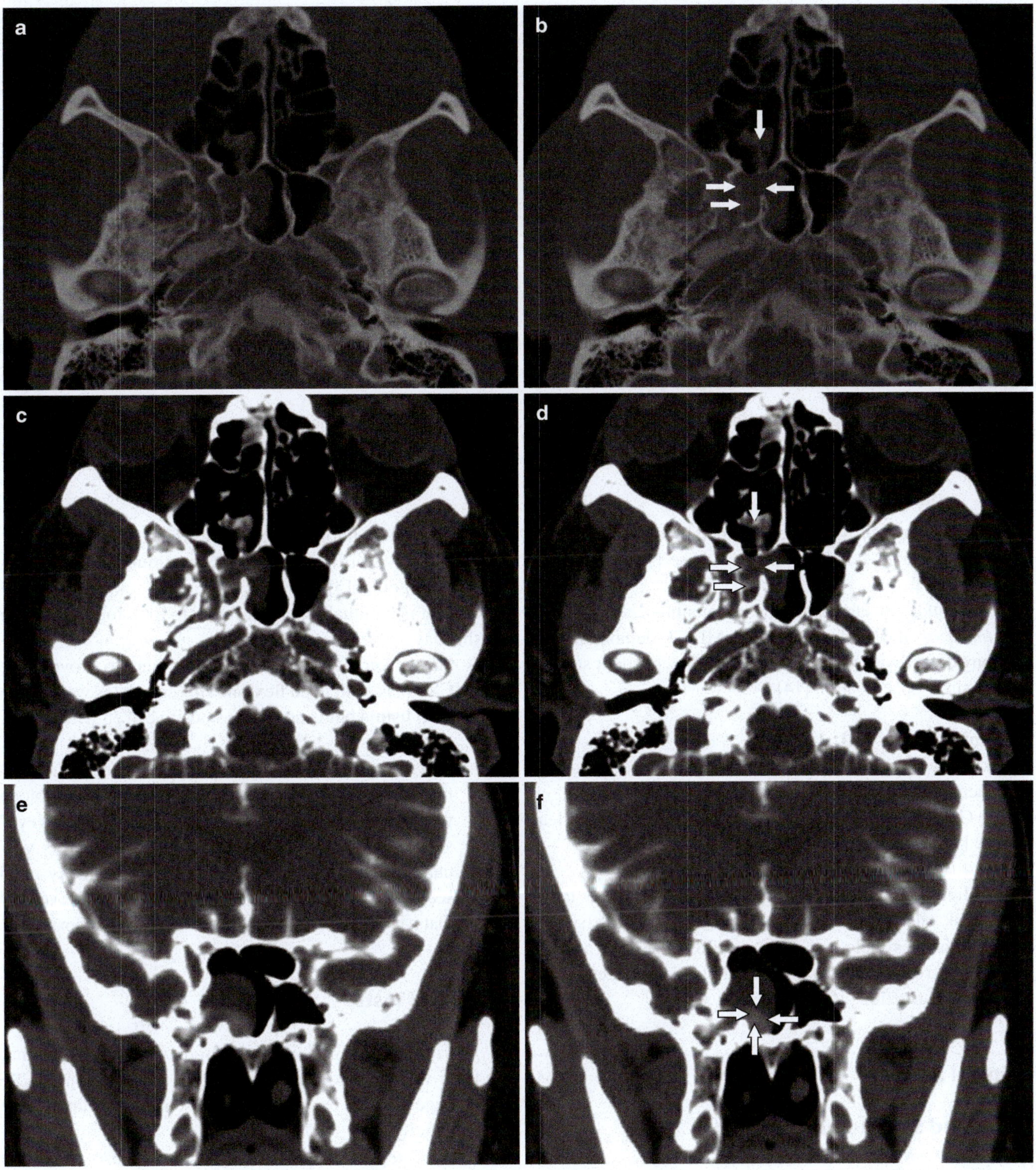

Fig. 27.1 Axial CTC without (**a**, **c**) and with (**b**, **d**) arrows shows a soft tissue mass filling the lateral recess of the right sphenoid sinus and a portion of the right sphenoid sinus. A similar density involves the posterior portion of the adjacent ethmoid sinus. There is a large bony defect (arrow ←) in the sinus wall. Shows subtle fingers of contrast in the right lateral recess (arrow →) and in the right ethmoid sinus (arrow ↓). Axial CTC without (**e**) and with (**f**) arrows show a soft tissue mass in the dependent portion of the right sphenoid sinus. Arrows define an area of higher attenuation contrast within an otherwise low attenuation mass

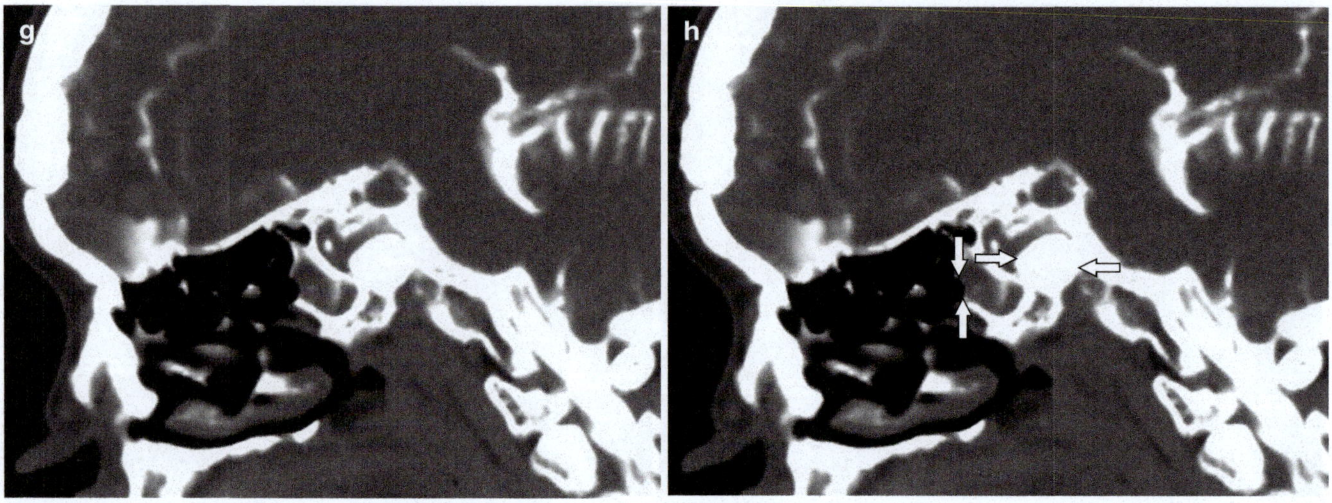

Fig. 27.1 (continued) Sagittal CTC without (**g**) and with (**h**) arrows show a contrast filled mass (arrows →←) in the dependent portion of the sphenoid sinus on somewhat delayed images. Large bony defect anteriorly (arrows ↓, ↑) shows sharp demarcation between air anteriorly and fluid posteriorly at the blatant bony defect (arrows ↓, ↑). Other areas of high signal contrast in the sinuses secondary to leak

- MRC does not provide fine bony detail necessary for surgical planning; however, most of these patients already had HRCT.
- To exclude an encephalocele or meningocele, MRC is *almost always* performed when MDCT demonstrates a bony defect with nearby lobular or nondependent soft tissue sinus opacification [14].

V. Conventional MRI

- Skull base multiplanar MRI and MRC are suggested when a meningoencephalocele is suspected.
- T1 GD: Frequently found dural enhancement at the leak site [14].
- T2
  - High-resolution T2 images may demonstrate larger leak sites, particularly when performed with special sequences including CISS or PROPELLER (periodically rotated overlapping parallel lines with enhanced reconstruction – GE Medical Systems).

Clinical Issues

Signs and Symptoms

- Separating CSF rhinorrhea from other spurious secretions is the foundation for CSF fistula diagnosis [5].
- While the diagnosis of profuse posttraumatic CSF leakage may seem overtly obvious, some patients forget to read the text, particularly when they are obtunded from severe head trauma.
- Problematic patients frequently present with a serosanguineous discharge from facial fractures, and it is not always the clinicians first thought that there may be a CSF component.
- It is not uncommon for CSF rhinorrhea to be intermittent, sometimes starting years after the traumatic event has been forgotten [5].
- And, it is habitually helpful for us to look for signs along the way:
  - "Reservoir sign": Ability of the patient to provoke the CSF leak with head flexion. This correlates well with a CSF fistula but is not always positive even when a leak exists.
  - "Target sign": CSF has the ability to migrate further on a filter paper (or gauze) than does accompanying blood which is heaver and less lithe. This creates a "bull's eye" stain with a bloody center. Some say this sign is very unreliable as it can occur with blood and watery nasal secretions. But this test doesn't cost much, and it is good that we were actually thinking about this diagnosis.

Chemical Tests

- *β_2 transferrin test*: Since its introduction in 1979, it has been widely used for the diagnosis of extracranial CSF leakage with reported 99% sensitivity and 97% specificity.
- *Glucose test*: Contemporary glucose oxidase assays are *too* sensitive, featuring frequent *false-positive* reactions. While it could be used to "rule out" a CSF leak, instead most clinicians currently consider it "obsolete."

Treatment and Prognosis

- Most CSF leaks (particularly those which are posttraumatic) respond to conservative treatment of bed rest, head elevation, and avoidance of straining [14].

- CSF leaks which are unresponsive to conservative management can be regularly repaired by endoscopy [3].
- CSF leaks vary from the patent posttraumatic (or post-surgical) lavish leak to a draining discontinuous discharge where the etiology is elusive [3].
- When in doubt as to the fluid's origin, β_2 transferrin (β_2 TF) assay confirms a CSF leak with 97% sensitivity and 99% specificity [3].
- Patients with posttraumatic narrow skull base fractures have a better prognosis.
- Patients with large or multiple fractures from a broad or multifocal injury, as well as those with penetrating injury with significant skull base comminution, are the most difficult to treat.
- The key to management of CSF leaks is prompt, accurate diagnosis and treatment, thereby minimizing meningitis with its resultant neurologic complications.

Differential Diagnosis

A. Classic Encephalocele

- A characteristic sac-like protrusion of brain and meninges through an osseous cranial defect usually results from incomplete neural tube closure during fetal development.
- An encephalocele consists of brain herniated through cranial bone. Meningocele means herniated dura. When both brain *and* dura are herniated, the proper term is meningoencephalocele.
- 15% of encephaloceles are frontoethmoidal. A transsphenoidal encephalocele may present as a nasopharyngeal mass.
- Encephaloceles typically show a CSF attenuation midline hypo-attenuating soft tissue mass with a thin wall which scallops the adjacent intact bony cortex.
- T1 and T2 show a fluid-filled midline abnormality outside the calvarium which is isointense to CSF. This can contain a component of brain which is isointense to intracranial brain.
- Most encephaloceles are found soon after birth or even during fetal ultrasound.
- At birth, sphenoidal encephaloceles are classically clinically occult usually revealing their presence during the first year of life.
- Children with transsphenoidal encephaloceles may present with nasal obstruction but are frequently occult until found by the clinician using a nasoscope.
- See Chap. 17, Nasofrontal Encephalocele and Chap. 33, Basal Encephalocele.

B. Sternberg's Canal Encephalocele (SCE) [15]

- Intrasphenoidal encephaloceles are extremely rare.
- Sternberg's canal results from incomplete fusion of the basisphenoid and greater sphenoid wing creating a craniopharyngeal canal laterally.
- Sternberg's canal causes a weakness which may possibly promote protrusion of a temporal lobe encephalocele into the nearby lateral sphenoid sinus recess.
- Located medial to the foramen rotundum, congenital intrasphenoidal encephaloceles are believed to be due to persistent Sternberg's canals.
- Detractors like to point out that a "congenital" origin seems unlikely since most of these encephaloceles are first found in adults and anatomic studies are "inconsistent" in the exact location of Sternberg's canal.
- Nevertheless, encephaloceles should be suspected in patients presenting with spontaneous CSF rhinorrhea since singular surgical solutions apply for this uncommon conundrum.

A Closer Look

I. Paradoxical Rhinorrhea [5]

- And, just to mention that nothing in medicine is ever as easy as it seems, we frequently face paradoxical rhinorrhea.
- Traumatic CSF leaks involving the anterior skull base may paradoxically exit through the naris contralateral to the leakage site.
- This may occur with displaced fractures involving midline structures including the crista galli and vomer.
- Paradoxical rhinorrhea may occur when a mucocele blocks the ipsilateral naris.
- It also occurs with temporal bone fractures where the temporal dura is torn and CSF escapes via the Eustachian tube travelling into the nasopharynx to exit through the contralateral naris.
- Fortunately for both patients and physicians, most paradoxical CSF leaks are successfully managed conservatively.

II. Statistical Soup

- The risk of recurrent meningitis after posttraumatic CSF leakage has been reported to range up to 50% and carries a neurological complication rate of almost 30% [5].
- This is clearly a situation where time is of the essence for diagnosis with post-fracture/pretreatment meningitis risk approximating 1.3% per day for the first 2 weeks after injury, 7.4% per week in the first month after injury, and a cumulative risk of 85% at the 10-year follow-up. This is a little like having compound interest working against you.

III. Historic Highlights

- Galen described CSF leaks in the second century, proposing periodic nasal CSF leakage via the sella and ethmoids was "normal" [1, 2].
- In 1745 Bidloo the Elder was the first to describe and correlate CSF rhinorrhea after a traumatic skull fracture [5, 8].

- In 1888, anatomist Maximilian Sternberg described the lateral craniopharyngeal canal currently carrying his name.
- In 1899, St. Clair Thompson described a series of abnormal, nontraumatic CSF leaks which he termed "rhinorrhea," challenging Galen's theory that this was a "normal" physiologic pathway [1, 2, 14].
- In 1926, Dandy described the first successful *intradural* closure of a CSF leak using fascia lata [5].
- In 1937, British neurosurgeon Cairns showed surgical repair of CSF leaks could be made using *extradural* suturing of the fascia lata [5, 9].
- In 1944, Dandy demanded a 2-week window for surgical repair of CSF leaks to prevent meningitis [5, 10].
- In 1948, Dohlman performed the first *extracranial* repair of spontaneous CSF rhinorrhea [5, 11].
- In 1960, Ommaya classified CSF leaks into traumatic and nontraumatic etiologies [14].
- In 1981, Wigand was the first to use the *endoscope* for *extracranial* CSF leak repair [5, 13].
- In 1985, Di Chiro first described intrathecal injection of Gd in monkeys [5, 6]. (And animal rights groups are still up in arms about that).
- In 1990, Mattox and Kennedy employed the endoscope to *both diagnose and repair* CSF rhinorrhea in fortuitous fractures [5, 12].
- In 1994, Gammal and Brooks developed Di Chiro's method for Magnetic Resonance Cisternography (MRC) in humans [5, 7].

Selected References

1. Stone JA, Castillo M, Neelon B, Mukherji SK. Evaluation of CSF leaks: high-resolution CT compared with contrast-enhanced ct and radionuclide cisternography. AJNR Am J Neuroradiol. 1999;20:706–12.
2. Zlab MK, Moore GF, Daly DT, Yonkers AJ. Cerebrospinal fluid rhinorrhea: a review of the literature. Ear Nose Throat J. 1992;71:314–7.
3. La Fata V, McALean N, Wise SK, et al. CSF leaks: correlation of high-resolution CT and multiplanar reformations with intraoperative endoscopic findings. AJNR. 2008;29:536–41.
4. Shetty PG, Schroff MM, Sahani DV, et al. Evaluation of high-resolution CT and MR cisternography in the diagnosis of cerebrospinal fluid fistula. AJNR Am J Neuroradiol. 1989;19:633–9.
5. Ziu M, Savage JG, Jimenez DF. Diagnosis and treatment of cerebrospinal fluid rhinorrhea following accidental traumatic anterior skull base fractures. Neurosurg Focus. 2012;32(6):e2.
6. Di Chiro G, Knop RH, Girton ME, et al. MR cisternography and myelography with Gd-DTPA in monkeys. Radiology. 1985;157:373–7, 35.
7. el Gammal T, Brooks BS. MR cisternography: initial experience in 41 cases. AJNR Am J Neuroradiol. 1994;15:1647–56.
8. Dagi FT. Management of cerebrospinal fluid leaks. In: Schmidek HH, Roberts DW, editors. Schmidek & sweet operative neurosurgical techniques: indications, methods, and results, vol. 1. 5th ed. Philadelphia: Saunders Elsevier; 2006. p. 130–45.
9. Cairns H. Injuries of the frontal and ethmoidal sinuses with special reference to cerebrospinal fluid rhinorrhea and aeroceles. J Laryngol Otol. 1937;52:589–623.
10. Dandy WE. Treatment of rhinorrhea and otorrhea. Arch Surg. 1944;49:75–85.
11. Dohlman G. Spontaneous cerebrospinal rhinorrhoea; case operated by rhinologic methods. Acta Otolaryngol Suppl. 1948;67:20–3.
12. Mattox DE, Kennedy DW. Endoscopic management of cerebrospinal fluid leaks and cephaloceles. Laryngoscope. 1990;100:857–62.
13. Wigand ME. Transnasal ethmoidectomy under endoscopical control. Rhinology. 1981;19:7–15.
14. Lloyd KM, DelGaudio JM, Hudgins PA. Imaging of skull base cerebrospinal fluid leaks in adults. Radiology. 2008;248(3):725–36.
15. Bendersky DC, Landriel FA, Ajler PM, et al. Sternberg's canal as a cause of encephalocele within the lateral recess of the sphenoid sinus: a report of two cases. Surg Neurol Int. 2011;2:171.
16. Alonso RC, de la Pena MJ, Caicoya AG, et al. Spontaneous skull base meningoencephaloceles and cerebrospinal fluid fistulas. Radiographics. 2013;33(2):553–70. https://doi.org/10.1148/rg.332125028.

28 Esthesioneuroblastoma

Pertinent Points

- *Definition*: Esthesioneuroblastoma is a rare neuroendocrine malignancy of neural crest origin which arises from olfactory epithelium near the cribriform plate and nearby the nasal cavity [5, 20].
- *Classic Clue*: An unfortunate patient presents following many months of vague indicators including one or more of the following: headache, stuffy nose, epistaxis, rhinorrhea, anosmia, facial pain, diplopia, or proptosis [2, 3, 20]. Frequently find an avidly enhancing "dumbbell"-shaped mass with its "waist" collocated at the cribriform plate protruding into the nasal cavity, ACF, and orbit [20].
- *AKA*: Olfactory neuroblastoma.
- *Age*: Although esthesioneuroblastoma arises in all age groups, it presents bimodal peaks at the second and sixth decades [3].

Imaging

General Imaging Features

- Demonstrates "dumbbell or figure 8"-shaped mass with its "waist" at the cribriform plate.
- Usually a unilateral mass with an established epicenter near the superior nasal margin.
- On CT, an opacified obstructed paranasal sinus can be misconstrued as tumor progression [3, 20].
- Esthesioneuroblastoma portrays a predictable pattern of metastasis to cervical nodes, frequently first favoring level II but consistently choosing levels I, III, and RPN (retropharyngeal nodes) for runner-up destinations [21, 22] (see Figs. 28.1a, b and 28.2a–d).

CT Features

- See *General Imaging Features* [20].
- NECT shows a soft tissue nasal cavity mass resulting in remodeling and enlargement.
- Varying with the tumor's age, esthesioneuroblastoma may breed bone destruction while concurrently cultivating calcifications sometimes showing a somewhat "speckled" configuration.
- Hyperostosis suggesting slow growth is sometimes seen [3, 20].
- The cribriform plate is a frequent site for finding bony changes.
- CECT exhibits an enhancing homogeneous soft tissue mass.
- CTA (CT angiography) parades a prominent vascular blush.
- See Fig. 28.3a, b.

MRI Features [20]

- See *General Imaging Features*.
- Unlike the perpetual problem for CT, MRI should easily separate a simple sinus obstruction from a tumor-filled sinus [3, 20].
- Characteristic cystic areas at tumor/brain margins declare the diagnosis and are probably pathognomonic, although it is not completely clear whether these cysts are part of the tumor or the brain's reaction to the tumor [2].
- Frequently found both T1, T2, and proton density show intermediate signal similar to brain [2, 3]. Associated *peripheral marginal cysts* [1] cause heterogeneity, in general showing focal ↓ T1 and ↑ T2 signal.

F. A. Midyett, S. K. Mukherji, *Skull Base Imaging*, https://doi.org/10.1007/978-3-030-46447-9_28

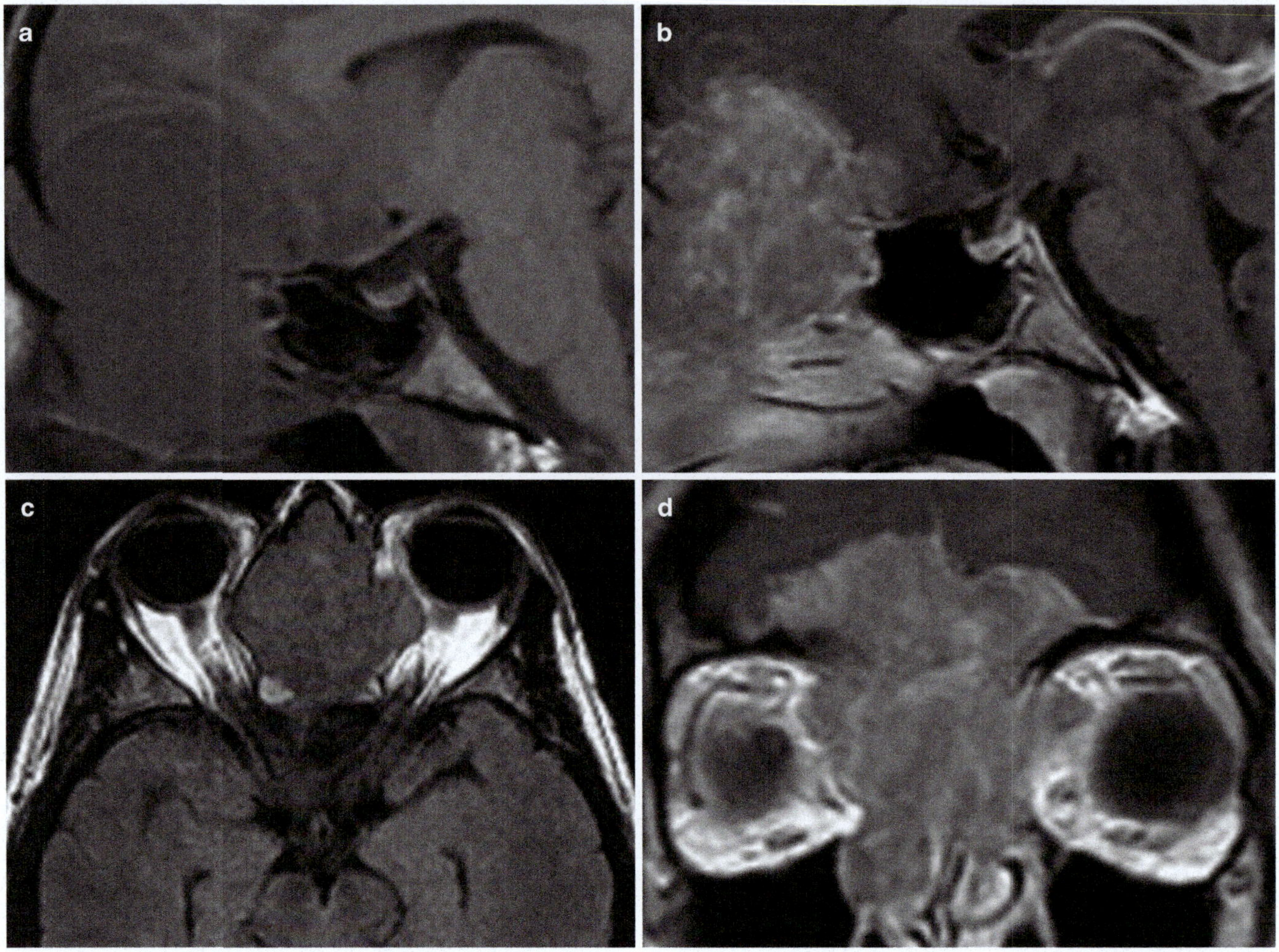

Fig. 28.1 Sagittal T1 without (**a**) and with Gd (**b**) show a huge soft tissue mass somewhat "dumbbell" shaped with its waist near the now destroyed cribriform plate. There is a huge hole in the floor of the anterior cranial fossa with conspicuous loss of its characteristic linear dark signal. The tumor is mildly heterogeneous and relatively isointense to brain before Gd demonstrates avid heterogeneous enhancement. Tumor extends cranially into the frontal lobes, caudally and anteriorly into the nasal cavity, and posteriorly into the sphenoid bone. The adjacent brain exhibits edema. **Question: What other important imaging finding is displayed on these two images (Figures 1a, b)? After reviewing Case 2, Figures 2a–d, please return to confirm that you identified this important finding.** (**c**) Axial T1 depicts huge ACF skull base and nasal cavity mass extending into both orbits displacing their contents laterally. The tumor is mildly heterogeneous, relatively isointense to brain, and distinctly lower in signal than nearby orbital fat. (**d**) Coronal T1 Gd depicts huge mass overrunning orbits displacing their contents laterally. Tumor enhancement is extensively heterogeneous. There is dramatic destruction of the floor of the anterior cranial fossa as well as portions of the bony orbits. The tumor displaces both frontal lobes and extends caudally into the nasal cavity. Demonstrates "dural tails" in the interhemispheric and left supraorbital regions

- T1 Gd:
  - Although variable and heterogeneous, solid components usually exhibit eager (moderate to intense) enhancement. However, the "classic cysts" exhibit erratic enhancement, sometimes showing enhancement of cyst margins [2].
  - See Fig. 28.1b, d.
  - Sometimes suggests meningioma with enhancement evoking the distinctive "dural tail" sign (see Fig. 28.1d).
- DWI demonstrates moderate restricted diffusion with ↑ DWI signal and corresponding ↓ signal on ADC map.
- MRI is the ideal imaging modality for evaluating esthesioneuroblastoma, possessing the power to readily reveal retropharyngeal nodal extension, a preferred path for esthesioneuroblastoma (see Figs. 28.2a–d; then 28.1a, b).

Nuclear Medicine Features

- MIBG (metaiodobenzylguanidine) is a functional analog of the neurotransmitter norepinephrine and has been shown in specific storage and uptake systems for neuroblastoma [21].
- In the differential diagnosis of ENB, a scintigraphic study using MIBIG (metaiodobenzylguanidine) labeled with radioactive iodine (^{123}I or ^{131}I) is helpful because ENBs are markedly avid for MIBG [8].
- Initial cases suggest significantly higher uptake of ^{123}I MIBG by ENB than many other tumors often considered in the differential [8].

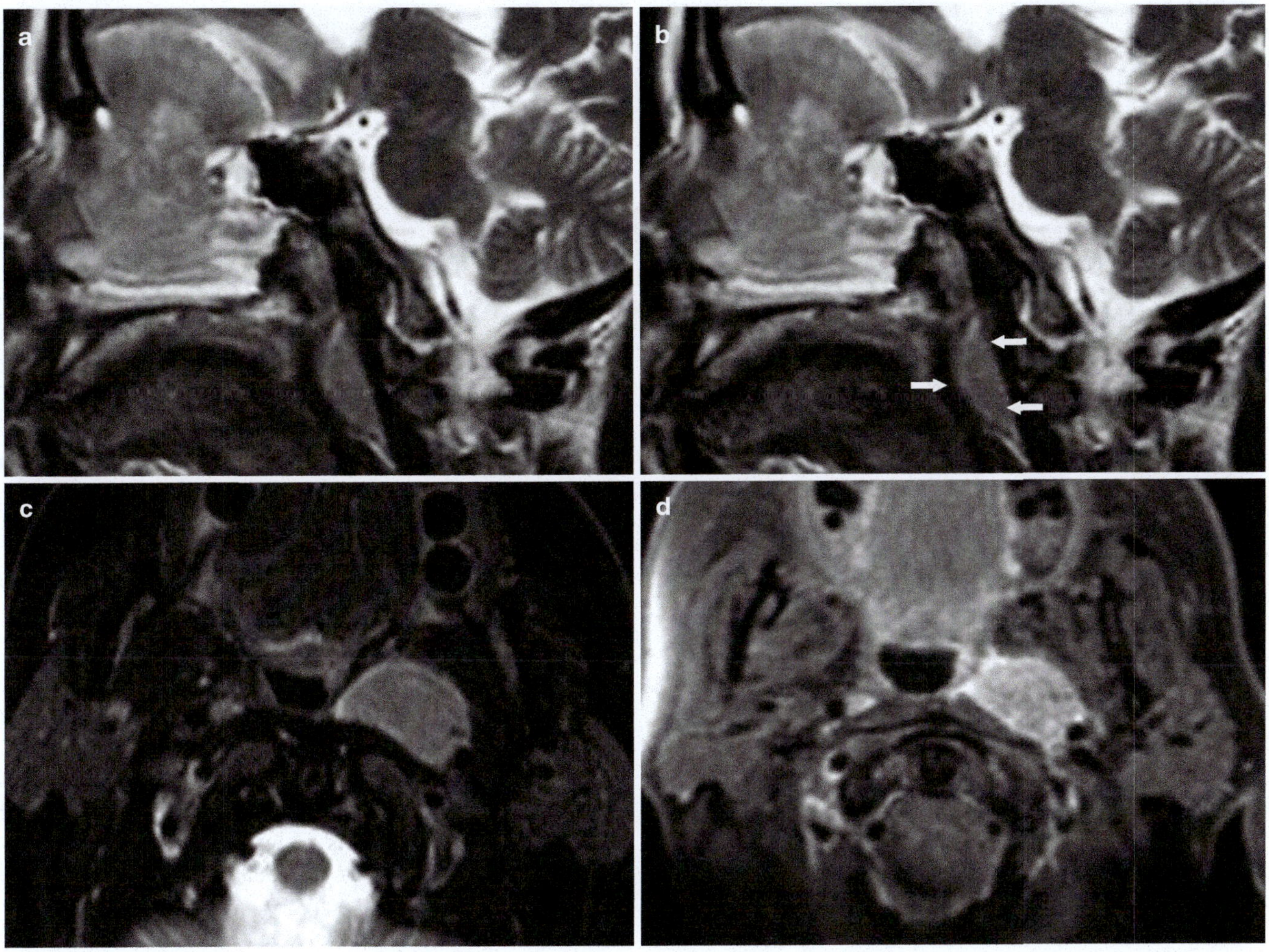

Fig. 28.2 Sagittal T2 without (**a**) and with arrows (**b**). There is a huge soft tissue mass overtly "dumbbell" shaped with its waist near the now destroyed cribriform plate. There is a huge hole in the floor of the anterior cranial fossa with conspicuous loss of its dark signal. The tumor is moderately heterogeneous and hyperintense to brain. Tumor extends cranially into the frontal lobes and caudally into the nasal cavity. [Note: 2a–d is a different (although strikingly similar) patient than 1a–d]. There is a semilunar retropharyngeal mass demonstrating tumor spread to this large retropharyngeal node (defined by arrows on Fig. 28.2b). Axial T2 (**c**) and T1 Gd (**d**) again depict the large left retropharyngeal lymph node. It is moderately heterogeneous with conspicuous increased signal on T2 and T1 Gd images

- Some authors have suggested strategies for preoperative radiochemotherapy to convert inoperable lesions to resectable ones [8].
- Demonstration of metastasis is critical to staging, and MIBG imaging may be very helpful [8].
- Metastatic nodes from esthesioneuroblastoma are also strongly FDG avid [22].

Clinical Issues

Presentation

- Patients sometimes show symptoms over many months which are nonspecific including stuffy nose, epistaxis, rhinorrhea, anosmia, headache, facial pain, diplopia, and proptosis [2, 3, 20].
- Symptoms seem confusing but can be categorized into diverse groups including:
  - Eye symptoms

    ENB often involves the orbit and can cause blindness [5].

    Eye-specific signs and symptoms include proptosis, periorbital pain, ↓ visual acuity, ↓ EOM, and chemosis [5].
  - Ear symptoms: Pain and serous otitis media frequently follow Eustachian tube blockage.
  - Nasal symptoms: Obstruction, epistaxis, discharge, anosmia and polyps.
  - Neurologic symptoms: Headache and nausea
  - Mouth symptoms: Ulceration, non-healing extraction site, ill-fitting dental prosthesis, and occasionally a mobile tooth.

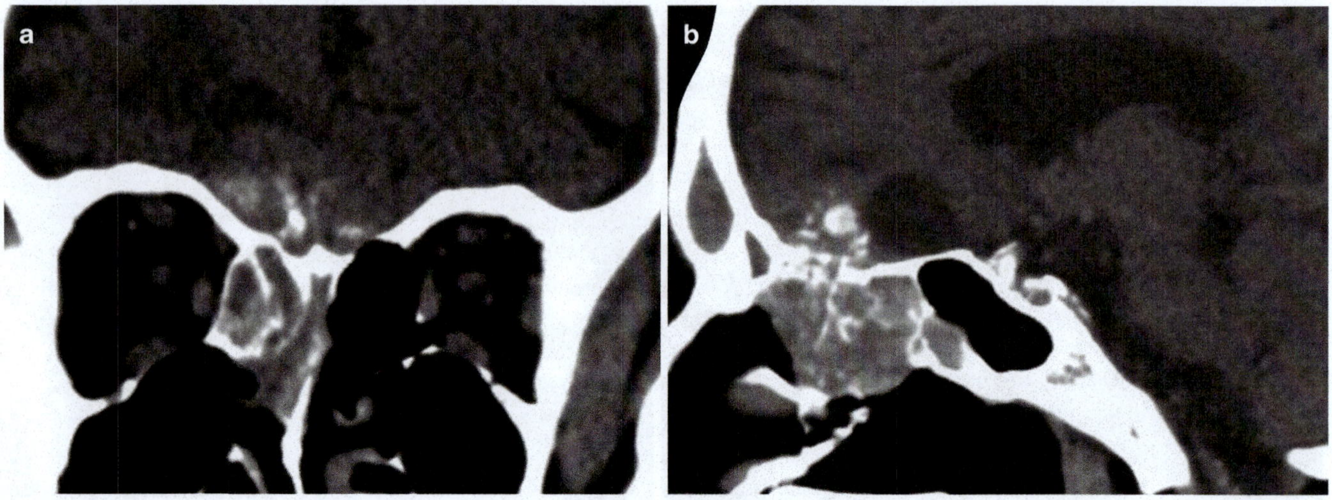

Fig. 28.3 NECT coronal A and sagittal B show a huge anterior skull base ENB with its epicenter near the cribriform plate. The tumor is predominately isointense with the brain, but it is filled with innumerable high attenuation calcific foci. The cribriform plate has been clearly breached as well as the roof of the left sphenoid sinus. A large low attenuation cystic component abuts the posterior aspect of the intracranial mass

  - Facial symptoms: Swelling, pain, anesthesia, and rarely trismus.
  - Cervical symptoms: Adenopathy with palpable mass.
- Because symptoms seem subtle, we tend to first find ENBs when they are already advanced with most having associated adjacent microscopic dural depositions and 30% displaying gross intracranial intrusions [2].
- Diagnostic delay in some series shows the mean time from onset of symptoms to diagnosis is approximately 17 months [5].
- Surfacing secondary symptoms sometimes cause the clinician to first be concerned for an occult malignancy.

Treatment

- Robust craniofacial resection is regularly recommended, even in the presence of intracranial involvement [3].
- Typical treatment by a combination of anterior skull base resection, radiation, and/or chemotherapy results in a 70% overall cure rate [2].
- Sometimes see cure rates of 85–90% for small tumors with limited intracranial involvement.
- Larger high-grade tumors more frequently receive chemotherapy.

Prognosis

- Esthesioneuroblastoma boasts an 80% 8-year disease-free survival and carries an overall cure rate of approximately 70% [2].
- Early diagnosis and treatment are particularly important as patients with small lesions showing limited intracranial involvement who have energetic en bloc craniofacial resections frequently flaunt cure rates ≤90% [2, 3, 20].
- Distant spread is perpetually problematic with ≤35% of ENB patients experiencing one or more bouts of metastatic disease. Metastasis occurs with lymphatic involvement of cervical nodes or hematogenous spread to the brain, liver, lung, or bone [2, 3].
- Potential pessimistic prognostic pointers include [4]:

1. Female	worse prognosis
2. Age: <20 or >50	worse prognosis
3. Tumor grade:	
(a) Low-grade tumors:	80% 5-year survival
(b) High-grade tumors:	40% 5-year survival
4. Significant intracranial spread	worse prognosis
5. Metastasis	
(a) No distant metastasis	60% 5-year survival
(b) Distal metastasis	0% 5-year survival
6. Recurrence	worse prognosis

- Hyams: The Hyams histologic grading system generally is also a reliable prognostic predictor. Grade I tumors habitually have a very favorable forecast, whereas Grade IV is fundamentally fatal with Grades II and III seemingly somewhere in between [13].

Pathology

General Pathology

- ENBs arise from neuroectodermal stem cells found in mucosa lining the cribriform plate, superior turbinates, and anterior ethmoids, as well as the nasal cavity's roof and septum [3].

- ENB shows slow growth generally demonstrating destruction, bony expansion, or erosion.

Gross and Microscopic Pathology

- *Gross*: Friable multilobulated grayish-pink tumors which tend to blatantly bleed despite timorous touching.
- *Microscopically* ENB seems to be swarming with small round cells [2]. Both histologic and radiologic appearances can cause confusion with several sinonasal neoplasms [3].
- Definitive diagnosis may eventually entail electron microscopy and immunohistochemistry [3].
- "Typical" imaging may point the pathologist toward the proper path. Sadly, some tumors "don't read the book" and fail to show "typical" findings.
- Most manifest microscopic dural invasion adjacent to the cribriform plate. Regrettably, 30% display gross intracranial spread at presentation [2].
- Light microscopy frequently features the following: multiple small, round cells showing small nucleoli containing coarsely granular chromatin, scant cytoplasm, and prominent nuclear membranes with fibrous septa and pseudo- or Homer-Wright *rosettes.*
- When light microscopy is inconclusive, the electron microscope may definitely decide the diagnosis by revealing neurosecretory granules.
- Currently, ENBs are probably in a pathologic "gray zone" as some suggest they belong better with Ewing's sarcomas than neuroblastomas [12]. Stay tuned; classifications pivot on the pathologist's "state of mind."

Staging

- Cross-sectional imaging is invaluable for preoperative staging which poses a premier predictor of clinical outcome [3, 7].
- Local disease habitually has an outstanding prognosis after treatment [3].
- Staging systems used for ENB include the more typical TMN and the less common (but potentially more helpful) Kadish systems [3].

TNM

- T1 – Tumor involves the nasal cavity and/or paranasal sinuses, sparing superior ethmoid cells, and *excludes the sphenoid sinus.*
- T2 – Tumor involves the nasal cavity and/or paranasal sinuses with extension to and/or erosion of the cribriform plate and also *involves the sphenoid sinus.*
- T3 –Tumor involves the orbit and/or anterior cranial fossa, *without dural invasion.*
- T4 – Tumor involves the brain.
- N and M indicate nodal involvement and metastasis, respectively (see Figs. 28.1a, b and 28.2a–d).

Kadish

- Kadish A: Tumor is confined to the nasal cavity.
- Kadish B: Tumor is confined to the nasal cavity and the paranasal sinuses.
- Kadish C: Tumor extends beyond the nasal cavity and paranasal sinuses to additionally involve one of following: orbit, skull base, anterior cranial fossa, or cervical nodes ± distant metastasis.
  - Unfortunately, Kadish C is the most common category because of patients' propensity for perpetually late presentations.
  - By definition orbital involvement places the patient in Kadish C (see Fig. 28.1c, d).

Differential Diagnosis

A. Olfactory Groove Meningioma (OGM) [20]

- OGM is a rare entity also associated with anosmia and headache like ENB.
- OGM patients habitually have symptoms 6–36 months prior to detection with delinquent diagnoses including frontal sinusitis, migraine, and neuralgia [15]. ENB patients usually show symptoms for many months prior to diagnosis.
- A skull base mass which has hyperostosis is highly suggestive of OGM. However, hyperostosis with ENBs has been rarely reported [14].
- A broad dural base with a "dural tail" comprises classic OGM findings. ENBs frequently develop "dural tails" (see Fig. 28.1d).
- OGM occurs from 33 to 91 years with a mean age of 58 years [23]. ENBs arise in all age groups depicting bona fide bimodal peaks in the second and sixth decades [3].
- T1 is usually isointense, although occasionally hypointense to gray matter in OGM.
- OGM T2: Compared to gray matter, T2 is isointense in 50%, hyperintense in 40%, and hypointense in 10%.
- OGM: Atypical and malignant subtypes sometimes show ↑ restricted diffusion on DWI. ENB: Moderate restriction of diffusion.
- OGM: T1 Gd habitually has homogenous avid enhancement. ENB: Also avid enhancement but often contains "classic cysts" which show erratic enhancement.

- Nuclear Medicine Features: Both OGM and ENB show ↑ uptake on bone scans. However, *ENB's exceptional affinity for MIBG may be helpful in the DDx.*
- See Chap. 13, Anterior Fossa Meningioma.

B. Inverted Papilloma (IP) [20]

- IP is frequently found in patients age 40–60 [11]. ENB occurs in all age groups bearing bimodal peaks in the second and sixth decades [3].
- IP's epicenter is near the middle meatus. ENB's epicenter is near the cribriform plate.
- IP exhibits expansile, benign appearing bone changes. ENB sometimes shows hyperostosis suggesting slow growth [3, 14].
- ENB frequently features a "dumbbell"-shaped mass with its "waist" at the cribriform plate. This is not a feature for IP.
- Depending on the tumor phase, ENB may demonstrate destruction of bone with calcifications sometimes showing a "speckled" pattern. This is not a feature for IP.
- ENB is particularly prone to involve the cribriform plate, not an attribute of IP.
- ENB's characteristic cystic areas at tumor/brain margin may be pathognomonic. This is not an attribute of IP.
- ENB's concomitant cysts show ↑ T2 signal and variable enhancement [2]. This is not an attribute of IP.
- IP demonstrates a *dramatic male preference* with M:F = 10:1 [10]. ENB exhibits no gender preference.
- ENB exhibits a T1 signal iso- to slightly hyperintense to muscle. T2 shows an intermediate signal. There is seemingly "no signature MRI appearance" for IP [11].
- IP often exhibits its distinctive CCP ("onvoluted cerebriform pattern") of enhancement, particularly in its maxillary sinus component. This is a reliable although not pathognomonic feature [24]. CCP is not a feature for ENB.
- Nuclear Medicine Features: Both IP and ENB shows ↑ uptake on bone scans. However, *ENB's exceptional affinity for MIBG may be helpful in the DDx.*
- See Chap. 14, Inverted Papilloma.

C. Rhabdomyosarcoma (RMS)

- RMS is more often found in *children* <15 years of age and is the most common childhood soft tissue sarcoma. ENB occurs in all age groups featuring bimodal peaks in the second and sixth decades [3].
- RMS classically appears as a homogeneous well-circumscribed non-calcified soft tissue mass with irregular margins isodense to muscle. Rarely resembles a cystic mass with hemorrhagic foci [8, 9].
- NECT shows a mass which is isodense to muscle. CECT shows the mass to be slightly hyperintense to surrounding muscle [24].
- RMS classically erodes and destroys adjacent bone but usually does not contain calcifications or provoke hyperostosis from adjacent bone [8, 9, 24].
- CT and FDG PET/CT play primary roles in assessing metastatic disease.
- MRI is the preferred modality for assessment of skull-based RMS.
- T1: Isointense to muscle but hypointense to orbital fat.
- T2: Heterogeneous hyperintense to muscle with multiple foci of high T2 signal.
- ENB typically shows intermediate signal on both T1 and T2 [2].
- T1 Gd: Demonstrates *avid* heterogeneous enhancement as does ENB [2].
- DWI: Both RMS and ENB demonstrate *restricted diffusion* with *bright DWI* images and corresponding *dark ADC* images.
- Nuclear Medicine Features: Both RMS and ENB show ↑ uptake on bone scans. However, *ENB's exceptional affinity for MIBG may be helpful in the DDx.*
- See Chap. 49, Rhabdomyhosarcoma.

D. Paranasal Sinus Cancer

- Malignant tumors arising from paranasal sinus epithelium comprise the most common malignant tumors of the anterior skull base.
- Age: 50–70 years old. Gender: ↑ M > F prevalence probably related to occupational exposure. By comparison, ENB occurs in all age groups with bimodal peaks in the second and sixth decades.
- CT superbly portrays osseous involvement including cortical thickening, sclerosis, erosion, destruction, or remodeling.
- NECT shows a solid mass which with aggressive bone destruction. CECT shows moderate enhancement.
- Paranasal sinus SCCAs show gross bony destruction. ENBs show a soft tissue mass with slower bony growth causing nasal cavity expansion and remodeling with occasional hyperostosis. Depending on the tumor phase, NECT sometimes shows bone destruction with "speckled calcifications."
- T1: Superb at evaluating tumor extending into cortical bone or fatty marrow.
- T2: Shows intermediate signal mass and is useful in separating tumor from obstructed sinus secretions.
- T1 Gd: Exhibits moderate tumor enhancement.
- ADC (apparent diffusion coefficient) mapping shows significant promise for separating benign inflammatory lesions from malignant paranasal sinus tumors.
- STIR (Short Tau Inversion Recovery): Useful in looking for lymph nodes and marrow edema.
- ^{18}F FDG PET/CT has high sensitivity and moderate specificity.

- When SCCA starts high in the sinuses, separation from ENB by imaging may be nearly impossible.
- Nuclear Medicine Features: Both paranasal sinus cancer and ENB show ↑ uptake on bone scans. However, *ENB's exceptional affinity for MIBG may be helpful in the DDx.*
- See Chap. 22, Paranasal Sinus Cancer and Chap. 26, Sinonasal Undifferentiated Carcinoma.

E. Wegener's Granulomatosis (WG) [19]

- Wegener's Granulomatosis is a systemic vasculitis which causes granulomatous inflammation and necrosis. While typically presenting with a routine "runny nose," without modern medicine most patients perish within a few short months.
- WG may proffer a medial orbital mass in addition to adjacent ethmoid sinus disease.
- Intraorbital WG usually confers concomitant paranasal sinus involvement. Intraorbital ENB usually has a concomitant component with its epicenter near the cribriform plate.
- With WG the T1 is hyperintense to orbital fat. By contrast, ENB is typically *intermediate* on T1.
- WG shows ↓ T2 signal [relative to orbital fat], while ENB is typically *intermediate* on T2.
- WG has heterogeneous enhancement on T1 Gd with multiple tiny foci of ↓ signal. ENB exhibits *AVID* homogeneous T1 Gd enhancement [2, 3].
- ENB shows cystic areas at the tumor/brain margin which declare the diagnosis [2] and may be pathognomonic. Not a feature of WG.
- These cysts on ENB which show ↑ T2 signal and variable enhancement are not a feature of WG.
- Unlike ENB, 90% of WG patients are Caucasian.
- While WG prefers the middle aged, it has been reported in both younger and older patients. ENB is nondiscriminatory occurring in all age groups bringing bimodal peaks to the second and sixth decades.

F. Antrochoanal Polyp (AP)

- APs are "dumbbell"-shaped masses often observed to divide their domicile between a maxillary sinus and the nasal cavity. Although ENBs are also often "dumbbell" shaped, their much higher "waist" is near the cribriform plate where they extend into the cranial cavity.
- Antrochoanal polyps are non-enhancing masses with benign appearing bone changes. By contrast, ENBs exhibit *AVID* enhancement.
- Antrochoanal polyps sometimes show cystic changes. ENBs characteristically contain small cystic areas near their tumor/brain margins.
- Grossly, APs are glistening white polypoid masses. ENBs are friable multilobulated pink-gray/reddish-gray tumors which tend to blatantly bleed from timorous touching.

A Closer Look

I. Fast Facts

- Esthesioneuroblastoma accounts for ~2% of nasal neoplasms [3].

II. Historic Highlights

- Since 1924 when Berger and Luc first found ENB, approximately 1000 new cases have been recorded in the literature [6, 9].

III. Genetics

- Currently, no genuine genetic feature has been identified to accurately assist diagnosis or predict prognosis.
- Genetic alterations which have been associated and are currently being investigated include the following:
  – ENB is associated with trisomy eight [16].
  – Reported chromosomal aberrations include the reciprocal translocation at t (11;22) (q24; q12) which has also been reported in Ewing's sarcoma, Askin's tumor, and peripheral neuroepithelioma suggesting some common stem cell origin [17].
  – Chromosomal gains in 7q11 and 20q as well as chromosomal deletions in 2q, 5q, 6p, and 18q.
  – Abnormalities at 20q have been implicated in various other cancers including breast, ovary, and SCCA.
  – The HASH1 gene, involved in olfactory neuronal differentiation, may be useful in separating ENB from other poorly differentiated tumors with "small blue cells" [18].
  – Further research will be required to determine the role of genomic variants in esthesioneuroblastoma.

Selected References

1. Som PM, Lidov M, Brandwein M, et al. Sinonasal Esthesioneuroblastoma with intracranial extension: marginal tumoral cysts as a diagnostic MR finding. AJNR. 1994;15:1259–62.
2. Fischbein NJ, Dillon WP, Barkovich AJ. Teaching atlas of brain imaging. New York: Thieme; 2000. p. 532–4.
3. Lufkin R, Borges A, Villablanca P. Teaching atlas of head and neck imaging. New York: Thieme; 2000. p. 333–6.
4. Morita A, Ebersold MJ, Olsen KD, et al. Esthesioneuroblastoma: prognosis and management. Neurosurgery. 1993;32:706–15.
5. Laforest C, Selva D, Crompton J, et al. Orbital invasion by Esthesioneuroblastoma. Ophthal Plast Reconstr Surg. 2005;21(6):435–40.
6. Broich G, Pagliari A, Ottaviani F. Esthesioneuroblastoma: a general review of the cases published since the discovery of the tumour in 1924. Anticancer Res. 1997;17(4A):2683–706.
7. Zollinger LV, Wigging RH, Cornelius RS, et al. Retropharyngeal lymph node metastasis from Esthesioneuroblastoma: a review of the therapeutic and prognostic implications. AJNR Am J Neuroradiol. 2008;29(8):1561–3.

8. Sasajima T, Kinouchi H, Tomura N, et al. High uptake of ^{123}I-metaiodobenzylguanniding related to olfactory Neuroblastoma revealed by single photon emission CT. AJNR Am J Neuroradiol. 2000;2(4):717–20.
9. Berger L, Luc G, Richard D. L'esthesioneuroepitheliome olfact. Bull Assoc Fr Etud Cancer. 1924;13:410–21.
10. Saha SN, Ghosh A, Sen S, et al. Inverted papilloma: a clinicopathological dilemma with special reference to recurrence and malignant transformation. Indian J Otolaryngol Head Neck Surg. 2010;62(4):354–9.
11. Yousem DM, Fellows DW, Kennedy DW, et al. Inverted papillomas: evaluation with MR imaging. Radiology. 1992;185(2):501–5.
12. Sorensen PH, Wu JK, Berean KW, et al. Olfactory Neuroblastoma is a peripheral primitive neuroectodermal tumor related to Ewing Sarcoma. Proc Natl Acad Sci U S A. 1996;93(3):1038–43.
13. Miyamoto RC, Gleich LL, Biddinger PW, et al. Esthesioneuroblastoma and sinonasal undifferentiated carcinoma: impact of histological grading and clinical staging on survival and prognosis. Laryngoscope. 2000;110(8):1262–5.
14. Ramanathan M, Germanwala AV. Hyperostotic esthesioneuroblastoma. J Case Rep Med. 2013;2:Article ID 234779. https://doi.org/10.4303/jcrm/235779.
15. Tsikoudas A, Martin-Hirsch DP. Olfactory groove meningiomas. Clin Otolaryngol Allied Sci. 1999;24(6):507–9.
16. VanDevanter DR, George D, McNutt MA, et al. Trisomy 8 in primary esthesioneuroblastoma. Cancer Genet Cytogenet. 1991;57(1):133–6.
17. Whang-Peng J, Freter CE, Knutsen T, et al. Translocation t(11;22) in esthesioneuroblastoma. Cancer Genet Cytoqenet. 1987;l29(1):155–7.
18. Mhawech P, Berczy M, Assaly M, et al. Human achaete-scute homologue (hASH1) mRNA level as a diagnostic marker to distinguish esthesioneuroblastoma from poorly differentiated tumors arising in the sinonasal tract. Am J Clin Pathol. 2004;122(1):100–5.
19. Midyett FA, Mukherji SK. Chapter 48. Wegener's granulomatosis. In: Orbital imaging. Philadelphia: Elsevier; 2014. p. 227–30. ISBN 9780323340373.
20. Midyett FA, Mukherji SK. Chapter 22. Esthesioneuroblastoma. In: Orbital imaging. Philadelphia: Elsevier; 2014. p. 91–8. ISBN 9780323340373.
21. Wafelman AR, Hoefnagel CA, Maes RAA, Beijnen JH. Radioiodinated metaiodobenzylguanidine: a review of its biodistribution and pharmacokinetics, drug interactions, cytotoxicity and dosimetry. Eur J Nucl Med. 1994;21:545–59.
22. Howell MC, Branstetter BF, Snyderman CH. Patterns of regional spread for esthesioneuroblastoma. AJNR. 2011;32:929–33.
23. Nakamura M, Struck M, Roser F, et al. Olfactory groove meningiomas: clinical outcome and recurrence rates after tumor removal through the frontolateral and bifrontal approach. Neurosurgery. 2007;60(5):844–52.
24. Jeon TY, Kim HJ, Chung SK, et al. Sinonasal inverted papilloma: value of convoluted cerebriform pattern on MR imaging. AJNR. 2008;29:1558–60.

Part IV

Middle Cranial Fossa

29 Jugular Foramen Paraganglioma

Pertinent Points

- *Definition:* Jugular foramen paragangliomas (JFPs) are gradually growing highly vascular tumors typically arising from the temporal bone's jugular foramen at the jugular bulb's dome, from specialized neural crest chemoreceptor cells which readily respond to variations in BP and temperature [2].
- *Classic Clue*: Middle-aged patient presents with pulsatile tinnitus alleging a "family history" of hearing loss. He has an eagerly enhancing jagged jugular foramen mass peppered by high velocity flow voids portraying permeative bone destruction.
- *AKA:* Glomus jugulare paragangliomas, glomus jugulotympanicum, glomus tumors, paragangliomas, chemodectomas.
- Head and neck paragangliomas arise from five basic areas:
  - Type I: Glomus jugulare paragangliomas (GJP)
    Arise from the jugular bulb dome and are completely confined to the jugular foramen.
    Clinically, the glomus jugulare conveys a normal appearing TM (tympanic membrane).
  - Type II: Glomus tympanicum arises from the tympanic plexus of the middle ear cavity.
  - Type III: Glomus jugulotympanicum
    Combines Types I and II.
    The tumor involves BOTH the jugular foramen and the middle ear cavity.
    Clinically, the glomus jugulotympanicum reveals a reddish retrotympanic mass.
  - Type IV: Glomus vagale. <5% of paragangliomas arises from vagus nerve's nodose ganglion.
  - Type V: Carotid body tumors arise from the carotid body near the carotid artery bifurcation.
- Jugular foramen paragangliomas [JFPs] comprise two typical types, i.e., types I and III as listed above.
- While progress from neural crest cells with 96% being benign, unfortunately 4% are malignant [2].
- Sporadic paragangliomas are multicentric in ~3%. When familial, they are multicentric in ~25% [1].
- Incidence: F > M = 3:1. Age: Typically seen in adults, during fourth and fifth decades [13, 14].
- Jugular foramen paragangliomas are the most frequently found jugular foramen tumor and are usually unilateral but may be bilateral [14].

Imaging

General Imaging Features

- Jugular foramen paragangliomas are irregular marginated masses [2].
- Tumors >2 cm tend to show prominent intralesional flow voids [2].
- Irregular, permeative erosion of margins of the jugular foramen and jugular spine.
- Imaging features vary with tumor location type as described.

CT Features

- See *General Imaging Features.*
- HRCT (high-resolution CT) is often the initial imaging modality employed to show bony structures and access tumor extension [16].
- When a suspicious mass is demonstrated on noncontrast HRCT, a contrast-enhanced temporal bone CT may dif-

F. A. Midyett, S. K. Mukherji, *Skull Base Imaging*, https://doi.org/10.1007/978-3-030-46447-9_29

ferentiate an avidly enhancing paraganglioma from other benign and malignant skull base tumors [16].

- They expand and erode the jugular foramen and contiguous cortex [11]. Erosion of the jugular plate is very suggestive of a JFP. A "moth-eaten" pattern of bony destruction is typical [16] causing irregular permeative bone destruction [2] (See Fig. 29.1a, b and 29.2b, c).
- Large lesions may exhibit extensive skull base destruction [11].
- They typically show an avidly enhancing heterogeneous lobulated, specked mass [11] (See Figs. 29.1c, d and 29.2g).
- Temporal bone CT can demonstrate the glomus tympanicum engulfing but *not* destroying the ossicles. This may be helpful when the lesion is small with cholesteatoma in the differential diagnosis [12] (See Fig. 29.2b–e).

MRI Features

- See General Imaging Features.
- MRI shows superior soft tissue detail and importantly identifies intracranial tumor extension [16].
- T1: Intermediate signal with "salt and pepper" appearance. The dark "pepper" is caused by high velocity signal loss flow voids surrounded by tumor parenchyma. Less frequently seen, the "salt" is secondary to ↑signal from subacute hemorrhage [2, 3, 11, 12].
- T2: Isointense to mildly hyperintense [2] (see Fig. 29.2h).
- T1 Gd: Vigorous, heterogeneous enhancement (See Figs. 29.1c, d and 29.2f, g).

Angiographic Features

- Angiography is usually useful for identification of feeding vessels and preoperative embolization [2].
- Typically feed from the ascending pharyngeal branch of the ECA (external carotid artery).
- A characteristic hypervascular mass shows intense prolonged tumor blush with arteriovenous shunting showing early venous drainage [3] (See Fig. 29.1e, f).
- ~5% of glomus tumors secrete norepinephrine and may require α (alpha)-adrenergic blocking agents to prevent precipitation of a hypertensive angiographic crisis [12] (See Fig. 29.1e, f).

Nuclear Medicine Features

- Indium^{111} DTPA-D-Phe1-octreotide is currently the preferred radiotracer used to evaluate patients suspected of having multiple paragangliomas [16].

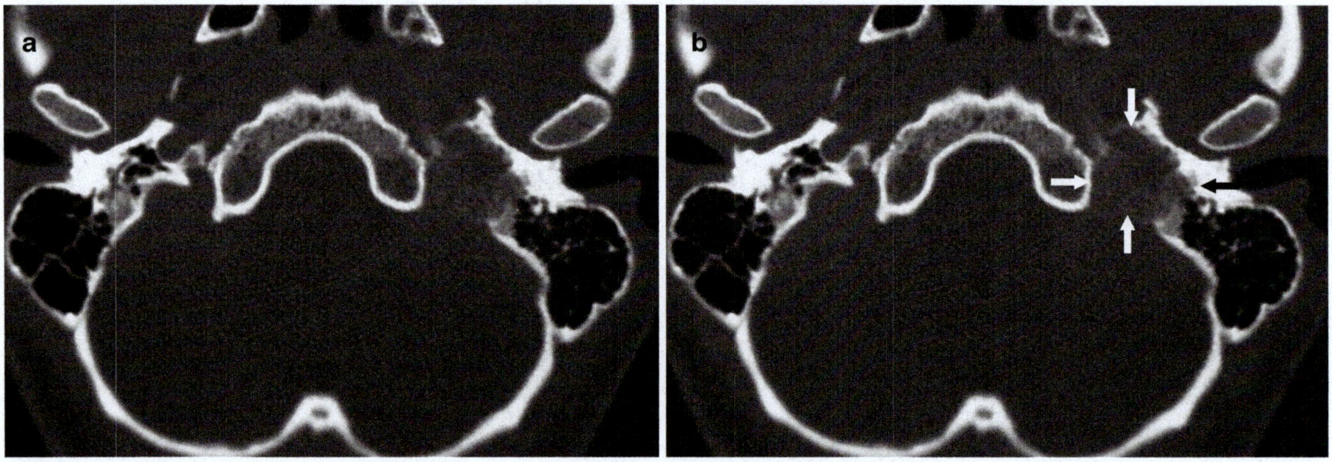

Fig. 29.1 (**a**, **b**) Axial NECT without (**a**) and with (**b**) arrows show irregular permeative destruction of the left jugular foramen and surrounding structures

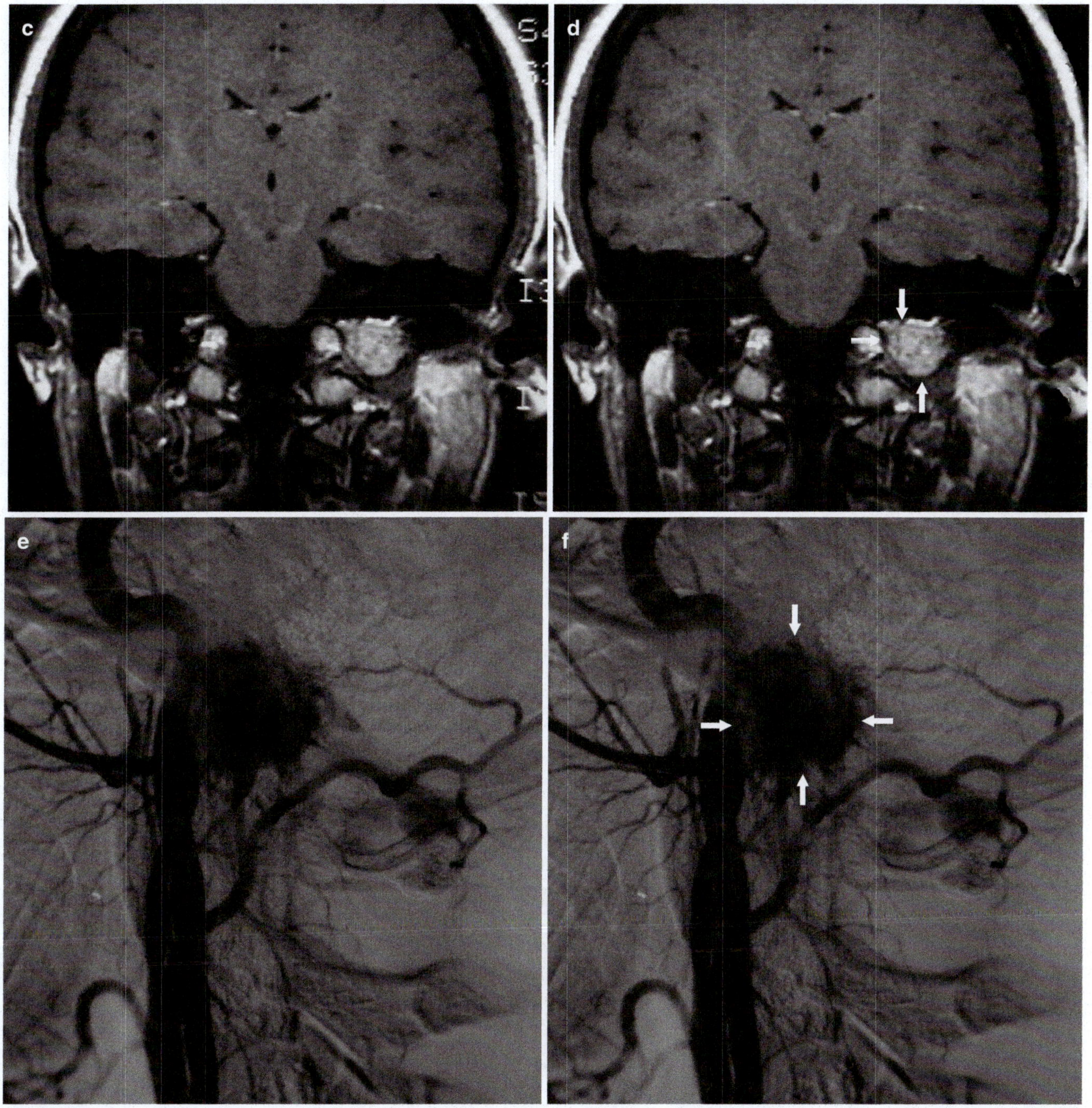

Fig. 29.1 (continued) (**c**, **d**) Coronal T1 Gd without (**c**) and with (**d**) arrows shows avidly enhancing left jugular foramen mass featuring frequent focal low signal "flow voids." (**e, f**) Left common carotid angiogram without (**e**) and with (**f**) arrows shows characteristic hypervascular tumor with tangled throng of enlarged arteries corresponding to demonstrated destructive defect in (**a**, **b**) and enhancing enlargement in (**c**, **d**)

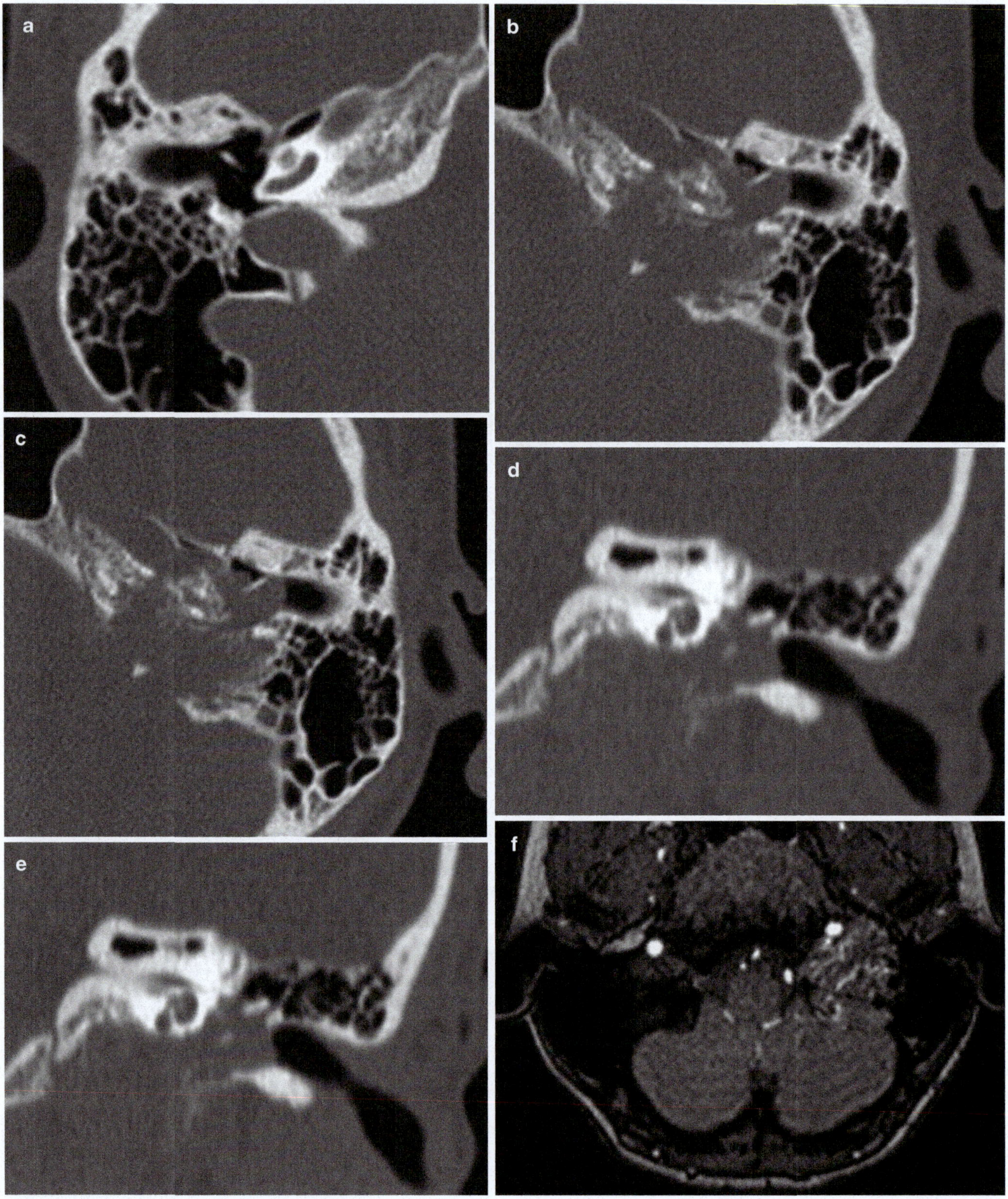

Fig. 29.2 (**a**) Axial NECT TB normal right for comparison depicting intact jugular foramen and ossicles (in a second patient). (**b**, **c**) Axial left TB without (**b**) and with (**c**) arrows show irregular permeative destruction of left jugular foramen with tumor extending into the middle ear. Note that the soft tissue mass surrounds but does *not* destroy the visualized ossicle (arrow). (**d**, **e**) Coronal left TB without (**d**) and with (**e**) arrow shows irregular permeative destruction of the left jugular foramen with extension into the middle ear. Again, note that the soft tissue mass surrounds but does *not* destroy the visualized ossicle (arrow). (**f**) Axial T1 Gd shows large left jugular foramen mass with worm-like collection of enhancing vessels

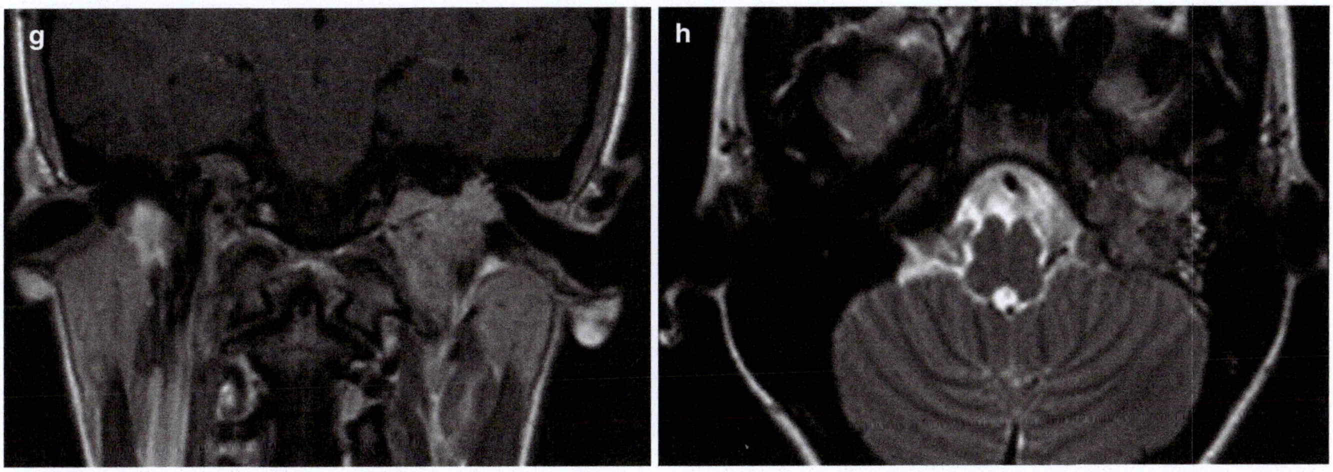

Fig. 29.2 (continued) (**g**) Coronal T1 Gd shows that the large left glomus jugulotympanicum with its epicenter in the jugular fossa clearly has invaded the middle ear cavity bulging into the EAC (external auditory canal). The clinician's otoscopic view truly tells only the tale of the "iceberg's tip". (**h**) Axial T2 shows heterogeneous mildly hyperintense left jugular foraminal mass with multiple "flow voids" truly corresponding to a tangled mass of vessels comprising this tumor

Clinical Issues

Presentation and Symptoms

- Can cause: pulsatile tinnitus, hearing loss (conductive or sensorineural), vertigo, facial weakness/paralysis, hoarseness, or swallowing difficulty [3].
- May involve CN IX, X, XI, and ± XII. Less frequently involves CN VII and VIII.
- Glomus Tumor Location Types:

I. Type I: Jugular Foramen Paraganglioma

- Refers to a glomus tumor confined to the jugular foramen.
- Arises from jugular bulb dome.
- The tumor may extend inferiorly into the jugular vein as well as sigmoid or transverse sinuses [12].

II. Type II: Glomus Tympanicum Paraganglioma

- Arises from the tympanic plexus in the middle ear cavity causing relatively early symptoms.
- Usually seen as a *small soft tissue mass*, bulging behind the tympanic membrane.
- Arises from *Jacobson's nerve*, the tympanic branch of CN IX.
- Best demonstrated by high-resolution temporal bone CT and tumor can encase but *does not erode ossicles* [12].
- Typically present early with well-defined soft tissue mass and *no bony involvement* [14].

III. Type III: Glomus Jugulotympanicum

- Describes glomus tumor which *involves both the jugular foramen and the middle ear cavity.*
- Combines types I and II described above.
- Arises from *Arnold's nerve* which is the auricular (or mastoid) branch of the vagus nerve (CN X).
- When a type I JFP extends cranially from the jugular bulb into the middle ear cavity, it can clinically simulate a (type II) glomus tympanicum. In reality, this tumor has become type III glomus jugulotympanicum.
- This is problematic for the clinician who without imaging only sees the tip of the iceberg (See Fig. 29.2g).
- Typical middle-aged patient presents late in disease process with painless slow-growing mass [3].

Natural History

- The natural history of the disease varies with tumor location types as listed above.
- The outcome varies according to tumor cell type with 96% being benign and 4% malignant [2]. See section on Treatment.
- Treatment options vary with tumor location types, tumor cell type, and stage at time of disease presentation.
- Outcome varies with all the above listed factors.

Epidemiology and Pathology

- Gross Pathology: A tangled mass of enlarged arteries form a lobulated reddish-purple tumor covered by a fibrous pseudocapsule.
- Microscopic:
  - Light microscopy shows sustentacular and chief cells with fibromuscular stroma parading a unique "zellballen" whorled pattern [3].
  - Electron microscopy shows neurosecretory granules [3].

- Extension into the tympanic cavity causes pulsatile tinnitus [1].
- JPFs may be multiple and familial. They rarely metastasize [2].
- Overall, <10% of head and neck paragangliomas are malignant with the incidence of malignancy highest in vagal paragangliomas, less in carotid body tumors, and least in jugulotympanic tumors [16].
- As there are currently no accepted histopathologic criteria for malignancy in paragangliomas that diagnosis is reserved for demonstrated metastasis to nonneuroendocrine tissue [17].
- ≤5% of malignant paragangliomas spread to regional nodes or demonstrate distant metastasis [13].

Treatment

Current treatment options include watchful waiting, embolization, conventional surgical excision, radiotherapy, and stereotactic radiosurgery [16].

Surgical Treatment

- Surgical treatment is usually definitive [3].
  - Here, size makes a definite difference:
    Small lesions are more often treated with surgery.
    Larger lesions may require surgery and radiation therapy.
  - Surgery shows 60% incidence of postoperative cranial neuropathy.

Radiation Therapy

- Patients of advancing age are often offered palliative radiation therapy.
- Palliative adjunctive treatment is available for atypical tumors not suited to surgery [3].
- Posttreatment response sometimes shows ↓ size, ↓ flow voids, and ↓ enhancement [1].
- Malignant paragangliomas should probably have preoperative embolization, maximal safe surgical resection, and postoperative radiotherapy [13].

Differential Diagnosis

Paragangliomas comprise 90% of jugular foramen tumors [14].

The other 10% of jugular foramen masses include:

A. Jugular Foramen Meningioma [2]
- Meningioma may have hyperostotic bony changes. This is *not* a feature for jugular foramen paraganglioma (JFP).
- Meningiomas have a broad dural base. *Not* a feature for JFPs.
- When larger, JFPs show characteristic *flow voids*. *Not* a feature for meningiomas [2].
- Frequently find enhancing "dural tail(s)" with meningioma. *Not* a feature for JFP.

B. Jugular Foramen Schwannoma [2]
- Schwannomas show *smooth* bone erosion or remodeling. Paragangliomas portray permeative destruction on CT.
- Larger jugular foramen paragangliomas (JFPs) have hypervascularity with *flow voids* showing the "salt and pepper" appearance. *Not* a feature for schwannoma [2].
- Schwannomas show a dumbbell-shaped spread along CN IX, X, and XII. This is *not* a feature for JFP.
- Schwannomas show smooth fusiform enhancing masses. Paragangliomas portray lobulated enhancing masses.

C. Metastasis
- Hypervascular metastasis may *also* sometimes show a salt and pepper appearance.
- However, metastasis usually shows somewhat more erosive invasion than JFP [2].

D. Jugular Bulb Variants
- Enlarged jugular bulb
  - Normal variant
  - Smooth, uneroded cortex of jugular foramen
- High-riding jugular foramen
  - Normal variant.
  - Margins of jugular foramen are intact with normal appearing cortex.
  - MR signal transient in high-riding bulb.
- Dehiscent jugular bulb
  - Normal variant.
- Focal defect in sigmoid plate.
- Jugular bulb extends into the middle ear through a sigmoid plate defect.

A Closer Look

I. Genetics
- Paragangliomas are both sporadic and familial.
- Associated genetic mutations have been currently identified in the SDHB, SDHC, and SDHD genes. Multiple newly discovered genes have yet to be completely studied for their connection with the hereditary paraganglioma-pheochromocytoma syndrome.

- The incidence of paragangliomas is prominent in several syndromes including NF1, MEN II, and VHL.
- All individuals having head and neck paragangliomas should seek genetic counseling as 30% are found to have genetic mutations despite not being associated with the "usual" syndromes [16].

II. Fast Facts

- Glomus tumors are associated with thyroid carcinoma, neurofibromatosis, and multiple endocrine neoplasia (MEN) syndromes [13].
- Arnold's nerve was first found by and named after German anatomist Friedrich Arnold (1803–1890) [15].
- Arnold's nerve is also known as Alderman's nerve based on a belief that after gorging, Aldermen would wiggle a pinkie in their external auditory canal in an attempt to alleviate post prandial acquired abdominal aching.

III. Historic Highlights

- In 1941 Gild first reported the glomus "jugularis" as a "hitherto unrecognized structure in man" at the American Association of Anatomists in Chicago [4, 5].
- In 1945 Rosenwasser first identified the relationship between Gild's glomus "jugularis" and "carotid body like" tumors occurring in the temporal bone [4, 6].
- In 1953 Gild found glomus formations to occur in serially sectioned human temporal bones *only* along the nerves of *Jacobson* (tympanic branch of glossopharyngeal nerve) and *Arnold* (auricular branch of vagus) [4, 7].
- In 1953 Semmes pioneered the suboccipital approach to treat a patient with a paraganglioma [8].
- In 1969 House described preservation of the osseous ear canal during glomus jugulare tumor removal [9].
- In 1977 Gardner, Cocke, Robertson, et al. described a combined three phase lateral skull base approach performed by a multidisciplinary team [10]. The move to multidisciplinary teams ties together the best from several subspecialties to fight this formidable foe.

Selected References

1. Castillo M. Neuroradiology companion. Philadelphia, PA: J.B. Lippincott; 1995. p. 294.
2. Fischbein NJ, Dillon WP, Barkovich AJ. Teaching atlas of brain imaging. New York: Thieme; 2000. p. 610–2.
3. Rao AB, Koeller KK, Adair CF. From the archives of the AFIP. Paragangliomas of the head and neck: radiologic-pathologic correlation. Armed Forces Institute of Pathology. Radiographics. 1999;19(16):1605–32.
4. Michael LM, Robertson JH. Glomus jugulare tumors: historical overview of the management of this disease. Neurosurg Focus. 2004;17(2):1–5.
5. Gild SR. A hitherto unrecognized structure, the glomus jugularis in man. Anat Rec. 1941;79(Suppl 1):28m (Abstract).
6. Rosenwasser H. Carotid body tumor of the middle ear and mastoid. Arch Otolaryngol. 1945;41:64–8.
7. Gild SR. The glomus jugulare, a nonchromaffin paraganglion, in man. Ann Otol Rhinol Laryngol. 1952;62:1045–71.
8. Semmes RE: Discussion of Alexander E Jr, Beamer PR, Williams JO. Tumor of the glomus jugulare with extension into the middle ear. J Neurosurg. 1951;8:515–23.
9. House W: Discussion in McCabe BF, Rosenwasser H, House W, et al. Management of glomus tumors. Arch Otolaryngol. 1969;89:170–8.
10. Gardner G, Cocke EW, Robertson JT, et al. Combined approach for removal of glomus jugulare tumors. Laryngoscope. 1977;87:665–725.
11. Osborne AG. Diagnostic Neuroradiology. St. Louis: Mosby; 1994. p. 507–9.
12. Grossman RI, Yousem DM. Neuroradiology: the requisites. Philadelphia: Mosby; 1994. p. 345–7.
13. Hansen EK, Roach M. Handbook of evidence-based radiation oncology. 2nd ed. New York: Springer; 2010. p. 191–5.
14. Runge VM. Review of neuroradiology. Philadelphia: WB Saunders Company; 1996. p. 91.
15. Whonamedit. A dictionary of medical eponyms. Subject: Frederich Arnold: www.Whonamedit.com. No update date given. Accessed 08/11/2014.
16. Woolen S, Gemmete JJ. Paragangliomas of the head and neck. Neuroimaging Clin N Am. 2016;26(2):259–78. https://doi.org/10.1016/j.nic.2015.12.005. Epub 2016 Mar 5.
17. Lee JH, Barich F, Karnell LH, et al. National Cancer Data Base report on malignant paragangliomas of the head and neck. Cancer. 2002;94(3):730–7.

Clivus Chordoma

30

Pertinent Points

- Definition: Relatively rare malignant tumor arising from embryonic remnants of the primitive notochord. Embryologically, the notochord is the initial axial skeletal structure, a primitive cell line around which the skull base and vertebral column develop [1, 2].
- *Classic Clue*: Midline lobular tumor with bony destruction arising in or near the clivus which on T2 MRI is hyperintense to nearby intervertebral disks (see Fig. 30.2b).
- *AKA*: Intracranial chordomas
- While considered slow-growing low-grade neoplasms, they are locally aggressive and highly recurrent.
- Clival chordomas are rare representing <0.2% of all intracranial tumors.
- M:F = 2:1; Whites > Blacks
- Primarily in adults. Rarely occur <30 years old. Age ranged from 8 to 80 in Dahlin's series of 155 chordoma cases seen at the Mayo Clinic between 1910 and 1971 [2].
- A more recent review of 400 US patients seen between 1973 and 1995 found an approximately equal distribution of chordomas between the cranium, spine, and sacrum changing somewhat the distribution reported by Dahlin's earlier smaller series [2, 3].
- Intracranial chordomas most often originate from the clival spheno-occipital synchondrosis.

Imaging

General Imaging Features

- Lobulated midline mass causing conspicuous bony destruction.
- MRI and CT complete complimentary evaluation roles.

CT Features

- See *General Imaging Features.*
- *Midline* soft tissue mass arising from the clivus causing adjacent bone destruction [4].
- *Destructive lytic* bone lesion usually with *hypodense soft tissue mass.*
- CT is superior to scrutinize the degree of destruction of bone and display *amorphous intratumoral calcifications.*
- About 1/2 show abnormal bony sclerosis.
- Shows mild to moderate heterogeneous enhancement with IV contrast.
- *Cystic necrosis* causes variable areas of heterogeneity.
- Areas of low CT attenuation within the soft tissue mass correspond to myxoid and gelatinous material found on gross pathologic examination [5].
- CT is superior to MRI for depicting precise *osteolytic involvement* of the skull base and is particularly suited to showing skull base foramina [6, 7].
- See Fig. 30.2a.

F. A. Midyett, S. K. Mukherji, *Skull Base Imaging*, https://doi.org/10.1007/978-3-030-46447-9_30

MRI Features

- MRI is the *single best modality* for evaluating clival chordomas [8].
- T1: Heterogeneous hypo- to isointense signal compared to marrow.
  - *Small foci of hyperintensity* are related to intratumoral hemorrhage or mucus ponds.
- T2: Hyperintense to intervertebral discs and CSF (see Figs. 30.1a and 30.2b, c).
  - Sometimes shows low signal fibrous septae.
- T1 Gd: Heterogeneous enhancement with honeycomb pattern varies from barely blushing to avid light bulb bright (see Figs. 30.1b–d and 30.2e, f).
- *Gradient Echo: If hemorrhage is present, sometimes see "blooming."*
- *DWI:*
  - DWI may be useful in distinguishing classic chordoma from chondrosarcoma.
  - Chondrosarcoma is associated with statistically significant higher ADC values compared to classic chordoma.
  - The statistical differences do not appear to help to distinguish the more favorable chondroid chordoma.
  - Differences in T2 signal appear more clear-cut with classic chordoma brightest (hyperintense), chondrosarcoma (less bright), and poorly differentiated chordoma (even less bright) appearing isointense to the brain [9].
  - See General Imaging Features.

Other Modality Findings

- Plain Films
  - Most lesions are lytic with frequent intratumoral calcifications or sequestered bone fragments. Four frequent features include (1) expansion, (2) rarefaction, (3) trabeculation, and (4) intratumoral calcification.
  - Plain films tend to underestimate tumor size by not appreciating soft tissue components or portions of tumor without calcifications.
- Radionuclide Bone Scan: May be normal or show decreased uptake with "cold lesion."

Clinical Issues

Presentation

- Most commonly present with headache and diplopia from CN palsy [10]. Headache may be occipital or retro-orbital.
- Involvement of CN V and CN VIII is most frequent.

Natural History

- Clivus chordomas are characteristically slow-growing lesions.
- Approximately 10% demonstrate distant metastasis to the brain, lung, liver, bone, abdominal viscera, and lymph nodes.

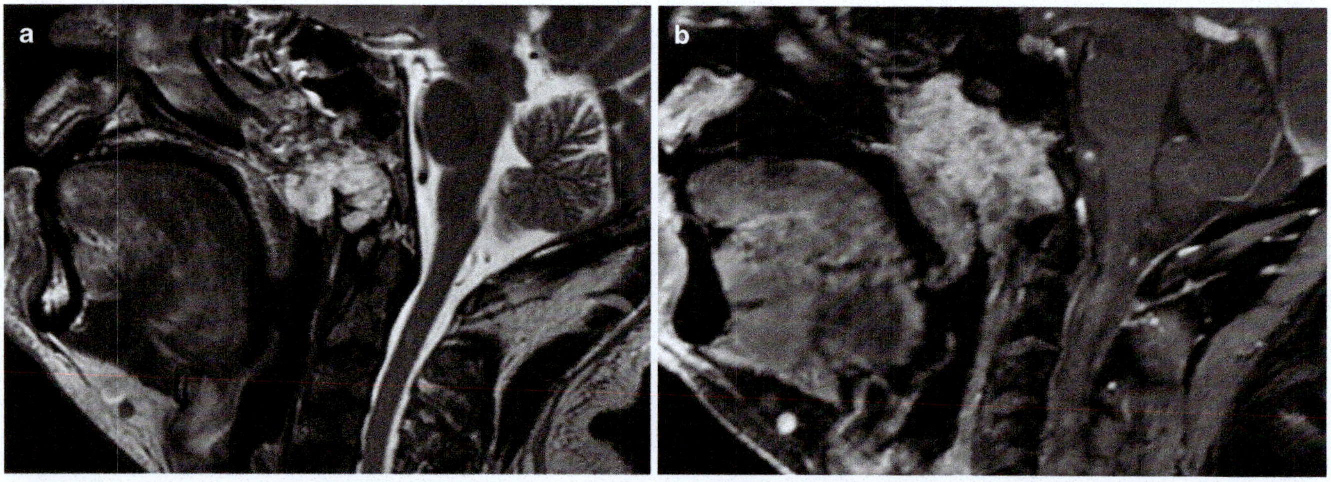

Fig. 30.1 (**a**) Sagittal T2 shows large heterogeneous mass exhibiting an epicenter anterior to the clivus. Some portions of the tumor are as bright as nearby CSF. Low signal vessels permeate the tumor. The black line from anterior clival cortex is clearly destroyed when compared to the posterior clivus and the planum sphenoidale. (**b**) Sagittal T1 Gd shows avid enhancement of large heterogeneous mass exhibiting an epicenter anterior to the clivus. Low signal vessels permeate the tumor. The anterior clival cortex is clearly destroyed with enhancing tumor invading clival marrow

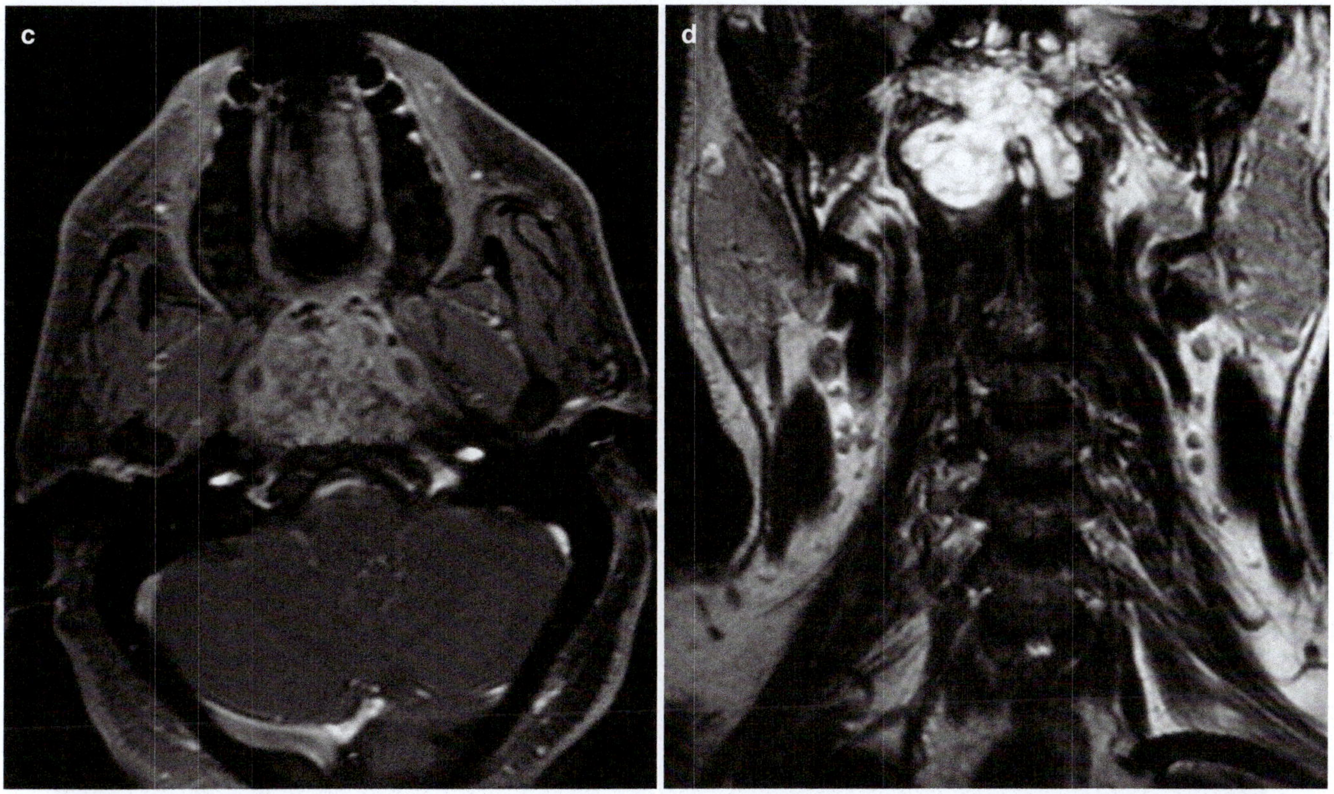

Fig. 30.1 (continued) (**c**) Axial T1 Gd shows avid enhancement of a large preclival mass. Low signal vessels permeate the tumor. The anterior clival cortex (black line) has been breached by this enhancing tumor. (**d**) Coronal T2 shows bright heterogeneous T2 signal from large clival mass flaunting a classic "grape-like" appearance of multiple high signal fluid filled foci

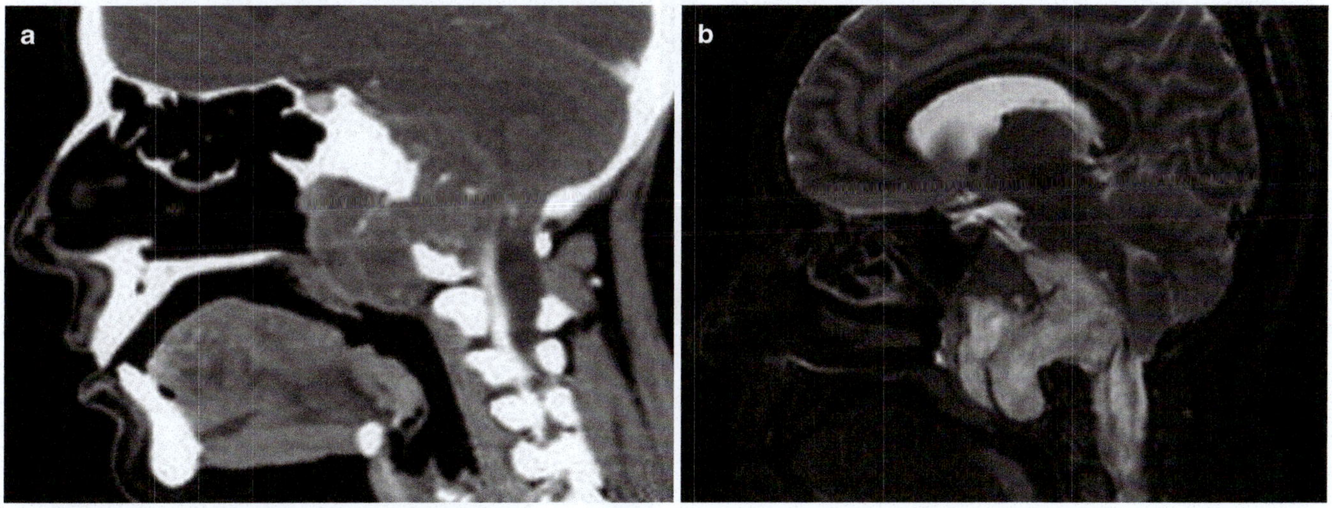

Fig. 30.2 (**a**) Sagittal CECT depicts devastating destruction of the distal clivus with a huge soft tissue mass extending both anteriorly and posteriorly. The soft tissue mass contains innumerable contrast containing serpiginous vascular channels. The tumor's epicenter is near the clival spheno-occipital synchondrosis. (**b**) Sagittal T2 shows huge heterogeneous clival mass extending more anteriorly than posteriorly. T2 signal is isointense with and is virtually indistinguishable from adjacent CSF. Clearly the clival cortex has been breached both anteriorly and posteriorly by this angry aggressive tumor

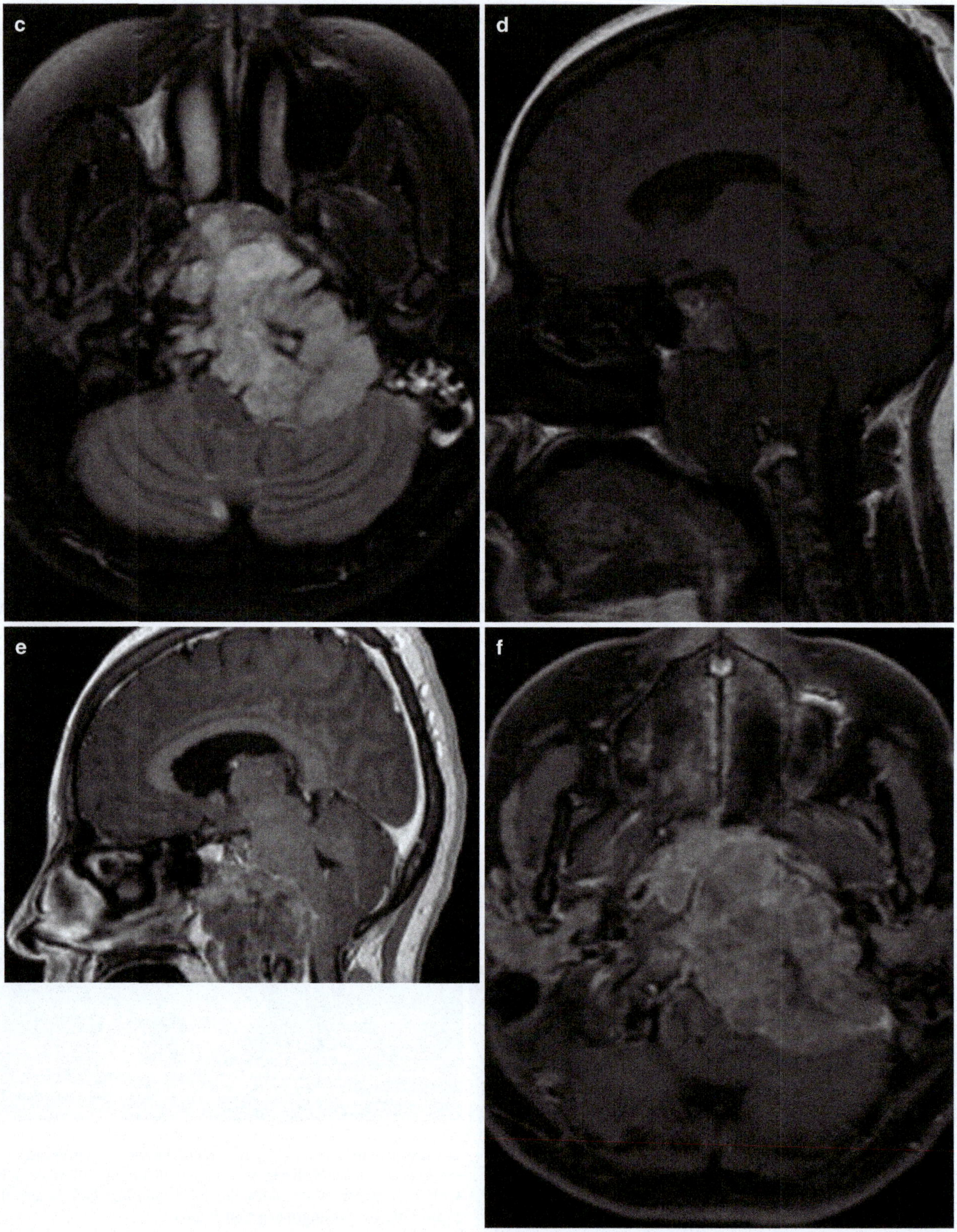

Fig. 30.2 (continued) (**c**) Axial T2 shows huge heterogeneous lobulated clival mass extending both anteriorly and posteriorly displacing and compressing critical structures including the pons and cerebellum. Fluid in the left mastoid air cells is probably related to compression of the Eustacean tube. (**d**) T1 sagittal shows a huge heterogeneous mass occupying the clivus extending more anteriorly than posteriorly. T1 signal is isointense with and virtually indistinguishable from adjacent muscle. Tumor has destroyed the distal clivus, portions of the skull base, and C1. It has breached some of the cortex of C2. (**e**) Sagittal T1 Gd shows huge heterogeneous mass occupying the clivus. Signal is heterogeneous with contrast in vessels extending through and around the tumor's periphery. The tumor itself is otherwise relatively isointense to brain. (**f**) Axial T1 Gd shows huge heterogeneous mass occupying clivus, extending both anteriorly and posteriorly, compressing and displacing the pons and cerebellum. Signal is heterogeneous with contrast in vessels extending through and around the tumor's periphery. The tumor itself is otherwise relatively isointense to brain

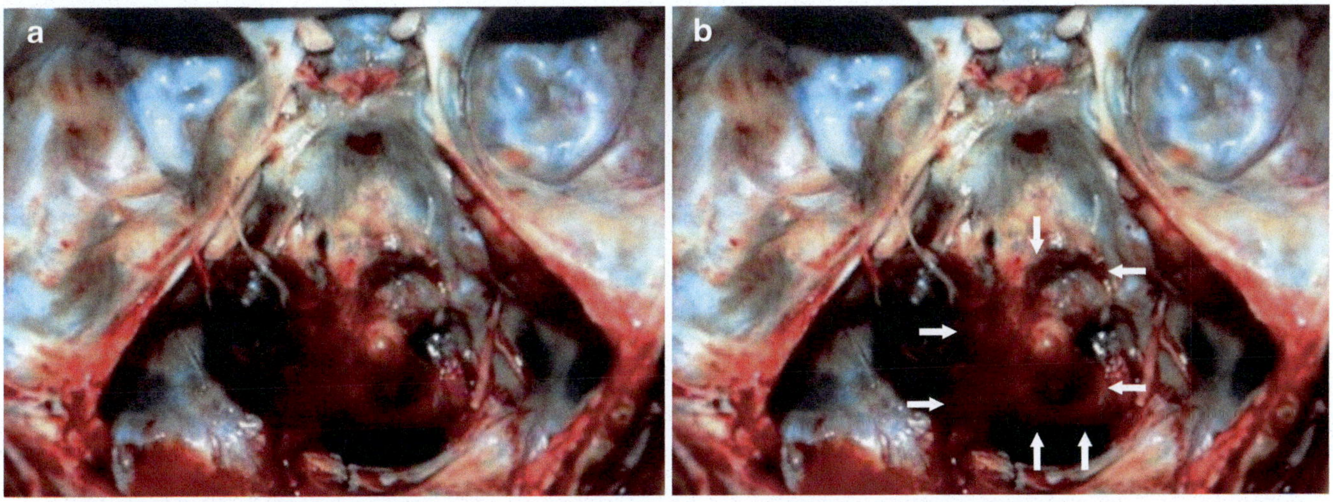

Fig. 30.3 (**a**) (without) and (**b**) (with arrows) depict the catastrophic consequence of a 5 cm clivus chordoma. Photograph of gross autopsy specimen views from above portions of the middle and posterior fossae. The lobulated mass arises from and involves the middle and lower clivus with its dural covering glistening for the photograph. The tumor has almost fully filled the foramen magnum providing a paltry crescent passageway posteriorly for the compressed brainstem which was extricated prior to this photograph. We gratefully acknowledge MedPix and its Chief Editor James G. Smirniotopoulos, M.D., for providing this genuinely graphic and informative image

Epidemiology and Pathology

- *Etiology*: Arise from remnants of the primitive notochord [1, 2].
- *Locations:* Approximately 1/3 cranial, 1/3 spinal, and 1/3 sacral [3]. (Yes, this is different than the numbers we all learned before based on older smaller studies.)
- *Incidence:* Chordomas are *rare* tumors with an estimated incidence of one case in two million. (So, some say when the incidence is one in a million, it can be called "common" but when one is in two million, it is now "rare."
- Clivus chordomas represent less than 0.2% of all intracranial tumors.
- M > F = 2:1; Whites > Blacks.
- Primarily occur in adults. Rarely occur <30 years old. Age ranged from 8 to 80 in Dahlin's series [2].
- *Histologic variants*: classic, chondroid, and dedifferentiated.
- Classic chordomas are 2–5 cm in size, semi-translucent grayish, gelatinous multilobulated with fibrous septa [11] See Fig. 30.3a, b.
- Histologically their round nuclei have abundant vacuolated cytoplasm described as *physaliferous* [12].

Treatment and Prognosis

Surgery and Radiotherapy

- Current preferred treatment is surgical resection combined with proton beam radiotherapy [11, 13].
- Newer types of radiation therapy are being used as well as radiosurgery [13].
- Recurrences are common and are related to poor prognostic factors including large size, subtotal resection, and microscopic necrosis.
  - Percutaneous radiofrequency ablation is being used in adjunctive treatment trials [14].
- *Chemotherapy*: Clivus chordomas are insensitive to current conventional chemotherapies. Targeted therapies using genetics and molecular biology will hopefully be helpful in the future [13].

Differential Diagnosis (DDx)

A. Chondrosarcoma

- Clival chordomas are located more *centrally* arising near the clival synchondrosis. Most chondrosarcomas originate more *laterally* in the petroclival fissure although overlap occurs in about 1/3 of cases [11].
- Immunohistochemistry facilitates separation of chordoma, chondroid chordoma, and chondrosarcoma [11]
- See Chap. 46, Skull Base Chondrosarcomas.

B. Clival Meningiomas

- Clival meningiomas demonstrate a dural attachment and usually display an *enhancing "dural tail"* with contrast.
- Clival meningiomas often show bone sclerosis *not* the lytic bone destruction displayed by chordomas.

- Clival meningiomas demonstrate more homogeneous enhancement [15]. Chordomas show heterogeneous enhancement having a *honeycomb pattern*.
- Chordomas are unusually *hyperintense on MRI T2* sequences and sometimes show *low signal fibrous septa*. Meningiomas' increased T2 is less pronounced and less frequent.

C. Plasmacytoma, Lymphoma, and Metastasis
- When located centrally these may mimic chordoma.
- The relative extra-osseous tumor component of metastasis is usually smaller than the extra-osseous tumor component of chordoma.

D. Rhabdomyosarcoma [RMS]
- Should be included in the diagnosis for pediatric patients.
- Originates from the nasopharynx often presenting with a large bulky intra- and extracranial tumor with lytic bone destruction [11].
- Not usually a problem as most chordomas are in adults, rarely <30 years old, whereas RMS is more frequently found in patients 1–5 years old.
- See Chap. 49, Rhabdomyosarcoma.

E. Ecchordosis Physaliphora (EP)
- *Definition*: Ecchordosis pysaliphora was once an obscure, relatively rare, notochordal remnant formerly found in 2% of autopsies, but now it repeatedly rears its head on conventional cross-sectional imaging.
- *Classic Clue*: Small smooth non-enhancing asymptomatic midline retro-clival mass with limited bony involvement which is hypointense on T1 and hyperintense on T2, showing an occasional osseous stalk.
- *Imaging*:
  - CT and MRI can play complimentary evaluation roles although EP's small size and CT's posterior fossa artifacts favor MRI over CT.
  - CT cisternography and magnified bone windows are usually more useful than conventional CT alone.
  - When MRI reveals a retro-clival mass requiring extra elucidation, an osseous stalk on thin-section CT can clinch the diagnosis [16].
- *Clinical Significance:*
  - Ecchordosis pysaliphora frequently flies under the conventional clinical radar because most cases are asymptomatic. Ecchordosis pysaliphora secures it standing for relative lack of symptoms with its small size and gentle growth pattern.
  - When sporadically symptomatic, its spectrum of scattered symptoms ranges from obscure to deadly serious including headache, diplopia, sudden sensorineural hearing loss, hemiparesis, hemi-hypoesthesia, CSF fistula, subarachnoid hemorrhage, and lethal pontine hemorrhage.
- *In Contrast*:
  - While chordomas are commonly extradural, the rare intradural chordoma tends to be encapsulated and well circumscribed without osseous involvement.
  - All reported cases of retroclival intradural chordoma exhibited brain stem symptoms or cranial nerve palsy.
- However, these lesions share the same embryonic etiology and may be difficult to distinguish from ecchordosis pysaliphora [16].

A Closer Look

I. Fast Facts
- *Rare:* Clival chordomas are really *rare* representing <0.2% of all intracranial tumors.
- *Incidence: Peak incidence is in the fifth to sixth decades and they are rare in children.*
- *Variant:*
  - Chondroid chordoma is a *variant* more commonly seen in 1/3 of skull-based chordomas, which habitually has a better prognosis than "classic chordomas" [1, 17].
  - Chondroid chordomas resemble low-grade chondrosarcomas requiring immunohistochemical studies for separation [1, 2].
- *Recurrences*: Patients who have both radiation and surgery suffer treatment failure with recurrence in about 5% [18].

II. Historic Highlights
- Chordomas' complicated history goes back over 150 years and is continually improving as we head into the future.
- In 1846 German physician and pathologist Rudolph Virchow described the lesion as an incidental small slimy growth on the dorsum sellae [19, 20].
- In 1856 German anatomist Hubert von Luschka described another "jelly-like" clival chordoma [21].
- Then in 1857 Virchow first fully described both the gross and histologic pathology of this entity [20].
- In 1858 Müller suggested these tumors were of notochord origin [22].
- In 1864 Krebs gave the first case report confirming their clinical importance.
- In 1894 Ribbert first coined the name "chordoma."
- In 1973 Dahlin published his landmark review of 155 skull-based chordomas seen at the Mayo Clinic between 1920 and 1971 and recognized a subgroup which looked like chondrosarcomas actually portrayed a paradoxically indolent course and he called them "chondroid"

chondromas [1]. This is *a happy paradox* in that *they looked worse but acted better.* We certainly need to find more of these happy paradoxes in medicine!

III. Genetics

- Most individuals with chordoma have *no* positive family history.
- However, various cases within families have been documented, suggesting some sort of genetic predisposition.
- Chordoma is currently linked to changes in the TBXT gene which provides instructions for making a T gene protein called *brachyury*.
- *Brachyury* is an associate in the T-box protein family which plays a pivotal part during notochordal development.
- The notochord normally disappears before birth but, in a small percentage of individuals, persists and gives rise to a spectrum of abnormalities associated with notochordal remnants.
- Duplication of the TBXT gene has been found in a few families which have an increased risk for chordoma as well as in individuals who show no familial tendency for chordoma.
- And, some individuals with chordomas show no changes in their TBXT gene, suggesting yet another unnamed genetic culprit is yet to be found [23].

Selected References

1. Heffelfinger MJ, Dahlin DC, MacCarty CS, Beabout JW. Chordomas and cartilaginous tumors at the skull base. Cancer. 1973;32:410–20.
2. Dahlin DC, Beabout JW. Dedifferentiation of low-grade chondrosarcomas. Cancer. 1971;28:461–6.
3. McMaster ML, Goldstein AM, Bromley CM, Ishibe N, Parry DM. Chordoma: incidence and survival patterns in the United States, 1973–1995. Cancer Causes Control. 2001;12:1–11.
4. Meyer JE, Oot RF, Lindfors KK. CT appearance of clival chordomas. J Comput Assist Tomogr. 1986;10(1):34–8.
5. Moore KA, Bohnstedt BN, Shah SU, Abdulkader MM, Bonnin JM, Ackerman LL, et al. Intracranial chordoma presenting as acute hemorrhage in a child: case report and literature review. Surg Neurol Int. 2015;6:63.
6. Fenerty KE, Patronas NJ, Heery CR, Gulley JL, Folio LR. Resources required for semi-automatic volumetric measurements in metastatic chordoma: is potentially improved tumor burden assessment worth the time burden? J Digit Imaging. 2015;29(3):357–64.
7. Müller U, Kubik-Huch RA, Ares C, Hug EB, Löw R, Valavanis A, et al. Is there a role for conventional MRI and MR diffusion-weighted imaging for distinction of skull base chordoma and chondrosarcoma? Acta Radiol. 2015;57(2):225–32.
8. Larson TC, Houser W, Laws ER. Imaging of cranial chordomas. Mayo Clin Proc. 1987;62:886–93.
9. Yeom KW, Lober RM, Mobley BC, et al. Diffusion-weighted MRI: distinction of skull base chordoma from chondrosarcoma. AJNR Am J Neuroradiol. 2013;34(5):1056–61.
10. Mizerny BR, Kost KM. Chordoma of the cranial base: the McGill experience. J Otolaryngol. 1995;24:14–9.
11. Weber AL, Liebsch NJ, Sanchez R, Sweriduk ST. Chordomas of the skull base. Radiologic and clinical evaluation. Neuroimaging Clin N Am. 1994;4(3):515–27.
12. Chugh R, Tawbi H, Lucas DR, Biermann JS, Schuetze SM, Baker LH. Chordoma: the nonsarcoma primary bone tumor. Oncologist. 2007;12(11):1344–50.
13. Walcott BP, Nahed BV, Mohyeldin A, Coumans JV, Kahle KT, Ferreira MJ. Chordoma: current concepts, management, and future directions. Lancet Oncol. 2012;13(2):e69–76.
14. Neeman Z, Patti JW, Wood BJ. Percutaneous radiofrequency ablation of chordoma. AJR Am J Roentgenol. 2002;179(5):1330–2.
15. Doucet V, Peretti-Viton P, Figarella-Branger D, Manera L, Salamon G. MRI of intracranial chordomas: extent of tumour and contrast enhancement—criteria for differential diagnosis. Neuroradiology. 1997;39:571–6.
16. Alkan O, Yildirim T, Kizilkilc O, et al. A case of ecchordosis physaliphora presenting with an intratumoral hemorrhage. Turk Neurosurg. 2009;19(3):293–6.
17. Clark WC, Robertson JH, Lara R. Chondroid chordoma. J Neurosurg. 1982;57:842–5.
18. Fischbein NJ, Kaplan MJ, Holliday RA, Dillon WP. Recurrence of clival chordoma along the surgical pathway. AJNR. 2000;21:578–83.
19. Virchow R. Untersuchungen uber die Entwickelug des Schadelgrundes. Berlin: G. Reimer; 1857.
20. Sahyouni R, Goshtasbi K, Mahmoodi A, Chen JW. A historical recount of chordoma. Historical vignette. J Neurosurg Spine. 2018;28:422–8.
21. Luschka H. Ueber gallertartige Auswuchse am Clivus Blumenbachii. Virchows Arch. 1857;11:8–11.
22. Muller H. Ueber das Verkommen von Resten der Chorda dorsalis bei Menschen nach der Geburt, und uber ihr Verhaltnis zu den Gallertgeschwulsten der Clivus. Z Rat Med. 1858;2:202–29.
23. Yang XR, Ng D, Alcorta DA, et al. T (Brachyury) gene duplication confers major susceptibility to family chordoma. Nat Genet. 2009;41(11):1176–8.

31 Lymphatic Malformations

Pertinent Points

- Definition: Lymphatic malformations (LMs) are rare non-malignant sponge-like masses consisting of fluid-filled channels or spaces thought to be caused by failure of the lymphatic system to properly connect to the venous system.
- *Classic Clue*: Insinuating non-encapsulated often multilocular cystic mass with fluid-fluid levels habitually extending into multiple adjoining spaces.
- *AKA*: Cystic hygroma, cystic lymphangioma, vasculolymphatic malformation.
- Lymphatic malformations have been seen everywhere except the brain; they are most common in the head and neck.
- They consist of cavernous lymphatic spaces with endothelial linings.

Imaging

General Imaging Features

- Lymphatic malformations may be unilocular or multilocular.

CT Features

- See *General Imaging Features*
- Ill-defined, hypodense, non-enhancing cystic mass.
- Most are homogeneous, but some appear heterogeneous because of blood, fat, or proteinaceous fluid.
- CT sometimes shows intrinsic septations.
- Displacement and compression of adjacent structures vary with lesion size (see Fig. 31.1a, b. This case clearly compresses and displaces the nearby nasopharynx and face).

MRI Features

- See General Imaging Features.
- MRI is the premier modality for classification of vascular anomalies [3].
- T1: Usually low signal but varies directly proportional to protein content, i.e., being brighter with more protein content.
- *Fluid-fluid levels* can be quite conspicuous (see Fig. 31.1a, d).
- T2: Slow-flow vascular malformations like LMs usually have high T2 signal (whereas high flow lesions contain signal voids) [3].
- T1 Gd: Occasionally find faint rim enhancement (see Fig. 31.1a–d).

Ultrasound Features

- Lymphatic malformations are frequently found on ultrasonic antenatal appraisals.

F. A. Midyett, S. K. Mukherji, *Skull Base Imaging*, https://doi.org/10.1007/978-3-030-46447-9_31

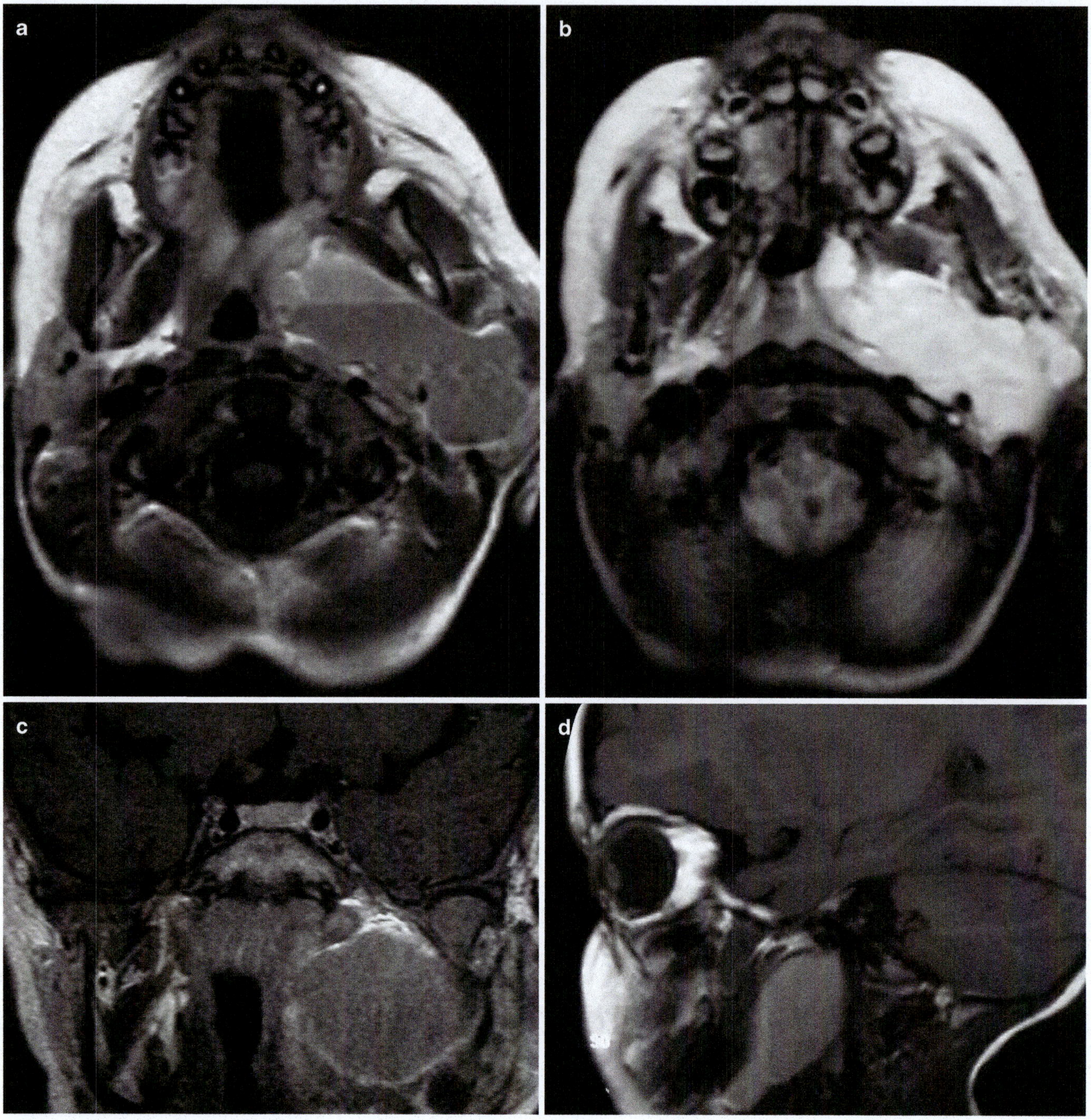

Fig. 31.1 (**a**) Axial T1 Gd shows large heterogeneous sausage-shaped cystic mass located just caudal to the left middle fossa. The periphery of the mass enhances. There is a fluid-fluid level with higher attenuation fluid layered on top of lower attenuation fluid. The mass extends medially displacing the nasopharyngeal air shadow and laterally displacing the left ear deforming the left side of the face. It extends anteriorly to the left mandibular angle and posteriorly to abut the left ICA. (**b**) Axial T2 shows bright T2 signal in large cystic mass described in image (A). The fluid-fluid level is not well appreciated on this sequence. (**c**) Coronal T1 Gd shows section through large left infratemporal mass which enhances around its periphery. Fluid within the mass is mildly heterogeneous with signal mildly hyperintense to brain. The mass extends laterally to the mandible, medially to displace the nasopharynx, and superiorly within a few millimeters of the temporal cortex. (Note this is not a plane to appreciate the fluid-fluid level.). (**d**) Sagittal T1 shows large heterogeneous sausage-shaped cystic mass located just caudal to the left middle fossa. Again demonstrated is the fluid-fluid level with higher attenuation fluid layered anteriorly

Clinical Issues

Presentation

- Symptoms arise from compression or obstruction of adjacent structures.
- Lymphatic malformations usually enlarge as the patient grows but sometimes spontaneously regress.
- Rapid enlargement is predominantly precipitated by trauma, hemorrhage, or infection.

Natural History

- Prevalence is approximately 1 in 4000 live births.
- No gender prevalence: M = F.
- 50% seen at birth, 90% evident by age two [4].
- 15% show spontaneous regression.

Epidemiology and Pathology [5]

- *Nomenclature:* The term "lymphatic malformation" is more commonly used since most are sponge-like collections containing lymph rather than totally cystic structures as the term cystic hygroma would imply.
- *Etiology:* They are thought to arise from failure of the lymphatic system to communicate with the cervical venous system.
- *Appearance:* They are frequently found during routine fetal ultrasound. When not apparent at birth, these malformations typically emerge by age two.
- *Location:* Most are stereotypically seen in the neck's posterior triangle and axilla, but remember ~10% may be cloaked in the chest.
- *Gross:*
  - Lymphatic malformations are soft, smooth, glistening, gray, non-encapsulated cystic masses containing lymphatic fluid.
  - They are endothelially lined cavernous lymphatic spaces.
  - Lymphatic malformations may mix with other types of vascular abnormalities, including capillary or venous malformations.

Treatment and Prognosis

Surgery [8]

- When possible, surgical resection is preferred.
- Multiloculation and association with major vascular and neural structures are complicating factors.
- High local recurrence rates are associated with incomplete resection.

Radiotherapy and Chemical Cautery

- Radiotherapy and chemical cautery are not as effective with lymphangioma as with hemangiomas.
- *Sclerosing agents*: In more complicated cases, sclerosing agents can be considered.
- *RF Ablation*: Radiofrequency ablation can be considered when lesions are superficialas.

Differential Diagnosis (DDx)

A. Dermoid

- Dermoids develop from germ cells in a spectrum of tumors between epidermoids and teratomas.
- CT shows well-circumscribed encapsulated fatty mass with areas of *very low* Hounsfield units.
- Commonly contained components include hair, blood, fat, bone, nails, teeth, eyes, cartilage, sebum, and thyroid tissue.
- The preferred imaging procedure is MRI with Gd and fat saturation.
- MRI reveals a well-circumscribed encapsulated mass filled with HIGH T1 signal material. LMs are *not* encapsulated.
- MRI well demonstrates a thick low signal dermis-like wall covering mass. Not a factor for LM.
- T1 is typically hyperintense (due to cholesterol components)
- T1 Gd: Dermoids typically exhibit a thin enhancing rim. This finding is occasionally observed with LM.
- T2 signal varies from hypo- to hyperintense.
- T2 sometimes shows chemical shift artifact at the fat-fluid interface.
- Dermoid cyst walls are lined by keratinizing squamous epithelium.
- Dermoid rupture sometimes sparks a severe inflammatory reaction [7].

B. Epidermoid Cyst (EC)

- Epidermoid cysts comprise <2% of all intracranial tumors.
- Epidermoid cysts are most commonly found in the CPA where they constitute 5% of CPA tumors.
- CT Features:
  - Usually non-enhancing hypodense mass.
  - 25% portray patchy peripheral calcifications.
  - Attenuation resembles CSF in most cases.

- MRI shows signal similar to CSF with telltale "dirty CSF" and characteristic restricted diffusion demonstrating *light bulb bright DWI and dark ADC map* insinuating itself by creeping into cisternal recesses.
- See Chap. 9, Epidermoid Cyst.

C. Basal Encephalocele
- Includes transethmoidal, sphenoethmoidal, transsphenoidal, and frontosphenoidal varieties.
- Important structures such as pituitary gland, hypothalamus, optic nerves, optic chiasm, and anterior third ventricle are typically involved with transphenoidal encephaloceles [6].
- See Chap. 17, Nasofrontal Encephalocele.

D. Second Branchial Cleft Cyst
- Non-enhancing, well-circumscribed ovoid unilocular cystic mass at the mandibular angle adjacent to the anterior margin of the sternocleidomastoid muscle.
- Located posterior to the submandibular gland and lateral to the carotid space.
- When infected their wall thickens and enhances along with the surrounding soft tissues.
- T1: Signal varies directly proportional to their protein content, i.e., being brighter with more protein content.
- T2: Hyperintense.
- T1 Gd: Unless infected, stereotypically shows *no enhancement.*

E. Thyroglossal Duct Cyst
- Midline oval unilocular cystic mass located at the level of hyoid bone.
- Encircled by contiguous infrahyoid muscles.

A Closer Look

I. Fast Facts
- Imaging findings support three subtypes:
  - (i) Macrocystic: Cysts >2 cm
  - (ii) Microcystic: Cysts <2 cm (or no appreciable cyst)
  - (iii) Mixed: Combined macrocystic and microcystic. Most lymphatic malformations are mixed

II. Historic Highlights

- 1828 Redenbacher first described a lymphangioma. No this is not the more familiar Orville Redenbacher who arrived almost a century later.
- 1843 Wernher gave the first case report of cystic hygroma combining Greek "hygroma" meaning fluid and "oma" meaning tumor.
- 1965 Bill and Summer submitted the supposition that cystic hygromas and lymphangiomas are variations of single entity.
- 1909 Sabin proposed that lymphatics are derived from primitive veins by budding endothelial cells.

III. Genetics and Environment
- May be sporadic or syndromal.
- *Turner and Down syndromes* are the most frequent associations.
- Aneuploidy is the presence of an abnormal number of chromosomes in a cell; in humans this normal is 46. Aneuploidy does not include a difference in one or more chromosome sets; that is known as euploidy [2].
- Aneuploidic associations include Turner and Down syndromes, trisomy 13 and 18, and triploidy [1].
- Non-aneuploidic associations include the following syndromes: Apert, Cornelia de Lange, fetal alcohol, Noonan, Fryns, Pena Shokeir, and the lethal multiple pterygium syndrome [1].

Selected References

1. Entezami M, Albig M, Knoll U, et al. Ultrasound diagnosis of fetal anomalies. New York: Thieme; 2003. ISBN: 1588902129.
2. Griffiths AJF, Miller JH, Suzuki DT. An introduction to genetic analysis. 7th ed. New York: W.H. Freeman & Company; 2000.
3. Hyodoh H, Hori M, Akiba H, Tamakawa M, Hyodoh K, Hareyama M. Peripheral vascular malformations: imaging, treatment approaches, and therapeutic issues. Radiographics. 2005;25(Suppl 1):S159–71.
4. Giguère CM, Bauman NM, Smith RJ. New treatment options for lymphangioma in infants and children. Ann Otol Rhinol Laryngol. 2002;111(12 Pt 1):1066–75.
5. Sabin FR. The lymphatic system in human embryos, with a consideration of the morphology of the system as a whole. Am J Anat. 1909;9:43–91.
6. Martinez-Lage JF, Poza M, Sola J, et al. The child with a cephalocele: etiology, neuroimaging, and outcome. Childs Nerv Syst. 1996;12:540–50.
7. Midyett FA, Mukherji SK. Orbital imaging. Amsterdam: Saunders/Elsevier; 2015. p. 54–6. ISBN: 978-0-323-34037-3
8. Sindou M. Practical handbook of neurosurgery: from leading neurosurgeons, vol. 1. Wien: Springer; 2009. p. 301.

32 Allergic Fungal Sinusitis

Pertinent Points

- *Definition*: Allergic fungal sinusitis (AFS) is a relatively recently appreciated, incompletely understood unique form of sinusitis which is often misdiagnosed. Although curable, physicians must understand its diagnosis and treatment [1].
- *Classic Clue*: Young immunocompetent patient from the Southwestern United States presents with therapy-resistant chronic sinusitis. Hypoattenuation on T2 MRI corresponds to *characteristically* hyperdense sinus with *characteristic serpiginous* pattern.
- *AKA*: Allergic fungal rhinosinusitis (AFRS).
- Hyperdense secretions on CT fall into three main causes:
  - Inspissated secretions
  - Fungal sinusitis
  - Hemorrhage
- Intrasinus hemorrhage is usually related to recent trauma, so in the absence of trauma, allergic fungal sinusitis must be considered.
- The *hyperdense* sinus is an *important* finding which may be the *only* clue to fungal sinusitis.
- Long-standing chronic sinusitis with bacterial infection is occasionally hyperdense, particularly in patients with cystic fibrosis.
- Allergic fungal sinusitis is a unique pathologic entity associated with allergic fungal mucin, a thick, tenacious eosinophilic secretion habitually having distinctive histologic features.
- Allergic fungal sinusitis is more common in 20–30 y/o males [10].
- Despite being the most common form of fungal sinusitis, allergic fungal sinusitis continues to be underdiagnosed because it is not fully recognized and treated as a distinct clinical entity [10].
- Since nasal polyposis is present in up to 100% of these cases [3], it is not enough to diagnose nasal polyposis and overlook the concomitant allergic fungal sinusitis.

Imaging

General Imaging Features

- CT and MRI findings taken together are remarkably specific for this diagnosis [2].
- When a *hyperdense* sinus on CT corresponds to a *hypointense* sinus on MRI, an inspissated accumulation with paramagnetic material and/or fungal sinusitis should be suspected.

CT Features

- See *General Imaging Features*.
- NECT: The majority of sinuses show near-complete opacification which centrally has hyperdense material surrounded by a peripheral rim of *hypodense mucosa*. The hyperdense central opacification is *characteristically serpiginous* [9].
- Sinus expansion is typical with 25% exhibiting erosion and some showing extension into surrounding structures.
- See Fig. 32.1a, c.

F. A. Midyett, S. K. Mukherji, *Skull Base Imaging*, https://doi.org/10.1007/978-3-030-46447-9_32

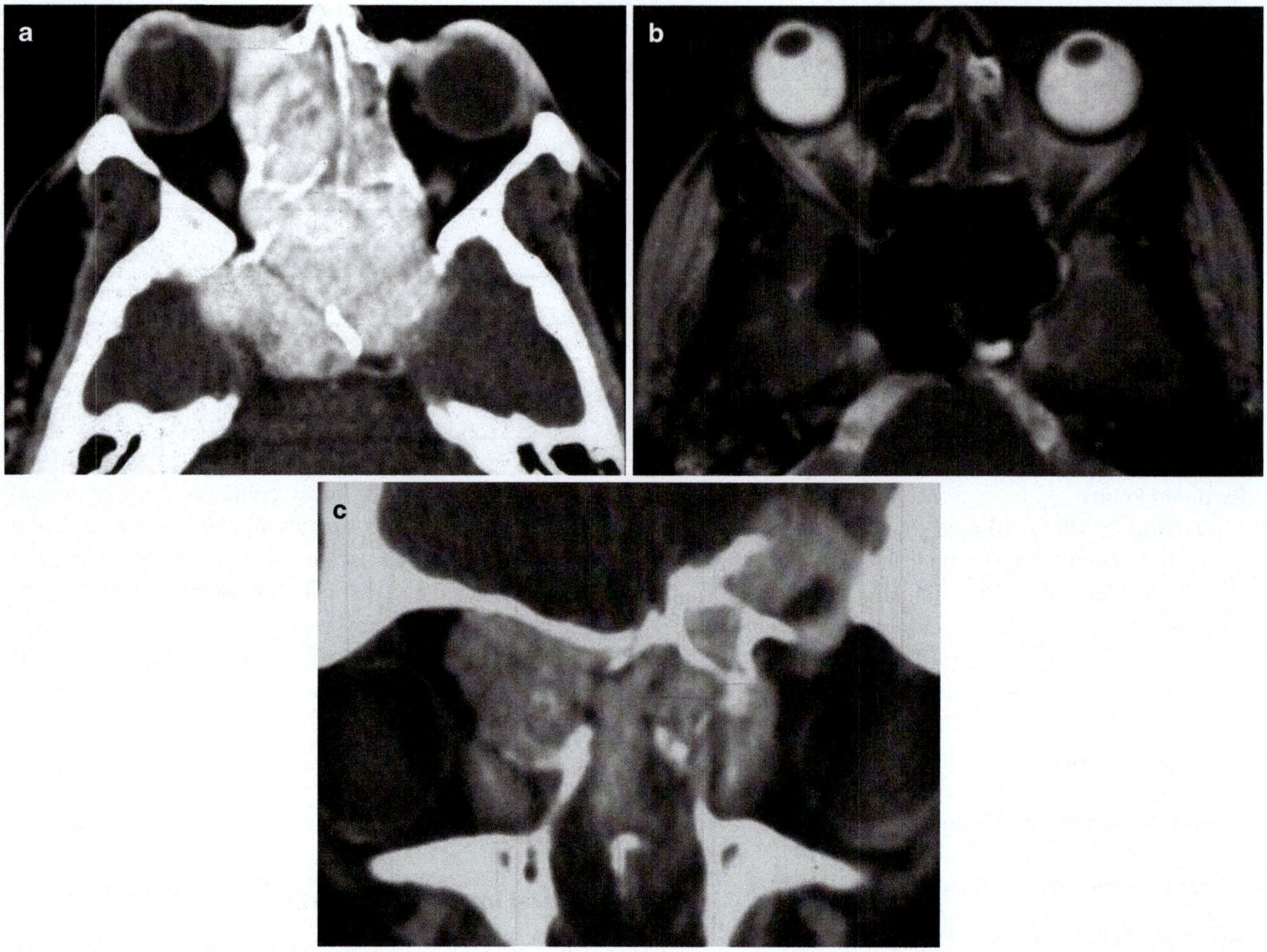

Fig. 32.1 (**a**) Axial NECT with soft tissue algorithm shows diffuse intrasinus increased attenuation. Even without bone algorithms, it is obvious that the process has breached bony borders extending into the middle cranial fossae and orbits. While neoplasm is certainly suggested, further analysis suggests the definitive diagnosis. Note how the mass clearly invades the right orbit through the lamina papyracea exhibiting exophthalmos. (**b**) Axial T2 shows huge "black hole" from diffuse hypo-attenuation having its epicenter in the sphenoid and right ethmoid sinuses. While potentially pathognomonic, MRI sometimes substantially underestimates disease portrayed on CT. (**c**) Coronal NECT with soft tissue algorithm shows diffuse intrasinus increased attenuation. Even without bone algorithms, it is obvious that the process has eroded and breached the bony borders extending into the left anterior cranial fossa and both orbits creating intraorbital masses. Attenuation is heterogeneous and increased

MRI Features

- See *General Imaging Features*.
- T1: Variable, although hypointensity is most common. T1 is optimal for evaluating interruption of the black signal void of cortical bone or low signal invasion of high signal fatty bone marrow of the skull base. Around the sinuses, however, some bony cortex can be too thin for adequate MRI evaluation [12, 13].
- T2: Hypointense signal or signal void is secondary to high concentrations of metals, high protein, and low free water in mucin. Fungal organisms concentrate various metals including iron, magnesium, and manganese.
- *Potential Pitfall*: Looking at *only* the MRI is a potential pitfall as the abnormal hypointense sinus may mimic a normal air-filled sinus (see Figs. 32.1b and 32.2a).
- T1 Gd: Exhibits enhancement of inflamed mucosa (often corresponding to hypodense rim seen on CT). However, most of the sinus content does *not* enhance.

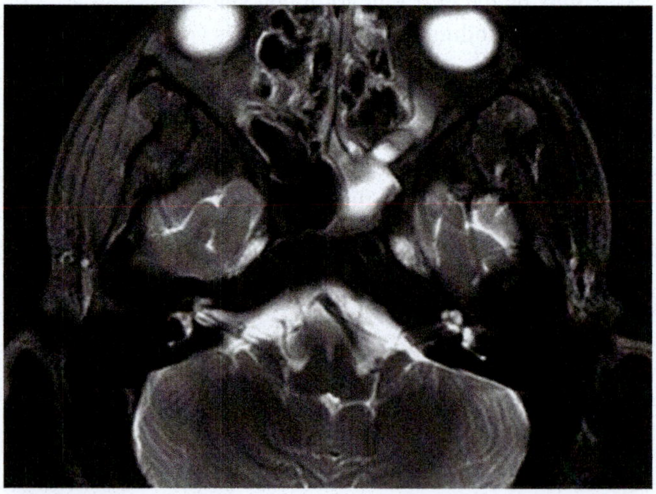

Fig. 32.2 (**a**) Axial T2 (in a different patient) shows hypo-attenuation within the sphenoid and ethmoid sinuses. This "mimics" sinuses which contain air and fluid. Allergic fungal sinusitis is often overlooked when MRI is the only imaging study

Clinical Issues

Presentation

- Most patients present with chronic headaches, allergic rhinitis, nasal airway obstruction, chronic sinusitis, and often prior sinus surgery.
- *Pain* is an *uncommon* presenting symptom.
- Usually unresponsive to antihistamines, intranasal steroids, and even immunotherapy.
- Most patients are immunocompetent young adults with nasal polyposis.
- Allergic fungal sinusitis prefers warmer environs including the Mississippi River basin as well as the Southeastern and Southwestern United States.
- Some see the Southwestern United States as a "hot spot" for the disease, particularly when the offending organism is *B. spicifera* [3].
- *Immune Status:* While patients with allergic fungal sinusitis are usually immunocompetent, patients with invasive fungal sinusitis are often immunocompromised.

Natural History

- Allergic fungal sinusitis is the most common form of fungal sinusitis [10].
- Patients primarily present with a story of sinus disease robustly resistant to conventional surgical and medical management meant for bacterial rhinosinusitis [7].
- Accurate diagnosis is important, as treatment is substantially different from other forms of fungal sinusitis [10].
- Allergic fungal sinusitis accounts for 6–8% of all chronic sinusitis requiring surgical intervention [9].

Epidemiology and Pathology

- Allergic fungal sinusitis is an immune-modulated disease entity [1].
- Mucosal inflammation illustrates increased lymphocytes and eosinophils.
- Cultures from children and adults show mainly *Bipolaris* and *Curvularia* species.
- Adults, however, habitually have a greater incidence of *Aspergillus* species than children [5].
- Extramucosal allergic mucin seen at surgery is characteristically a "peanut-buttery" material. Less appealing descriptions cite this as brown or greenish black with the consistency of cottage cheese [10]. Actually seeing this is sufficient to turn some against both peanut butter *and* cottage cheese!
- In addition to finding fungal elements and allergic mucin in an involved sinus, other important findings include Charcot-Leyden crystals, Type I hypersensitivity, and CT showing sinus expansion and bony erosion by a heterogeneous opacity [8].

Treatment and Prognosis

- Aggressive traditional surgery has evolved to incorporate almost exclusively endoscopic tissue-sparing techniques described as conservative but complete [1, 12, 13].
- Sinus surgery should be followed with allergen immunotherapy, systemic and topical corticosteroids, antihistamines, and antileukotrienes [4].

Differential Diagnosis

A. Acute Invasive Fungal Sinusitis

- Patients habitually have an acute onset fever, cough, nasal mucosal ulceration, epistaxis, and headache.
- Usually found in immunocompromised individuals.
- Associated conditions include diabetes mellitus, malignancy, neutropenia, and severe malnutrition.
- See Chap. 45, Invasive Fungal Sinusitis.

B. Acute Fulminant Fungal Sinusitis

- Invasion of mucosa, submucosa, or blood vessels by fungal hyphae.
- *Mucorales* genus and species *Aspergillus fumigatus* predominate.
- Patients require radical debridement, antifungal therapy, and treatment of their underlying causal condition.

C. Granulomatous Invasive Fungal Sinusitis

- AKA indolent fungal sinusitis.
- Rare condition chiefly reported in Africa and Southeast Asia and uncommonly in the United States.
- Characterized by copious fungal growth with regional tissue invasion.
- *A. fumigatus* is the most frequently isolated organism.
- Involves immunocompetent individuals.
- Histology portrays plasma and giant cells in noncaseating granulomas.
- Therapy requires antifungal treatment following surgical debridement.

D. Chronic Invasive Fungal Sinusitis

- Characterized by prolonged course.
- Typically associated with orbital apex syndrome.
- *Aspergillus flavus* is the most commonly isolated organism.
- Usually involves immunocompromised individuals.
- Requires treatment similar to acute invasive sinusitis.

E. Noninvasive Fungal Sinusitis

- Presents with chronic sinusitis refractory to prior medical and surgical treatment.

F. Sinonasal Polyposis with Fungal Colonization

- Diffuse sinonasal polyposis with fungal colonization may mimic allergic fungal sinusitis.
- CT shows complete opacification of the involved sinus with thickened sinus walls.
- There are intrasinus areas of high attenuation similar to those seen with allergic fungal sinusitis.
- Because of the polyposis, most of these cases will come to endoscopy where the absence of allergic mucin will provide the correct diagnosis.

G. Paranasal Sinus Cancer

- Squamous cell carcinoma is the most common malignant sinonasal tumor (80%), followed by adenocarcinoma [12].
- When extensive and slow growing, paranasal sinus cancer could initially cause a diagnostic dilemma.
- T2 typically shows intermediate signal neoplasm. This contrasts sharply with allergic fungal sinusitis where T2 hypo-attenuation causes a *characteristic black hole*.
- See Chap. 22, Paranasal Sinus Cancer.

A Closer Look

I. Genetics and Environment

- Patients with AFS (allergic fungal sinusitis) and HSD (hypertrophic sinus disease) have HLA-DQB1 *03 as a risk factor for disease [11].

II. Common spread patterns in advanced AFS:

- Intraorbital extension through the lamina papyracea (see Fig. 32.1a, c).
- Intracranial extension occurs by means of erosion of the sphenoid sinus, planum sphenoidale, and posterior wall of the frontal sinus [10].

III. Historic Highlights

- 1976 Safirstein first reported AFS as a distinct clinical entity [6].
- 1991 Allphin described features differentiating AFS from other forms of fungal sinusitis.
- 1993 Loury and Schaefer proposed diagnostic criteria including eosinophilia, antibodies to fungal antigen, nasal mucosal edema or polyposis, and characteristic CT or MRI findings.
- 1994 Cody simplified the diagnostic criteria.
- 1994 Bent and Kuhn's redefined the diagnostic criteria most commonly in use today [1].
- 1997 deShazo proposed five diagnostic criteria including radiographic evidence of sinusitis, allergic mucin, positive fungal stain/culture, absence of fungal invasion, and absence of contributory factors (i.e., diabetes, immunodeficiency).
- 1998 Mukherji et al. drew attention to the entity describing CT findings found from a large multi-institutional series. They pointed out that this underappreciated unusual entity was really the most common cause of fungal sinusitis.

Selected References

1. Glass D, Amedee RG. Allergic fungal rhinosinusitis: a review. Ochsner J. 2011;11(3):271–5.
2. Zinreich SJ, Kennedy DW, Malat J, Curtin HD, Epstein JI, Huff LC, Kumar AJ, Johns ME, Rosenbaum AE. Fungal sinusitis: diagnosis with CT and MR imaging. Radiology. 1988;169(2):439–44.
3. Schubert MS, Goetz DW. Evaluation and treatment of allergic fungal sinusitis. I. Demographics and diagnosis. J Allergy Clin Immunol. 1998;102(3):387–94.
4. Schubert MS. Allergic fungal sinusitis: pathogenesis and management strategies. Drugs. 2004;64(4):363–74.
5. McClay JE, Marple B, Kapadia L, et al. Clinical presentation of allergic fungal sinusitis in children. Laryngoscope. 2002;112(3):565–9.
6. Safirstein B. Allergic bronchopulmonary aspergillosis with obstruction of the upper respiratory tract. Chest. 1976;70:788–90.
7. Kuhn FA, Javer AR. Allergic fungal rhinosinusitis: perioperative management, prevention of recurrence, and role of steroids and antifungal agents. Otolaryngol Clin N Am. 2000;33(2):419–33.
8. Saravanan K, Panda NK, Chakrabarti A, et al. Allergic fungal rhinosinusitis: an attempt to resolve the diagnostic dilemma. Arch Otolaryngol Head Neck Surg. 2006;132(2):173–8.
9. Bent JP, Kuhn FA. Diagnosis of allergic fungal sinusitis. Otolaryngol Head Neck Surg. 1994;111(5):580–8.
10. Mukherji SK, Figueroa RE, Ginsberg LE, et al. Allergic fungal sinusitis: CT findings. Radiology. 1998;207(2):417–22.
11. Schubert MS, Hutcheson PS, Graff RJ, et al. HLA-DQB1 *03 in allergic fungal sinusitis and other chronic hypertrophic rhinosinusitis disorders. J Allergy Clin Immunol. 2004;114(6):1376–83.
12. Eggesbo HB. Imaging of sinonasal tumors. Cancer Imaging. 2013;12:136–52.
13. Casselman JW. The skull base: tumoral lesions. Eur Radiol. 2005;15:534–42.

Basal Encephalocele

33

Pertinent Points

- Definition: Extracranial herniation of the meninges and/or brain that maintains a subarachnoid connection.
- The term encephalocele covers the characteristic sac-like protrusions of the brain and meninges through osseous cranial defects resulting from incomplete neural tube closure during fetal development.
- An encephalocele which has lost its intracranial connection is a nasal glioma (see Chap. 20, Nasal Glioma).
- *AKA:* Cranium bifidum (Latin), meningocele, meningoencephalocele, transsphenoidal encephalocele, cephalocele [3].
- *Classic Clue*: Patient sent for evaluation having a history of clear rhinorrhea and a nasopharyngeal mass. The ophthalmologist subsequently confides that the patient has an optic nerve abnormality, hypertelorism, and morning glory syndrome. Imaging illustrates an unusual skull base mass with CT depicting osseous changes and MRI showing CSF signal.
- *Etiology:* Encephaloceles can be congenital or acquired with the latter related to trauma, surgery, tumors, osteoradionecrosis, or sphenoid dysplasia in NF 2 [18].
- These protrusions can be classified as meningoceles or meningoencephaloceles depending on the presence of neural components within the herniation.
- Encephaloceles are usually classified as anterior (frontoethmoidal or sincipital), basal, and posterior occipital types.
- *Prevalence:* Encephaloceles involving the skull base are rare with a prevalence of 1 in 35,000 births. The transsphenoidal encephalocele is the least frequent, comprising approximately 5% of those [10, 11].
- *Scope:* This chapter concentrates on basal encephaloceles (see Chap. 17, Nasofrontal Encephalocele for more information on anterior encephaloceles).
- *Classification:*
  - Basal encephaloceles protrude through anterior and central skull base defects and can be classified into the following subtypes: sphenoethmoidal, sphenomaxillary, spheno-occipital, transethmoidal, and transsphenoidal.
  - Posterior encephaloceles occur in occipital or craniocervical locations with abnormalities often involving the occipital bone, atlas, and hindbrain. They are frequently found associated with Chiari and Dandy-Walker malformations.
- An encephalocele consists of the brain herniated through a cranial bone. Meningocele means herniated dura. When *both the brain and dura* are herniated, the proper term is meningoencephalocele. But, alas, simply too many syllables for some, so we commonly call them all encephaloceles.
- The neural tube is the embryonic tissue which develops into the brain, spinal cord, and surrounding bone. This narrow structure folds and closes during the third and fourth weeks of fetal development during brain and spinal cord development. Rare neural tube defects (NTDs) develop when this process goes awry with the tube failing to close completely. Of late, this fourth week faux pas is currently called a "late neurulation defect." [1]
- Locations and incidences of encephaloceles [4]:
  - 75% occipital
  - 15% frontoethmoidal
  - 10% basal:
    - Transethmoidal
      - Most frequent accounting for 1–5% of encephaloceles [16]
    - Sphenoethmoidal

F. A. Midyett, S. K. Mukherji, *Skull Base Imaging*, https://doi.org/10.1007/978-3-030-46447-9_33

  - Sphenoethmoidal (and nasofrontal) encephaloceles are most frequently found in Southeast Asian Women.
- Transsphenoidal
  - Rarest form of basal encephalocele, estimated at 1 in 700,000 live births [11]
  - Associated with visual and hormonal disturbances
- Frontosphenoidal [4]

Sternberg's Canal [24]

- In 1888 anatomist Maximilian Sternberg described the lateral craniopharyngeal canal currently bearing his name.
- The sphenoid bone develops from separate ossification centers which form its body as well as its lesser and greater wings.
- Sternberg's canal is a congenital fusion plane defect resulting from incomplete fusion between the body and greater wings.
- Sternberg's canal is a structural skull base "soft spot" through which temporal lobe encephaloceles potentially protrude into the lateral recess of the sphenoid sinus [19, 21].
- Sternberg's canal was previously thought to be present in ≤4% of adults but more recently could be confirmed in only 1 in 1000 by CT.
- Sternberg's canal was proposed to be *lateral* to the foramen rotundum, while CT analysis suggests it is *medial* to the foramen rotundum (see Chap. 51/Foramen Rotundum).
- Well over a century since Sternberg's description, his canal certainly continues to be connected to controversy [20].
- From a practical standpoint, the current controversy appears to be related to nomenclature rather than treatment philosophy, as management of lateral recess encephaloceles (and leaks whether medial or lateral to the foramen rotundum) is well defined.
- Currently, the etiology of lateral CSF leaks is more frequently felt to be a consequence of a combination of anatomic and physiologic factors including a change in CSF dynamics with aberrant arachnoid granulations [18, 22].
- Perhaps, we as twenty-first century clinicians, with our state-of-the-art scanners, should simply stand in awe of an anatomist who found and described this entity almost a century before we were able to routinely execute these elaborate examinations.

Imaging

General Imaging Features

- Ocular hypertelorism which is usually associated with basal encephaloceles in children is not always found in adults exhibiting this entity [12].
- Meninges may herniate into the nasal cavity, nasopharynx, pterygopalatine fossa, or orbit as well as the sphenoid or ethmoid sinuses [15].
- Transsphenoidal encephaloceles typically traverse a sellar floor defect into the nasal cavity. They may also project into the oral cavity and are often associated with a cleft palate [4].
- Transethmoidal encephaloceles project through a midline or cribriform plate defect into the nasal cavity [4].
- When located anterior to the dorsum sella, transsphenoidal encephaloceles splay the sphenoid and may displace the cavernous sinus laterally.

CT Features

- *See General Imaging Features.*
- Typically shows CSF attenuation midline soft tissue mass and depicts bony changes as outlined in *General Imaging Features.*
- Frequently find a midline hypo-attenuating mass with a thin wall which sometimes scallops adjacent intact bony cortex.
- We sometimes see gross bony destruction when lesions are long standing. While devastating, the features favor slow growth over aggressive malignant destruction (see Fig. 33.1a–c).
- CTC (CT cisternography) [9]
  - CTC is habitually helpful for evaluation of CSF leaks.
  - CTC is usually reserved for patients where high-resolution CT does not identify a bony defect or those unfortunate patients where there are multiple defects and it is not clear which one is leaking.
  - See Chap. 27, Skull Base CSF Leaks.

MRI Features

- *See General Imaging Features.*
- T1 and T2 show a midline, extracranial, fluid-filled CSF isointense, abnormality which can contain a component of the brain that is isointense to intracranial brain (see Fig. 33.1d).
- *T1 Gd:* Typically follows signal of intracranial CSF and brain (see Fig. 33.1e, f).
- *DWI*: Shows *no* restricted diffusion.

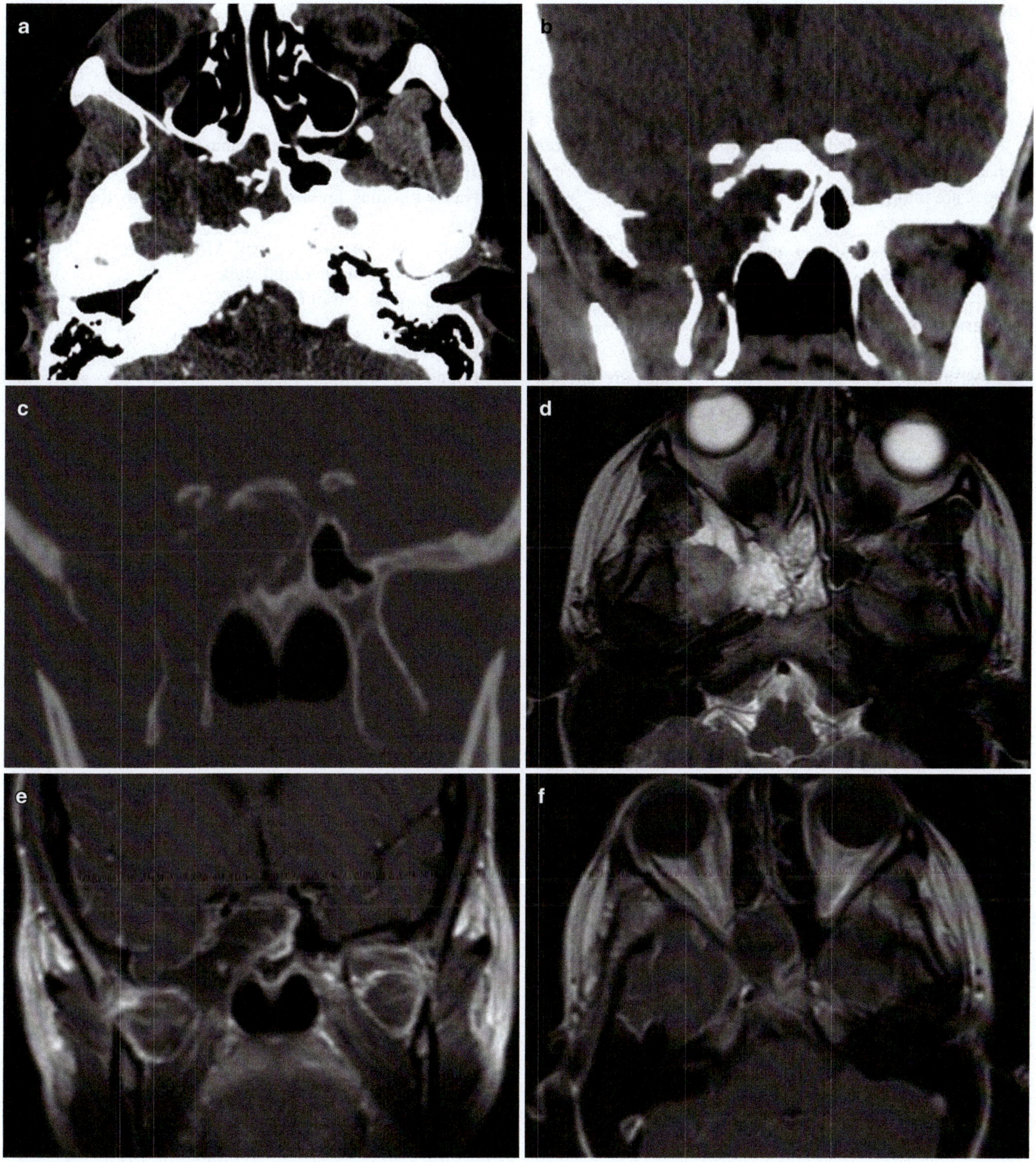

Fig. 33.1 (**a**, **b**) Soft tissue algorithm Axial (**a**) and Coronal CECT (**b**) show huge destructive process involving the right central skull base. The soft issue component is mildly heterogeneous with no demonstrable enhancement. (**c**) Bone algorithm Coronal CECT shows huge destructive process involving the right central skull base. The floor of the middle cranial fossa is absent with destruction of the pterygoid sparing only portions of the pterygoid plates. The lateral wall of the right sphenoid sinus, foramen rotundum, and lateral recess have been totally destroyed. The lesser sphenoid wings are largely intact, including the anterior clinoids. While devastating, the features favor slow growth over aggressive malignant destruction. (**d**) Axial T2 shows the large right central skull base mass presents predominately CSF intensity. It extends anteriorly to the orbit crossing the midline to abut an intact contralateral bony cortex. Its posterior extension almost touches clival marrow. The mass has thinned and breached neighboring cortical margins at multiple sites. (**e**, **f**) Coronal (**e**) and Axial (**f**) T1 Gd show the large right central skull base mass again exhibiting predominately CSF intensity without abnormal enhancement, although it has some prominent contrast containing veins around its periphery. This is massive destruction by what appears to be a slow growing, most likely benign process. Although rare, this is not an uncommon consequence of a long standing basal encephalocele

Ultrasound Features

- May encounter these entities incidentally on routine prenatal ultrasound.
- Habitually have herniation through a calvarial defect by a spherical, fluid-filled structure which can contain brain parenchyma.
- 90% are midline.

Clinical Issues

Presentation

- Most anterior and posterior encephaloceles are encountered soon after birth or even during antenatal fetal ultrasound.
- Basal encephaloceles may present as intranasal or nasopharyngeal masses.
- They can cause nasal airway obstruction, CSF rhinorrhea, recurrent meningitis, or seizures.
- Encephaloceles may increase in size with a Valsalva maneuver, i.e., Furstenberg sign.
- Encephaloceles may transilluminate.
- Encephaloceles may come to imaging for evaluation of a nasopharyngeal mass.
- They may masquerade as nasal polyps or enlarged adenoids and may be associated with a cleft palate.
- Unfortunate attempts to repair a cleft palate and/or biopsy an associated mass have resulted in CSF rhinorrhea, meningitis, and death [15].
- Associated osseous dysplasia suggests NF.
- See Chap. 17, Nasofrontal Encephalocele.

Treatment

- Therapy involves resection, closure of the dural defect, and reconstruction of an associated bony defect [1].
- The prognosis is better for frontoethmoidal encephaloceles than for occipital or parietal encephaloceles.
- This is because frontoethmoidal encephaloceles are not typically related to the various anomalies [4] where their prognosis is chiefly contingent on these associated abnormalities [1, 2].

Differential Diagnosis [1]

A. Nasal Glioma [4, 5]

- Nasal glioma is a congenital heterotopic non-neoplastic mass which occurs near nasal root.
- Nasal gliomas are composed of dysplastic glial tissue.
- 15% connect to the brain by a stalk but do *not* communicate with the CSF-filled subarachnoid space.
- Nasal gliomas are distinctly different from encephaloceles which *do connect with the subarachnoid space and do contain CSF.*
- Nasal gliomas are 30% intranasal, 60% extranasal, and 10% mixed.
- Nasal gliomas are usually isointense to the brain on MRI.
- High-resolution surface coil MR imaging is useful in illustrating an intracranial stalk.
- See Chap. 20, Nasal Glioma.

B. Dermoid and Epidermoid Cysts

- Found in various locations around the skull and midface.
- Dermoids contain ectoderm and skin elements. Epidermoids contain ectoderm with *no* skin elements.
- CT attenuation varies depending on fat content *showing fat with dermoids* and *fluid with epidermoids*.
- MRI signal varies with fluid content ranging from pure fluid (isointense with CSF on T1 and T2 in epidermoids to a more complex intensity for dermoids (T1 hyperintense, T2 hypointense).
- A key factor here is that *epidermoid cysts typically show restricted diffusion* and are bright on DWI with a dark area on corresponding ADC map. This is NOT a feature for encephaloceles.
- See Chaps. 9, Epidermoid Cyst and 19, Nasal Dermoid.

C. Nasal Teratomas [6, 7]

- Teratomas are neoplasms containing all three germ layers.
- In general, H&N teratomas tend to be benign in children whereas in adults appear to be mostly malignant.
- Most H&N teratomas contain *calcifications* which are not features of encephaloceles.

A Closer Look

I. Fast Facts [13–16]

- Basal encephaloceles are associated with the morning glory syndrome [MGS].
- MGS is an uncommon anomaly in which the optic disc resembles a morning glory flower on fundoscopy and imaging.
- Both basal encephaloceles and the morning glory syndrome have common associations including:
  - Agenesis of the corpus callosum
  - Hypertelorism
  - Coloboma

II. Historic Highlights [2, 8]

- Encephaloceles have been recorded since the sixteenth century [2].
- In 1755, Corvinus described draining CSF and resecting the surrounding membrane.
- In 1774, Freeand published an article on "hernia of brain" and advocated supporting the surgical repair with boiled leather to facilitate firm scar formation.
- In 1827, Geoffroy Saint-Hilaire published his "adhesive theory" of basal encephalocele formation, attributing its bony defect to faulty separation of neural from surface ectoderm during neural tube formation. This presumably prevented mesoderm (which forms the bone), from inserting itself between those adherent germ layers. This is an admirable insight for 1827 but does not answer all the questions raised by inquiring minds in the twenty-first century [10, 11].
- In 1888, Anatomist Maximilian Sternberg described the lateral craniopharyngeal canal currently carrying his name.
- In 1970, Kindler reported ten cases of morning glory syndrome [13, 17].

III. Genetics and Associations

- Encephaloceles are rare types of neural tube defects (NTDs).
  - The CDC estimates that 1 of 10,000 babies born in the United States will exhibit an encephalocele [23]. The worldwide rate is higher at 1 in 5000 live births.
  - Encephaloceles have a genetic component and often occur in families having a history of spina bifida and anencephaly.
  - A clival encephalocele has been reported with a 5q15 chromosome deletion [24].
  - Specific genes currently linked to spina bifida include:
    MTHFR and SHMT1 which are involved in folic acid metabolism
    VANGL1 gene which encodes for glucose metabolism
- Associations [16]:
  - Hypertelorism is usually present but may be mild or inconspicuous.
  - Cleft lip, cleft palate.
  - Agenesis of corpus callosum.
  - Spina bifida.
  - Morning glory syndrome.
  - Coloboma.
  - Sphenoid dysplasia is associated with NF.

Selected References

1. Hoving EW. Nasal encephaloceles. Childs Nerv Syst. 2000;16:702–6.
2. Tirumandas M, Gbenimacho SA, Shoja MM, et al. Nasal encephaloceles: a review of etiology, pathophysiology, clinical presentations, diagnosis, treatment, and complications. Childs Nerv Syst. 2013;29(5):739–44.
3. Koral K, Geffner ME, Curran JG. Australas Radiol. 2000;44(2):220–4.
4. Moron FE, Morriss MC, Jones JJ, Hunter JJ. Lumps and bumps on the head in children: use of CT and MR imaging in solving the clinical diagnostic dilemma. Radiographics. 2004;24(6):1655–74. https://doi.org/10.1148/rg.246045034.
5. Lowe LH, Booth TN, Joglar JM, Rollins NK. Midface anomalies in children. Radiographics. 2000;20:907–22.
6. Cukurova I, Gumusssoy M, Yaz A, et al. A benign teratoma presenting as an obstruction of the nasal cavity: a case report. J Med Case Rep. 2012;6:147. https://doi.org/10.1186/1752-1947-6-147.
7. Barnes L, Eveson J, Reichart P, Sidransky D. Germ cell tumours. In: Cardesa A, Luna M, editors. Pathology and genetics of head and neck tumors. Lyon: IARC Press; 2005. p. 76–9.
8. McGee JDF. The history of nasofrontal encephaloceles. Am Assoc Neurol Surg. 2004.
9. Stone JA, Castillo M, Neelon B, Mukherji SK. Evaluation of CSF leaks: high-resolution CT compared with contrast-enhanced CT and radionuclide cisternography. AJNR Am J Neuroradiol. 1999;20(4):706–12.
10. Blustajn J, Netchine I, Fredy D, et al. Dysgenesit of the internal carotid artery associated with transsphenoidal encephalocele: a neural crest syndrome? AJNR. 1999;20:1154–7.
11. Smith D, Murphy M, Hitchon P, Babin R, Abu-Yousef M. Transsphenoidal encephaloceles. Surg Neurol. 1983;20:471–80.
12. Harada N, Nemoto M, Miyazaki C, et al. Basal encephalocele in an adult patient presenting with minor anomalies: a case report. J Med Case Rep. 2014;8:24.
13. Midyett FA, Mukherji SK. Chapter 24, Coloboma. In: Orbital imaging. Amsterdam: Elsevier/Saunders; 2015. p. 107. ISBN: 978-0-323-34037-3.
14. Minotto I, Abdala N, Miachon AAS, et al. Basal encephalocele associated with morning glory syndrome: case report. Arq Neuropsiquiatr. 2007;65(4):988–91. https://doi.org/10.1590/S0004-282X2007000600013. Available from: http://www.scielo.br/scielo.php?script=sci_arttext&pid=S0004-282X2007000600013&lng=en&nrm=iso. ISSN: 1678-4227.
15. Pollock JA, Newton TH, Hoyt WF. Transsphenoidal and transethmoidal encephaloceles. Radiology. 1968;90:44253.
16. Caprioli J, Lesser RL. Basal encephalocele and morning glory syndrome. Br J Ophthalmol. 1983;67:349–51.
17. Kindler P. Morning glory syndrome: unusual congenital optic disc anomaly. Am J Ophthalmol. 1970;69:376–84.
18. Settecase F, Harnsberger HR, Michel MA, et al. Spontaneous lateral sphenoid cephaloceles: anatomic factors contributing to pathogenesis and proposed classification. AJNR. 2014;35(4):784–9. https://doi.org/10.3174/ajnr.A3744.
19. Bendersky DC, Landriel FA, Ajler PM, et al. Sternberg's canal as a cause of encephalocele within the lateral recess of the sphenoid sinus: a report of two cases. Surg Neurol Int. 2011;2:171.
20. Baranano CF, Cure J, Palmer JN, Woodworth BA. Sternberg's canal: fact or fiction? Am J Rhinol Allergy. 2009;23:167–71. https://doi.org/10.2500/ajra.2009.23.3290.
21. Sternberg M. Ein bisher noch nich beschrieben Kanal im Keilben des Menschen. Anat Anz. 1888;3:225–53.
22. Schlosser RJ, Woodworth BA, Wilensky EM, et al. Spontaneous cerebrospinal fluid leaks: a variant of benign intracranial hypertension. Ann Otol Rhinol Laryngol. 2006;115:495–500.
23. Canfield MA, Honein MA, Yuskiv N, Xing J, Mai CT, Collins JS, et al. National estimates and race/ethnic-specific variation of selected birth defects in the United States, 1999–2001. Birth Defects Res A Clin Mol Teratol. 2006;76(11):747–56.
24. Puvabanditsin S, Malik I, Garrow E, et al. Clival encephalocele and 5q15 deletion: a case report. J Child Nerurol. 2015;30(4):505–8.

34 Cavernous Carotid Aneurysm

Pertinent Points

- *Definition*: Cavernous carotid aneurysms involve the cavernous portion of the internal carotid artery as it passes through the cavernous sinus. While typically benign, an astute clinician can help these patients select the specialized medical treatment needed to avoid very serious consequences including subarachnoid hemorrhage (SAH) or exsanguination from epistaxis.
- *Classic Clue*: Patient presenting with diplopia and CN palsies has an imaging study showing cavernous sinus enlargement. Vascular studies show abnormal enlargement of the cavernous carotid but no abnormality of the SOV (superior ophthalmic vein) or observed cavernous sinus thrombi.
- *AKA*: Cavernous sinus aneurysm
- While most CCAs are berry aneurysms, some are posttraumatic, and others are mycotic.
- *Average Age*: Non-traumatic, 52 years; traumatic aneurysms, 29 years [15].
- *Incidence*: CCAs account for 5% of all intracranial aneurysms.
- *Location*: CCAs arise from the cavernous portion of the internal carotid artery as it passes through the cavernous sinus.
- The cavernous sinus consists of a complex of paired venous channels. Along the lateral walls run CN III (oculomotor), CN IV (trochlear), and V_1 and V_2 (first and second divisions of the trigeminal nerve).
- *Usual Course*: CCAs are, as a rule, considered relatively benign lesions likely showing a languid course with a low risk of life-threatening complications. However, large lesions sometimes show growth, mass effect, bone erosion, thrombosis, inflammation, or rupture with resultant SAH or CCF (carotid cavernous fistula) [2, 4].
- This chapter considers the facts necessary to answer the question of which CCA should be treated and which should simply be scrutinized [1].

Imaging

General Imaging Features

- The C4 segment of the ICA (AKA cavernous portion) begins at the superior margin of the petrolingual ligament and extends to the PDR (proximal dural ring).
- CCAs show different imaging signals depending on a number of factors including:
  - Whether the aneurysm contains clot or dissection and, if clotted, the stage of clot development.
  - Incompletely thrombosed giant aneurysms show mixed signal intensity from various stages of intramural and intraluminal thrombus.

CT Features

- *See General Imaging Features.*
- The appearance depends primarily on the presence (or absence) of thrombus.
- NECT: Usually shows asymmetric widening of the ipsilateral cavernous sinus (see Fig. 34.1a, b).
- CCAs are well-defined, usually round, and slightly hyperattenuating and can contain calcifications.
- CECT
  - If patent, CCAs appear bright showing uniform enhancement.

F. A. Midyett, S. K. Mukherji, *Skull Base Imaging*, https://doi.org/10.1007/978-3-030-46447-9_34

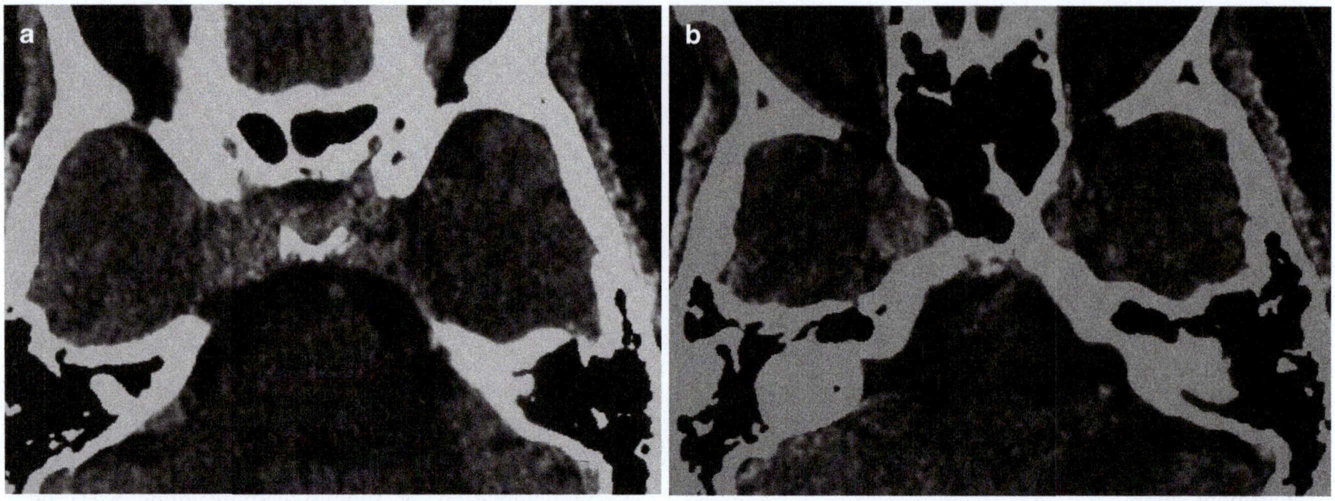

Fig. 34.1 (**a**, **b**) Axial NECT images display asymmetric enlargement of the right cavernous sinus. Although somewhat striking, in this setting, these findings didn't attract much attention from initial observers

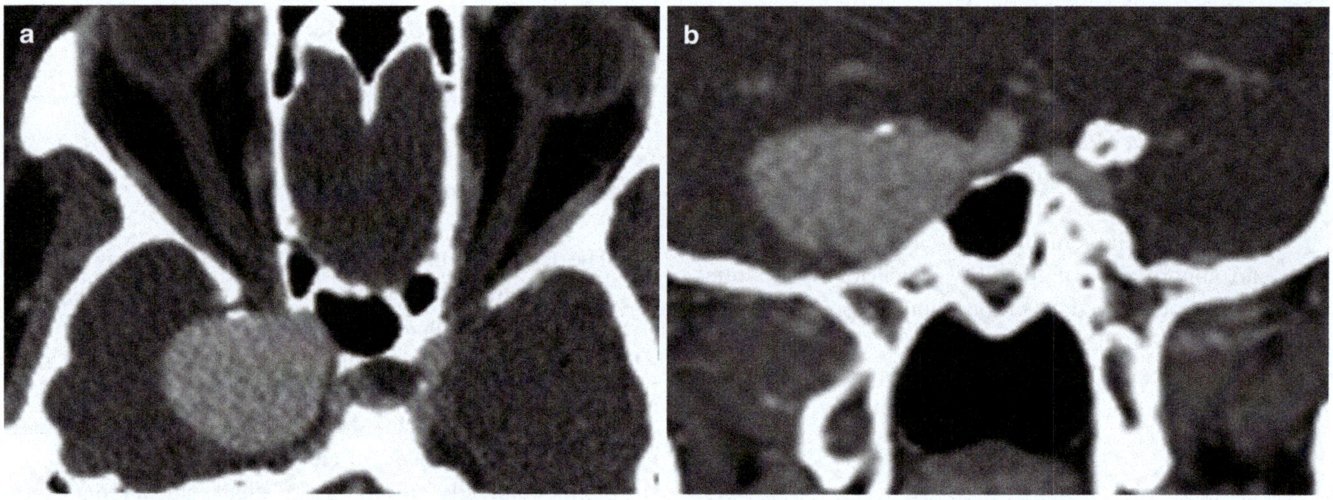

Fig. 34.2 Axial (**a**) and coronal (**b**) CTA (of a second patient) showing a giant right cavernous carotid aneurysm homogeneously filled with contrast and eroding the bony wall of the adjacent sphenoid sinus

  – If thrombosed, sometimes see rim enhancement with filling defects.
- CTA is the standard imaging procedure provided in most of these cases (see Fig. 34.2a, b).
- Post treatment with GDC coiling shows "mass of metal" balled at the aneurysm site causing massive metallic artifact streaking (see Fig. 34.3a, b).
- CTAs can be coupled with 3D reconstructions to portray elegant angiographic detail in unlimited projections (see Fig. 34.4a).

MRI Features

- *See General Imaging Features.*
- The lumen of a patent aneurysm is usually depicted as signal intensity flow void on spin echo imaging and high signal intensity on GRE (gradient echo) imaging [4].
- Pulsating patent aneurysms sometimes show ring-like flow artifacts.

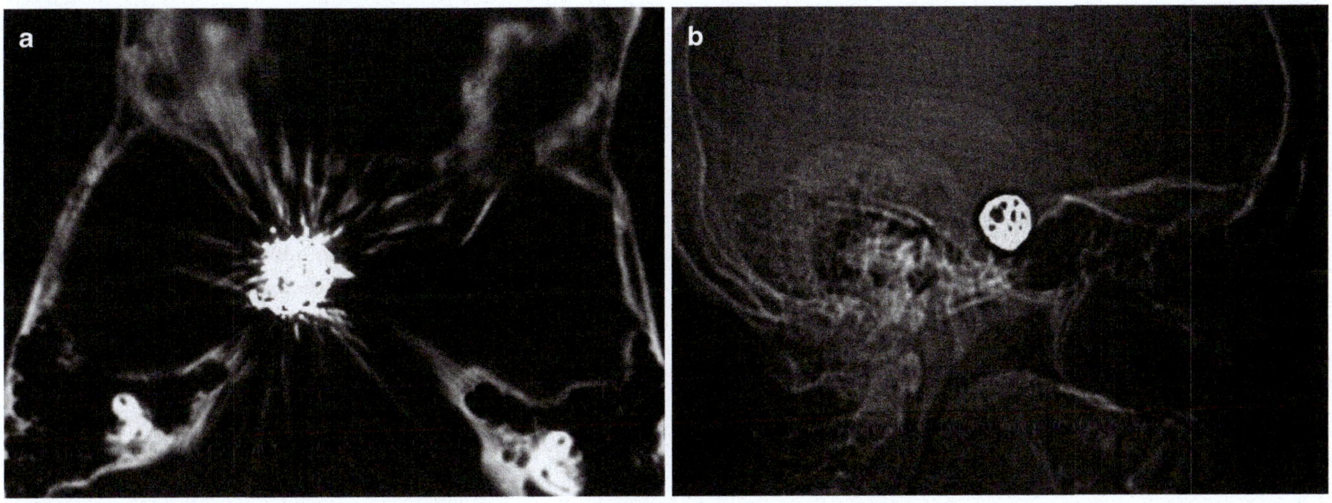

Fig. 34.3 Axial NECT (**a**) and lateral plain film (**b**) show large ball of platinum GDC coils after successful endovascular treatment of CCA aneurysm in yet a different patient. This causes colossal beam hardening artifact on the axial CT image (3**a**)

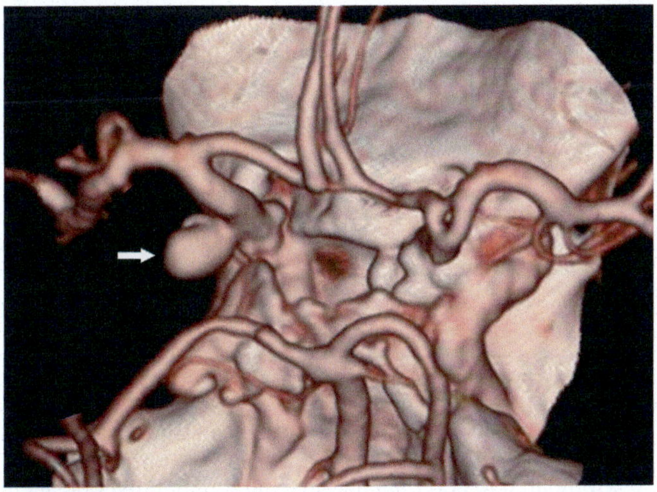

Fig. 34.4 (**a**) Shows smaller right CCA (→ arrow) elegantly exhibited using 3D reconstruction from a CTA (CT angiogram)

- T1
  - Most patent aneurysms appear as a flow void.
  - The appearance of a thrombosed aneurysm depends on the clot's age.
  - Hyperintensity may be flow related or secondary to subacute thrombosis [7].
- T2
  - Heterogeneous signal depends on flow (low signal flow voids), calcifications, and intracellular deoxy- or methemoglobin [7].
  - When patent, CCAs typically have hypointense internal signal secondary to flow voids.
  - Laminated thrombus can have a hyperintense rim.
  - Hypointense T2 signal *surrounding* a CCA should raise the suspicion for a mycotic aneurysm [8].
- T1 Gd
  - *Fat saturation* techniques are very helpful in separating enhancing tissue from adjacent normal fatty tissue.
  - Enhancement surrounding a CCA should raise the suspicion for a mycotic aneurysm.
- Digital Subtraction Angiography (DSA)
  - The sensitivity for small aneurysm detection is reported to be increased with 3D DSA over 2D DSA [11].
  - 3D DSA, however, has a propensity for false-negative and false-positive results related to vascular pulsations and volume averaging.
  - 3D DSA can cause underestimation of an aneurysm's size by as much as 20%.
  - 3D DSA has been reported to overestimate an aneurysm's neck size, a discrepancy which can change the choice of current treatment options.
  - Because volume averaging produces spatial resolution less than conventional DSA, it is recommended that reconstructed images be compared to native 2D images [11].
- MRA
  - Time-of-flight MRA (TOF-MRA) is typically used to detect and evaluate CCAs.

Clinical Issues

Presentation

- Because of the small risk for severe complications, most small asymptomatic CCAs do not require treatment. Because symptomatic CCAs present with a mean size of

~17 mm, some recommend treatment of all asymptomatic CCAs ≥15 mm. A minimum recommended size for treatment has, however, not yet been established.

- ~25% of CCAs present with diplopia from cranial nerve palsies, and ~2.5% present with subarachnoid hemorrhage (SAH) [12].
- Recommendations for treatment include larger aneurysms, aneurysms demonstrating serial enlargement, or those extending into the maxillary sinus or subarachnoid space [12].
- Erosion of a CCA through the sphenoid into the maxillary sinus can cause catastrophic epistaxis [12].

Pathology/Pathogenesis

- Most aneurysms are "basic" berry aneurysms and when involving the cavernous carotid present a predictably benign course.
- However, mycotic aneurysms (MAs) have high rates of spontaneous hemorrhage resulting in significant morbidity and mortality.
- Containment of CSA (cavernous sinus aneurysm) hemorrhage within the cavernous sinus usually causes CCF (carotid cavernous fistula).
- Sometimes see SAH, intracerebral hemorrhage, or even exsanguination into the paranasal sinuses.

Treatment and Prognosis

Surgery

- Conventional open surgical treatment with direct clipping is difficult because of contiguous cavernous sinus structures.
- Prior surgical therapies have included ICA ligation and direct microsurgical exposure of cavernous aneurysms.
- Some surgical centers currently perform bypass grafts before endovascular treatment in an attempt to decrease post endovascular complications [3].

Endovascular Treatment

- Since 1974 detachable balloons have been used to perform endovascular parent vessel occlusion [6].
- Since 1991 GDC (Guglielmi Detachable Coils) have been used to fill aneurysms via an endovascular approach [6].
- Conventional surgery has largely been replaced by less invasive endovascular treatment methods which foster fewer complications, as well as lower post treatment and recovery times [6].
- The incidence of CCF from ruptured cavernous sinus aneurysm is 1.5%, while the incidence of CCF from *treated symptomatic* cavernous sinus aneurysms is approximately 25% [3].
- Clearly, when considering treatment options for a cavernous sinus aneurysm, the risk for permanent post-surgical complications must be carefully weighed against their relatively benign natural history [1, 6].
- Factors promoting treatment recommendations include larger aneurysms, enlarging aneurysms, or extension into the maxillary sinus or subarachnoid space [12].

Complications

- While associated mass effect causing cranial neuropathy often progresses, it also spontaneously disappears in 20% of affected patients.
- Erosion of a CCA through the sphenoid into the maxillary sinus can cause catastrophic epistaxis [12].
- Endoscopic debridement of the sphenoid sinus can cause fatality in cases of fungal sinusitis with a mycotic CCA [16] (see Fig. 34.2a, b where aneurysm is clearly eroding into the sphenoid sinus).
- The 5-year SAH rupture risk relative to CCA size is as follows:

<12 mm	0%
13–24 mm	3%
>25 mm	6.4%

Differential Diagnosis

A. Mycotic Aneurysm (MA)

- Compared to berry aneurysms, intracranial mycotic aneurysms are rare, comprising ≤5% of all cerebral aneurysms [13].
- Mycotic aneurysms are so named because of their resemblance to fungal vegetation. While occasionally fungal in origin, they are more commonly caused by bacterial infections.
- Mycotic aneurysms are often caused by vessel wall necrosis following showering by bacterial emboli from endocarditis.
- Findings suggesting mycotic aneurysm include fusiform shape, multiplicity, distal location, and change in shape on follow-up.
- Other indicators include concomitant endocarditis, positive blood culture, leukocytosis, ↑ ESR, ↑ CRP (C-reactive protein) [13].
- Identification of a mycotic aneurysm is important as treatment course and thresholds are different from the more common berry aneurysm.
- While a fusiform shape should suggest the possibility of a mycotic aneurysm, they should also be considered when

we see significant perianeurysmal inflammatory change surrounding a saccular aneurysm [8, 9].
- *Hypointense T2 signal* surrounding a CCA should raise suspicion for a mycotic aneurysm [8].

B. Cavernous Sinus Thrombosis (CST) [5]
- Patient presents with recent onset HA, photophobia, periorbital edema, proptosis, ophthalmoplegia, and vision loss demonstrating dilated SOV (superior ophthalmic vein) and CS (cavernous sinus) thrombi.
- Although frequently the first imaging study, CT is negative in 1/3 of cases.
- CECT shows multiple low attenuation filling defects within the cavernous sinus and the superior orbital vein.
- Sporadically see narrowing or occlusion of the cavernous ICA causing associated cerebral infarction.
- MRI sometimes shows changes in the cavernous sinus including contour, size, or signal.
- MRI signal varies with oxidation of intracellular and extracellular hemoglobin.
  – Stages of intracranial thrombus develop as follows:
    1. *Acute Stage*
       - During its first week, an acute thrombosis is often subtle.
       - Paramagnetic deoxyhemoglobin is found in RBCs.
       - T1 is *isointense* and may be *difficult to diagnose.*
       - T2 is *hypointense showing an expected flow void.*
       - Marginal enhancement of the cavernous sinus is often the first sign of thrombus.
       - Indirect signs include dilated superior ophthalmic vein, exophthalmos, and abnormal dural enhancement.
    2. *Subacute Stage*
       - Occurs between 7 and 14 days.
       - Early subacute stage.
         – ↑ T1, ↓ T2 secondary to *intracellular methemoglobin*
         – Subacute thrombus may signal its presence with ↑ T1 *bright* signal secondary to methemoglobin.
       - Late subacute stage.
         – Exhibits extracellular methemoglobin with ↑ *T1 and T2* being *both bright.*
    3. *Chronic Stage*
       - Chronic thrombus conspicuously has high signal on all pulse sequences.
       - DWI reveals restricted diffusion.

C. Tolosa-Hunt Syndrome [THS] [5]
- Retro-orbital pseudotumor progresses to involve the cavernous sinus (CS).
- Clinical triad includes (1) ophthalmoplegia, (2) CN palsies, (3) dramatic steroid response.
- Location: While 95% of cases are unilateral, 5% are bilateral.
- CT and MRI of the orbits and CS (cavernous sinus) are often normal.
- When positive, most cases exhibit mild enlargement of the cavernous sinus by abnormal soft tissues isointense to muscle on T1. T2 signal varies from dark to bright.
- Usually see avid postcontrast enhancement sometimes showing an enhancing "dural tail" ascending from the cavernous sinus.
- May extend into the orbital apex or narrow the cavernous ICA.
- Histology shows a low-grade nonspecific inflammatory process with plasma cells and lymphocytes.

D. Metastasis
1. *Hematogenous Metastasis*
   - The most likely sources include renal, gastric, thyroid, lung, or breast.
   - Cavernous sinus enlargement bows the lateral sinus wall with homogeneously enhancing tissue extending into Meckel's cave.
2. *Perineural Metastasis*
   - Usually extends along CN V branches.
   - Adenoid cystic carcinoma and SCC comprise the most frequent primaries to show perineural spread.
   - Can also be found with lymphoma, melanoma, basal cell carcinoma, and rhabdomyosarcoma.
   - MRI exhibits enlargement and enhancement of nerve with concurrent destructive foraminal enlargement [5].

E. Carotid Cavernous Fistula (CCF)
- Constitutes an abnormal connection between the cavernous sinus (CS) and carotid arterial systems.
- MRI Findings:
  – Frequently find dilation of the CSs and the SOVs.
  – Also find flow related enhancement of dilated CS and SOV in patients presenting with proptosis.
  – Sometimes shows "dirty" appearing retro-orbital fat with enlarged EOMs.
  – CCFs are sometimes subdivided into the following types:
    1. *Type A Direct CCF*
       - High-flow connection between ICA and CS.
       - Usually secondary to trauma or ruptured ICA aneurysm.

- Typically shows acute presentation with pulsatile exophthalmos, chemosis, and carotid sinus syndrome.

2. *Type B, C, and D Indirect Dural CCF*
   - Comprise low-flow fistulas between meningeal branches of the carotid artery and the CS.
   - Tend to show fewer symptoms than the direct CCF [5].

F. Sarcoidosis [5]
- While sarcoidosis can exclusively involve the cavernous sinus (CS), it customarily concurrently involves other areas as well.
- Sarcoidosis sometimes shows one or more of the following: multiple dural-based lesions, pachymeningitis, leptomeningeal enhancement, scattered brain lesions, and multifocal periventricular white matter lesions.
- While imaging is nonspecific, as a rule an abnormality appears dark on T2-weighted images.

G. Wegner's Granulomatosis (WG) [5]
- Wegner's granulomatosis is a rare disease of unknown etiology characterized by necrotizing granulomas involving the nasal cavity, paranasal sinuses, orbits, or very rarely the cavernous sinus.
- T1 Gd demonstrates thickened, enhancing meninges sometimes involving the CS.
- Characteristically low T2 signal is related to the entities propensity to promote extensive fibrosis.
- Most Wegener's patients have a known diagnosis before neuroimaging and are less likely to be confused clinically with other types of CST.

H. Tuberculosis [5]
- Tuberculosis typically shows pachymeningitis featuring focal or diffuse extra-axial nodular masses which can involve the cavernous sinus.
- T1 Gd lesions exhibit avid homogeneous enhancement.
- Tuberculosis shows dark lesions with ↓ T2.
- TB typically does not limit its involvement to the cavernous sinus and imagers frequently find concomitant basal meningitis.
- Tuberculosis sometimes seems indistinguishable from sarcoidosis on imaging studies.

I. Fungal Infection [5]
- Aspergillosis, mucormycosis, and actinomycosis can continue from the paranasal sinuses into the cavernous sinus.
- Mucormycosis can cause cavernous sinus thrombosis [CST] with carotid arterial wall thickening and luminal narrowing.
- Aspergillosis contributes ferromagnetic and calcium-containing molecules which can cause a *characteristic low signal on both T1 and T2 images.*
- Actinomycosis shows nonspecific MRI features.
- Despite the facility for fungal infections to cause CST, they tend to typically not be confused with the classic causes of CST.

A Closer Look

I. Fast Facts
- *Anatomy:* The specific anatomy of the cavernous carotid is vastly variable depending on the size and shape of the cavernous sinus.
- The cavernous carotid segment ends when the ICA passes through an opening in the anterior cavernous sinus wall called the proximal dural ring (PDR).
- Beyond the PDR, the transitional segment changes from being intracavernous to intradural/subarachnoid.
- The transitional segment ends when it passes through the distal dural ring (DDR) adjacent to the superior surface of the anterior clinoid.
- Despite numerous attempts to classify all the various carotid artery segments, the endlessly variable cavernous carotid consistently contains three subsegments:
  - Posterior ascending (vertical) segment
  - Horizontal (longer) segment
  - Anterior vertical (short) segment
- The low SAH risk (of 0.4% per patient per year) is probably related to the reliability of the proximal and distal dural rings, which while not depicted by angiography are clearly seen at surgical and anatomic analysis (Fig. 34.5a, b).

II. Etiology
- Most CCAs are idiopathic, but we sporadically see mycotic or traumatic types.
- While an archetypal fusiform shape should surely suggest the possibility of a mycotic aneurysm (MA), they should be considered whenever we see significant perianeurysmal inflammation, even if the aneurysm is saccular shaped [8, 9].
- Hypointense T2 signal surrounding a CCA should also elicit suspicion for a mycotic aneurysm [8].
- Cavernous carotid aneurysm 5% rule:
  - CCAs account for 5% of intracranial aneurysms.
  - CCAs account for 5% of giant aneurysms >2.5 cm [4].
  - Mycotic aneurysms account for 5% of intracranial carotid artery aneurysms.

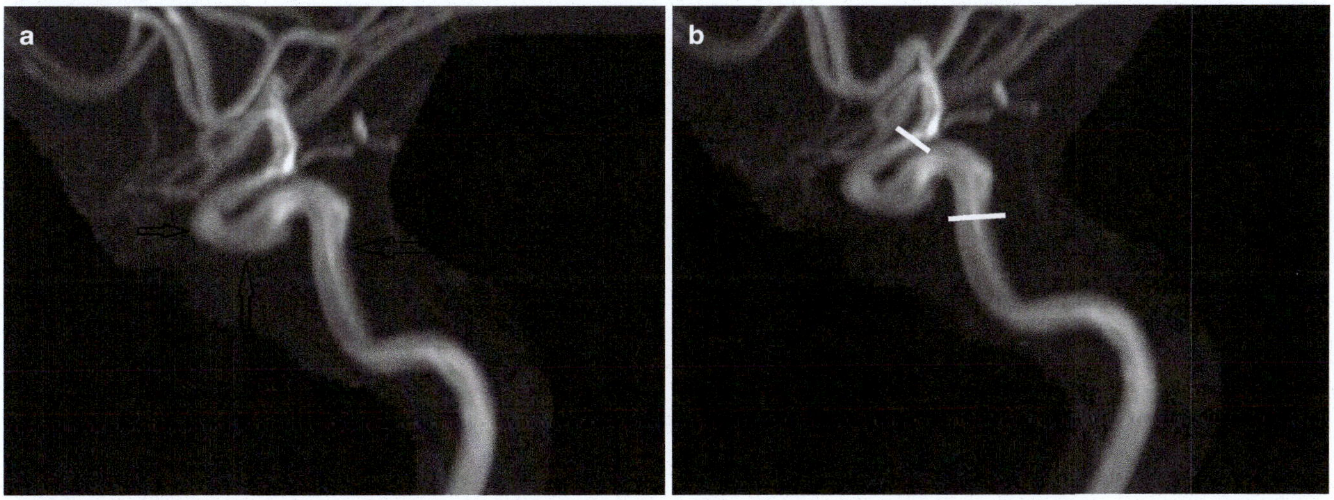

Fig. 34.5 (**a**, **b**) Lateral ICA angiogram depicting normal anatomy of the cavernous carotid artery. Posterior ascending vertical portion (←), longer horizontal segment (↑), short anterior vertical portion (→), caudal horizontal line depicts proximal dural ring (PDR), cranial angled line depicts location of distal dural ring (DDR)

III. Historic Highlights

- In the sixteenth century, Pare' revealed a relationship between infection and aneurysmal arterial dilation [9].
- In 1885 Sir William Osler, pathologist and "father of modern medicine," first coined the term "mycotic aneurysm" [9].
- In 1990 Dr. Guido Guglielmi, Italian neurosurgeon, released a revolutionary endovascular approach to treat aneurysms using platinum Guglielmi detachable coils (GDCs) [6, 14].
- Working with a UCLA team in 1990, the first human patient treated with a GDC was treated for CCA (Fig. 34.3a, b show a successfully treated CCA patient post GDC coiling).

IV. Genetics and Associations

- Familial tendencies toward aneurysms are acknowledged as patients who have more than one close relative with an aneurysm stand a 30% chance of also acquiring an aneurysm [10].

Selected References

1. Eddleman CS, Hurley MC, Bendok BR, et al. Cavernous carotid aneurysms: to treat or not to treat? Neurosurgical focus. JNS J Neurosurg. 2009;26(5):E4.
2. Ambekar S, Madhugiri V, Sharma M, et al. Evolution of management strategies for cavernous carotid aneurysms: a review. World Neurosurg. 2014;82(6):1077–85. https://doi.org/10.1016/j.wneu.2014.03.042.
3. van Rooij WJ, Sluzewski M, Beute GN, et al. Ruptured cavernous sinus aneurysms causing carotid cavernous fistula: incidence, clinical presentation, treatment and outcome. AJNR. 2006;27:185–9.
4. Razek AAAKA, Castillo M. Imaging lesions of the cavernous sinus. AJNR Am J Neurol. 2009;30:444–52.
5. Midyett FA, Mukherji SK. Chapter 29, cavernous sinus thrombosis. In: Orbital imaging. Amsterdam: Elsevier/Saunders; 2015. p. 133–8. ISBN : 978-0-323-34037-3.
6. van der Schaaf I, Brilstra EH, Buskens E, et al. Endovascular treatment of aneurysms in the cavernous sinus. Stroke. 2002;33:313–8.
7. Korchi AM, Cuvinciuc V, Caetano J, et al. Imaging of the cavernous sinus lesions. Diagn Interv Imaging. 2014;95:849–59.
8. Deltomme M, Schroeven M, Lawson TM, et al. MRI and MRA features of saccular mycotic aneurysm of the cavernous carotid artery resulting from invasive Aspergillus sinusitis. Belgian J Radiol. 2015;99(2):76–9. https://doi.org/10.5334/jbr-btr.886.
9. Cloud GC, Rich PM, Markus HS. Serial MRI of a mycotic aneurysm of the cavernous carotid artery. Neuroradiology. 2003;45:546–9. https://doi.org/10.1007/s00234-003-1021-1.
10. Takahashi S. MRI & microangiography, neurovascular imaging. Berlin: Springer Verlag; 2010. ISBN:1848821336.
11. Cieściński J, Serafin Z, Strześniewski P, et al. DSA volumetric 3D reconstructions of intracranial aneurysms: a pictorial essay. Pol J Radiol. 2012;77(2):47–53.
12. Choulakian A, Drazin D, Alexander MJ. Endosaccular treatment of 113 cavernous carotid artery aneurysm. J NeuroIntervent Surg. 2010;2:359–62. https://doi.org/10.1136/jnis.2010.003137.
13. Zanaty M, Chalouhi N, Starke RM, et al. Endovascular treatment of cerebral mycotic aneurysm: a review of the literature and single center experience. Bio Med Res Int. 2013;2013:8. https://doi.org/10.1155/2013/151643. Article ID 151643.
14. Gugliemi G, Vinuela F, Duckwiler G, et al. Endovascular treatment of posterior circulation aneurysms by electrothrombosis using electrically detachable coil. J Neurosurg. 1992;77:515–24.
15. Keane JR. Cavernous sinus syndrome. Analysis of 151 cases. Arch Neurol. 1996;53(10):967–71.
16. Hurst RW, Judkins A, Bolger W, et al. Mycotic aneurysm and cerebral infarction resulting from fungal sinusitis: imaging and pathologic correlation. AJNR Am J Neuroradiol. 2001;22(5):858–63.

Selected References

Cholesterol Granuloma of the Petrous Apex

35

Pertinent Points

- *Definition*: Classically considered to be an expansile cystic mass arising in petrous apex air cells which have undergone cycles of obstruction, edema, and hemorrhage. They contain cholesterol crystals surrounded by foreign body giant cells, fibrous tissue, and chronic inflammation [1].
- *Classic Clue:* The patient presents with headache, hearing loss, dizziness, and tinnitus showing an expansile petrous apex lesion with both ↑ T1 and T2 signals but *no* enhancement.
- *AKA*: Petrous apex cholesterol granuloma, petrous apex granuloma, cholesterol cyst, "chocolate cyst."
- *Age:* Young to middle-aged adults.
- *Locations*: The petrous apex (PA) is the pyramidal, medial projection of the petrous portion of the temporal bone [5].
- *Occurrence*: CGPA is the most common petrous apex (PA) abnormality to require surgical intervention. Fully one third of normal adults show some petrous apex pneumatization.
- *Prevalence*: While 1/3 of normal patients have pneumatized petrous apices, PA lesions are (fortunately) uncommon [3].
- Evaluation of asymmetric petrous apex fatty marrow and effusions is aided by close inspection of imaging findings which eventually establish an accurate diagnosis [3].
- Intermediate or high T1 signal in effusions are most frequently confused with CGPA. Since surgery is offered only to symptomatic patients, it seems sensible to follow these patients on a long-term basis, as long as they are asymptomatic.
- Petrous apex lesions are really rare, and clinicians rely heavily on radiologists to help sort these "rare birds" into categories of those to be treated and those which can safely be ignored [3].
- The petrous apex occupies a unique position between the suprahyoid neck and the calvarial compartment [5].
- As with most skull base lesions, pathologic processes can arise above, below, or intrinsic to the skull base, making symptom-based diagnosis difficult. And as usual, imaging is vitally important [5].

Imaging

General Imaging Features

- CGPA's mass shows features suggesting it is slow growing with smooth margins.
- Smaller lesions tend to show unilocular smooth expansion, while larger lesions tend toward being multilocular.
- CGPAs may eventually extend medially into the clivus, laterally into the inner and middle ear, and posteriorly into the prepontine and cerebellopontine cisterns.

CT Features

- *See General Imaging Features.*
- Typically depicts well-defined smooth sharply marginated, expansile petrous apex mass causing trabecular eradication with subsequent cortical thinning and dehiscence. [See noninvolved aerated petrous apex margins Fig. 35.1a (↓ arrow)].
- Often exhibits "eggshell" thin medial margins (see Fig. 35.1a (↑ arrow)).
- Larger lesions eventually erode the adjacent petrous bone (see Fig. 35.1a, b).

F. A. Midyett, S. K. Mukherji, *Skull Base Imaging*, https://doi.org/10.1007/978-3-030-46447-9_35

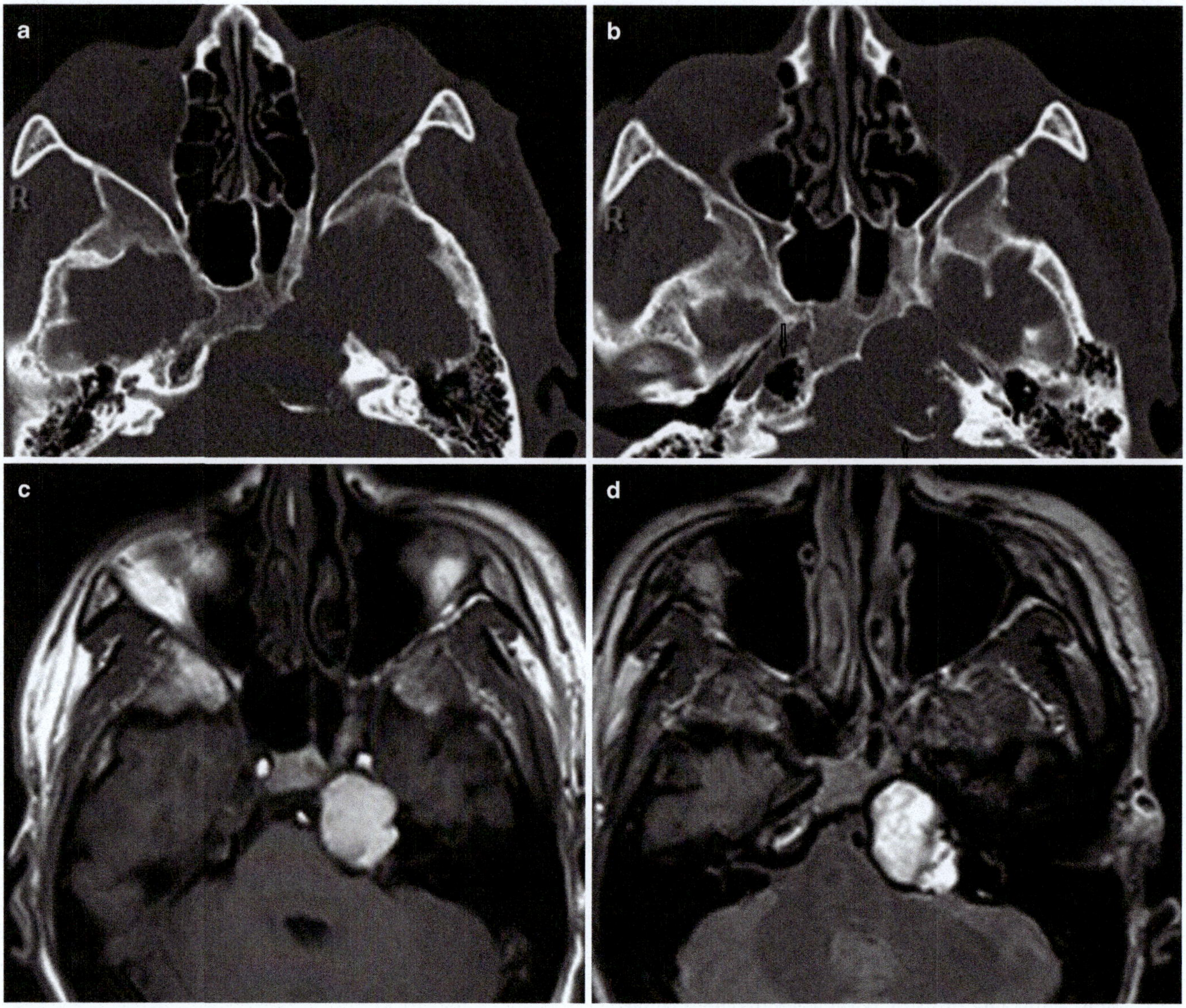

Fig. 35.1 (**a**, **b**) Skull base NECT demonstrates a huge expansile lesion involving and almost completely destroying the left petrous apex. A thin "eggshell rim" remains inferiorly on the left (depicted by ↑ arrow). By comparison, the ↓ arrow depicts the uninvolved area of aeration in the normal right petrous apex. (**c**) Axial T1 shows a very bright, somewhat heterogeneous signal within a large left CGPA. Lower signal from more viscous material is clearly surrounded by less viscous, higher signal material. The well-circumscribed lesion extends anteriorly to the clivus and medially into the CPA where it displaces and deforms the pons. (**d**) Axial FLAIR shows very bright, somewhat heterogeneous signal within the large left CGPA which is partially surrounded by a dark peripheral hemosiderin rim. The lesion is well-circumscribed extending anteriorly to the clivus and medially into the CPA to displace and deform the pons and cerebellum

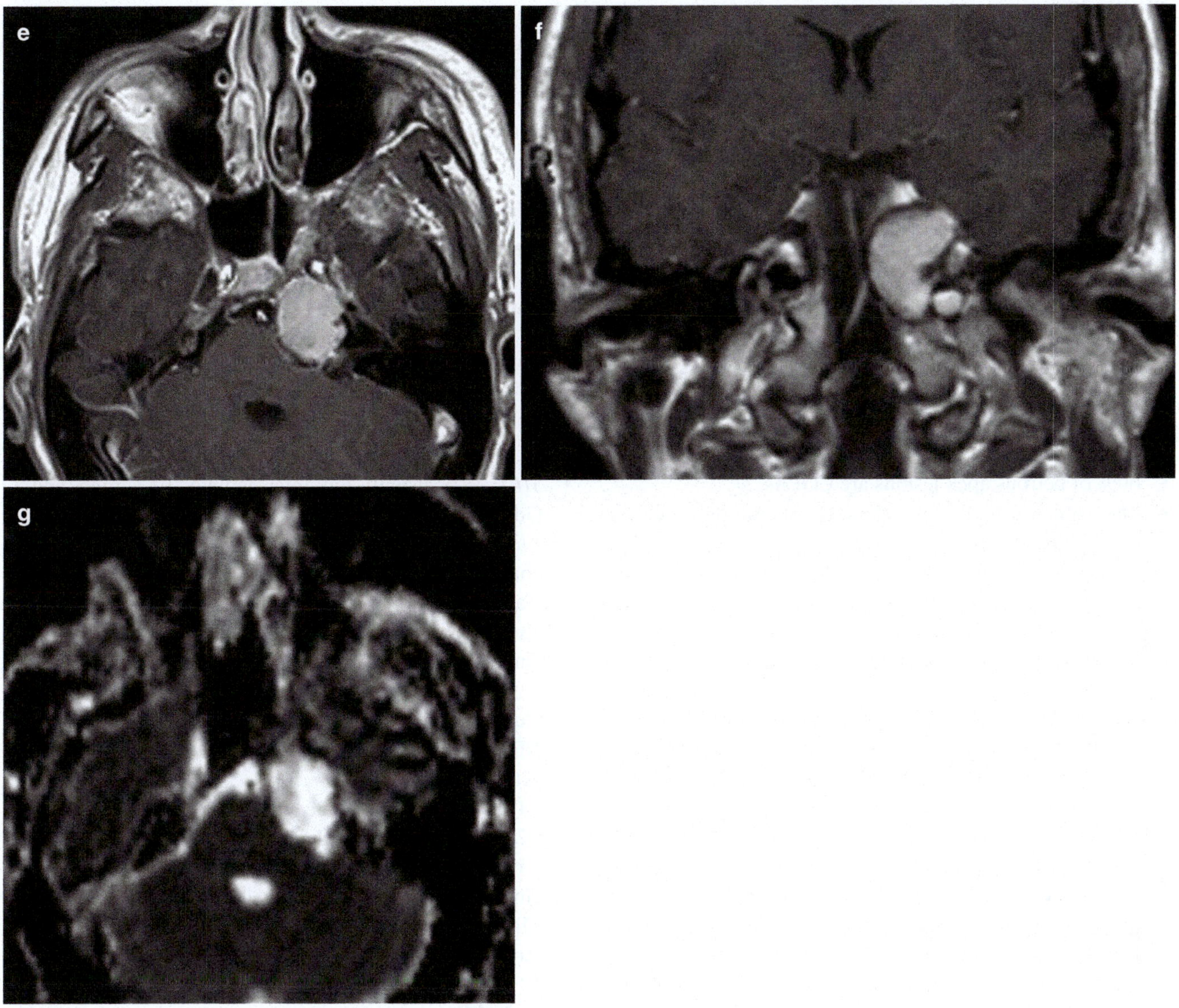

Fig. 35.1 (continued) Axial (**e**) and coronal (**f**) T1 Gd shows very bright, somewhat heterogeneous signal within a large left CGPA which is partially surrounded by a very dark peripheral rim. The well-circumscribed lesion extends anteriorly to the clivus and medially into the CPA to distort and displace the pons and cerebellum. It extends medially to abut the basilar artery. This lesion does not demonstrate enhancement of any of the cyst's contents. Other than making the surrounding vascular structures more conspicuous, Gd is habitually *not* helpful. (**g**) Axial DWI demonstrates bright signal arising from the lesion. Corresponding ADC map (not shown) should show low signal

MRI Features

- See *General Imaging Features.*
- T1 and T2: Characteristic elevated T1 and T2 signal stems from hemorrhagic blood products and cholesterol crystals.
- T2: Often depicts distinct *hypointense peripheral rim* related to hemosiderin deposition [5].
- T1 GD: Sometimes see subtle peripheral enhancement secondary to inflammation but *no* central solid tissue enhancement [5] (see Fig. 35.1d, e, f).
- DWI: Moderate restricted diffusion with bright DWI signal (see Fig. 35.1g). They typically show an associated low ADC map signal (not shown here) [5].
- FLAIR: Exhibits elevated signal interior with sharp *hypo-attenuating hemosiderin rim* [see Fig. 35.1d] [2].

Clinical Issues

Presentation

- Most CGPA patients present with SNHL. Sensorineural hearing loss (SNHL) accounts for ~90% of all hearing loss implying that the root cause is related to the inner ear, cochlea, or vestibulocochlear nerve.
- Other initial indicators include vestibular symptoms, tinnitus, headache, facial numbness or spasm, trigeminal neuralgia, CN VI (abducens) palsy, otorrhea, diplopia, and facial weakness.

Pathophysiology

- 60% of petrous apex lesions are CGPAs.
- *Theories:* Currently two theories of etiologies of this entity exist [1, 2]:
  I. Classic obstruction/vacuum hypothesis: This "older theory" maintains that mucosal swelling combines with gas resorption to cause negative pressure and hemorrhage in temporal bone air cells.
  II. Exposed marrow hypothesis: This "newer theory" avers that prolific pneumatization exposes marrow-filled spaces producing a tendency toward hemorrhage. Hemorrhage → thrombus → obstruction of petrous apex outflow tract.
- *Comment:* If this class of controversy is captivating to you, recent releases regarding Nevada's Area 51 may eventually enlist your reading genre. Otherwise, you will probably just join the majority of us who are content to believe that this could happen to any of the plethora of patients whose imaging studies routinely reveal their patently pneumatized petrous apices.

Treatment

Watchful Waiting

- Asymptomatic patients can be safely followed by careful clinicians who employ excellent imaging with watchful waiting.

Surgery

- Advocated surgery for symptomatic patients demands drainage with surgeons frequently favoring an infracochlear approach.
- The primary surgical aim is to establish a permanent outflow drainage pathway to prevent recurrence.
- Post-surgical histopathologic sampling shows fibrous tissue, granulomatous reaction, and new bone formation which tend to obstruct surgical drains.
- Some suggest stenting the surgically created drainage pathway to prolong its effective useful life, decreasing the likelihood of symptomatic recurrence [1].

Differential Diagnosis

A. Petrous Apex Effusion [1]

- *NECT*:
  – Fluid fills and opacifies air cells in the petrous apex.
  – The air cells are NOT expanded.
  – The bony trabeculae and cortex are intact.
- *MRI:* T1 is usually low-intermediate, T2 is high, and T1 Gd exhibits *no* enhancement.
- *Fluid*: Sterile, clear, or xanthochromic containing a few chronic inflammatory cells but *no* bacteria.
- Can be misconstrued by an unwary radiologist as a cholesterol granuloma of the petrous apex.
- One of the "Leave Me Alone" *Lesions* of the petrous apex [3].

B. Congenital Cholesteatoma [1]

- NECT: Shows smooth margins with lesion expanding the petrous apex.
- T1: Low to intermediate signal intensity
- T2: Intermediate to high signal intensity
- T1 Gd: Exhibits enhancement of rim
- Gross pathology: Pearly white lesions
- Microscopic pathology: Desquamated keratin with squamous epithelium

C. Apical Petrositis [1]

- NECT: Demonstrates permeative destruction of both cortical and trabecular bone
- T1: Low signal in petrous apex
- T2: High signal in petrous apex
- T1 Gd: Enhancement of peripheral rim and adjacent meninges which appear thickened.
- Gross: Really "gross" with yellow green pus!
- Microscopic: Mostly white blood cells. Sometimes see bacteria when patient is not on an appropriate antibiotic.

D. Petrous Apex Cephalocele [1]

- NECT: Shows nonspecific findings. Sometimes shows smooth erosion, pointing to a site of origin such as Meckel's cave
- T1: Low signal intensity in the petrous apex
- T2: High signal intensity in the petrous apex
- T1 Gd: Non-enhancing petrous apex lesion
- FLAIR and DWI: Low signal intensity

E. Petrous Apex Arachnoid Cyst [1]

- Incidence: Extremely rare in contrast to their comparable CPA counterparts
- NECT: Nonspecific imaging
- T1: Low signal in the petrous apex
- T2: High signal in the petrous apex
- T1 Gd: Non-enhancing petrous apex lesion
- FLAIR and DWI: Low signal intensity

F. Asymmetric Fatty Marrow [3]

- One of the "Leave Me Alone" Lesions of the petrous apex [3].
- Signal follows marrow on all sequences.
- While the T1 signal is high, T2 is lower showing the same signal as orbital fat.
- Can be construed by an unwary radiologist to be a CGPA.

A Closer Look

I. Anatomy: For anatomic purposes, the petrous apex is that pyramidal portion of the temporal bone anteromedial to the inner ear, between the basisphenoid anteriorly and the occipital bone posteriorly with the extreme apex terminating at the foramen lacerum [3, 4, 5] (see Anatomic Skull Base Fig. 35.2a, b).
   - The anterior petrous apex is filled with marrow in 60%, pneumatized in 33%, and sclerotic in 7% of patients.
   - Petrous apex pneumatization is asymmetric in 5–10% of patients.
   - The petrous apex extends to the inner ear structures laterally, the petro-occipital fissure medially, the petrosphenoidal fissure and ICA anteriorly, as well as the posterior cranial fossa posteriorly [6].

II. Historic Highlights
   - Cholesterol granuloma was first described by Manasse in 1894 [7].

III. Genetics
   - Cholesterol granuloma of the petrous apex is not usually attributed to a genetic link.
   - A rare case of intracranial cerebral cholesterol granuloma has been reported in homozygous familial hypercholesterolemia, although not related to the petrous apex [8].

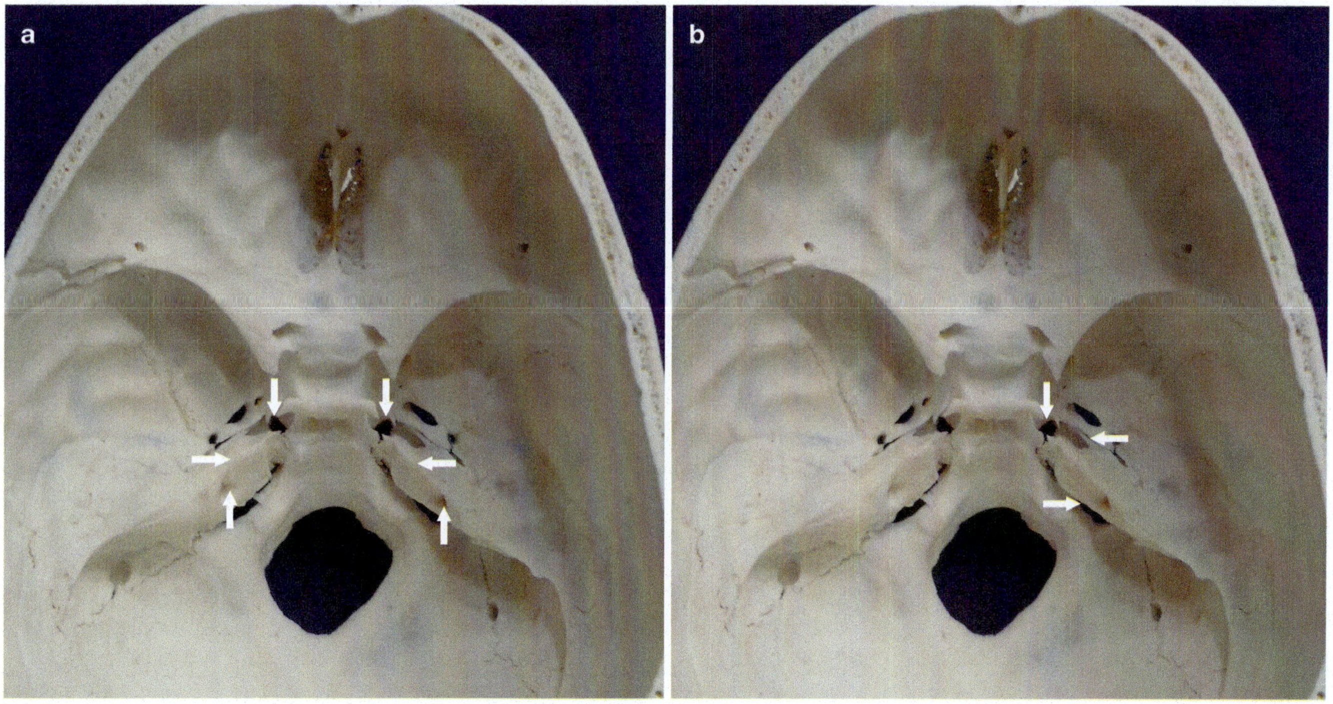

Fig. 35.2 (**a**) View of endocranial anatomic skull base depicts: (1) petrous apex → ← arrows, (2) foramen lacerum ↓ arrows, (3) internal acoustic meatus ↑ arrows. (**b**) View of endocranial anatomic skull base depicts: (1) petrosphenoidal fissure (← arrow), (2) foramen lacerum (↓ arrows), (3) petro-occipital fissure (→ arrow)

Selected References

1. Hoa M, House JW, Linthicum FH, Go JL. Petrous apex cholesterol granuloma: pictorial review of radiological considerations in diagnosis and surgical histopathology. J Laryngol Otol. 2013;127(4):339–48. https://doi.org/10.1017/S0022215113000091.
2. Jackler RK, Cho M. A new theory to explain the genesis of petrous apex cholesterol granulomas. Otol Neurotol. 2003;24:96–106.
3. Moore KR, Harnsberger HR, Shelton C, Davidson HC. Leave me alone. Lesions of the Petrous Apex AJNR Am J Neuroradiol. 1998;19:733–8.
4. Larson T. Petrous apex and cavernous sinus: anatomy and pathology. Semin Ultrasound CT MR. 1993;14:232–46.
5. Chapman PR, Shah R, Cure JK, Bag AK. Petrous apex lesions: pictorial review. AJR Integrative Imaging, Lifelong Learning For Radiology. 2011:196. https://doi.org/10.2214/AJR.10.7229.
6. Razek AA, Huang BY. Lesions of the petrous apex: classification of findings at CT and MR imaging. Radiographics. 2012;32(1):151–73. https://doi.org/10.1148/rg.321105758.
7. Tringali S, Linthicum FH. Cholesterol granuloma of the petrous apex: temporal bone histopathology case of the month. Otol Neurotol. 2010;31(9):1518–9. https://doi.org/10.1097/MAO.0b013e3181d279c3.
8. Francis GA, Johnson RL, Findlay JM, et al. Cerebral cholesterol granuloma in homozygous familial hypercholesterolemia. CMAJ. 2005;172(4):495–7.

Skull Base Lymphoma

36

Pertinent Points

- Definition: Skull base lymphoma (SBL) is a rare tumor which is increasing in incidence as the prevalence of CNS lymphoma rises. It is known to be a master "mimic" of the other "usual suspects" often implicated in the region [2].
- *Classic Clues:*
  - Children: A 9-year-old boy comes in with (one or more of) the following symptoms: cranial neuropathy, facial pain, hearing loss, vertigo, proptosis, visual symptoms, and facial weakness. He has an avidly enhancing skull base abnormality which sometimes shows cavernous sinus involvement.
  - Adults: *An immunocompetent* adult presents with visual disturbance and ophthalmoplegia, and imaging shows an avidly enhancing skull base abnormality which can involve the cavernous sinus.
- *AKA*: Non-Hodgkin's lymphoma (NHL), non-CNS lymphoma, extracerebral lymphoma, atypical intracerebral lymphoma, primary CNS lymphoma (PCNSL).
- *Preferences and Prevalences*:
  - Age: Peak incidence of NHL is between 7 and 11.
  - Sex: M: F = 3:1 [1]. The incidence of reported skull base lymphoma is: M: F = 1.7:1 [1].
  - Prevalence: Although lymphoma is the third most common pediatric cancer and accounts for 12% of childhood cancers, primary skull base lymphoma remains relatively rare comprising a mere 1–2% of skull base tumors [1, 3, 9].
- The incrementally increasing incidence of primary CNS lymphoma has apparently augmented the amount of skull base lymphoma.
- Although lymphoma can implicate any head and neck structure, it prefers to involve nodes. However, extranodal involvement is more frequent in children than adults with 60% of pediatric lymphoma being NHL [1].

Imaging

General Imaging Features

- As with most skull base lesions, pathologic processes can arise above, below, or intrinsic to the skull base, making symptom-based diagnosis difficult. As usual, imaging is critically important with both CT and MRI being essential for their evaluation [1].
- MRI with Gd is, however, the imaging method of choice for the diagnosis of intracranial lymphoma.
- *No Arterial Narrowing:* Frequently find involvement of the cavernous sinus without carotid artery luminal narrowing [2] (see Fig. 36.1e, f).
- *Master Mimic:* Skull base lymphoma is known to be a master "mimic" of the other "usual suspects" for this region [2].
- The definitive differential diagnosis resolution may require biopsy [2].

CT Features

- See *General Imaging Features.*
- CT sometimes shows sclerotic or osteoblastic alterations with the permeated cortex convincingly portraying an intact outline [2].
- Less often CT depicts a destructive, lytic motif more typical for involvement by adjacent sinonasal cancer [2].

F. A. Midyett, S. K. Mukherji, *Skull Base Imaging*, https://doi.org/10.1007/978-3-030-46447-9_36

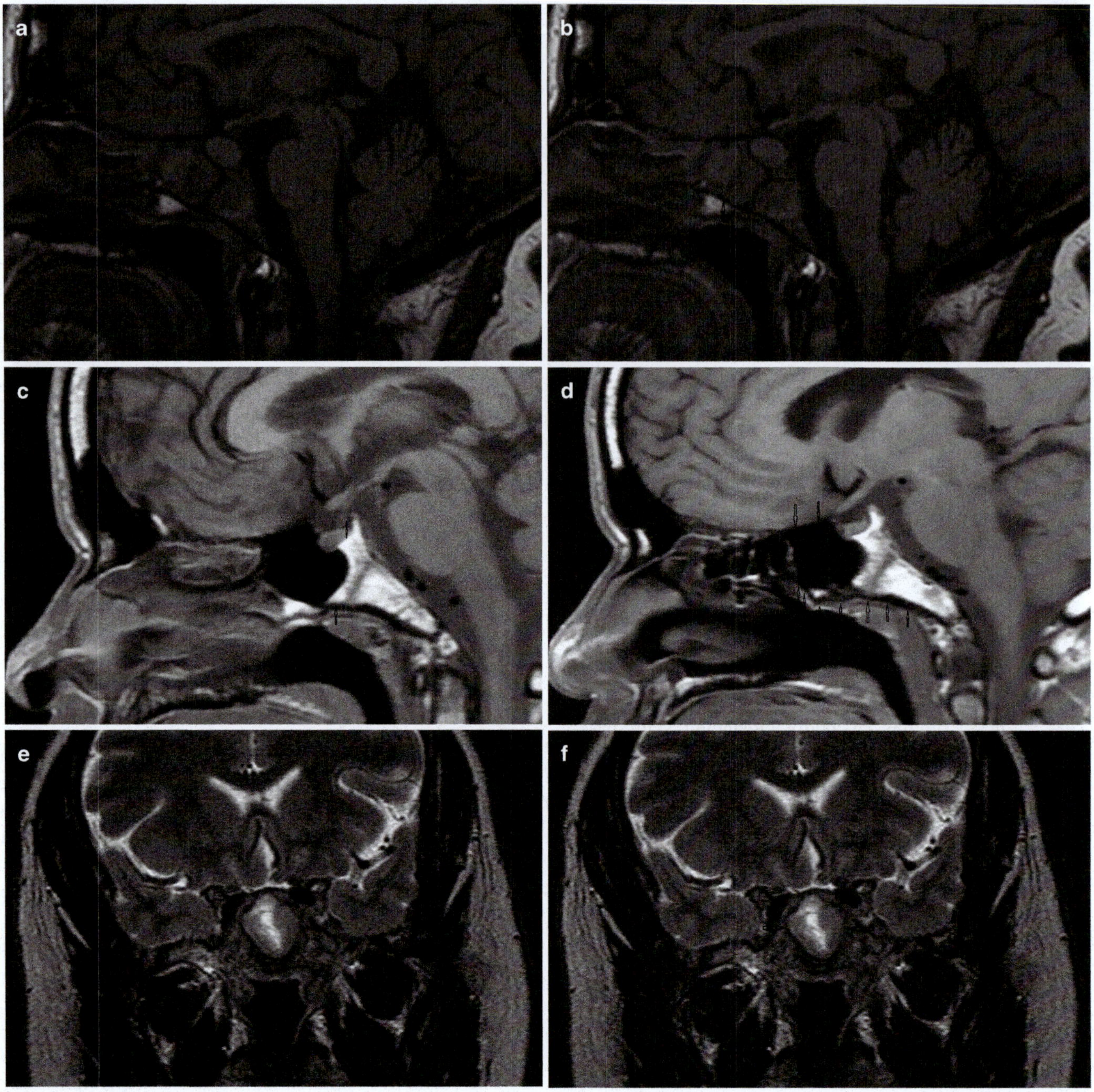

Fig. 36.1 (**a**) Without and (**b**) with arrows show somewhat high signal fluid (↓ arrow) within the sphenoid sinus of this young patient. The fluid has been limited by the soft tissue tumor within (← arrow) which fills a significant portion of the sphenoid sinus and has a T1 signal almost isointense to brain. Dark signal from the clival cortex is intact and continues to be contiguous with the floor of the sphenoid sinus (↑ arrow). The anterior margin of the sphenoid sinus floor (→ arrow) is not visualized and is demonstrably dehiscent. (**c**) Sagittal T1 of a normal patient depicts bright marrow (arrows) which is conspicuously absent on prior figures (**a**, **b**). This bright marrow is positioned just posterior to the well-aerated sphenoid sinus which contains tumor and fluid on the prior abnormal figures (**a**, **b**). (**d**) Sagittal T1 of a normal patient depicts dark signal from sphenoid sinus air (↓ arrows) and black line from cortex of sphenoid bone (↑ arrows) which has been compromised by infiltrative tumor on prior figures (**a**, **b**). Coronal T2 without (**e**) and with arrows (**f**) shows oval signal in center of image depicting sphenoid sinus containing tumor which is isointense to gray matter around its periphery with higher T2 signal fluid inside. Note the sphenoid sinus black cortical line is intact on the right (→ arrow) but missing along the comparable left margin (← arrow).

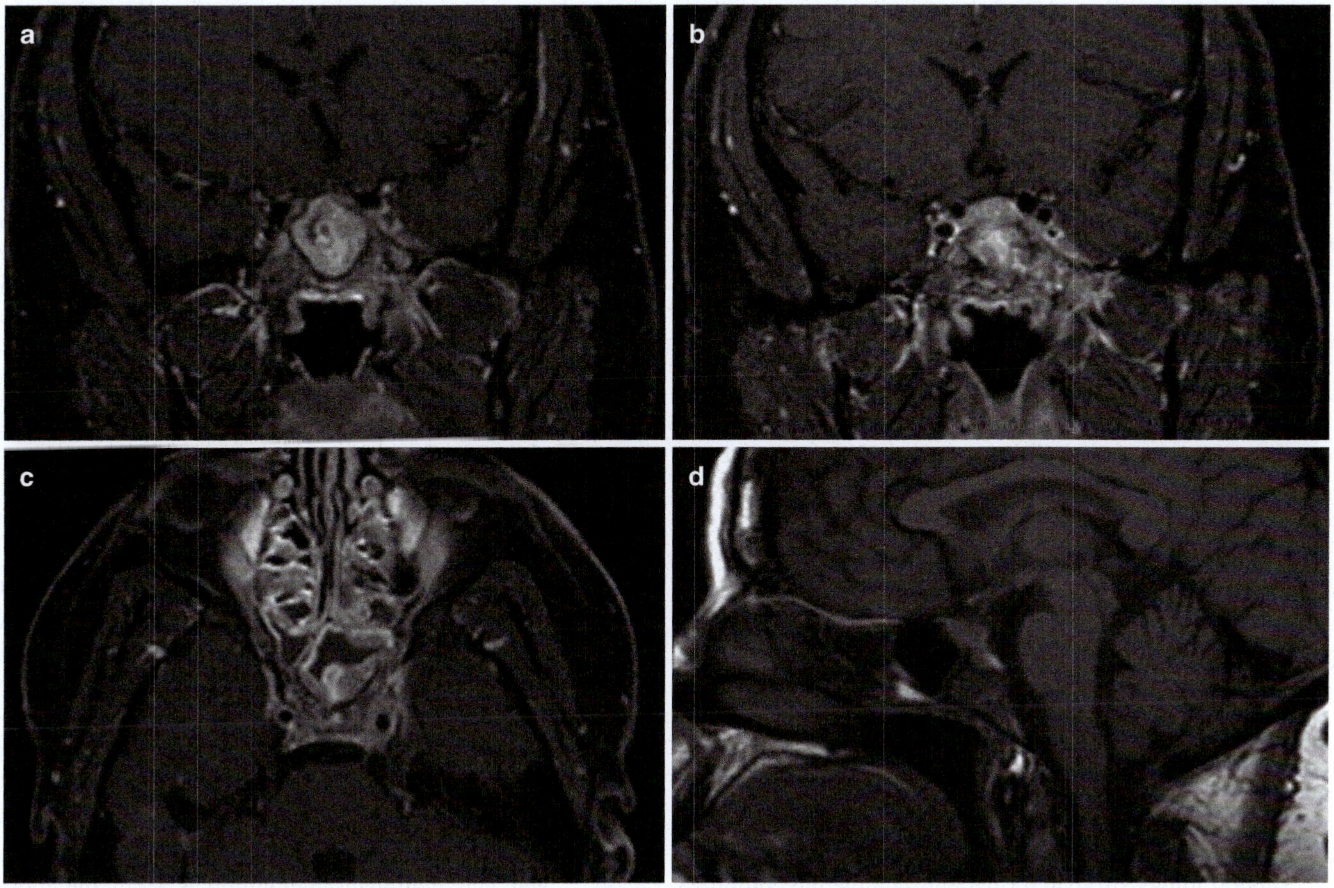

Fig. 36.1 (continued) Coronal T1 Gd Fat Sat (**a**,**b**) shows avidly enhancing tumor inside the sphenoid sinus and extending into the adjacent cavernous sinuses. Note that the carotid siphons (low signal flow voids) while clearly surrounded by abnormally enhancing infiltrative tumor *do not* demonstrate luminal narrowing. Axial T1 Gd Fat Sat (**c**) shows avid enhancement of an infiltrating tumor involving the sphenoid sinus, nasal cavity, nasolacrimal ducts, orbits, and cavernous sinus. The carotid siphon flow voids are *not narrowed*. Sagittal T1 (**d**) post treatment shows response to therapy including clearing of the sphenoid sinus compared to pretreatment figures (**a**, **b**)

MRI Features

- See *General Imaging Features.*
- T1: Isointense to gray matter [1, 2, 7] (see Fig. 36.1a, b).
- T2: May be variable but is often *isointense to gray matter* [1, 2] (see Fig. 36.1e, f).
- T1 Gd: Shows moderate heterogeneous or homogeneous enhancement. It may exhibit intracranial *en plaque* enhancement with/without a dural tail. Fat saturation is habitually helpful (see Fig. 36.1).
- DWI: Skull base lymphoma reveals *restricted diffusion*.
  - Because lymphoma is characteristically comparatively cellular, the space available for water molecules is constrained, causing skull base lymphoma to appear *hyperintense on DWI* and *hypointense on ADC maps* [8].

Clinical Issues

Presentation

- *Diagnostic Delays*: The interval from initial presentation to diagnosis varies from a week to a year [1].
- *Symptoms:*
  - Presenting symptoms include cranial neuropathy, facial pain, hearing loss, vertigo, proptosis, visual symptoms, and facial weakness.
  - Patients complaining of cranial nerve symptoms present earlier than those suffering symptoms from mass effect and increased intracranial pressure [1].
  - Systemic symptoms include cough, fever, pruritus, and abdominal masses.

  - Most pediatric patients presenting with NHL have disseminated disease and require a complete workup for staging [1].
- *Associations:*
  - Children with T-cell deficiency have ↑ risk for NHL [1].
  - Chiasmatic lymphoma has been reported with AIDS or immunosuppressive therapy [1].
  - Skull base lymphoma's incidence is ↑ with AIDS [1].

Treatment

A. Surgery [1]

- Because extensive skull base surgery can cause significant morbidity, its role is debatable [9]. However, biopsy is regularly required to confirm histology.
- Surgery has seldom, but occasionally, been used for complete resection of skull base lymphoma lesions.
- Aggressive skull base surgery may require grafts which in themselves can create complications including (but not limited to) CSF leaks [9]. Secondary surgery is sometimes required for CSF leak repair [3].

B. Chemotherapy and Radiotherapy

- While some clinicians classically consider multiagent chemotherapy to be NHL's curative citadel [1], statistics support longer survival for patients completing combined modalities [9].
- Chemotherapy and radiotherapy appear to have significantly increased survival for immunocompetent individuals suffering from primary CNS lymphoma [9].

Pathology

- *Gross*: Typically seen as soft tan-gray "fish-flesh" masses [6].
- *Microscopic*: Usually show sheets of atypical lymphoid cells infiltrating underlying connective tissue stroma [6].
- Most lymphoproliferative lesions arising from the skull base are B-cell lineage lymphomas and sinonasal NK/T--cell lymphoma, a rare type of non-Hodgkin lymphoma [6].

Differential Diagnosis

Skull base lymphoma is often a diagnostic dilemma because of its scarcity and similarity to other entities including the following:

A. Meningioma

- Meningiomas demonstrate a dural attachment, and post contrast usually exhibits an enhancing "dural tail."
- Frequently find bony hyperostosis with meningiomas. Not a feature for skull base lymphoma [2].
- Lymphoma can cause sclerotic or osteoblastic change with permeative bone involvement leaving the cortical outlines intact [2].
- Meningiomas usually have homogeneous enhancement.
- *Arterial Narrowing:* When invasive skull base lymphoma surrounds the intracavernous carotid artery, it typically does *not* cause luminal narrowing. This contrasts with meningioma which typically tends to cause luminal narrowing [2, 7].
- MRI Features:
  - T1: Most show heterogeneous low T1 signal.
  - T2: Most exhibit elevated signal on T2.
  - T1 Gd:
    All show enhancement (83% avid, 17% moderate).
    >50% demonstrate a "dural tail" sign.
    The "dural tail" sign is frequent but nonspecific as it may be seen with any tumor which invades the dura or provokes a dural reaction. Dural tails usually represent hypervascular dural reaction rather than tangible tumor involvement.
  - FLAIR: Most meningiomas show high signal on FLAIR.
  - DWI:
    DWI appears to be a useful tool for separating atypical and malignant meningiomas from the more common benign meningiomas.
    Most meningiomas are benign and typically isointense/slightly hyperintense on DWI with ADC isointense/slightly hyperintense.
    Restricted diffusion with markedly hyperintense (light bulb bright) DWI images which correspond to hypointense (black hole) ADC maps suggests atypical or malignant meningioma.
- Meningiomas' most frequent associated findings include dural tail sign and bone infiltration.
  See Chap. 13, ACF 1, Anterior Fossa Meningioma, and Chap. 43, PCF2, Posterior Fossa Meningioma.

B. Paranasal Sinus Carcinoma

- Malignant tumors arising from paranasal sinus epithelium comprise the most common malignant tumor of the anterior skull base but are frequently a diagnostic dilemma in the middle cranial fossa as well.
- Tumor Types: Squamous cell carcinoma is the most common malignant sinonasal tumor (80%), followed in frequency by adenocarcinoma.
- NECT: Superbly portrays osseous involvement including cortical thickening, sclerosis, erosion, destruction, and remodeling.

- T1: Intermediate signal mass. T1 is excellent for evaluation of tumor extending into cortical bone or fatty marrow with loss of dark (cortical bone) or bright (marrow) signals, respectively.
- T2: Intermediate signal mass. T2 is useful in separating tumor from obstructed sinus secretions which usually have higher signal.
- T1 Gd: Exhibit moderate tumor enhancement.
- ADCs of malignant tumors are consistently lower than benign tumors or inflammatory lesions.
- ^{18}F FDG PET/CT (^{18}F Fludeoxyglucose positron emission tomography CT) has high sensitivity with moderate specificity and seems superior to conventional CT and MR imaging for imaging residual/recurrent tumor.
- See Chap. 22, Paranasal Sinus Cancer.

C. Chordoma

- Relatively rare malignant tumor arising from embryonic remnants of the primitive notochord.
- Midline lobular tumor arising in or near the clivus which on MR T2 imaging is hyperintense to nearby intervertebral disks with bony destruction.
- NECT:
  - Midline soft tissue mass arising from the clivus causing adjacent bone destruction.
  - Destructive lytic bone lesion usually having a hypodense soft tissue mass.
- T1:
  - Heterogeneous hypo- to isointense signal compared to marrow.
  - Small foci of hyperintensity are related to intratumoral hemorrhage or mucus ponds.
- T2:
  - Hyperintense to intervertebral discs and CSF (see Chap. 30, Clivus Chordoma, Figure 1A).
  - Sometimes shows low signal fibrous septae.
- T1 Gd: Heterogeneous enhancement with honeycomb pattern varies from barely blushing to avid light bulb bright [see Chap. 30, Clivus Chordoma, Figs. 1B, C, D].
- Gradient Echo: If hemorrhage is present sometimes shows “blooming.”
- DWI: May be useful in distinguishing classic chordoma from chondrosarcoma.
- See Chap. 30, Clivus Chordoma.

D. Rhabdomyosarcoma (RMS)

- Should include RMS in the differential diagnosis for pediatric patients.
- Often originates from the nasopharynx with a large bulky intra- and extracranial tumor causing lytic bone destruction.
- NECT shows a mass which is isodense to muscle.
- CECT shows a mass slightly hyperdense to surrounding muscle.
- T1: Isointense to muscle but hypointense to orbital fat.
- T2: Heterogeneous hyperintense to muscle with multiple high signal foci.
- T1 Gd: Demonstrates avid heterogeneous enhancement.
- DWI:
  - ADC values are potentially useful in separating various benign and malignant tumors.
  - Demonstrates *restricted diffusion* with *bright DWI* images and corresponding *dark ADC* images.
- See Chap. 49, Skull Base Rhabdomyosarcoma.

E. Skull Base Osteomyelitis (SBO)

- Skull base osteomyelitis (SBO) is a potentially life-threatening disorder showing very aggressive severe skull base infection and is most frequently found in older diabetics (or immune suppressed of any age), and it can cause frequent fatalities in spite of vigorous antibiotic treatment.
- Clinical Findings: SBO can cause cranial neuropathies, obscure headaches, and ↑ erythrocyte sedimentation rate, with curious concomitant clival imaging findings.
- CT: Shows sclerosis, cortical discontinuity, and medullary expansion.
- MRI: Highly sensitive but nonspecific findings include ↓ T1 and ↑ T2.
- T1 Gd: Sometimes shows abnormal enhancement by both infection (SBO) and neoplasm (Skull Base Lymphoma).
- DWI may help to distinguish SBO from lymphoma and NPC [5].
- Technitium^{99m} and Ga^{67} gallium citrate scintigraphy is sometimes useful in initial diagnosis.
- See Chap. 44, Skull Base Osteomyelitis (SBO).

A Closer Look

- Lymphoma is the second most common primary head and neck malignancy.
- For children, lymphoma is the third most common cause for cancer and is responsible for 10–12% of all pediatric malignancies [4].
- The incidence of aggressive NHL is *increasing* in young and middle-aged patients.
- Lymphoma is typically divided into two main groups:
  1. Hodgkin’s disease (HD)
     - US prevalence: 0.3 cases/million.
     - *Incidence is decreasing.*
     - Age: Average 28 years with peaks 15–24 and second peak after age 55.
     - Involves 15% of all lymphoma cases.

  - Hodgkin's is characterized microscopically by Reed-Sternberg cells.
2. Non-Hodgkin's disease (NHL)
  - US prevalence: 1.6 cases/million.
  - *Incidence is increasing.*
  - Average age is ~67.
  - NHL comprises 85% of all lymphomas.
  - Extranodal involvement is more frequent in children [4].
- While CNS lymphoma is uncommon, its incidence is increasing in both immunocompetent and immunocompromised individuals [9].

Genetics

- *Associations:* Individuals inheriting genetic mutations which alter their immune system show substantially increased incidences of lymphoma.
- *Candidate Genes:*
  - Several studies suggest shared low penetrance genomic modifications impact the likelihood of lymphoma, although additional studies are essential to eliminate feasible false positives.
  - The pool of associated candidate genes is very deep with the current collection considered too long to list in this thesis [10].

Selected References

1. Belhoucha B, Aderdour L, Mohamed S, et al. Isolated primary malignant lymphoma arising from the skull base. Inter J Hematolog Disorders. 2015;2(1):1–3.
2. Dare AO, Datt RV, Loree TR, et al. Sinonasal non-Hodgkins's lymphoma with Skull Base involvement. Skull Base. 2001;11(2):129–35.
3. Teo M, Sam E. Skull Base in non-Hodgkin's lymphoma. Skull Base. 2009:19–A104. https://doi.org/10.1055/s-2009-1242381.
4. Choi HK, Cheon JE, Kim IO, et al. Central skull base lymphoma in children: MR and CT features. Pediatr Radiol. 2008;38:863–7.
5. Ozgen B, Ogua KK, Cila A. Diffusion MR imaging features of skull base osteomyelitis compared with Skull Base malignancy. AJNR Am J Neuroradiol. 2011;32:179–84.
6. Hanna EY, DeMonte F. Comprehensive management of skull base tumors: CRC Press; 2008. p. 57–8.
7. Han MH, Chang KH. Kim I0, et al. non-Hodgkin lymphoma of the central skull base: MR manifestations. J Comput AssistTomogr. 1993;17:567–71.
8. Haldorsen IS, Espeland A, Larsson E.-M. Central nervous system lymphoma: characteristic findings on traditional and advanced imaging. AJNR Am J Neuroradiol 2011;32:984–992.
9. Teo M, Martin S, Bowness J, Eljamel MS. Dural graft-induced fibrotic mass twelve years after successful treatment of Skull Base non-Hodgkin lymphoma mimicking recurrence: case report and literature review. Open J Mod Neurosurg. 2014;4:7–12.
10. Skibola CF, Curry JD, Nieters A. Genetic susceptibility to lymphoma. Hema. 2007;92(7):960.

Adenoid Cystic Carcinoma of the Skull Base

37

Pertinent Points

- *Definition:* Adenoid cystic carcinoma (ACC) is a gradually growing indolent cancer arising from exocrine gland origin possessing a particular propensity to invade adjacent structures via perineural pathways [1]. It has come to be known as a treacherous, unpredictable neoplasm with an affinity to recur at a new location.
- *Classic Clue:* An adult patient presents with a multi-month history of symptoms including stuffy nose, pain, epistaxis, or diplopia. Imaging shows an aggressive, slow-growing skull base lesion which can contain pseudocysts.
- AKA: Cylindroma, cylindroma-type adenocarcinoma.
- Age: Predominately occurs in adults with peak incidence in the fourth through sixth decades. Occasionally seen in children [19].
- Gender Preference: Shows no gender preference.
- *Significance:*
  - Adenoid cystic carcinomas display a seemingly slothful distinctive deliberate although aggressive clinical course and possess the propensity for premature perineural propagation. They flaunt a fondness for frequent local recurrence and a peculiar proclivity for late distant metastasis [18, 19].
  - They are unresponsive to current chemotherapy and are ostensibly "radioresistant" (albeit radiosensitive but not radiocurable).
  - Adenoid cystic carcinoma accounts for 1% of head and neck cancers.
- *Multi Fossae:* Adenoid cystic carcinoma is a classic entity which refuses to fit into a single cranial fossa. While some ACCs are clearly confined to the ACF, others involve the MCF, and some are seen in both. While separating by cranial fossa seems a good starting point, the enlightened reader is encouraged to look for ACC in both locations.
- *Submucosal Spread:* ACC's propensity for submucosal tumor spread enables it to slip in under the clinical diagnostic radar. Definitive diagnosis may prove to be problematic particularly at the skull base [1].
- Adenoid cystic carcinoma accounts for 1% of head and neck cancers.

Imaging

General Imaging Features

- As with most skull base lesions, pathologic processes can arise above, below, or intrinsic to the skull base, making symptom-based diagnosis difficult. As usual, imaging is critically important with both CT and MRI being essential for their evaluation.
- MRI with Gd is, however, the imaging method of choice for the diagnosis of skull base ACC.
- Invasion of both cavernous sinuses has been reported to "mimic" a meningioma both by imaging and histology [5].
- ACCs have been reported to assume a dumbbell shape centered at the planum sphenoidale [6], clearly involving the anterior cranial fossa (ACF).
- Patients with skull base ACC often have concomitant involvement in other areas including [18]:

Sphenoid sinus	61%
Nasopharynx	61%
Meckel's Cave	57%
Brain	52%

F. A. Midyett, S. K. Mukherji, *Skull Base Imaging*, https://doi.org/10.1007/978-3-030-46447-9_37

Clivus	48%
Orbital soft tissues	39%
Frontal sinus	17%

- Unencapsulated, enhancing, infiltrating mass often showing irregular outline adjacent non-bony margins [2].

MRI Features

- *See General Imaging Features.*
- MRI features vary, with tumor type as listed in "Histopathology" section [22].

I. Cribriform Pattern
  - May be heterogeneous showing septations or central necrosis
  - T1 isointense to adjacent muscle
  - T2 heterogeneous with hypointense septations
    - According to pathologists, the cyst-like spaces clearly shown on imaging are not true cysts because microscopically they do not demonstrate "true glandular" tissue and because these spaces are not separate from surrounding stroma [25].
    - Since pathologists pigeonhole them as "pseudocysts," we will follow their precedent.
      These pseudocysts vary in T2 signal depending on whether they contain more or less than 35% protein. Lesions with less than 35% protein are bright; >35% protein are dark.
  - T1 Gd has a heterogeneous appearance formed from avid solid component enhancement perforated by non-enhancing pseudocysts.
  - Not a surprising imaging facade for a tumor classically characterized as showing "Swiss cheese" appearance.

II. Tubular Pattern
  - Homogeneous on MRI [22].
  - T1 is isointense to adjacent muscle.
  - T2 is isointense to cortical brain.
  - T1 Gd exhibits moderate homogeneous enhancement.

III. Solid Pattern
  - May be heterogeneous with septations or show central necrosis.
  - T1 is isointense to adjacent muscle.
  - T2 is heterogeneous and isointense to cortical brain.
  - T1 Gd demonstrates avid heterogeneous enhancement.

- Presented Case (see Fig. 37.1).
  I. T1: Heterogeneous with solid components hypointense to orbital fat. Pseudocysts show signal similar to ocular vitreous (see Fig. 37.1a–d, i, j).
  II. T2: Heterogeneous with solid components similar to the cortical brain. Most of the pseudocysts have low T2 signal suggesting a high protein concentration >35%. One of the smaller juvenile pseudocysts shows signal similar to ocular vitreous, suggesting it (see star *) has not yet achieved a protein concentration >35% (see Fig. 37.1e, f).
  III. T1 Gd: Quite heterogeneous with moderate avid multifocal enhancement of solid components separated by areas of poorly enhancing pseudocysts (see Fig. 37.1g, h).
- See Discussion PNS below.

CT Features

- See *General Imaging Features.*
- NECT sometimes shows effects from slow tumor growth with bony bowing or destruction.
- CECT shows avid enhancement of solid components of tumor containing multiple non-enhancing areas.
- See Fig. 37.2a, b.

Clinical Issues

Presentation

- Diagnostic Delay: The median interval from initial presentation to correct clinical diagnosis is 12 months [1, 18].
- Patient's presenting symptoms include [18]:

Cranial nerve deficits	48%
Nasal congestion/obstruction	43%
Facial pain or numbness	35%
Headache	29%
Dental problems	29%
Visual impairment	22%

Treatment

- Few statistics are available to guide treatment of this aggressive tumor when it involves the skull base [4].
- Most agree that the patient's best hope lies in an aggressive multidisciplinary treatment approach [4].

Surgery [1]
- Surgery is typically the treatment of choice, although complete resection is often not possible because of diffuse infiltration and PNS (perineural spread) of tumor. This is particularly problematic for skull base tumors [1].
- As adenoid cystic carcinoma (ACC) does not tend to involve local nodes, neck dissections are not normally performed.

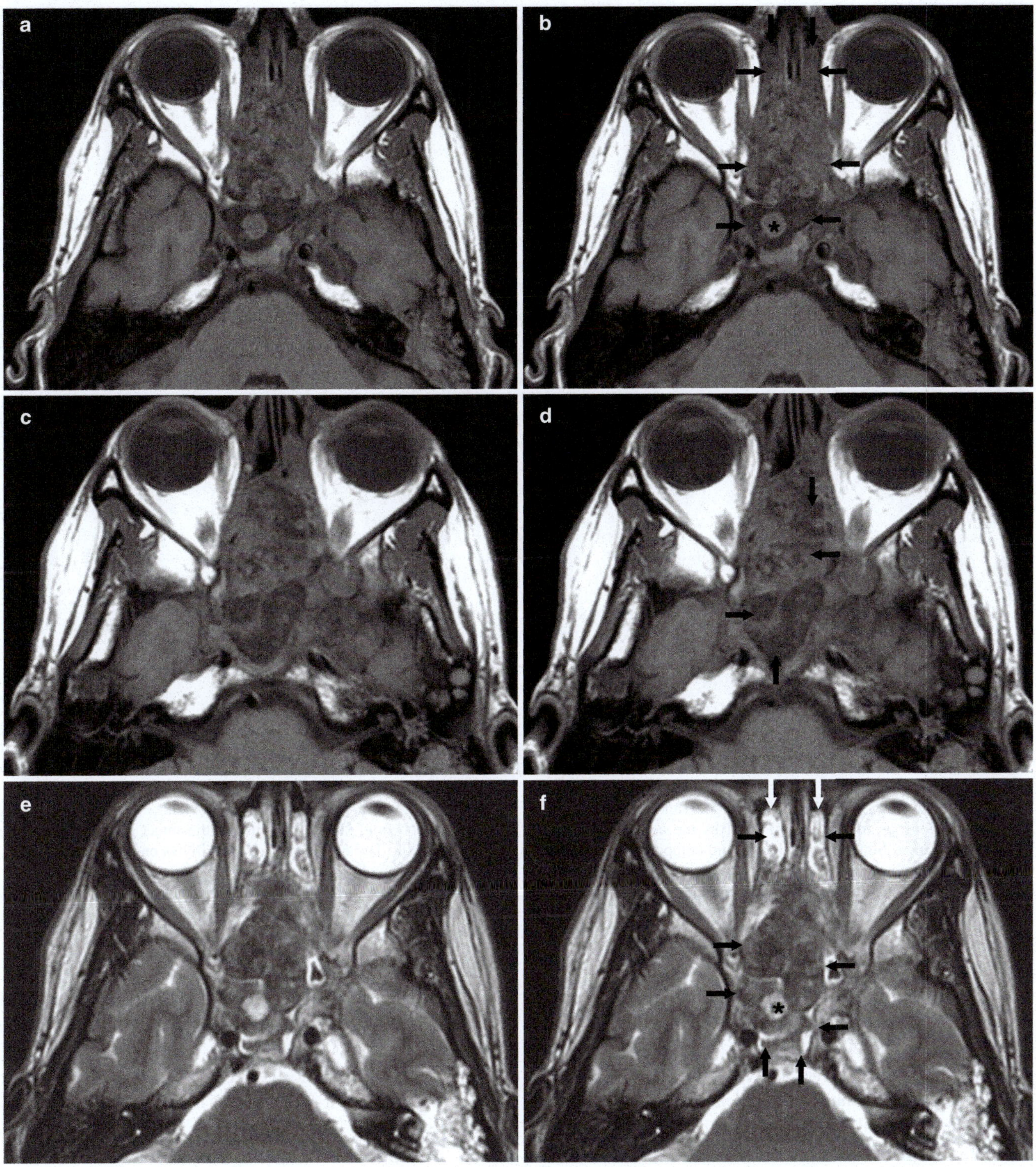

Fig. 37.1 Axial T1 (**a**) (without) and (**b**) (with) arrows. Huge heterogeneous mass involves the central middle and anterior skull base. Signal is predominately isointense to muscle with focal areas of lower signal interspersed. Small oval fluid-filled collection with low attenuation center and higher attenuation rim (star *). Axial T1 (**c**) (without) and (**d**) (with) arrows. Huge heterogeneous mass involves the central middle and anterior skull base. Signal in solid components is predominately isointense to muscle with focal areas of lower signal interspersed fluid (arrows). Axial T2 (**e**) (without) and (**f**) (with) arrows. Huge heterogeneous mass (arrows) involves the central middle and anterior skull base. Signal in peripheral solid components is predominately isointense to cortical brain. Most of the signal is low approximately isointense to muscle. Small oval fluid-filled collection has high T2 signal isointense to CSF (star *)

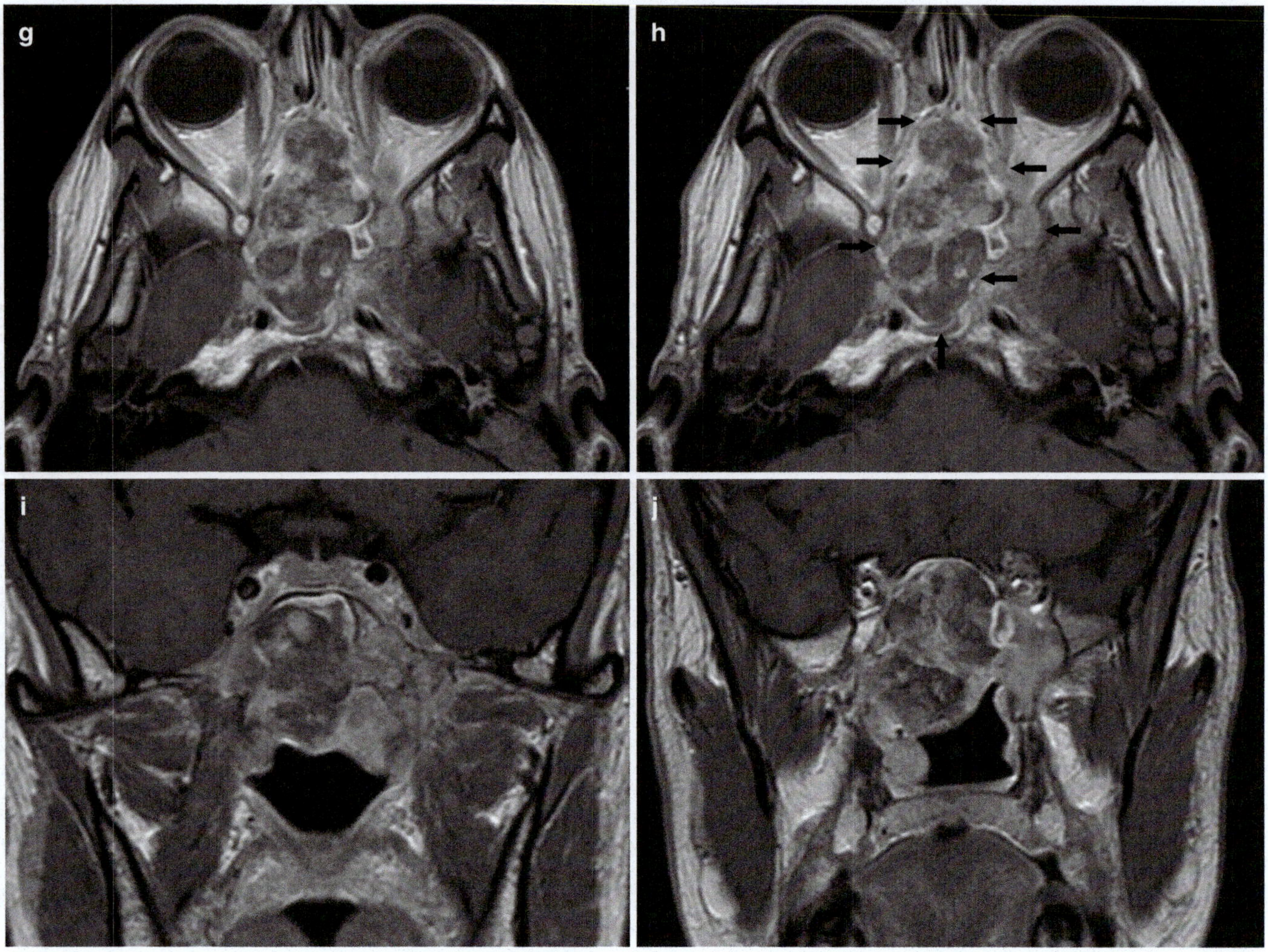

Fig. 37.1 (continued) Axial T1 Gd (**g**) (without) and (**h**) (with) arrows. Huge heterogeneous mass (arrows) involves the central middle and anterior skull base. Signal in peripheral solid components exhibit avid heterogeneous enhancement. Multiple loculated areas are predominantly non-enhancing but are filled with myriad small contrast containing vessels. Coronal T1 Gd (**i**, **j**) again show huge heterogeneous mass filling the sphenoid sinus extending to the intact cortex (black line) below the sella. The tumor extends caudally to encroach on the nasopharyngeal airway R>L (Image **j**)

Radiotherapy and Chemotherapy

- Some series suggest that clean surgical margins are only obtained in 1/3 to 1/2 of these cases [1, 4].
- Some consider ACC to be "radioresistant," while others call it "radiosensitive but not radiocurative" [19].
- Postoperative radiation is currently recommended for patients with infiltrated surgical margins [1, 4].
- Some recommend radiation therapy alone for elderly or multimorbid patients [1].
- High-dose conformal proton beam radiation therapy shows encouraging results for local control of skull base ACC [3, 18].
- While some authors advocate using chemotherapy for palliation [1, 19], other large center studies state flatly that current chemotherapy does not bestow benefit [4, 15].

Prognosis

- Early diagnosis and treatment of H&N ACC are essential as skull base involvement slashes average survival from 144 to 99 months [1].
- The principal prognostic predictor is the presence (or absence) of tumor-free surgical margins which are often attained in only 1/3 to 1/2 of these cases [1, 4].
- ACCs characteristic indolent growth pattern and propensity to recur following years of remission require lifelong follow-up [1].
- Skull base involvement by ACC conveys poor prognosis lowering local control and survival rates [18].
- Sphenoidal and clival involvement further patently portend poor prognosis for these patients [18].
- Involvement of the pterygopalatine fossa decreases disease-free survival but not overall survival [18].

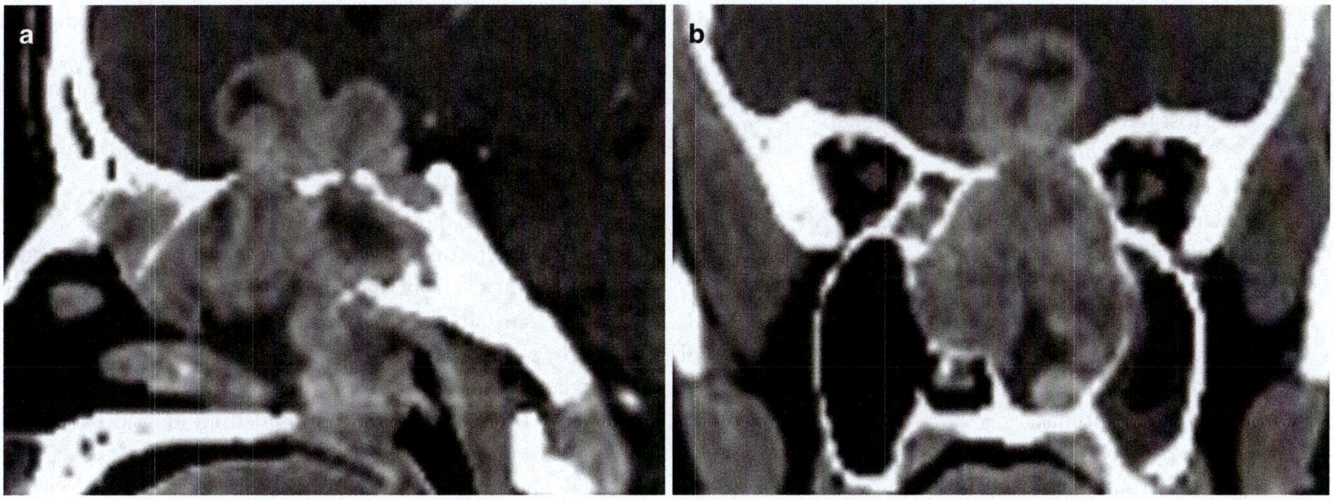

Fig. 37.2 CECT sagittal (**a**) and coronal (**b**) reconstructions show huge dumbbell-shaped tumor with heterogeneous enhancement extending above and below the skull base. The lobulated intracranial component has a fairly smooth outline with areas of central low attenuation pseudocystic components. While not bone algorithms, it is clear that the floor of the anterior cranial fossa and (anterior and inferior) sphenoid sinus walls have been blatantly breached. The massive tumor involves the nasal cavity and ethmoid sinus with a huge component filling the nasopharynx. Coronal (**b**) shows bowing of the left maxillary sinus wall from slow steady growth before the tumor breached this wall extending into the left maxillary antrum

- Surprisingly, some suggest that involvement of the cavernous sinus, infratemporal fossa, nasopharynx, frontal sinus, orbit, or brain does not seem to be of particular prognostic significance [18].
- Distant metastasis (which can come 10 to 15 years later) often defeats successful local disease control. Unlike pulmonary metastasis which may appear isolated, slowly progressive, and resectable, bony metastasis is frequently found to be rapidly fatal [19].

Pathology

- This uncommon tumor appears to arise from both major and minor salivary glands [18].

A. Gross

- Usually 2–4 cm but seldom larger than 6 cm [21]. ACCs >3 cm tend to metastasize more frequently [23].
- Firm grayish/yellowish-white circumscribed tumors showing incomplete encapsulation with features of infiltration [19, 21].
- ACCs show scant tendency toward cystic degeneration or hemorrhage [21] but when present should support suspicion for high-grade transformation [24].
- ACC's propensity for submucosal tumor spread enables it to surreptitiously slip in under the clinical diagnostic radar.

B. Histology

- The three commonly recognized histologic patterns of ACC include [22]:

I. Cribriform
  - Most common and easily recognized
  - Composed of compactly arranged sheets of cytoplasm-poor cells prominently punctured by large hyaline-filled spaces showing palisading cells creating a "Swiss cheese" appearance
  - Recurrence rate: 89%

II. Tubular
  - Second most frequent
  - Most differentiated
  - Recurrence rate: 59%

III. Solid
  - Least common
  - Recurrence rate: 100%

- Unlike most head and neck carcinomas, ACC rarely spreads to regional lymph nodes. However, 40% show distant metastasis with standard sites involving the lungs, liver, kidney, bones, and brain [17].

Differential Diagnosis

- The diagnostic dilemma caused by skull base ACC is often ultimately resolved by biopsy, because of its scarcity and similarity to other entities including the following:

A. Meningioma

- Meningiomas habitually have a dural attachment which frequently exhibit an enhancing "dural tail" after contrast.

- Frequently find bony hyperostosis and homogeneous enhancement.
- MRI Features:
  - T1: Most have *heterogeneous low* signal.
  - T2: Most have *high* signal.
  - T1 Gd:
    - I. Universally exhibit enhancement with 83% avid and 17% moderate.
    - II. >50% show "dural tail" sign
  - FLAIR: Most meningiomas show high signal on FLAIR.
  - DWI appears to be a useful tool for separating atypical and malignant meningiomas from the more common benign meningiomas.
- See Chap. 13, ACF 1, Anterior Fossa Meningioma, and Chap. 43, PCF2, Posterior Fossa Meningiomas.

B. Paranasal Sinus Carcinoma

- Malignant tumors arising from paranasal sinus epithelium comprise the most common malignant tumor of the anterior skull base but are frequently a diagnostic dilemma in the middle cranial fossa as well.
- Squamous cell carcinoma is the most common malignant sinonasal tumor (80%), followed by adenocarcinoma.
- NECT: Superbly portrays osseous involvement including cortical thickening, sclerosis, erosion, destruction, and remodeling.
- T1: Intermediate signal mass. T1 is excellent in evaluating tumor extension into cortical bone or fatty marrow with loss of dark (cortical bone) or bright (marrow) signal, respectively.
- T2: Intermediate signal mass. T2 is useful in separating tumor from (higher signal) obstructed sinus secretions.
- T1 Gd: Moderate tumor enhancement.
- ADCs of malignant tumors are consistently lower than benign tumors or inflammatory lesions.
- ^{18}F FDG PET/CT has high sensitivity (and moderate specificity) and seems superior to conventional CT and MR imaging for imaging residual/recurrent tumor.
- See Chap. 22, Paranasal Sinus Cancer.

C. Clivus Chordoma

- Relatively rare malignant tumor arising from embryonic remnants of the primitive notochord.
- Midline lobular tumor arising in or near the clivus which on MRI T2 is *hyperintense* to nearby intervertebral disks with bony destruction.
- NECT:
  - Midline soft tissue mass arising from the clivus causing adjacent bone destruction.
  - Destructive lytic bone lesion usually with hypodense soft tissue mass.
  - See Chap. 30, Clivus Chordoma, Fig. 30.2a.
- T1: Heterogeneous hypo- to isointense signal compared to marrow.
  - Small foci of hyperintensity are related to intratumoral hemorrhage or mucus ponds.
- T2: Hyperintense to intervertebral discs and CSF (see Chap. 30, Fig. 30.2b, c).
  - Sometimes shows low signal fibrous septae.
- T1 Gd: Heterogeneous enhancement with honeycomb pattern varies from barely blushing to avid light bulb bright (see Chap. 30, Clivus Chordoma, Figs. 30.1b, c, d, 30.2b, e, f).
- Gradient Echo: When hemorrhagic, can cause "blooming."
- DWI: May be useful in distinguishing classic chordoma from chondrosarcoma.
- See Chap. 30, Clivus Chordoma.

D. Skull Base Chondrosarcoma (SBC)

- Chondrosarcomas are chondroid malignancies which commonly select a synchondrosis when they rarely involve the skull base.
- *Classic Clue*: Skull base mass exhibiting an affinity for the POF (petro-occipital fissure) sometimes showing a chondroid matrix, characterized by low T1 and high T2 signals.
- Chondrosarcomas can occur de novo or from preexisting conditions including enchondromas, exostoses, osteochondromas, as well as Ollier's and Paget's disease.
- DWI with ADC appears useful in separating SBC from chordoma.
- Skull base chondrosarcomas (SBCs) have a markedly more favorable prognosis than chordoma and exhibit fewer recurrences.
- CT shows well-circumscribed, often scalloped, or lobulated lytic lesions exhibiting chondroid calcifications.
- T1 demonstrates ↓ hypointense (to intermediate) signal intensity.
- T2 has very high T2 signal.
- T1 Gd exhibits avid enhancement. Fat saturation is very helpful for definitive delineation.
- Chondrosarcoma is associated with statistically higher ADC values compared to classic chordoma.
- See Chap. 46, Skull Base Chondrosarcoma.

E. Skull Base Lymphoma (SBL)

- Skull base lymphoma (SBL) is a rare tumor which is increasing in incidence as the prevalence of CNS lymphoma intensifies.
- This master "mimic" of the other "usual suspects" is often implicated in the skull base region.
- While lymphoma is the third most common pediatric cancer accounting for 12% of childhood cancers, primary SBL remains relatively rare comprising a mere 1–2% of skull base tumors.

- CT sometimes shows sclerotic or osteoblastic alterations with permeated cortex convincingly portraying an intact outline.
- Less often CT depicts a destructive, lytic motif more typical for involvement by adjacent sinonasal cancer.
- T1: Isointense to gray matter (see Chap. 36, Skull Base Lymphoma, Figs. 36.1a, b).
- T2: May be variable but often is *isointense to gray matter* (see Chap. 36, Skull Base Lymphoma, Figs. 36.1e, f).
- T1 Gd: Shows moderate heterogeneous or homogeneous enhancement. It sometimes shows intracranial en plaque enhancement. Fat saturation is habitually helpful (see Chap. 36, Skull Base Lymphoma, Figs. 36.1 g, h, i).
- See Chap. 36, Skull Base Lymphoma.

A Closer Look

I. Genetics

- Currently the most frequently found genetic change is loss of 1p32-p36 and is a predictor of poor prognosis [12].
- The p53 tumor suppressor gene may be inactivated in advanced disease [13].
- The Ki-67 marker value is significantly higher in patients with treatment failure and wide topical spread [12, 16].
- ACC can be connected to a constant chromosomal translocation, t(6; 9) (q22–23; p23–24), with the fusion copy concerning genes MYB and NFIB [14].
- No consistent environmental factors have been found.

II. Perineural Spread (PNS)

- Perineural tumor spread is one of the most insidious, intimidating, and perplexing forms of cancer proliferation and is problematic for patients, clinicians, and radiologists [20].
- Perineural tumor spread entails extension of malignant cells along adjoining nerves to invade previously untarnished territory.
- Imaging is vital in assessment of potentially silent perineural spread and is often decisive for directing optimum treatment. Some show sensitivity to perineural spread as high as 95% [20].
- *PNS* vs. *PNI:* While perineural spread (PNS) and perineural invasion (PNI) are often used interchangeably, please remember that *PNI is a microscopic histologic diagnosis* and *PNS is a gross pathologic/radiologic diagnosis* [28, 30].
- Perineural tumor spread gives a grim prognosis and is an autonomous prognostic pointer for tumor staging [26]. It portends a profound negative effect on therapeutic options and prognosis [20].
- Perineural tumor spread causes ↑ nerve size, ↑ enhancement, and ↓ surrounding fat with enlargement/destruction of skull base foramina.
- Denervation from perineural spread first instigates ↓ intracellular and ↑ extracellular water and afterward muscular atrophy with fatty infiltration [27].
- It has become blatantly clear that ACC has a propensity for perineural spread not possessed by other more aggressive neoplasms which sometimes occur in similar regions.
- Perineural spread appears to result from intricate interactions between certain sorts of tumor cells, sustaining stroma and nerves [28].
- Certain crucial genetic alterations enable tumor cells to dissect collagenous supportive structures to spread along nerve sheaths.
- This aptitude is achieved by escalating actions of matrix metalloproteinase and cell surface receptors or their ligands (such as the chemokine CX3CL1 or its receptor CX3CR1) [28].
- Additional secreted molecules such as GDNF (glial cell line-derived neutrophic factor), NGF (neuron growth factor), and neutrotrophins promote PNS [28].
- Neutrotrophins comprise a family of proteins which stimulate neuronal survival, development, and function.
- NCAM (neural cell adhesion molecule), AKA CD56, is strongly associated with PNS and has been found in 89% of all ACCs and 93% of those with PNS [28, 29].

III. Historic Highlights

- 1842 Cruveilheir first reported neoplastic neural invasion [19].
- 1853, 1854 Frenchmen Charles Robin and Alexandre Laboulbene first described the "cylindrical" appearance of this tumor [1, 7, 8, 10, 18].
- 1859 Austrian surgeon Christian Albert Theodur Billroth coined the term "cylindroma" to describe this slow-growing, ostensibly benign tumor showing nonspecific symptoms and "a great tendency to recur" [7]. But the "rest of the story" is that this is a malignant epithelial neoplasm [2].
- 1930 Spies was probably the first to use the term ACC [7, 9].
- 1943 Dockerty and Mayo stressed that ACC is indeed malignant and reaffirmed its peculiar propensity for perineural spread [8, 10, 11].
- 1999 Issing et al. suggest Billroth "did not do justice" to ACC and almost certainly failed to appreciate the serious survival rates for patients with skull base ACC [1].

Selected References

1. Issing PR, Hemmanouil I, Stover T, et al. Adenoid cystic carcinoma of the skull base. Skull Base Surg. 1999;9(4):271–5.
2. Midyett FA, Mukherji SK. Chapter 42, adenoid cystic carcinoma of the lacrimal gland, orbital imaging: Elsevier/Saunders; 2015. p. 194–9. ISBN: 978-0-323-34037-3.

3. Pommier P, Liebsch NM, Deschler DG, et al. Proton beam radiation therapy for skull base adenoid cystic carcinoma. Arch Otolaryngol Head Neck Surg. 2006;132(11):1242–9.
4. Ramakrishna R, Raza SM, Kupferman M, et al. Adenoid cystic carcinoma of the skull base: results with an aggressive multidisciplinary approach. J Neurosurg. 2016;124(1):115–21.
5. Arsene D, Ardeleanu C, Danaila L. Skull base tumor invading both cavernous sinuses. Adenoid cystic carcinoma mimicking a meningioma. Romanian J Morphol Embryol. 2006;47(4):367–71.
6. Brunori A, Scarano P, Iannetti G, Chiappetta F. Dumbbell tumor of the anterior skull base: meningioma? No, adenoid cystic carcinoma! Surg Neurol. 1998;50(5):470–4.
7. Bradley PJ. Adenoid cystic carcinoma of the head and neck: a review. Curr Opin Otolaryng Head Neck Surg Lippincott Williams & Wilkins. 2004;12:127–32.
8. Stell PM. Adenoid cystic carcinoma. Clin Otolaryngol. 1986;11:267–91.
9. Spies JW. Adenoid cystic carcinoma. Arch Surg. 1930;21:365–404.
10. Tauxe WN, McDonald JR, Devine KD. A century of cylindromas. Arch Otolaryngol. 1962;75:1–6.
11. Dockerty MB, Mayo CW. "Cylindroma" (adenocarcinoma, cylindroma type); report of 2 cases with metastasis. Surgery. 1943;13:416–22.
12. Rao PH, Roberts D, Zhao YJ, et al. Deletion of 1p32-p36 is the Most frequent genetic change and poor prognostic marker in adenoid cystic carcinoma of the salivary glands. Clin Cancer Res. 2008;14(16):5181–7.
13. Edwards PC, Bhuiya T, Kelsch RD. Assessment of p63 expression in the salivary gland neoplasms adenoid cystic carcinoma, polymorphous low-grade adenocarcinoma, and basal cell and canalicular adenomas. Oral Surg Oral Med Oral Pathol Oral Radiol Endod. 2004;97(5):613–9.
14. Bell D, Hanna EY. Head and neck adenoid cystic carcinoma: what is new in biological markers and treatment? Curr Opin Otolaryngol Head Neck Surg. 2013;21(2):124–9. https://doi.org/10.1097/MOO.0b013e32835c05f.
15. Terashima K, Shioyama Y, Nakamura K, et al. Long-term local control of recurrent adenoid cystic carcinoma in the parotid gland with radiotherapy and intra-arterial infusion chemotherapy. Radiat Med. 2006;24(4):287–91.
16. Triantafillidou K, Dimitrakopoulos J, Iordanidis F, et al. Management of adenoid cystic carcinoma of minor salivary glands. J Oral Maxillofac Surg. 2006;64(7):1114–20.
17. Moskaluk CA. Adenoid cystic carcinoma: clinical and molecular features. Head Neck Pathol. 2013;7(1):17–22. https://doi.org/10.1007/s12105-013-0426-3. Epub 2013 Mar 5.
18. Pommier P, Liebsch NJ, Deschler DG, et al. Proton beam radiation therapy for skull base adenoid cystic carcinoma. Arch Otolaryngol Head Neck Surg. 2006;132(11):1242–9. https://doi.org/10.1001/archotol.132.11.1242.
19. Pinakapani R, Chaitanya NC, Lavanya R, et al. Adenoid cystic carcinoma of the head and neck- literature review. Qual Prim Care. 2015;23(5):309–14.
20. Nemzek WR, Hecht S, Gandour-Edwards R, et al. Perineural spread of head and neck tumors: how accurate is MR imaging? AJNR Am J Neuroradiol. 1998;19:701–6.
21. Foote FW, Frazell EL. Tumours of the major salivary glands. Cancer. 1953;6:1065–133.
22. Liu XW, Xie CM, Li H, et al. Nasopharyngeal adenoid cystic carcinoma: magnetic resonance imaging in ten cases. Chin J Cancer. 2012;31(1):19–28. https://doi.org/10.5732/cjc.011.10242.
23. Spiro RH. Distant metastasis in adenoid cystic carcinoma of salivary origin. Am J Surg. 1997;174(5):495–8.
24. Seethala RR, Hunt JL, Baloch ZW, et al. Adenoid cystic carcinoma with high-grade transformation: a report of 11 cases and review of the literature. Am J Surg Pathol. 2007;31(11):1683–94.
25. Ellis GL, Auclair PL. Tumors of the salivary glands. Washington, DC: American Registry of Pathology; 2008. p. 225–59. Atlas of Tumor Pathology; 4th series, fascicle 9
26. Sobin LH, Gospodarowicz MK, Wittekind C. TNM classification of malignant tumours. 7th ed: Wiley-Blackwell; 2009.
27. Russo CP, Smoker WR, Weissman JL. MR appearance of trigeminal and hypoglossal motor denervation. AJNR Am J Neuroradiol. 1997;18:1375–83.
28. Paes FM, Singer AD, Checkver AN, et al. Perineural spread in head and neck malignancies: clinical significance and elevation with ^{18}FDG PET/CT. Radiographics. 2013;33(6):1717–36. https://doi.org/10.1148/rg.336135501.
29. Barrett AW, Speight PM. Perineural invasion in adenoid cystic carcinoma of the salivary glands: a valid prognostic indicator? Oral Oncol. 2009;45(11):936–40.
30. Ginsberg LE. Imaging of perineural tumor spread in head and neck cancer. Semin Ultrasound CT MR. 1999;20(3):175–86.

38 Aneurysmal Bone Cyst

Pertinent Points

- Definition: Aneurysmal bone cysts (ABCs) are benign, osteolytic, expansile, occasionally locally destructive lesions which more frequently involve long bones; however, when rarely involving the skull base, we frequently find features we have come to expect with extracranial involvement [1].
- *Classic Clues:* Young patient presents with focal neurologic deficit exhibiting enhancing multi-cystic mass with fluid-fluid levels showing "soap bubble" appearance. Slim, distinctly defined cyst borders seem somewhat unlike other similar entities which we encounter in the differential diagnosis.
- Preferences:
  - Age: Frequently found in the first and second decades [1].
  - Gender Preference: F>M.
  - Locations:

    We expect to encounter ABCs in the extremities, pelvis, thorax, and vertebrae but should not be so surprised when we happen upon them in the head and neck where they show a preference for the paranasal sinuses and mandible [8, 12].

    ABCs commonly involve the metaphysis of long bones, flat bones, and posterior vertebral elements [1, 2].

    2–6% of ABCs involve the skull with involvement of the vault > skull base [1, 3].
- Frequency: ABCs are uncommon, accounting for 1–2% of all primary bone tumors [7, 8].
- Pathologic Diagnosis and Etiology:
  - This tumor was first described almost 75 years ago [6]. Since 1942 when Jaffe and Lichtenstein first described and coined the term ABC, that has been their moniker. While they resemble aneurysms on imaging, they clearly are not aneurysms. Some say ABCs are neither cysts nor neoplasms [11, 16]. So they are not really aneurysms, cysts, nor neoplasms, what are they? All agree however, that they involve bone. Jaffe and Copeland agreed in 1963 that the term "ABC represents a state of mind when used in classifying the end result of a variety of disease processes" [11].
- Well, we always somehow knew that the final diagnosis rested with the pathologist's "state of mind" on the day he/she signed out the case.
- Etiology:
  - While the short answer is that while we don't really know what causes ABCs [24], it is currently convenient to speculate that they are some sort of bony anomalous vascular malformation. In the interim we await the pathologist's next "state of mind" for further clarification.
  - Recently, pathologists reacted to the elephant in the room and raised the obvious question: is ABC a primary or secondary lesion [23]? The short answer is "yes." The current "state of mind" for pathologists classifies the 1/3 of ABCs which are found in the presence of other tumors to be "secondary" and the 2/3 of ABCs which arise de novo to be "primary" ABCs [23].

Imaging

General Imaging Features

- Enhancing multi-cystic mass with fluid-fluid levels [4].
- Imaging often exhibits an eccentric area of well-defined osteolysis with periosteal elevation.
- Typically, rapidly growing with progressive destruction.

F. A. Midyett, S. K. Mukherji, *Skull Base Imaging*, https://doi.org/10.1007/978-3-030-46447-9_38

- Usually find an expanding lesion in an eccentric location expanding or blowing out bony contour causing characteristic "aneurysmal" appearance [10].
- Calcification and ossification follow "soap bubble" stage and may progress to a firm dense mass.
- T1 MRI is more likely to show fluid-fluid levels than CT [10].

CT Features

- *See General Imaging Features.*
- Bone algorithms typically show a lytic, expansile mass surrounded by a thin bony shell, frequently focally eroded or almost totally invisible (see Fig. 38.1a).
- Soft tissue algorithms depict many of changes described above and also show "Swiss cheese" pattern of multiloculated higher attenuation septae filled with lower attenuation fluid (see Fig. 38.1b).
- Habitually shows smooth, sharp, curving peripheral rim signifying periosteal restraint [4].
- CT often exhibits expansion of bone with widened diploic spaces, narrowed neural and vascular foramina, "ground-glass" opacity, and post contrast enhancement [7, 10].
- About 1/3 of cases show fluid-fluid levels with lower attenuation liquid floating atop higher attenuation fluid [7].
- Fluid-fluid levels are more frequently demonstrated following a period of prescanning patient immobilization and the use of narrow viewing windows [4].
- ABC's "soap bubble" appearance is associated with lesion stability [10] (see Fig. 38.1a, b).

MRI Features

- *See General Imaging Features.*
- Typically exhibits expansile, multiloculated lytic lesion bordered by a thin low signal rim [4].
- Frequently find multiple cysts which contain fluid-fluid levels with individual cysts confirming their own thin well-defined low signal surrounding rim [4].
- Characteristic fluid-fluid levels are seemingly secondary to settling and layering of breakdown blood products.
- T1:
  - Solid components show heterogeneous signal similar to cortical brain.
  - Multiple septations separate cystic components (see Fig. 38.2a, b).
  - Multiple internal cystic components contain blood depicting diverse signals which vary according to differing ages of their degradation products [7, 10].
  - Fluid levels are found in 1/3.
  - Habitually have a demarcating *hypointense rim* separating the lesion from surrounding structures.
- T1 Gd:
  - Avid heterogeneous enhancement of solid components including septa surrounding non-enhancing cysts. Sometimes shows "soap bubble" appearance [7, 10].
  - See Fig. 38.2c, d, e, f.
- T2:
  - Solid components are isointense to cortical brain.
  - Cystic components show high signal isointense to ocular vitreous.
  - Sometimes shows fluid-fluid levels.

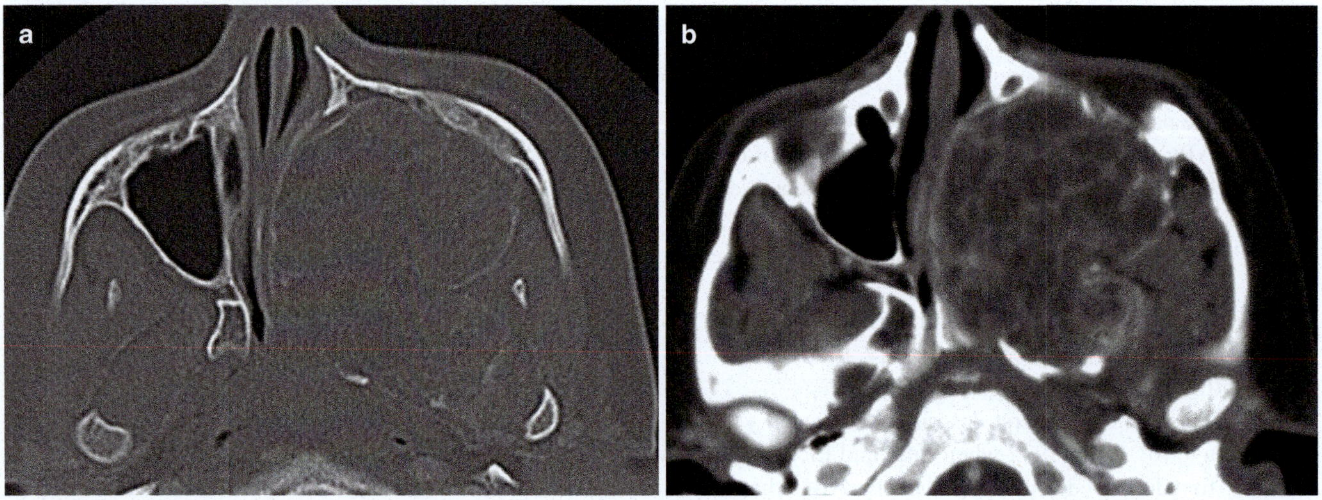

Fig. 38.1 CECT axial bone (**a**) and soft tissue (**b**) algorithms show huge ABC in the left maxilla. The maxillary sinus has been massively enlarged by this slow-growing tumor which retains much of its smooth, curving peripheral bony shell. The tumor exhibits a "Swiss cheese" or "soap bubble" pattern of multiloculated septations filled with lower attenuation material

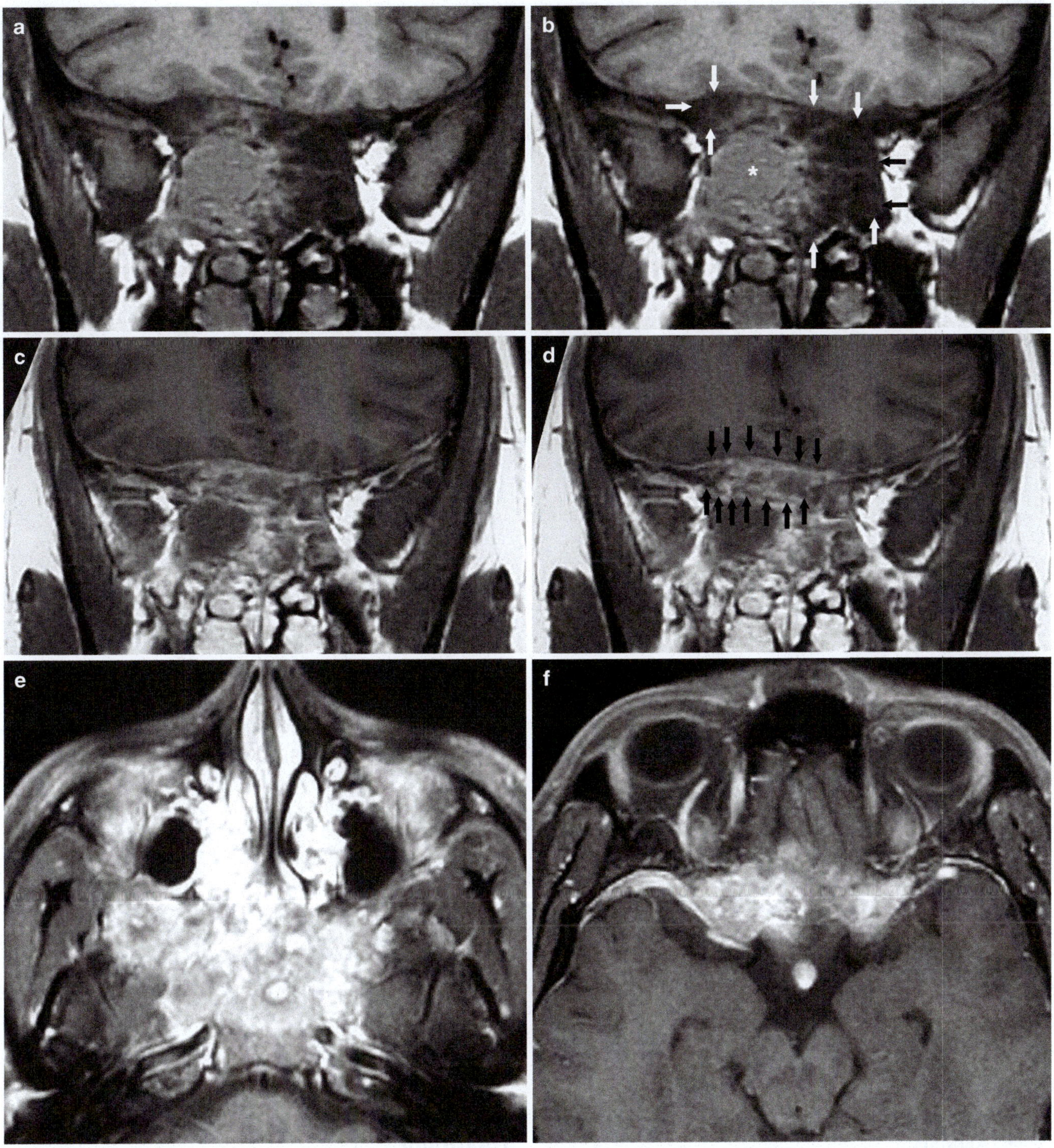

Fig. 38.2 (**a**, **b**) Coronal T1 (**a**) without and (**b**) with arrows. Huge heterogeneous mass abuts the inferior aspect of the anterior skull base. Signal in solid components (star *) is predominately isointense to brain with focal areas of interspersed lower signal. Multiple oval fluid-filled collections (arrows) with low attenuation center and higher attenuation rims. (**c**, **d**) Coronal T1 Gd (**c**) without and (**d**) with arrows. Huge heterogeneous mass involves the inferior aspect of the anterior skull base. The right (and to a lesser extent the center) anterior skull base is ellipsoid from intradiploic tumor expansion. The intracranial margin of the anterior cranial floor shows cephalic bowing (↓ arrows) and has been replaced by enhancing tumor which creates a "dural tail." The caudal cortex of the right anterior cranial floor has been bowed caudally (↑ arrows) as well as having been breached by tumor which extends caudally into the adjacent nasal cavity and paranasal sinuses. (**e**, **f**) Axial T1 Gd. Huge heterogeneous mass involves the anterior and middle skull base exhibiting avid enhancement. The margins are extremely irregular and indistinct (**e**). There is abnormal asymmetric enhancing dural thickening involving the anterior aspect of the right temporal fossa. Enhancing tumor infiltrates both lesser sphenoid wings (**f**)

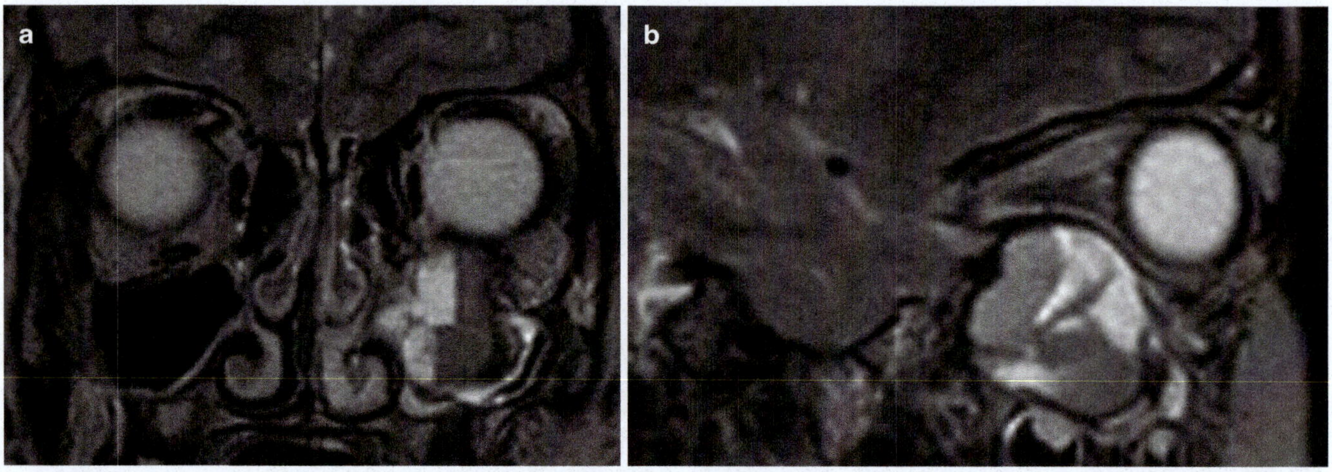

Fig. 38.3 (**a**, **b**) T2 coronal (**a**) and sagittal (**b**) show large ABC filling and expanding the left maxillary sinus bowing but not destroying the adjacent orbital floor. Solid components are isointense to the cortex and fluid is isointense to ocular vitreous. (Unlike many cases in this textbook, the cranial fossae floors are impressively intact)

  – May have a hypointense peripheral rim demarcating the lesion from surrounding structures.
  – See Fig. 38.3a, b.
- STIR [short tau inversion recovery] is a fat suppression technique which often improves imaging of bony lesions.

Angiography

- Commonly can confirm characteristic tumor blush with a very vascular periphery surrounding an avascular center [7].
- However, sometimes shows no blush but mass effect displaces surrounding normal vessels [7].

Clinical Issues

Presentation

- Skull base ABCs possess the possibility of presenting with myriad maladies including [7]:

I. Focal neurologic deficits causing:
  - Anosmia
  - Visual deficits
  - Facial numbness and weakness
  - Diplopia with ocular motility defects
  - ↓ hearing
  - Jugular foramen syndrome
  - Ataxia

II. Signs and symptoms from:
  - ↑ ICP (increased intracranial pressure)
  - ICH (intracranial hemorrhage)
  - Seizures
  - Hydrocephalus
  - Proptosis
  - Nasal obstruction and epistaxis
  - Otalgia, otitis media, and ear mass

- Diagnostic Delay: Pain and swelling are often present up to 6 months before diagnosis [10].
- 2/3 of ABCs appear to arise de novo.
- 1/3 of ABCs are associated with prior trauma or preexisting conditions including [10, 11]:
  – Giant cell tumor
  – Chondroblastoma
  – Chondromyxoid fibroma
  – Nonossifying fibroma
  – Osteoblastoma
  – Osteosarcoma
  – Fibrous dysplasia
  – Angioma
- Because of the propensity for ABC to coexist with a preexisting condition, it is essential to establish the proper pathologic diagnosis to rule out an underlying malignancy.

Treatment

I. Surgery

- While gross total resection is the treatment of choice, this is often difficult to achieve for large or skull base lesions.
- Surgical procedures range from conservative curettage to radical enucleation with various variations in between including endoscopic surgery, paralateral rhinotomy, and bifrontal craniotomy [4].

II. Endovascular Embolization

- Preoperative selective endovascular embolism of arterial feeders often helps to significantly improve hemostasis and reduce intraoperative hemorrhage in this very vascular neoplasm [3, 4].

III. Other Therapies for Unresectable Lesions [4]

- Medical management with interferon alfa-2a
- Radiation therapy

Pathology

- First described in 1942 by Jaffe and Lichtenstein as benign, expansile lytic bone lesions [6].
- They are formed from thin-walled cavities which lack normal vascular intima, characteristically containing blood [4].

A. Gross

- At surgery they seem soft, pulsatile, and friable [5].
- Typically, they are reddish tan with cut section showing multiple blood containing cystic cavities.

B. Histology

- Microscopically the tumor is separated by fibrous septa into multiple blood containing cavities.
- The septae are capillary rich and filled with foci of fibroblasts, reactive bone, chronic inflammatory infiltrates, and scattered giant cells [7].

Differential Diagnosis (DDx)

- For ABCs, there is a real requirement for an actual radiologic and pathologic differential diagnosis, as ABCs are often mistaken for other significant tumors including osteogenic malignancies [13].
- While fluid-fluid levels are distinctive ABC features, they are frequently found in other lesions like giant cell tumor, chondroblastoma, telangiectatic osteosarcoma, cystic hygroma, soft tissue cavernous hemangioma, and simple bone cysts.
- ABCs' unique slim, distinctly defined borders tend to differentiate it from similar entities.
- Lesions which perpetually prove problematic for the radiologic differential diagnosis of ABC include:

A. Fibrous Dysplasia (FD) [15]

- Frequently find expansile fibrous dysplasia in the ethmoid sinuses where it classically cavalcades its characteristic "ground-glass" appearance. Not a feature for ABC.
- Unlike in ABC, fibrous dysplasia's cortical margins are intact with minimal thinning.
- Fibrous dysplasia sometimes shows bubbly blistering cysts with hemorrhage but habitually find few fluid levels to cause confusion with ABC.
- Fibrous dysplasia is more prevalent in children and young adults, an age group similar to ABC.
- We find fibrous dysplasia in three basic varieties: sclerotic, lytic, and mixed with sclerotic lesions leading in the skull base.
- T1 Gd shows avid enhancement for FD.
- Fibrous dysplasia shows no known gender preference.
- See Chap. 25, Fibrous Dysplasia

B. Plasmocytoma [14]

- CT shows focal lytic lesions which expand bone with soft tissue components which can cause bone remodeling or erosion.
- Solitary bone plasmacytomas arising in the marrow cause characteristic bony destruction.
- T1 and T2 show a homogeneous appearance of pure soft tissue components while having a markedly heterogeneous appearance in calcified/ossified portions of the tumor.
- T1 is isointense to muscle and brain but hypointense to orbital fat.
- T2 is isointense to muscle and brain. May be quite heterogeneous, depending on amount of calcification/bone formation.
- T1 Gd is variable. Often shows significant contrast enhancement with central heterogeneity. This heterogeneity correlates with calcification/ossification (often shown on CT).
- Sometimes shows "grapefruit-like" septations.
- Unlike other lesions in the differential like FD which stops at sutures, plasmacytoma can cross most anything in its path.
- Plasmacytoma may progress to erosion, expansion, and destruction of bone cortex with thick peripheral ridging causing characteristic "soap bubble" appearance. This "soap bubble" appearance is shared with ABCs and can clearly create confusion for the clinician and radiologist.

C. Giant Cell Tumor (GCT) [19]

- Giant cell tumors are frequently found in an older age group.
- Giant cell tumors may also show fluid-fluid levels.
- Giant cell tumors usually appear as nonspecific expansile lytic lesions lacking a sclerotic border.
- T1 and T2 typically show ↓ signal secondary to hemosiderin and/or fibrous components.
- Enhancement varies from slight to strong.

- Giant cell tumors are habitually histologically benign but locally aggressive. They may, however, undergo malignant transformation and may metastasize.
- See Chap. 24, Giant Cell Tumor (GCT).

D. Giant Cell Granuloma (GCG) [17]
- Jaffe coined the term "giant cell reparative granuloma" in 1953.
- He described GCG as a local reparative reaction to trauma-induced intra-osseous hemorrhage.
- Most have a history of prior trauma [4]. However, GCTs were subsequently found to occur without antecedent trauma, and pathologists promptly omitted the term "reparative."
- Giant cell granulomas are uncommon benign masses seen in a small segment of H&N tumors.
- Giant cell granulomas are slow-growing masses which typically show significant delay in diagnosis.
- CT usually shows expansion, remodeling, and lytic destruction of adjacent bone with intralesional mineralization.
- Giant cell granulomas sometimes show fluid-fluid levels [19].
- T1 Gd demonstrates marked homogeneous enhancement [17].
- T1 and T2 sometimes show ↓ signal secondary to hemosiderin and/or high collagen content [4, 18–20].
- GCG is radiologically indistinguishable from and frequently misdiagnosed as GCT [19].
- GCG undergoes neither malignant transformation nor metastasis [19].

E. Telangietatic Osteosarcoma (TO) [13]
- Telangiectatic osteosarcoma (TO) is an uncommon osteosarcoma variant.
- TO is characterized by dilated, blood-filled vascular spaces lined by malignant osteoblasts. These spaces are separated by fibrous septa which contain tumor osteoid and multinucleated giant cells.
- Tumor margins show a spectrum from well-defined borders to permeative destruction. This is potentially problematic for the differential diagnosis of ABC.
- TO has lytic lesions showing fluid-filled spaces. Also, potentially problematic for the differential diagnosis of ABC.
- Imaging, rapid growth, and aggressive behavior can cause confusion with ABCs.
- TO is actually *more aggressive* than ABC and occurs in an older age group.

F. Metastasis
- Most cases of metastasis show more than one lesion.
- While approximately half of patients with metastatic breast cancer are aware that they have cancer, most patients with metastatic lung cancer are unaware of the cancer. A chest radiograph is recommended for workup [22].
- T1:
  - T1 is the "go to" sequence for excluding bone marrow metastasis.
  - Metastatic carcinoma is graphically hypointense when compared to normal "bright" marrow signal.
  - A high homogeneous fatty signal excludes metastasis. Problematic areas may be further evaluated with T2 fat saturation or fast STIR sequences.
- T2: Usually hyperintense signal.

T1 Gd: Most metastatic lesions show avid enhancement of bone and soft tissue components [21].

A Closer Look

I. Genetics
- For purposes of pathologic diagnosis, it is often very important to distinguish primary from secondary ABC [7].
  - Primary ABC

    Frequently find a t (16;17) (q22; p13) translocation [7]. This anomaly is *only found in the fibroblasts* and does not affect the other cell types within these tumors [7].
  - Secondary ABC

    Secondary ABCs arising in the background of another proliferative process do not show the aforementioned translocation [7].

    Secondary ABCs occasionally show less frequent translocations like t(X;9) (q26; q32) [7].

II. Potpourri
- ABCs are uncommon, accounting for 1–2% of all primary bone tumors [7, 8].
- Only 3–6% of ABCs involve the skull [7, 9].

III. Historic Highlights
- 1942 Jaffe and Lichtenstein first described and coined the term aneurysmal bone cyst for a specific entity consisting of an expanding bony lesion with a vascular lining showing a soap bubble radiographic appearance [6].

Selected References

1. Aghaghazvini L, Sedighi N, Karami P, Yeganeh O. Skull Base aneurysmal bone cyst presented with foramen jugular syndrome and multi-osseous involvement. 2012 Iran J Radiol. 2012;9(3):157–60. https://doi.org/10.5812/iranjradiol.7952.
2. Resnick D. Tumor and tumor-like lesion of bone: imaging and pathology of specific lesions. In: Resnick D, editor. Bone & joint imaging. 3th ed: Elsevier/Saunders; 2003. p. 1187–9.
3. Sheikh BY, Kanaan I, AlWatban J, et al. Aneurysmal bone cyst involving the skull base. Skull base surgery. 1999;9(2):145–8.
4. Sinha NR, Szmigielski W, Khanna M. Aneurysmal bone cyst of the ethmoid sinus: a case report. Pol J Radiol. 2010;75(3):65–71.
5. Lin SP, Fang YC, Chu DC, et al. Characteristics of cranial aneurysmal bone cyst on computed tomography and magnetic resonance imaging. J Formos Med Assoc. 2007;106(3):255–9.
6. Jaffe HL, Lichtenstein L. Solitary unicameral bone cyst with emphasis on the roentgen picture, the pathologic appearance and the pathogenesis. Arch Surg. 1942;44:1004–25.
7. Hnenny L, Roundy N, Zherebitskiy V, et al. Giant aneurysmal bone cyst of the anterior cranial fossa and paranasal sinuses presenting in pregnancy: case report and literature review. J Neurol Surg Rep. 2015;76(2):e216–21. https://doi.org/10.1055/s-0035-1555017.
8. Leithner A, Windhager R, Lang S, et al. Aneurysmal bone cyst. A population based epidemiologic study and literature review. Clin Orthop Relat Res. 1999;363:176–9.
9. Guida F, Rapanà A, Conti C, et. al. Cranial aneurysmal bone cyst: a diagnostic problem. With a review of the literature. Childs Nerv Syst 2001; 17 (4–5) 297–301.
10. Senol U, Karaali K, Akyüz M, et. al. Aneurysmal bone cyst of the orbit. AJNR Am J Neuroradiol 2002; 23 (2) 319–321.
11. Kransdorf MJ, Sweet DE. Aneurysmal bone cyst: concept, controversy, clinical presentation, and imaging. AJR Am J Roentgenol. 1995;164:573–80.
12. Baker HL, Papsidero MJ, Batsakis JG, Krause CJ. Aneurysmal bone cyst of the ethmoid. Head Neck Surg. 1982;5(2):177–80.
13. Lee HM, Cho KS, Choi KU, Roh HJ. Aggressive aneurysmal bone cyst of maxilla confused with telangiectatic osteosarcoma. Auris Nasus Larynx. 2012;39(3):337–40. https://doi.org/10.1016/j.anl.2011.05.002. Epub 2011 Sep 8
14. Midyett FA, Mukherji SK. Orbital plasmacytoma and myeloma. Orbital imaging: Elsevier/Saunders; 2015. p. 233–40. ISBN: 978-0-323-34037-3.
15. Midyett FA, Mukherji SK. Fibrous dysplasia. Orbital imaging: Elsevier/Saunders; 2015. p. 241–6. ISBN : 978-0-323-34037-3
16. Mirra JM. Bone tumors: clinical, radiologic and pathologic correlations. Philadelpha: Lea & Fibiger; 1989. p. 1233–4.
17. Nackos JS, Wiggins RH III, Harnsberger HR. CT and MR imaging of Giant cell granuloma of the craniofacial bones. AJNR. 2006;27:1651–3.
18. Hrishikesh KA, Narlawar RS, Deasi SB, et al. Aneurysmal bone cyst of the ethmoid bone. BJR. 2002;75:916–8.
19. Aralasmak A, Aygun N, Westra WH, Yousem DM. Giant cell reparative granuloma of the sphenoid bone. AJNR Am J Neuroradiol. 2006;27:1675–7.
20. Aoki J, Tanikawa H, Ishii K, et al. MR findings indicative of hemosiderin in giant-cell tumor of bone: frequency, cause, and diagnostic significance. AJR Am J Roentgenol. 1996;166:145–8.
21. Vanel D. MRI of bone metastasis: the choice of the sequence. Cancer Imaging. 2004;4(1):30–4. https://doi.org/10.1102/1470-7330.2003.0029.
22. Midyett FA, Mukherji SK. Optic nerve metastasis. Orbital imaging: Elsevier/Saunders; 2015. p. 87–90. ISBN : 978-0-323-34037-3.
23. Saheeb BD, Ojo MA, Obuekwe ON. Aneurysmal bone cyst: a primary or secondary lesion. Niger J Clin Pract. 2007;10(3):243–6.
24. Tedesco N, Gellman H. Aneurysmal bone cyst: Background, history of the procedure, problem. http://emedicine.medscape.com/article/1254784-overview#a8. Accessed 20 April 2016.

Trigeminal Schwannoma

39

Pertinent Points

- Definition: Trigeminal schwannomas (TSs) are slow-growing, usually benign, encapsulated tumors arising from Schwann cells surrounding the trigeminal nerve.
- Classic Clue: Fortyish patient presents with "burning" facial pain, and imaging shows avidly enhancing, well-circumscribed "dumbbell" lesion involving middle cranial fossa causing curious denervation atrophy involving muscles of mastication.
- AKA: Trigeminal nerve schwannoma, schwannoma of CN V.
- The trigeminal nerve is the largest and most complex cranial nerve [16].
- Incidence:
  - Intracranial schwannomas are relatively common, comprising 8% of all intracranial tumors [12].
  - Trigeminal schwannomas account for 3% of intracranial schwannomas [1].
    While 95% of intracranial schwannomas involve CN VIII, TS is the second most common intracranial schwannoma.
    CN V is the most commonly involved nerve in the central skull base [12].
  - Benign trigeminal schwannomas accounts for <0.4% of all intracranial tumors [1, 13].
  - Malignant trigeminal schwannomas are fortunately very rare but have been reported and must be considered when evaluating this entity [13].
- *Age*: Peak incidence is in the fourth decade [12].
- *Gender:* No gender preference, F=M [12].
- Locations:
  - While TSs may arise along any nerve segment, most materialize near the Gasserian ganglion [1]. (AKA trigeminal ganglion, semilunar ganglion, or Gasser's ganglion).
  - From their common site of origin near the Gasserian ganglion, trigeminal schwannomas may extend posteriorly into the posterior fossa or anteriorly via skull base foramina to slip on schwannoma's classic "dumbbell" configuration [1].

Imaging

General Imaging Features

- CT and MRI are complimentary for evaluating bony and soft tissue changes.
- Trigeminal schwannomas can contain cysts, calcifications, or hemorrhage.
- *Denervation Atrophy:* Atrophy of mastication muscles can be crucial clues with progressive pterygoid and temporalis muscle atrophy the most common to suggest underlying denervation [18].
- Plain film or bone algorithm CT may exhibit enlargement, erosion, or remodeling of skull base foramina by relevant divisions [12]:

Superior orbital fissure	V_1
Foramen rotundum	V_2
Foramen ovale	V_3

- Benign vs. Malignant Trigeminal Schwannoma
  - Malignant trigeminal schwannomas tend to cause earlier erosion of the basilar foramina often out of proportion to the schwannoma's size [13].
  - Sometimes suggest a malignant diagnosis based on rapid growth or extensive nerve involvement [13].

F. A. Midyett, S. K. Mukherji, *Skull Base Imaging*, https://doi.org/10.1007/978-3-030-46447-9_39

- Confirmation of malignancy regularly requires a tissue diagnosis [13].
- After treatment by radiation or gamma knife surgery (GKS), imaging shows typical tumor necrosis with cystic degeneration.

CT Features

- *See General Imaging Features.*
- Smoothly marginated, round, oblong mass.
- Sometimes show schwannomas' classic "dumbbell"- or saddle-shaped configuration [1].
- Bone algorithms may exhibit enlargement of the superior orbital fissure, foramen ovale, and foramen rotundum or erosion of the petrous apex or floor of the middle cranial fossa.

MRI Features

- *See General Imaging Features.*
- T1 Signal:
  - T1 signal is slightly hypointense to brain parenchyma in ~2/3 and isointense in ~1/3 [9].
  - May have hemorrhage, cyst formation, or necrosis which are heterogeneous and often hypointense to brain.
  - See Fig. 39.1a.
- T2:
  - T2 signal is iso- to hyperintense to the brain with larger lesions more heterogeneous than smaller ones.
  - Cystic changes are hyperintense and cause significant heterogeneity.
  - See Fig. 39.1b.
- FLAIR:
  - Highly heterogeneous with fluid/degenerative components hyperintense to the brain.
  - See Fig. 39.1c.
- T1 Gd:
  - *Enhancement:*
    Avid post-contrast enhancement of solid components with heterogeneity varying directly proportional to degree of cystic degeneration and/or tumor necrosis.
    T1 Gd may demonstrate relative signal void in areas of cysts or cystic necrosis. These areas of tumor necrosis are particularly prominent after gamma knife surgery.
  - See Fig. 39.1d.
- CISS Imaging [17]:
  - While CN V does not normally enhance, it may be visualized as a linear low signal intensity adjacent high signal intensity from the adjacent enhancing venous plexus.
  - Contrast-enhanced 3D CISS sequences excel in depicting the Gasserian ganglion.
  - Contrast-enhanced 3D TOF is superior for showing cranial and foraminal segments of V1, V2, and V3.
  - Complete MRI evaluation of the Gasserian ganglion and its roots is best accomplished using both of these specialized sequences [17].
- DWI:
  - May see "T2 shine through" with ↑DWI and ↑ ADC, but TS typically *does not reveal restricted diffusion.*
- fMRI: [2]
  - Functional magnetic resonance imaging (fMRI) measures brain activity by discerning differences in blood flow.
  - fMRI exploits the fact that neuronal activation is inexorably connected to cerebral blood flow.
  - fMRI primarily uses images developed by BOLD (blood oxygen level-dependent) sequencing.
  - Diffusion tensor imaging (DTI) has emerged as a technique for quantification of water diffusion and can be used to visualize neural fibers.
  - These techniques may demonstrate abnormalities of tracts including displacement by tumor and are often useful for surgical planning.
  - Currently, while some fMRI images may seem less sharp than their pure anatomic counterparts, we embrace them for their valuable, previously undemonstrated "functional" information. We embrace them as momentous milestones and expectantly look forward to future software innovations [5].
  - See Fig. 39.1e, f, g.

Clinical Issues

Presentation

- Trigeminal schwannomas predominately present with "burning" facial pain [13].
- Patients are regularly referred to imaging with symptoms from sensory disturbances or abnormal corneal reflexes. Sensory symptoms often involve numbness, hypesthesia, or hypalgesia [1].
- Later, patients portray weakness involving muscles of mastication as the tumor enlarges to involve V_3 [13].
- *Diagnostic Delay*: Although symptoms are sometimes present for several months before diagnosis, tumor size is typically large because subtle symptoms sometimes make diagnosis difficult [18].
- Cavernous sinus involvement can cause further dysfunction of CN III, IV, and VI.
- Enlargement within the prepontine cistern can compress CN VII, VIII, and IX.

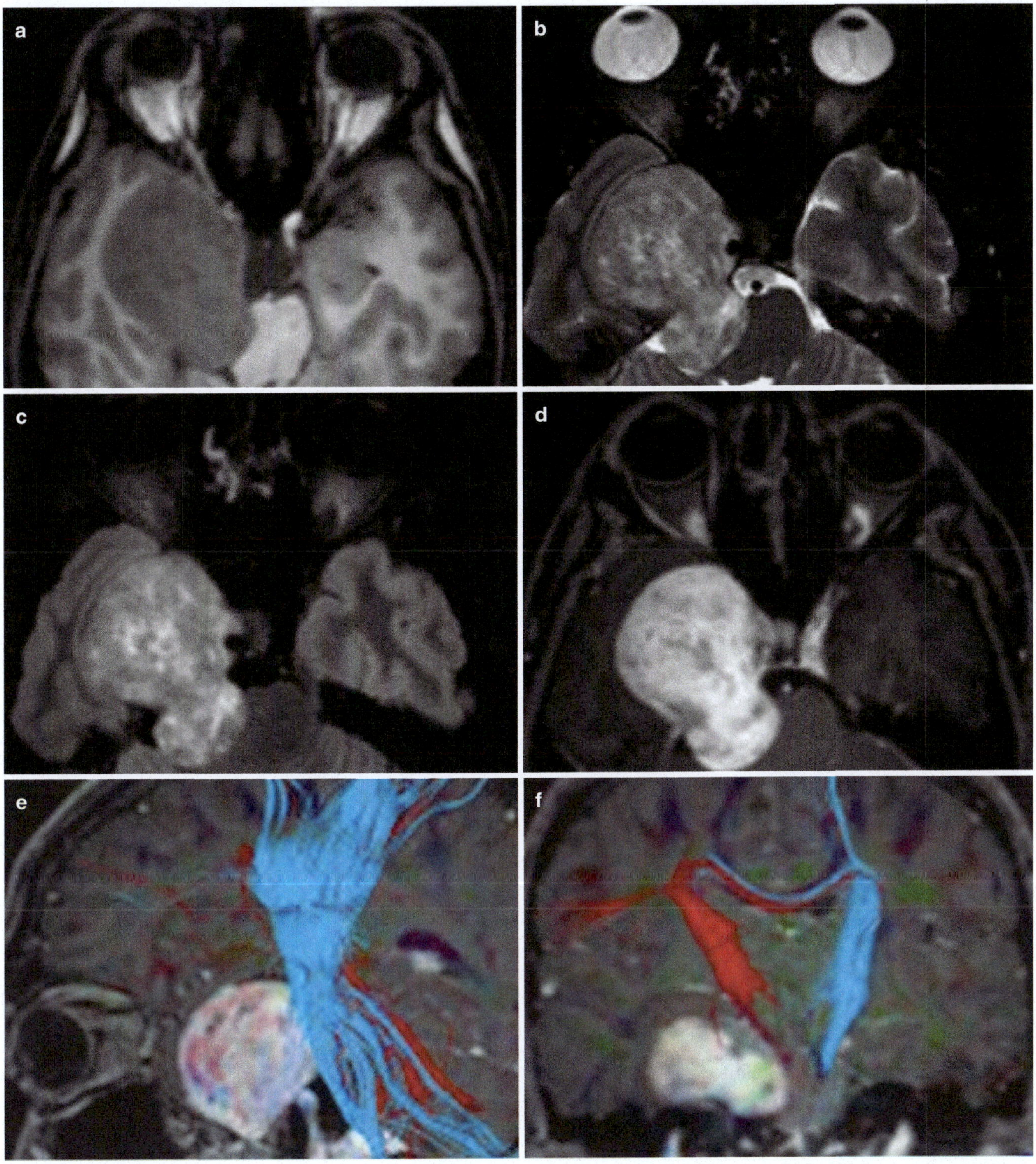

Fig. 39.1 (**a**) Axial T1 shows large right central skull base tumor causing considerable mass effect on the right temporal lobe and pons. Its signal is moderately heterogeneous and similar to gray matter. (**b**) Axial T2 exhibits a large dumbbell-shaped central skull base abnormality causing considerable mass effect on the right temporal lobe and pons. Its signal is highly heterogeneous with solid components similar to gray matter. It is laced with fluid components similar to CSF. The tumor is draped across the dark triangular petrous pyramid causing its sometimes suggested "saddle shape." (**c**) Axial FLAIR shows a large right "dumbbell-shaped" central skull base mass causing considerable mass effect on the right temporal lobe and pons. Its signal is highly heterogeneous with solid components similar to the brain. It is laced with multiple hyperintense foci. Axial T1 Gd (**d**) shows large right "dumbbell-shaped" central skull base mass exhibiting highly heterogeneous enhancement of solid components. It clearly contains significant non-enhancing components consistent with cystic fluid-containing areas demonstrated on other sequences. Sagittal (**e**), coronal (**f**), and axial

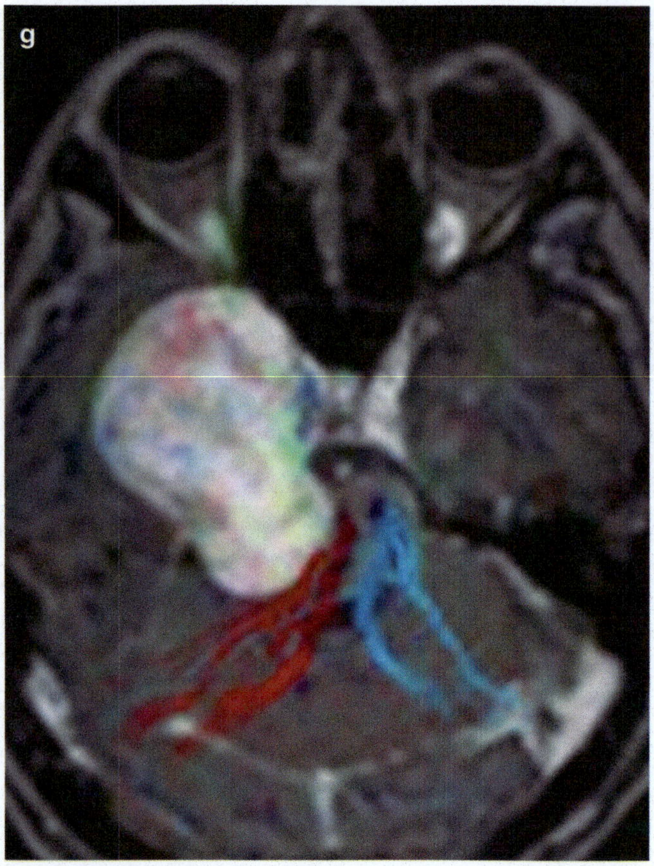

Fig. 39.1 (continued) (**g**) fMRI demonstrates "dumbbell-shaped" central skull base mass exhibiting highly heterogeneous post Gd enhancement. fMRI depicts in color the displacement of functioning nerve tracts by this large trigeminal schwannoma.While some fMRI images seem less sharp than their anatomic counterparts, we embrace them for their valuable, previously undemonstrated, "functional" information. We welcome them as momentous milestones, and expectantly look forward to future software innovations

Treatment and Prognosis [3, 5, 6, 10, 11]

Benign Trigeminal Schwannomas

- The superior solution is surgical excision, with benign Trigeminal Schwannomas showing a slight tendency for recurrence following fastidious removal [1].

Malignant Trigeminal Schwannomas

A. Surgery

I. Conventional Neurosurgery

- While some suggest that complete microsurgical excision should be the therapeutic "gold standard" [16], complete surgical resection is often not possible [3, 13].
- Neck dissection is not normally necessary as lymphatic spread is rare.

Gamma Knife Surgery (GKS)

- GKS (gamma knife surgery) affords a favorable risk to benefit profile for trigeminal schwannomas [14].
- GKS is a safe and effective treatment when used in selected trigeminal schwannoma patients [15].
- Patients showing mass effect on brainstem or fourth ventricle should initially undergo conventional surgery before battling residual tumor with GKS [15].

B. Radiation Therapy

- Currently conveys capricious results.

C. Chemotherapy

- Currently conveys a very limited role in management of unfortunate patients with this entity.

D. Prognosis

- 1/3 of malignant head and neck schwannomas develop late pulmonary or osseous metastasis [13].
- $\leq$ 50% of malignant schwannomas recur locally despite having negative surgical margins and receiving adjuvant radiotherapy [13].
- Despite our best clinical efforts, 5-year survival rates for malignant schwannomas struggle near a common coin chuck at 50% [13].

Pathology

Gross

- Ovoid, tan, encapsulated mass arising asymmetrically from the nerve.
- Commonly contains cystic degeneration with occasional hemorrhage.
- Untreated, usually has hemorrhage and intramural cysts.
- Post gamma knife surgery shows additional necrosis with cystic change.

Microscopic

I. Benign

- Contains two microscopically distinct tissue types:
  - Antoni A

    Dense mature collagen with ↑ cellularity.

    Cells are elongated and bipolar with indistinct borders.

    Arranged in palisades, parallel to each other.

– Antoni B
  Looser mucoid matrix with ↓ cellularity.
  Cellular nuclei resemble lymphocytes.
  Structure appears reticular with highly myxoid matrix.

II. Malignant [13]

- Mixture of plump spindle and polyhedral cells with large hyperchromatic pleomorphic nuclei.
- ↑ mitotic figures, necrosis, perineural extension, and perineural invasion.
- Immunohistochemical markers include S-100 protein, leucine 7, and myelin basic protein.
- Electron microscopy sometimes shows interdigitating cytoplasmic processes, scanty intercellular junctions, focal basal lamina, and interstitial collagen fibers.

Differential Diagnosis (DDx)

Definitely, the differential for trigeminal schwannomas varies with lesion size depending on whether the mass is small confined to Meckel's cave, clearly co-located within CN V, a large lesion extending into the CPA, or an absolutely huge lesion which appears to extend everywhere. While we can usually sort out the odd aneurysm, lipoma, epidermoid, and cephalocele, we are frequently left with difficult decisions involving one or more of the following choices:

A. Meningioma

- NECT:
  - Meningiomas can cause bony hyperostosis.
  - 75% show hyperdense mass.
  - 25% show sand-like calcifications.
- CECT:
  - 90% exhibit avid enhancement.
- T1:
  - Extra-axial mass, with 75% isointense and 25% hypointense to brain parenchyma.
  - 25% have hemorrhage, necrosis, or cyst formation.
- T2:
  - Extra-axial mass iso- or hyperintense to brain parenchyma.
  - *CSF Cleft*: Sometimes see CSF vascular cleft between brain and tumor.
- T1 Gd: 95% show *avid* enhancement of broad-based tumor frequently flaunting its "dural tail."
- While most meningiomas tend to be typical, considering their prevalence, statistics suggest we can probably predict a noteworthy number of "atypical" cases.
- Some unusual features which can be misleading include "ring enhancement," large cysts, and fatty transformation [4].
- See Chap. 10, Meningioma.

B. Skull Base Chondrosarcoma (SBC)

- Skull base mass exhibiting an affinity for the petro-occipital fissure sometimes showing a chondroid matrix, characterized by low T1 and high T2 signals.
- Appear as well-circumscribed, often scalloped, or lobulated lytic lesions exhibiting chondroid calcifications.
- Most SBCs occur *off midline*, commonly causing local extension with paranasal sinus and cavernous sinus invasion.
- T1: Hypointense (to intermediate) signal intensity.
- T2:
  - Very high signal.
  - Areas having heterogeneity can correspond to calcifications on CT.
- T1 Gd: Avid post-contrast enhancement.
- See Chap. 46, Skull Base Chondrosarcoma.

C. Perineural Tumor Spread (PNS)

- Perineural tumor spread propagates along the nerve sheath by uninterrupted extension as a solitary large lesion [12].
- An eccentric enhancing "skip" area along the trigeminal nerve constitutes a virtual "red flag" characteristic of PNS and should forthwith prompt pursuit for an underlying primary malignant neoplasm [12].
- Tumors particularly prone to present PNS include adenoid cystic carcinoma, mucoepidermoid carcinoma, lymphoma, and squamous cell carcinoma [12].
- PNS typically travels from secondary branches back toward the nerve's root [12].
- It is important to image all segments of the trigeminal nerve.
- PNS is one of the most insidious, intimidating, and perplexing forms of cancer proliferation and is problematic for patients, clinicians, and radiologists.
- Some suggest the sensitivity for detecting PNS is as high as 95%.
- PNS portends a profound negative effect on therapeutic options and prognosis.
- V_3's extensive branching network renders it especially exposed to PNS and shows significant signs including:
  - Nerve thickening
  - Neural foraminal enlargement
  - Meckel's cave mass
  - Cavernous sinus mass
  - Denervation atrophy of masticator muscles
- See Chap. 37, Adenoid Cystic Carcinoma of the Skull Base.

D. Other Schwannomas

- When large, schwannomas involving other cranial nerves can cause confusion with the differential diagnosis [12].

- Schwannomas involving the cisternal segments of CN VII and VIII are located more laterally in the prepontine cistern and track toward the IAC which is frequently enlarged [12].
- Schwannomas are more frequently found involving sensory rather than pure motor nerves.
- While schwannomas have been reported on CN III, IV, and VI, they are truly medical "zebras," really rarer than zebras at a local farmer's rodeo.

E. Neurosarcoidosis (NS)

- It is rare to see neurosarcoidosis (NS) without systemic disease, but patients with NS are frequently the first sarcoidosis patients to show symptoms.
- Frequently find multiple dural-based foci with neurosarcoidosis.
- Look for idiosyncratic involvement of the pituitary infundibulum.
- T1 is usually isointense to brain.
- T2 is often *hypointense*! This a ***key*** feature!
- T1 Gd shows *avid enhancement* varying from homogeneous to heterogeneous.
- Sometimes shows concomitant cerebral edema.
- 90% of sarcoidosis patients have pulmonary involvement including interstitial infiltrates with pulmonary fibrosis, hypertension, and restrictive pulmonary disease as well as the reliably recognizable hilar adenopathy.
- 30% of patients have dermatologic involvement including cutaneous sarcoidosis and erythema nodosum.
- 25% of patients have cardiac involvement including dysrhythmias and cardiomyopathy.
- See Chap. 6, Neurohypophyseal Sarcoidosis.

F. Metastasis

- Metastasis may occur via neurotropic, subarachnoid, or hematogenous spread.
- Hematogenous metastasis to the trigeminal nerve more commonly occurs from melanoma, breast, and lung carcinoma [12].
- Metastasis may display bilateral nerve involvement and/or multifocal meningeal involvement.

A Closer Look

Potpourri

Tumor Classification

- Trigeminal schwannoma can conveniently be classified according to its location along the trigeminal nerve [12].
- One classification useful in evaluating symptoms and determining surgical approach includes the following types [12]:
  - Type I. Arises in the middle cranial fossa from the Gasserian ganglion (most common).
  - Type II. Involves the nerve's cisternal component in the posterior cranial fossa.
  - Type III. Classic "dumbbell-shaped" lesion with one module in Meckel's cave and the other part in the posterior fossa's prepontine cistern. The two major sections are separated by a "waist" near the opening to Meckel's cave, the porus trigeminus. Type IIIs comprise the second most common type.
  - Type IV is primarily extracranial but may manifest intracranial components.

Historic Highlights

- 1833 Sir Charles Bell first authenticated a Meckel's cave neuroma [8].

Genetics and Associations

- Trigeminal schwannoma can develop de novo or in alliance with neurofibromatosis [12].
- Schwannomas show an association with NF II, which is related to mutation of the membrane-cytoskeleton scaffolding protein merlin (AKA neurofibromin 2 or schwannomin) [19].
- Malignant schwannomas of peripheral and cranial nerves are often associated with NF II [20]. This association has, however, not been found with malignant trigeminal schwannomas [13].
- The precise prevalence of malignant trigeminal schwannoma is difficult to determine because of its infrequent occurrence and its many monikers including malignant neurofibroma, neurofibrosarcoma, neurosarcoma, neurogenic sarcoma, malignant neurilemmoma, and malignant nerve sheath tumor [13].
- Schwannomas are universally positive for S-100 which is a marker for cells of neural crest origin.

Selected References

1. Fischbein NJ, Dillon WP, Barkovich AJ. Teaching atlas of brain imaging. New York: Thieme; 2000. p. 568–70.
2. Hakyemez B, Erdogan C, Bolca N, et al. Evaluation of different cerebral mass lesions by perfusion-weighted MR imaging. J Magn Reson Imaging. 2006;(24):817–24.
3. Wigand ME, Rettinger G, Haid T, et al. The removal of VIIIth nerve neurinomas from the cerebellopontine angle by enlarged middle fossa approach. HNO. 1985;33:11–6.
4. Buetow MP, Buetow PC, Smirniotopoulos JG. Typical, atypical, and misleading features in meningioma. Radiographics. 1991;11(6):1087–106.

5. Salzman KL, Childs AM, Davidson HC, et al. Intralabyrinthine Schwannomas: imaging diagnosis and classification. AJNR Am J Neuroradiol. 2012;33:104–9.
6. Koerbel A, Gharabaghi A, Safavi-Abasi S, et al. Evolution of vestibular schwannoma surgery: the long journey to current success. Neurosurg Focus. 2005;18(4):E10.
7. Wishart JH. Case of tumours in the skull, dura mater, and brain. Edin Med Surg J. 1822;18:393.
8. Bell C. The nervous system of the human body; embracing the papers delivered to the Royal Society on the subject of the nerves. Washington, DC: Duff Green; 1833.
9. Mulkens TH, Parizel PM, Martin JJ, et al. Acoustic schwannoma: MR findings in 84 tumors. AJR Am J Roentgenol. 1993;160(2):395–8.
10. Silk PS, Jl L, Driscoll CL. Surgical approaches to vestibular schwannomas: what the radiologist needs to know. Radiographics. 2009;29(7):1955–70.
11. Shelton C. Unilateral acoustic tumors: how often do they recur after translabyrinthine removal? Laryngoscope. 1995;105(9 pt 1):958–66.
12. Lufkin R, Borges A, Villablanca P. Teaching atlas of head and neck imaging. New York: Thieme; 2000. p. 8–12.
13. Stone JA, Cooper H, Castillo M, Mukherji SK. Malignant Schwannoma of the trigeminal nerve. AJNR. 2001;22:505–7.
14. Sheehan J, Yen CP, Arkha Y, et al. Gamma knife surgery for trigeminal schwannoma. J Neurosurg. 2007;106(5):839–45.
15. Haseqawa T, Kida Y, Yoshimoto M. Trigeminal schwannomas: results of gamma knife surgery in 37 cases. J Neurosurg. 2007;106(1):18–23.
16. Sutiono AB, Glady A, Zafrullah M, et. al. Three subtypes of trigeminal Schwannoma in relation with meninges pattern for surgical consideration: anatomy and histological study. JSM Neurosurgery Spine 2015; 3(2): 1056–1062.
17. Yousry I, Moriggl B, Schmid UD, et al. Trigeminal ganglion and its divisions: detailed anatomic MR imaging with contrast-enhanced 3D constructive interference in the steady state sequences. AJNR. 2005;26:1128–35.
18. Coniglio AJ, Miller MC, Walter KA, et al. Trigeminal Schwannoma with extracranial extension and brainstem compression. Otol Neurotol. 2013;34(6) https://doi.org/10.1097/MAO.0b013e318287f21b.
19. Hanemann CO. News on the genetics, epidemiology, medical care and translational research of Schwannomas. J Neurol. 2006;253(12):1533–41.
20. Majoie CBLM, Hulsmans FJH, Castelijns JA, et al. Primary nerve-sheath tumours of the trigeminal nerve: clinical and MRI findings. Neuroradiology. 1999;41:100–8.

Part V

Craniovertebral Junction

Atlanto-Occipital Dissociations

40

Pertinent Points

- *Definition:* Traumatic dislocation of the craniovertebral junction involves disruption of strong ligamentous attachments holding the atlas, axis, and occiput together. Atlanto-occipital dissociations (AODs) are severe injuries which include atlanto-occipital dislocation and atlanto-occipital subluxation.
- These injuries seriously threaten the adjacent critical neurovascular structures and life itself with atlanto-occipital dislocation usually being fatal.
- *Classic Clue*: The trauma service requests head and neck imaging for a patient who received multiple traumas as a pedestrian hit by a motor vehicle, who continues to complain of neck pain, although "no fracture" was identified on examination at an outside hospital which treated the patients other not insignificant injuries.
- *Synonyms:* Craniovertebral dissociation, atlanto-occipital dissociation, AOJ dislocation.
- The craniovertebral junction is a highly complex specialized mobile transition between the skull and the cervical spine and as such is quite vulnerable to trauma.
- The inherent vulnerability of the CVJ is because its design traded mobility for stability and relies on ligaments instead of intrinsic bony stability [2].
- Injuries to the CVJ disrupt structural integrity and vital neurovascular functions displaying a disproportionate danger of death [2].
- While traumatic osteoligamentous injuries of the CVJ are uncommon, early diagnosis and treatment is crucial to conservation of neurologic function.
- The unique anatomical features of the CVJ require specialized care when traumatic disruption occurs.
- Injuries to the craniovertebral junction are among a few skeletal injuries holding a high probability of impending death [2–5].

Imaging

General Imaging Features

- Atlanto-occipital Dissociation is often difficult to diagnose on initial imaging studies [2].
- Normal measurements for CT studies are distinctly different than for plain films, particularly in children [10]. If you even suspect a problem, get a CT.
- Even a tiny avulsion fracture in the cervical occipital region can be a harbinger of serious ligamentous injury or instability.
- Distance between occipital condyles and condylar surface of atlas >5 mm is a red flag.
- Harris Criteria or Harris Rule of 12's:
  - >12 mm from basion to odontoid tip
  - >12 mm from basion to posterior line drawn along posterior cortex of atlas body [17]
- The primary mechanism is hyperextension, but lateral flexion may be a complimentary component [13].

Traynelis Types of Atlanto-Occipital Dissociation [15]:

Type I
- Anterior displacement of head relative to spine
- Most common

Type II
- Longitudinal distraction with cephalic distraction of head relative to spine
- Most unstable

Type III
- Posterior displacement of head relative to spine
- Extremely rare

Plain Film Radiography

- A look at the accompanying plain films suggests they may be quite helpful *if* you know what to look for (see Fig. 40.1a, b).

F. A. Midyett, S. K. Mukherji, *Skull Base Imaging*, https://doi.org/10.1007/978-3-030-46447-9_40

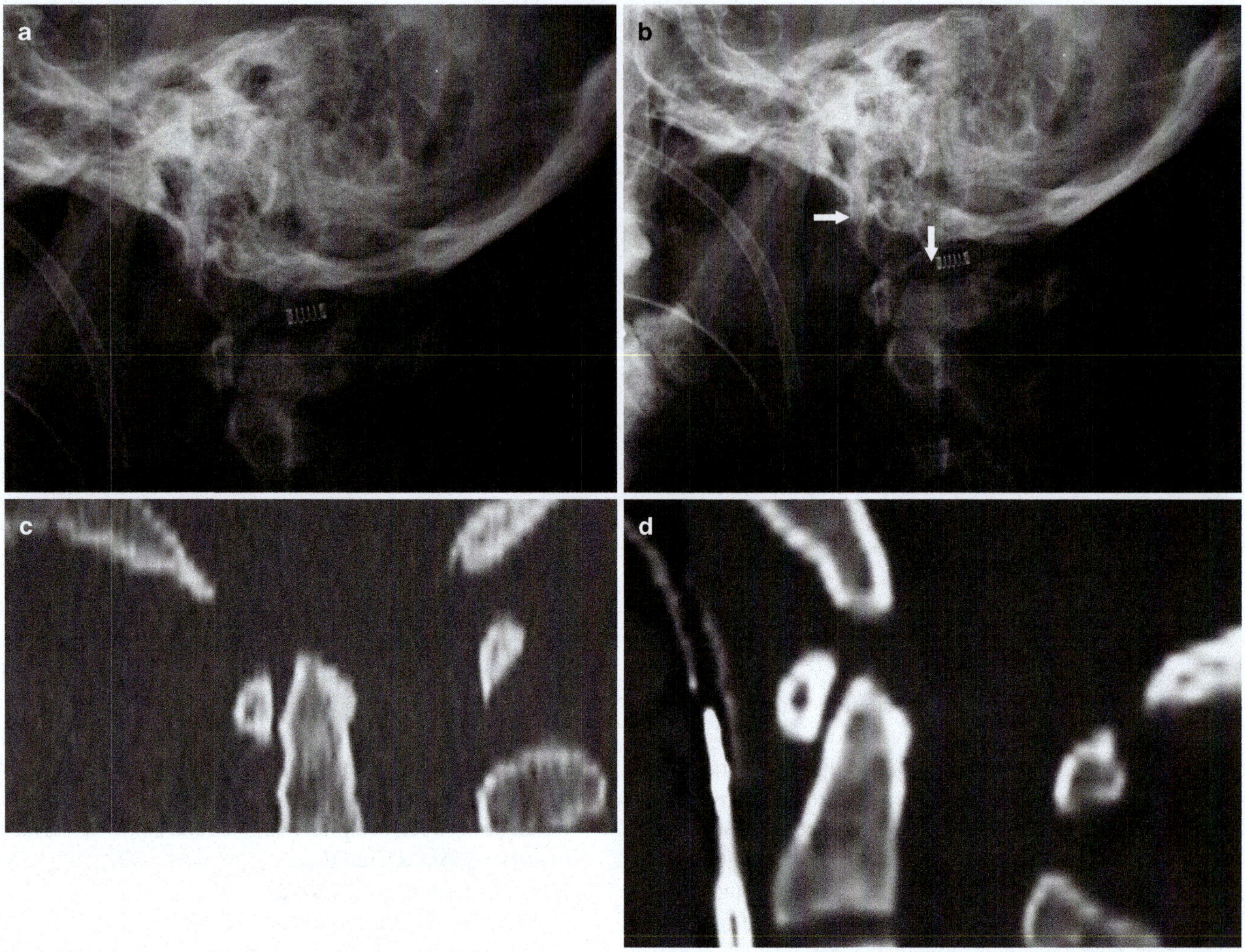

Fig. 40.1 (**a**) Portion of a lateral cervical spine where several observers said "No Fracture or Dislocation Seen." But the "expert" witness for the plaintiff (the patient's widow) said the abnormality was obvious. Do you see it? (**b**) Same view with arrows. The horizontal arrow points to the tip of the clivus. The vertical arrow points to the odontoid tip. But a line drawn down the posterior aspect of the clivus (Wackenheim's clivus line) typically falls tangent to the posterior aspect of the odontoid process. This is AOD. (**c**) Sagittal CT shows "No Fracture." Do you see the problem now? A line drawn down the posterior aspect of the clivus (Wackenheim's clivus line) does not have a normal relation to the odontoid. Take a look at the next image which is normal. (**d**) Sagittal CT shows a "normal" patient for comparison. Note the relationship of the clival and odontoid tips. Remember Wackenheim's clivus line typically falls tangent to the posterior aspect of the odontoid process

- There is no question that a higher level of imaging is imperative once AOD is *even* suspected.
- The following plain film findings suggest AOD:
  - Displacement of >10 mm between basion and dens [16]
  - Abnormal "Powers Ratio" >1
  - A distance of >13 mm between post mandible and anterior atlas or 20 mm between posterior mandible and dens
  - Failure of a line from basion to axis of spinolaminar junction to intersect C2 or a line from opisthion to posterior corner of the body of C2 to intersect C1
- Reported missed posttraumatic spine fractures by radiography vary from 15–30% [20, 21].
- This literature and other experience led some at a well-known neurologic institute to call plain films "essentially useless" in evaluating the craniovertebral junction [1], particularly in children.
- Some suggest plain films be used as tools for this rare but survivable injury [2], but relying on them may well be to the detriment of both the patient and the practitioner.
- The legal profession clearly tells us that anyone reading these plain film studies will be held to the highest standards for interpretation of these high-stakes cases.
- Logically, if plain films are positive, a higher level of imaging is required. If plain films are negative, higher level of imaging can be critical.
- So, in this day and age, plain films should probably ONLY be considered in those emergent cases in which more sophisticated imaging is NOT available.

CT Features

- For many of these AODs, the "eyeball test" is sufficient (See Fig. 40.2a–d).
- But we can and do use measurements to make us and the clinicians feel better (see Fig. 40.3a, b).
- The fact that there are so many measurements in use gives you an idea of the degree of confidence folks have placed in them.
- And remember these patients have a spectrum of injuries. Those with the most severe trauma are already in the morgue. Those with the least trauma are outside arguing with our staff. And we are looking at patients whose trauma is somewhere in the middle between those two extremes. And their findings may be subtle.
- Currently SIX measurements are currently in vogue including the following:

I. BAI

- Basion-axial interval.
- Distance from the clival tip (basion) to a line drawn along the posterior axial line drawn along the posterior cortex of the body of C2 (axis) and extended cranially.
- >12 mm in adults is abnormal.
- Basion-posterior axial line is reliable in children and <12 mm [17].

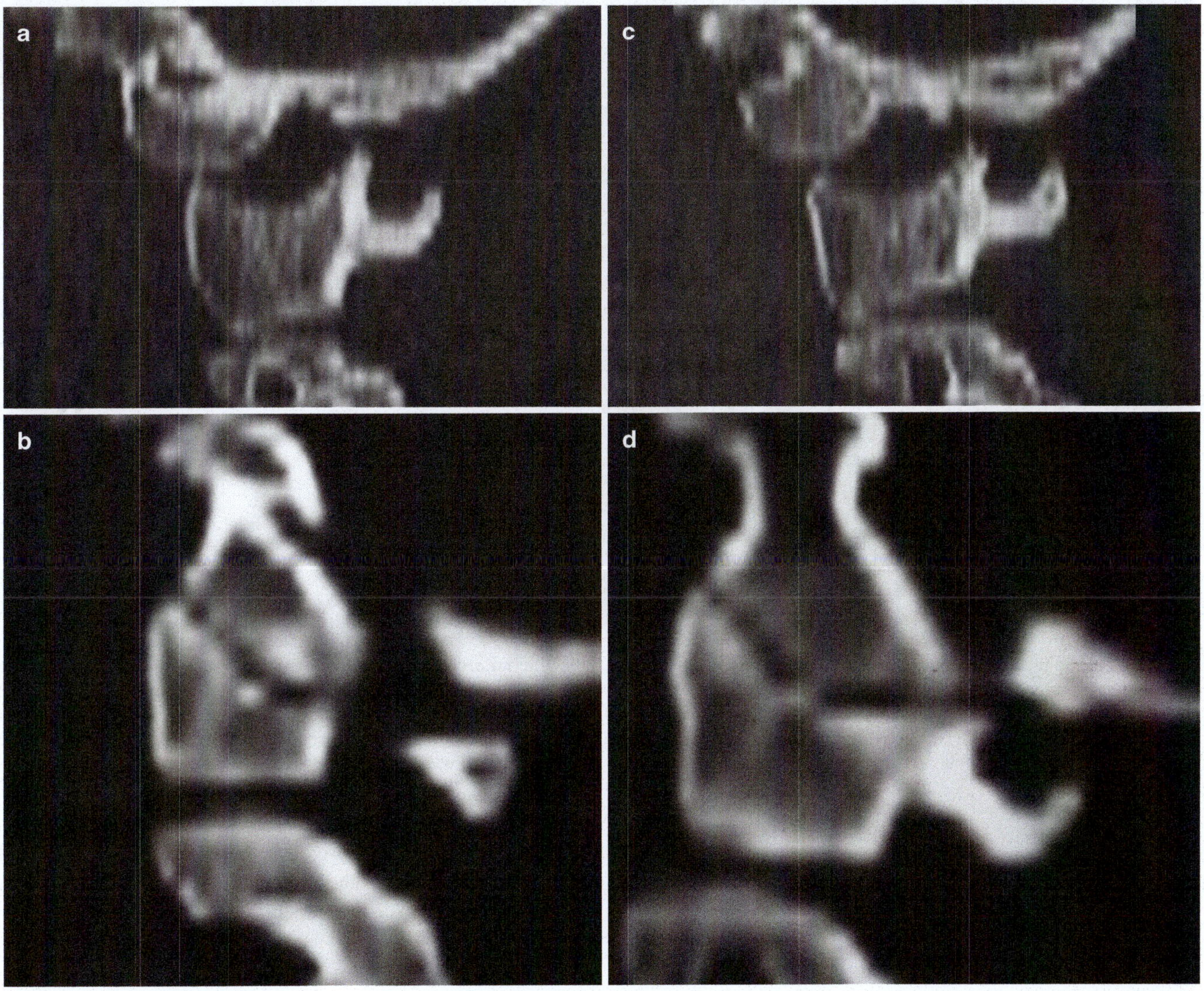

Fig. 40.2 (**a**) Parasagittal CT clearly shows dislocated left atlanto-occipital junction. Compare to "normal" next image. (**b**) Parasagittal CT shows a "normal" patient for comparison. Note the relationship of the occipital condyle above to the atlas below. (**c**) Right parasagittal CT clearly shows dislocated atlanto-occipital junction. Compare to "normal" next image. (**d**) Parasagittal CT shows a "normal" patient for comparison. Note the relationship of the occipital condyle above to the atlas below

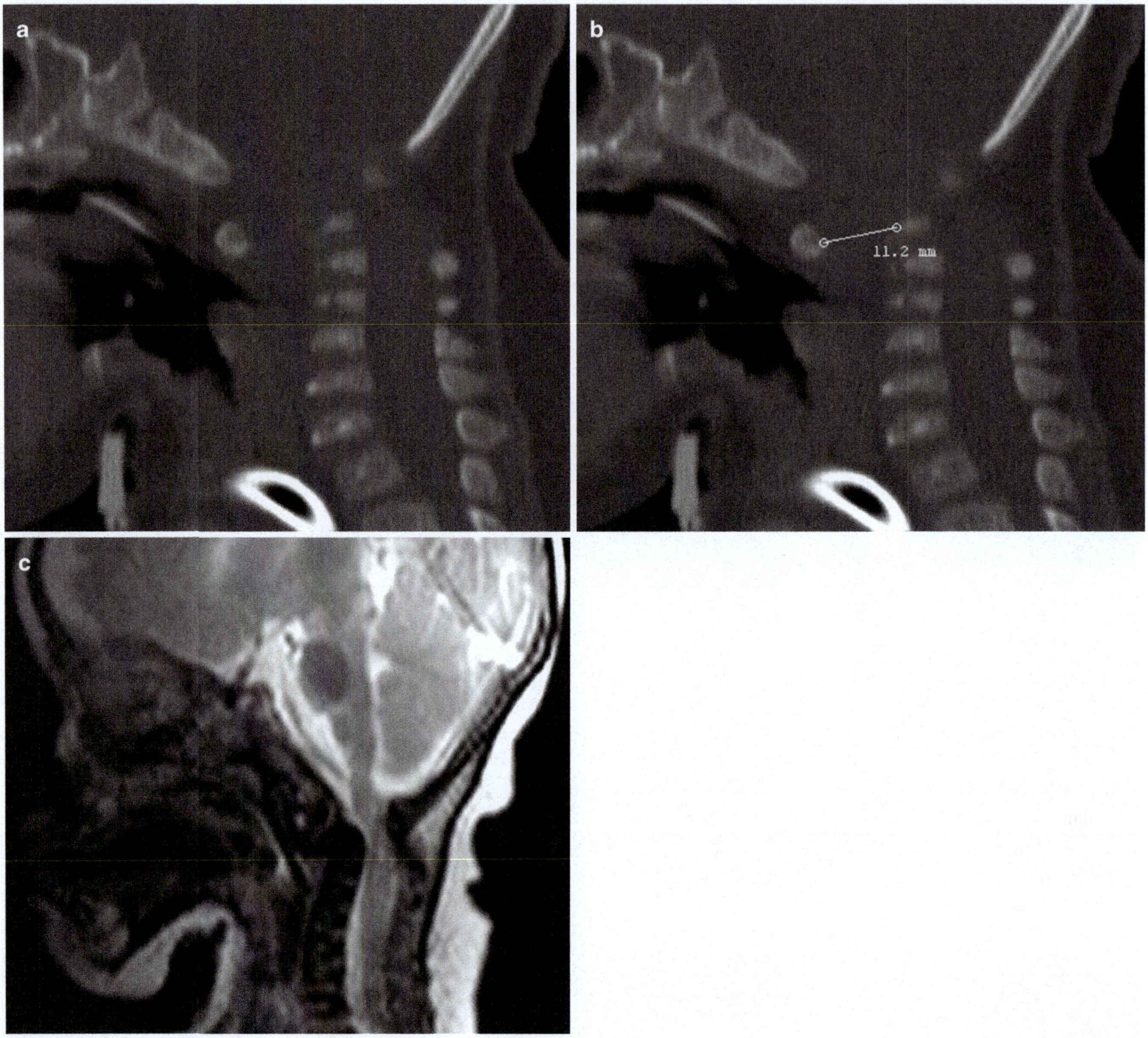

Fig. 40.3 (**a**) Sagittal CT. A quick "eyeball test" tells the observer that the relationship of the skull to the cervical spine is not right! The skull is dislocated anteriorly placing the odontoid near the foramen magnum. The distance between the anterior arch of C1 and the odontoid is grossly widened. (**b**) Sagittal CT. Well, no surprise here! The distance between the anterior arch of C1 and the odontoid is >11 mm. The normal ADI (atlantodental interval) is 2.6 mm on CT for children. (**c**) Sagittal T2 confirms craniovertebral dislocation causing compression of the thecal sac and cord. No surprise either that trials to wean this child off the ventilator were unsuccessful over the prior 6 weeks!

II. BDI

- Basion-dens interval.
- Distance from clival tip (basion) to odontoid tip (dens).
- > 12 mm in adults is abnormal.
- Some say BDI is unreliable in children <13 years old [17].
- Others feel that this measurement is clearly consistent although distinctly different than that reported for plain films. In children, BDI on CT is <10.5 mm compared with 12 mm on plain film radiographs in 97.5% of patients [10]. If we separate the pediatric population into two groups with those whose os terminale have [and have not] ossified, it changes the upper limit of normal by 2 mm [from 9.5 to 11.6 mm, respectively] [10].

III. Powers Ratio

- In 1979 Powers et al. described what is now known as the Powers Ratio for the evaluation of atlanto-occipital dissociation, and it is considered normal when <1 [8, 9].
- Divide the distance from the tip of the basion to the spinolaminar line by the distance from the tip of the opisthion

to the midpoint of the posterior aspect of the anterior arch of C1.

- >1 is abnormal.
- The Powers Ratio is insensitive to type II or type III [vertical or posterior] dissociations.

IV. ADI

- Atlantodental interval.
  - Synonyms: Predentate space, predental space, atlantodental distance.
- Perpendicular line from the anterior arch of C1 to the most anterior aspect of the odontoid (dens) at the craniocaudal midpoint of the arch.
- >3 mm in adult males, > 2.5 mm in adult females.
- In children the ADI is <2.6 mm on CT compared to 4–5 mm on plain film radiographs.
- Disruption of the transverse ligament may permit anterior subluxation at C1–C2. This type of subluxation may occur with an intact transverse ligament with fractures of odontoid or os odontoideum [27].
- The ADI measurement may be normal when the neck is neutral or extended and only be abnormal when the neck is flexed.

V. AOI (Left and Right)

- Draw a line perpendicular to the articular surfaces of the occipital condyle and the lateral mass of C1. This line is drawn at the center of the articulation ideally using a multiplanar work station.
- Atlanto-occipital interval in children on CT is <2.5 mm in 97.5% of population compared to accepted value of 5 mm on radiographs [10].
- Harris Rule of 12's:
  - The distance from the tip of the dens to the basion (clival tip) or from the basion (clival tip) to the posterior line (of C2) should not exceed 12 mm in an adult.

MRI Features

- In addition to all the relationships and measurements described above (which are extremely important but will NOT be repeated in this section), MRI has the unique ability to deftly demonstrate soft tissues including ligaments and the spinal cord (see Fig. 40.3c).
- Pertinent MRI finding include [23]:
  - Prevertebral soft tissue abnormalities
    Retropharyngeal hematoma is *invariably present* with AOD [26].
    Retropharyngeal emphysema occasionally present [26]:
  - Ligamentous injury
    MRI may demonstrate injury to major ligamentous structures at the CVJ including the tectorial membrane as well as the apical, transverse, cruciform, and interspinous ligaments [22].
    Sometimes see loss of anatomic continuity, high signal within incompletely ruptured ligament, or blood at ligament's bony insertion [27].
    T2 Fat Sat images may facilitate demonstrating disruption of ligaments which usually provide stability [6].
    Transverse ligament injuries are divided into two types, each requiring different treatment and having different prognosis:
    - Type I: Disruptions substance of transverse atlantal ligament
      - These all require early surgery.
    - Type II: Avulsion [or fracture] involving ligamentous attachment of transverse ligament to lateral mass of C1
      - Three fourths can be treated with rigid halo brace.
      - One fourth fail treatment by immobilization and require surgery [27].
  - Tectorial membrane elevation or tear:
    - The tectorial membrane is a broad, strong band which covers the dens and its ligaments and is an upward prolongation of the PLL (posterior longitudinal ligament).
    - Its anterior surface should relate to the transverse ligament of the atlas and its posterior surface to the dura.
    - It attaches inferiorly to the posterior body of the axis ascending to attach to the basilar groove of the occipital bone.
  - Retroclival hematoma.
  - Abnormal cord signal. This is *the most significant negative prognostic sign.*
- Associated imaging features in fatal cases:
  - Lacerations of pontomedullary junction in ¾
  - Laceration and/or contusion of caudal medulla or rostral spinal cord in 1/2
  - Laceration and/or stretching of midbrain in 1/3
- May be associated with:
  - SDH in 1/6
  - SAH (usually minimal quantity)
  - Vasospasm or dissection of ICA or vertebral arteries (unknown frequency)

Clinical Issues

Presentation

- Significant injury disrupts ligaments at CVJ.
- The types of trauma vary but correlate with the types of AOD.

- Sudden deceleration injuries comprise a significant component of cases.
- Clinical patterns vary, usually comprising cardiovascular or neurologic components.
- Neurologic presentations vary from no deficit to tetraplegia with ventilator dependency [11, 14].

Epidemiology and Pathology

- AOD causes severe ligamentous injury.
- Atlanto-occipital dissociation (AOD) injuries can be divided into two general groups: (I) dislocations and (II) subluxations.
- Atlanto-occipital dislocations are frequently fatal and not a diagnostic problem for the radiologist.
- Atlanto-occipital subluxations occur less often than dislocations and are rarely fatal [8].

Treatment and Prognosis

- Since first reported in 1908, AOD has been associated with very poor prognosis [24].
- CVJ fracture-dislocations have been shown by autopsy to be a leading cause of death in motor vehicle crashes [2, 4, 5, 7].
- It is essential to avoid C-spine flexion, particularly when placing children on adult trauma boards.
- Ensure the head is held in anatomic position by immobilizing sand bags.
- Traction is contraindicated with AOD.
- Rigid immobilization by halo is required to maintain position before and after surgery.
- A halo brace alone is inadequate to maintain permanent alignment, and acute internal fixation is required [27].
- Recommended treatment is craniocervical fusion of C2 to the occiput with internal fixation.
- Its frequency of fatality is associated with vascular injuries of the vertebral and carotid arteries and/or neurogenic injuries to the cervicomedullary region with phrenic or bulbar nerve palsy causing asphyxia [24].
- Many patients with traumatic AOD will die immediately or within the first few hours after trauma.
- Since first reported by Blackwood [25] in 1908, AOD's main advances involve ↑ index of suspicion, new diagnostic techniques, and changes in initial management.
- Paradoxically, on-scene intubation sorts these patients into two groups: Group I: those it saves and Group II: those it kills [24].
- Cervical spine trauma is rare in children accounting for only 1.5% of pediatric trauma admissions.
- Severe pediatric cervical spine trauma, however, clearly causes disproportionate medical and social expense compared to its low frequency [1].

Differential Diagnosis (DDx)

Nontraumatic causes of atlanto-occipital and atlanto-axial instability include:

I. Various arthritidies
- Rheumatoid arthritis
- Psoriasis
- Lupus

II. Various syndromes
- Down syndrome
- Morquio syndrome
- Larsen syndrome
- Grisel syndrome
- Kniest Syndrome

III. Neurofibromatosis
IV. Osteogenesis imperfecta
V. Metatropic dysplasia

A Closer Look

I. Fast Facts

- AOD is a rare medical condition accounting for ~1% of cervical spine injuries but ~15% of fatal spine trauma [11, 12].
- AOD is more common in children, probably because of their small, horizontally oriented occipital condyles, the flat surface of the lateral masses of C1, and a relatively "loose" ligamentous capsule.
- This architecture lacks sufficient structural stability to withstand significant trauma [24].
- Types I, II, and III AOD are clearly caused by different mechanisms including anterior translation (hyperflexion), longitudinal distraction, and posterior translation (hyperextension).
- These injuries are usually, but fortunately not invariably, fatal with lower brainstem injury causing respiratory arrest.

II. Historic Highlights

- 1871–1938: James Weldon Johnson, African-American author and songwriter composed "Dem Dry Bones" and may have been one of the first to talk/sing publically about AOD by vowing in verse 1 "Neck bone connected to the head bone" and in verse 2 "Head bone disconnected from the neck bone."
- 1908: Blackwood first more formally reported AOD in the *Annals of Surgery* [25].

- 1958: Wholey, Bruwer, and Baker described findings in lateral cervical spine with AOD dislocation [16].
- 1974: Wackenheim published an entire volume on *Roentgen diagnosis of the craniovertebral region* and is now remembered by "Wackenheim's clival line" [18] later specifically addressing "cervico-occipital joint" [19].
- 1979: Powers et al. published what is now known as "Powers Ratio" in traumatic AOD [9].
- 1994: Harris et al. compared three methods of detecting occipitovertebral relationships giving rise to "Harris Criteria" or "Harris Rule of 12's" [17].
- 2009: Berzotti, Rojas, and Martinez published standard measurements for CT of the CVJ in children demonstrating differences from adults and plain film measurements.

Selected References

1. Oppenlandr ME, Clark JC, VKH S, Nicholas T. Pediatric craniovertebral junction trauma: Springer; 2014.
2. Bellabarba C, Mirza SK, Chapman JR. Chapter 28 injuries of the craniocervical junction. In: Rockwood & green's fractures in adults. 6th ed: Lippincott Williams & Wilkins; 2006. p. 1436.
3. Ahuja A, Glasauer FE, Alker GJ Jr, et al. Radiology in survivors of traumatic atlanto-occipital dislocation. Surg Neurol. 1994;41:112–8.
4. Alker GJ, Oh YS, Leslie EV, et al. Postmortem radiology of head neck injuries in fatal traffic accidents. Radiology. 1975;114:611–7.
5. Bucholz RW, Burkhead WZ. The pathological anatomy of fatal atlanto-occipital dislocations. J Bone Joint Surg Am. 1979;61:248–50.
6. Kathol MH. Cervical spine trauma. What is new? Radiol Clin N Am. 1997;35:507–32.
7. Alker GJ Jr, Oh YS, Leslie EV. High cervical spine and craniocervical junction injuries in fatal traffic accidents: a radiological study. Orthop Clin North Am. 1978;9:1003–10.
8. Rojas CA, Bertozzi JC, Martinez CR. Et-al. Reassessment of the craniocervical junction: normal values on CT. AJNR Am J Neuroradiol. 2007;28(9):1819–23.
9. Powers B, Miller MD, Kramer RS, et al. Traumatic anterior atlanto-occipital dislocation. Neurosurgery. 1979;4:12–7.
10. Bertozi JC, Rojas CA, Martinez CR. Evaluation of the pediatric craniocervical junction on MDCT. Am J Roentgenol. 2009;192(1):26–31.
11. Labler L, Eid K, Platz A, Trentz O, Kossmann T. Atlanto-occipital dislocation: four case reports of survival in adults and review of the literature. Eur Spine J. 2004;13(2):172–80.
12. Van Den Bout AH, Dommisse GF. Traumatic occipito-atlantal dislocation. J Spinal Discord. 1986;11(2):174–6.
13. Woodring JJ, Selke AL, Duff DE. Traumatic atlanto-occipital dislocation with survival. AJR Am J Roentgenol. 1981;137(1):21–4.
14. Przybylski GJ, Clyde BL, Fitz CR. Cranio-cervical junction subarachnoid hemorrhage associated with atlanto-occipital dislocation. Spine. 1996;21(15):1761–8.
15. Traynelis VC, Marano GD, Dunker RO, Kaufman HH. Traumatic atlanto-occipital dislocation. Case report. J Neurosurg. 1986;65(6):863–70.
16. Wholey MH, Bruwer AJ, Baker HL. The lateral roentgenogram of the neck (with comments on the atlanto-odontoid-basion relationship). Radiology. 1958;71(3):350–6.
17. Harris JH Jr, Carson GC, Wagner LK, Kerr N. Radiologic diagnosis of traumatic occipitovertebral dissociation: part 2—comparison of three methods of detecting occipitovertebral relationships on lateral radiographs of supine subjects. Am J Radiol. 1994;162(4):887–92.
18. Wackenheim A. Roentgen diagnosis of the craniovertebral region. New York, NY: Springer; 1974.
19. Wackenheim A. Cervico-occipital joint. Berlin, Germany: Springer; 1985.
20. Reid DC, Henderson R, Saboe L, Miller JD. Etiology and clinical course of missed spine fractures. J Trauma. 1987;27:980–6.
21. Davis JW, Phreaner DL, Hoyt DB, Mackersie RC. The etiology of missed cervical spine injuries. J Trauma. 1993;34:342–6.
22. Grabb BC, Frye TA, Hedlund GL, et al. MRI diagnosis of suspected atlanto-occipital dissociation in childhood. Pediatr Radiology. 1999;29(4):275–81.
23. du Plessis JP, Dix-Peek S, Hoffman EB, et al. Pediatric atlanto-occiptial dissolution: radiographic findings and clinical outcome. Evid Based Spine Care J Feb. 2012;3(1):19–20.
24. Ehlinger M, Charles YP, Adam P, et al. Survivor of a traumatic atlanto-occipital dislocation. Orthopad Traumatol Surg Res. 2011;97(3):335–40.
25. Blackwood NJ. Atlanto-occipital dislocation. Ann Surg. 1908;47:654–8.
26. Winn HR. Chapter 313: evaluation and management of craniocervical disociation from youmans neurological surgery.
27. Dickman CA, Spetzler R, Sonntag VKH. Surgery of the Craniovertebral junction, vol. 180. New York: Thieme; 1998.

Paget's Disease Involving the Skull Base

41

Key Points

- *Definition*: A chronic progressive problem where aberrant osteoclasts and osteoblasts result in radical remodeling of bone. This hodgepodge of osteoclastic and osteoblastic commotion creates a surprising dichotomy showing simultaneous osseous enlargement and weakening.
- *Classic Clue*: Older patient presents with enlarging hat size, and examination may exhibit one of the following: loss of hearing, vision, and other sensory and motor functions including weakness, paralysis, or incontinence.
- *AKA*: Osteitis deformans, Paget's disease of bone, Paget disease.
- Osteoporosis circumscripta is frequently found in the frontal bone.
- Prevalence of Paget's disease (PD):
  - I. Its prevalence of 4% over age 40 increases to >10% by age 80 [7].
  - II. Interestingly, the demographic distribution of Paget's disease is exceptionally elevated in Great Britain where it was originally described with its pathologic prevalence clearly tracking into countries colonized by the British, including Australia, New Zealand, and the United States [7].
  - III. In contradistinction, Paget's was unknown in Japan until 1921 and has shown interim increasing incidence. Well, travel actually does more than broaden horizons, doesn't it? [7]
- Age: Usually >40.
- Gender preference: M>F=3:2.
- Locations.
  - I. Paget's predominately involves the axial skeleton with most commonly affected sites being pelvis, spine, and skull.
  - II. Skull involvement:
    - ~50% of patients with PD show skull involvement [11].
    - Paget's originates in the occipital or frontal regions initially sparing the skull's vertex.
    - The osteolytic phase of osteoporosis circumscripta is frequently found in the frontal bone.
    - Paget's disease involves both inner and outer tables [1].

Complications

- Pathologic fractures.
- Malignant degeneration.
  - M>F=2:1 [7]. Age: 55–80 [7]
  - <1% of monostotic disease, ≤10% polyostotic Paget's disease
  - 60% osteosarcoma, 25% fibrosarcoma, 10% chondrosarcoma, <5% lymphoma and angiosarcoma [7]
- Associated GCT (giant cell tumors).
- Bone deformity secondary to chronic stress insufficiency with basilar impression.
- Paget's vascular shunting can cause high-output CHF.
- Paget's neurologic complications include [11]:
  - Basilar invagination causing hydrocephalus with dementia, gait apraxia, and urinary incontinence.
  - Epilepsy may result from compression of the cerebral hemispheres.
  - While Paget's can compromise any cranial nerve, involvement of olfactory and auditory nerves is most frequent:

    CN I: Paget's affecting the cribriform plate can cause anosmia.

    CN II. Compression of the optic nerves' vasa nervorum can cause papilledema, retinal hemor-

F. A. Midyett, S. K. Mukherji, *Skull Base Imaging*, https://doi.org/10.1007/978-3-030-46447-9_41

rhage, optic atrophy, angioid streaking, and blindness.

CN III, IV, and VI: Involvement of these nerves as they pass through the superior orbital fissure impairs eye movement producing pupillary abnormalities and diplopia.

CN V: Lesions involving the trigeminal nerve can cause facial numbness and trigeminal neuralgia.

CN VII: Involvement of the facial nerve can cause hemifacial spasm or paresis.

CN VIII: Irreversible hearing loss is found in 13% of patients with Paget's involving the skull base.

CN IX, X, XI, and XII may be involved with basilar invagination.

Etiology

I. Sir James Paget proposed in 1877 an inflammatory etiology.
II. Subsequently, many proposed a "viral" etiology using the presence (in Paget's disease specimens) of osteoclastic intranuclear inclusion bodies as a "smoking gun." Yet, well over a century later, no offending virus has been discovered.
III. But genetic connections have been recognized, and while they seem somewhat complicated, we are finally beginning to "connect the dots."
IV. See section entitled "Genetics and Associations".

Imaging

General Imaging Features

- Paget's can produce a plethora of imaging patterns related to the various pathologic states of this complex process.
- Because Paget's can concurrently cause differing disease phases, it can cause a disorganized thickened trabecular "mosaic" or "jigsaw" pattern [7].
- Paget's displays diploic widening with involvement of *BOTH* inner and outer tables.
- Bone softening promotes basilar impression in about one third of patients with PD of the skull [10].
- Paget's healing phase promotes mixed lytic-sclerotic lesions which frequently flaunt their conspicuous *cotton wool* facade [1].
- The external auditory canal can become stenotic and tortuous.
- Although uncommon, facial bone involvement can occur with PD [1].
- Paget's disease demonstrates three distinct phases:
  I. Lytic Phase
    - Early lytic Paget's disease reflects unopposed osteoclastic activity.
    - Diminished osteoblastic activity causes well-defined lucent lytic lesions to lack sclerotic margins, particularly in the calvarium.
    - Most frequently found in the frontal and occipital bones.
    - Both inner and outer calvarial tables are affected, more extensively involving the inner tables. (This is in complete contradistinction to FD which predominately affects the outer table.)
    - Early changes consisting of *trabecular coarsening* and prominence may be seen in the late incipient or active lytic phases [7].

  II. Mixed Phase
    - Most Paget's disease discerned by radiologists is mixed phase.
    - Frequent findings consist of characteristic cortical coarsening and trabecular thickening [7].
    - Paget's presents its prototypical "picture frame" appearance in the spine during its mixed phase.

  III. Blastic Phase
    - Bony enlargement is particularly prominent in the blastic phase.
    - Sclerotic sections sometimes become distinguishing features with osteoblastic areas crossing some skull sutures.
    - Edges of prior osteoporosis circumscripta may become sclerotic progressing to focal opacity portraying the classic "cotton wool" appearance.
    - The "Tam O'Shanter skull" demonstrates dramatic calvarial enlargement featuring dramatic diploic space widening, particularly involving the inner table [7].
    - The "Tam O'Shanter" Scottish hat was made famous by Robert Burn's namesake poem. Patients afflicted with advanced Paget's often appear reminiscent of those hats [7].
    - Skull base softening produces *platybasia*, which when combined with conspicuous calvarial enlargement creates an appearance that the skull is falling down over face, much like a Tam O'Shanter hat falling over someone's head.

CT Findings

- *See General Imaging Features.*
  - Radiology forms the foundation for Paget's disease diagnosis portraying pathognomonic findings which reflect this predictable pathologic process [7].
- Skull Base and Calvarium:
  - Lytic lesions display a dearth of normal trabeculae.
  - Classically causes conspicuous cortical and trabecular thickening.
  - Osteoporosis circumscripta is more frequently found in the frontal bone.
  - Paget's healing phase frequently flaunts its conspicuous "cotton wool" facade [1].
  - "Pagetoid" changes classically avoid the anterior and central skull base, nose, sinuses, and mandible.
  - Frequently find frenzied cortical and trabecular thickening with scattered sclerosis in the blastic phase.
  - Paget's marrow can contain more fat than the adjacent uninvolved marrow.
  - Typically shows no cortical destruction or associated soft tissue mass.
- Temporal Bone:
  - As is frequently found with Paget's Disease, appearances change over time.
  - Early changes depict a diffuse lytic labyrinthine process. In later phases, these same areas show ↑ attenuation.
  - The lytic phase commences medially in the petrous apex, proceeding laterally.
  - There is thinning of the otic capsule (see Fig. 41.1a).
  - The middle ear cavity can be contracted by Paget's Disease.

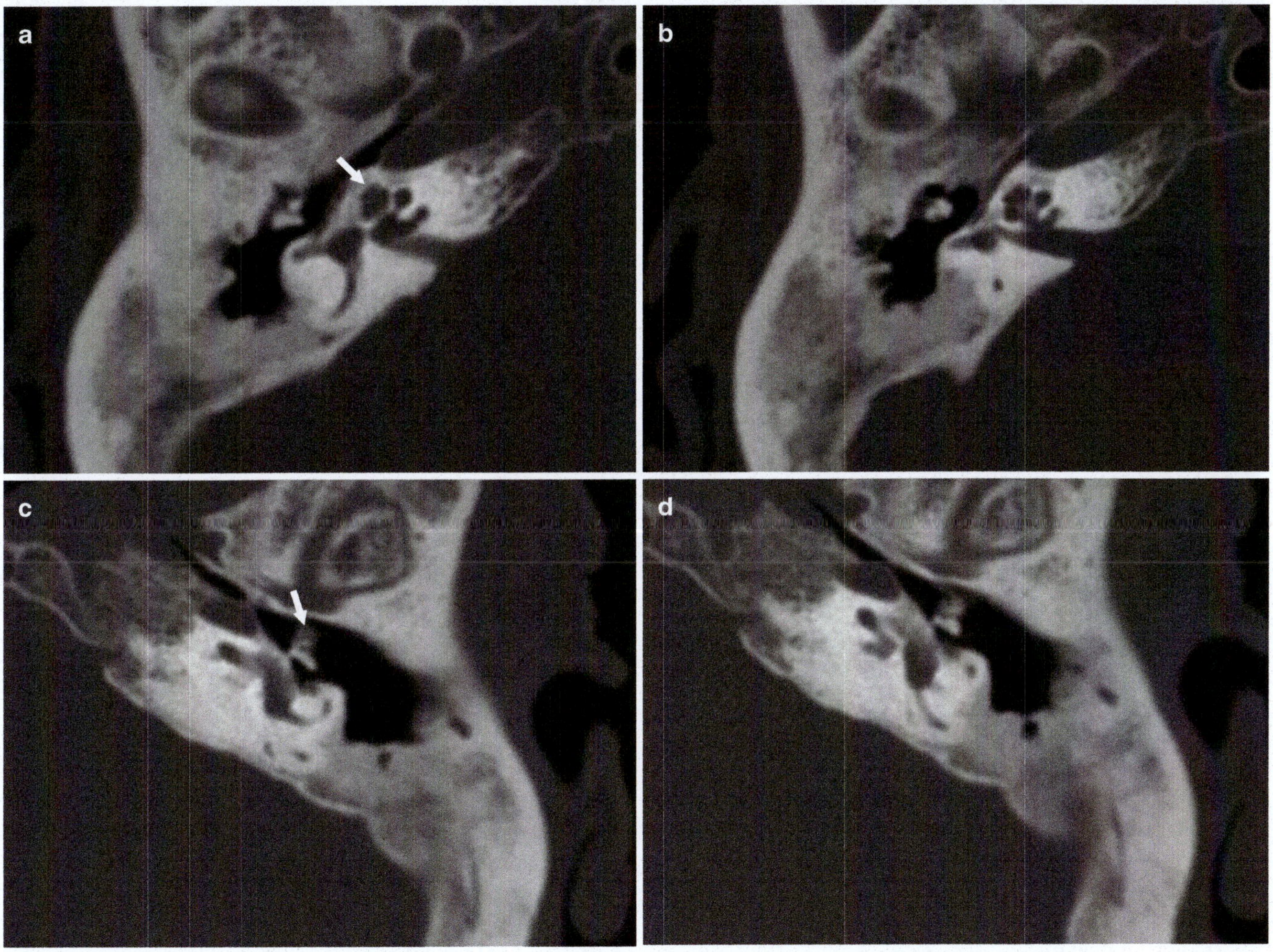

Fig. 41.1 (**a-d**) Axial temporal bone CT shows diffuse, uniform thickening of the squamous and petrous temporal bones typical for Paget's disease of bone. The otic capsule is indistinct and thinned anteriorly on right on Figure (**a**) (at lightning bolt). The ossicles confirm pagetoid changes best appreciated on Figure (**c**) (at lightning bolt)

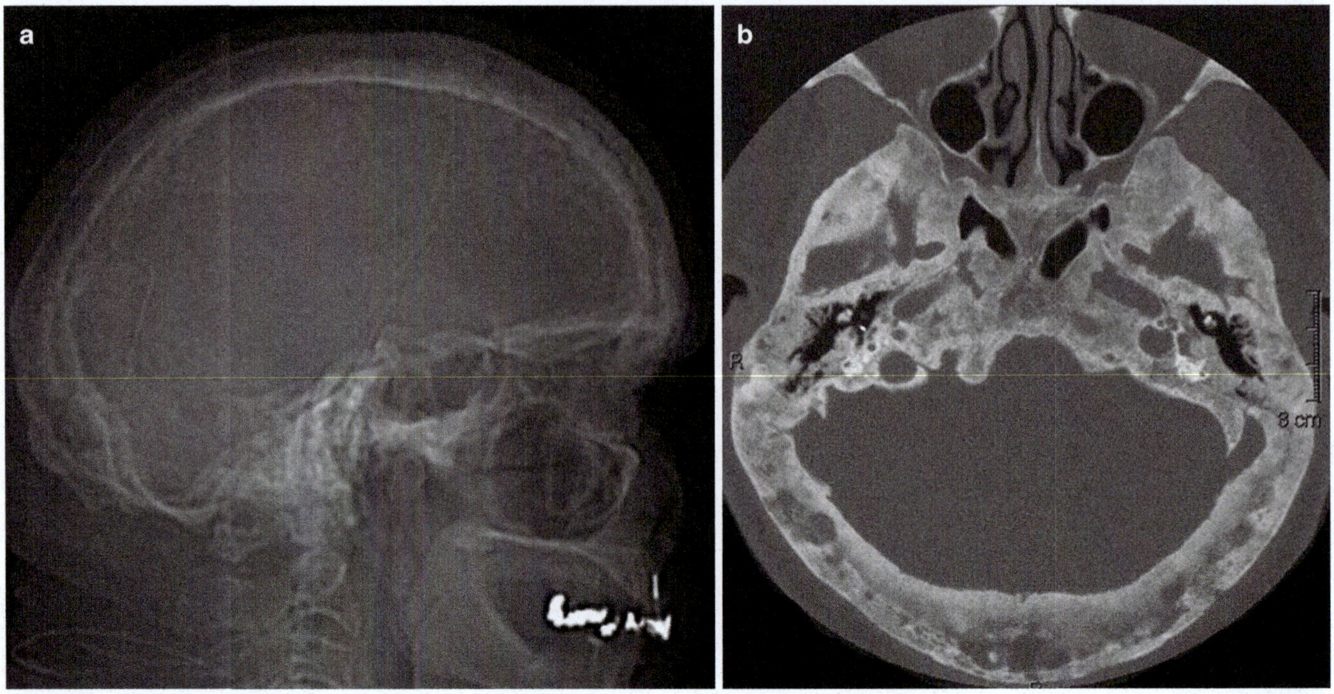

Fig. 41.2 (**a**) Lateral skull radiograph shows classic generalized pagetoid changes causing characteristic skull base softening with basilar impression. We could further evaluate this patient with a midline sagittal CT using conventional Chamberlain, McGregor, and McRae's lines. This patient already has an enlarging head circumference with pulsatile tinnitus and appears headed to development of a classic Tam O'Shanter as he ages. (**b**) Axial CT through the skull base showing classic pagetoid changes exhibiting dramatic diploic space expansion, with generalized cortical and trabecular thickening but without cortical destruction. For Figure (**a**) and (**b**), we wish to thank. C. Douglas Phillips, MD, FACR, Professor of Radiology, Director of Head and Neck Imaging, Weill Cornell Medicine, Department of Radiology, NewYork-Presbyterian Hospital

- Just remember Paget's begins peripherally proceeding centrally whereas cochlear otosclerosis starts centrally spreading outwardly.
- Sometimes see pagetoid changes involving the ossicles (see Fig. 41.1a–d).

MRI

- *See General Imaging Features.*

T1:

- T1 signal of Paget's varies depending on disease stage hinging on histologic marrow composition.
- Three general stages for non-complicated Paget's include:
  - I. Yellow Marrow Stage
    - "Atrophic marrow" of pagetoid bone can contain more fat than nearby normal bone.
  - II. "Speckled" Stage
    - Lytic to early mixed active phase.
    - Heterogeneous T1 and T2.
    - T1 ↓, similar to muscle with foci of normal and maintained yellow marrow. Finding this feature is important in excluding malignant transformation.
  - III. Sclerotic Stage
    - Late blastic phase.
    - Sclerotic marrow space shows low signal on all sequences.

T2:

- T2 has high heterogeneous signal, accentuated with water-sensitive pulse sequences.
- Corresponds to fibrovascular marrow replacement during more active phases.

FLAIR:

- Depends on disease phase. Mixed phase is heterogeneously hyperintense; blastic phase is hypointense.
- Paget's propensity for concurrent different disease phases can cause a potpourri of imaging signals.

T1 Gd:

- Increased blood flow causes increased enhancement compared to normal marrow.
- The active disease phase demonstrates more prominent enhancement favoring intracortical components.
- Intramedullary enhancement shows "speckled" enhancement.

Nuclear Medicine (NM):

- Radionuclide bone scans are useful in determining the disease's entire extent. Scintigraphy seems most valuable for detecting polyostotic disease distribution [7].
- Classically, scintigraphy shows increased uptake on all phases including blood flow, blood pool, and static images. While these findings are superbly sensitive, they are not significantly specific.
- Paget's is extremely "hot" in its lytic phase. However, inactive lesions can occasionally be "cold."
- Foci of Paget's tend to be *elongated* (as opposed to more characteristic circular myeloma or metastasis) [7].
- Scintigraphy sometimes seems "normal" while patients simultaneously show "abnormal" radiographic findings. These quiescent late phase lesions are asymptomatic in ≤75%.

Clinical Issues

Presentation

- 20% of all Paget's patients are initially asymptomatic [7].
- Some patients encounter an unexplained enlarging hat size, seemingly unassociated with an entry into politics.
- Patients usually show elevated serum alkaline phosphatase and urine hydroxyproline [7].
- Basilar impression narrows the foramen magnum and can cause cord compression, hydrocephalus, and/or brainstem/cerebellar compressive syndromes.
- Neural foraminal narrowing causes loss of hearing and vision as well as other sensory and motor functions including weakness, paralysis, and incontinence [7].
  - Can cause conductive or sensorineural hearing loss.
  - ~25% of patients with cranial Paget's suffer tinnitus or vertigo.

Treatment and Prognosis

Medical Treatments

1. Chelating Agents

- The word "chelation" is derived from Greek meaning "claw" and was used in 1920 by Morgan and Drew to liken a chelate to a great crustacean claw which grabbed hold and held on firmly.
- Bisphosphonates (diphosphonates) are frequently the first choice for Paget's. They encourage osteoclastic cell death inhibiting bone absorption and slowing bone loss. Oddly, patients responding to this therapy for osteoporosis often initially show little if any change in number of osteoclasts, and patients on long-term therapy often develop "giant osteoclasts" [8].
- Multiple bisphosphonates are currently available including etidronate disodium, pamidronate disodium, alendronate sodium, tiludronate disodium, risedronate sodium, and zoledronic acid.
- The principal differences between these medications involve the frequency and route of administration. All, however, are contraindicated in patients suffering severe renal disease.

2. Hormones

- Calcitonin is a hormone which inhibits osteoclastic activity and calcium resorption (both by the intestine and the renal tubules). Previously in common use, its application has decreased and is now employed primarily when hypocalcemia could be exacerbated by bisphosphonates.

3. Cytotoxic Agents

- Mithramycin is a cytotoxic antibiotic which inhibits RNA synthesis and is primarily toxic to osteoclasts. While useful in treating Paget's, it is typically toxic to other organs [6].
- Cytoxan is a cytotoxic chemotherapy "alkylating agent" which blocks production of cellular DNA acting as an immunosuppressant.

Surgery

- Prosthetic stapedectomies show inauspicious outcomes.
- Surgery for IAC stenosis has been hazardous.

Prognosis

- Temporal bone Paget's exhibits mixed conductive and sensorineural hearing deficits which may progress to total deafness.

Pathology

- Paget's exemplifies excessive, aberrant bone remodeling exhibiting both energetic and smoldering stages [7].
- Although histology provides us glances at the underlying complex changes, from the perspective of the areas involved, these changes can look more like the "War of the Worlds." And that doesn't include genetic and biochemical changes.
- While Paget's pathologic process probably proceeds in a comparative continuum, three typical phases have habitually been described including the following:

Lytic Phase

- Incipient → active.
- Osteoclasts predominate.
- Fibrovascular tissue begins to replace normal yellow marrow.
- Almost like in a science fiction story, we learn that the active phase of Paget's disease is characterized by "giant osteoclasts" which contain numerous nuclei.

Mixed Phase

- Active.
- Osteoblasts swarm the scene and eventually overcome the osteoclasts.
- Fibrovascular tissue marrow replacement ↓ in the early mixed phase.
- Normal yellow marrow gradually returns in the late mixed phase.

Blastic Phase

- Late → inactive.
- Osteoblastic activity gradually declines.
- The final inactive phase coincides with "atrophic marrow" having an actual ↑ marrow fat [7].

Differential Diagnosis

Clearly the differential diagnosis for Paget's disease varies with lesion size and depends on whether the mass is small confined to a limited skull base area (such as the temporal bone lesion shown), or a huge lesion boasting bizarre imaging features. For those later lesions, we must recollect that while sarcomatous transformation of Paget's is rare, it does occur. Furthermore, other lesions can be co-located with (or develop in) Paget's. Radiologists frequently face difficult decisions involving one or more of the following choices:

A. Fibrous Dysplasia [FD] [1]

- Fibrous dysplasia is a slowly progressing tumor-like process in which normal cancellous bone is replaced by immature woven bone and fibrous tissue.
- Fibrous dysplasia's fondness for the skull can cause serious skull base and orbital problems.
- Fibrous dysplasia falls into in three basic types: sclerotic, lytic, and mixed.
- Sclerotic lesions dominate the skull base with lytic lesions least likely. Fibrous dysplasia frequently demonstrates diffuse homogeneous osseous thickening.
- Fibrous dysplasia's matchless medullary cavity expansion conserves original bone shape while concurrently sparing its cortex.
- Classically, fibrous dysplasia displays a "ground-glass" appearance.
- While the cortex is classically preserved, severe expansion may cause the cortex to virtually *vanish.*
- Periosteal reaction raises a "red flag" for a pathological fracture or underlying malignant metamorphosis.
- Associated cystic degeneration near the orbit is a *red flag* foretelling a high incidence of visual impairment.
- Progressive lytic lesions suggest malignant degeneration.
- Tc^{99m} bone scans show ↑ uptake.
- CT:
  - FD expands bone keeping original shape while sparing the cortex.
  - Ground-glass appearance is "classic." When not classic "ground-glass" lesions may appear quite heterogeneous.
  - Clinicians frequently find 3D CT reconstructions to be useful pre-surgical planning roadmaps.

MRI:

- T1 is heterogeneous low to intermediate signal often isointense to brain.
- T2 is heterogeneous, usually low, often isointense to brain but may have regions of higher signal.
- T1 Gd exhibits *avid enhancement.*
- Cysts and hemorrhage can cause heterogeneous signals which vary depending on protein content and age of blood products.
- (See Chap. 25, Fibrous Dysplasia.)

B. Osteosarcoma (OSA)

- In 60% of Paget's sarcomatous transformations, the unfortunate outcome is osteosarcoma (OSA).
- After multiple myeloma, OSA is the second most frequent primary bone malignancy.
- Age: 10–30 years.
- Large lytic lesion with aggressive periosteal reaction sometimes showing a "sunburst sign" or "Codman's triangle."
- Cystic cavities can contain blood and/or necrosis which may mimic ABC (see Chap. 38, Aneurysmal Bone Cyst).
- Radiographic features include:
  - *No* medullary involvement!
  - Cortical thickening showing saucerization
  - Juxtacortical configuration with tumor closely connected to cortex
  - (See Chap. 50, Osteosarcoma)

C. Fibrosarcoma (FS)

- 25% of Paget's sarcomatous transformations fabricate fibrosarcomas.
- *Incidence:* FSs comprise <5% of all primary bone sarcomas. Comprising the second most common H&N sarcoma, they encompass ≤10% of that entire group, sometimes involving the skull base.
- *Distributions*: Mean age at diagnosis is 35 years, M>F.
- While typically osteolytic, depending on tumor stage, FSs can range from well-defined to ragged and moth-eaten.
- Periosteal reaction progresses to cortical destruction commonly extending into adjacent soft tissues.
- Fibrosarcoma attenuation is similar to nearby muscle.
- Most fibrosarcomas are well-circumscribed with 50% showing internal fibrous septae.
- Fibrosarcoma may be homogenous or heterogeneous.
- T1: Isointense to muscle.
- T2: Heterogeneous hyperintense to muscle with multiple foci of high T2 signal conceivably correlating to collagen collections.
- T1 Gd: *Avid enhancement* may be homogeneous or heterogeneous.
- NM: Scintigraphy shows ↑ uptake on bone scans.
- (See Chap. 48, Skull Base Fibrosarcoma.)

D. Chondrosarcoma (CS)

- 10% of Paget's sarcomatous transformations cause chondrosarcoma.
- Chondrosarcomas are chondroid malignancies which commonly select a synchondrosis when involving the skull base.
- *Classic Clue*: Skull base mass exhibiting an affinity for the POF (petro-occipital fissure) sometimes showing chondroid matrix, characterized by low T1 and high T2 signals.
- Chondrosarcomas appear as well-circumscribed, often scalloped, or lobulated lytic lesions exhibiting chondroid calcifications.
- Age: 10–79 years (mean 39).
- Low attenuation may make them subtle on brain soft tissue algorithms.
- T2: *Very high T2 signal.*
- (See Chap. 46, S1, Skull Base Chondrosarcoma.)

E. Giant Cell Tumor (GCT)

- Giant cell tumors are lytic, locally aggressive expansile tumors characterized by regular recurrence and sporadic metastasis. While mostly benign, 5–10% are malignant.
- Age: GCTs are frequently found in third and fourth decades.
- Gender preference: F>M. When 5–10% undergo malignant transformation, the sex preference shifts to males with M>F=3:1.
- Cranial GCTs often omit their characteristic "soap bubble" appearance seen in long bones.
  - GCTs generally appear as nonspecific expansile lytic lesions lacking a sclerotic margin with their contiguous cortex thinned, expanded, or breached. Periosteal reaction is present in ~25%.
  - GCT exhibits no bony matrix mineralization or calcification.
  - CECT shows slightly hyperdense homogeneous postcontrast enhancement.
  - Frequently find a soft tissue mass with nearly half exhibiting extraosseous involvement.
- T1 and T2 typically are isointense to gray matter, but signal sometimes is ↓ by hemosiderin and/or fibrous components.
- T1:
  - Solid components show heterogeneous signal similar to cortical brain.
  - Frequently find multiple cystic components flaunting fluid-fluid levels.
- T2:
  - Solid components are isointense to cortical brain.
  - Cystic components may show high signal (similar to vitreous) which may layer on top of lower signal fluid. Typically, adjacent brain *shows no edema.*
- T1 Gd:
  - Enhancement varies but often exhibits avid enhancement of solid components. Heterogeneity varies proportional to the cystic component content.
- DWI: Demonstrates restricted diffusion.
- NM: Uptake characteristically involves the lesions periphery and contains central photopenia demonstrating a *doughnut sign.*
- See Chap. 24, Giant Cell Tumor

F. Metastatic Neoplasm

- Metastatic neoplasm can cause a destructive mass anywhere along the skull base.
- Frequently find *multiple metastases* in patients having recognized primary neoplasms.
- In children, metastatic neuroblastoma should be considered in the differential.

G. Hyperparathyroidism (HPT)

- Sometimes shows a "ground-glass" appearance with mottled demineralization.
- Indistinct cortical margins of vascular grooves.
- HPT's "brown tumor" is rare but can cause focal destruction.
- HPT habitually has multiple skull defects.
- Radiologists must conscientiously search for subperiosteal absorption on hand radiographs and loss of lamina dura on images which include teeth.

A Closer Look

I. Genetics and Associations

- Two genes, SQSTM1 and RANK, as well as specific regions of chromosomes 5 and 6 are associated with Paget's disease of bone [3, 4].
- Paget's patients may or may not possess a positive family history (FH) for the disease.
- While 50% of patients with an inherited type of Paget's have a mutation of SQSTM1 [which encodes protein (p52) involved in regulation of osteoclastic function], 10–15% of patients with a negative FH also harbor an analogous mutation [2].
- Paget's is also associated with mutations in RANK (receptor activator of nuclear factor kappa B) [5].
- RANKL is an osteoclastic cell surface receptor that binds to RANK. RANKL is a type II membrane protein and a member of the tumor necrosis factor superfamily. RANKL controls bone regeneration and remodeling [5].
- Perspective: So, try not to be confused. Paget's is associated with RANK mutations. RANK is normally bound to RANKL which controls bone regeneration and remodeling. Sounds like a confirmed conspiracy here. And it looks like we have come a long way since 1877 when Sir James Paget first described this disease and thought it was inflammatory. Sure, many seem slow to look past a potential "slow virus" etiology, even though no one has yet found an associated virus, either fast or slow. Just hang on for a while folks; we are getting there!

II. Potpourri

A. Basilar Invagination, Basilar Impression, and Platybasia
   - While the terms basilar invagination and basilar impression are regularly employed interchangeably, purists want us to know: basilar invagination causes cephalic relocation of the vertebral elements into a foramen magnum with "normal bone," while basilar impression signifies similar displacement secondary to skull base softening.
   - Platybasia is abnormal skull base flattening (with a skull base angle >143^0 using lateral skull radiography).
   - Modified MRI technique [12]:
   - This technique is probably more pertinent for today's neuroradiologists.
   - Normal values 116^0–118^0 for adults and 113^0–115^0 for children.
   - Angle is formed by two easy lines:
     1. Line across anterior cranial fossa to dorsum's tip
     2. Line across posterior margin of clivus

B. Changing Prevalence

- Well, now for the good news/bad news section. We will start with the bad news first.
- Bad News: Paget's disease is second only to osteoporosis, as the bone disease most frequently found in the escalating elderly US population [9].
- Good News: The prevalence of Paget's disease appears to be decreasing around the world with a 50% decline over the last two decades [9].

III. Historic Highlights

- 1865: Boogaard extensively examined platybasia using angular measurements while studying basilar invagination [12].
- 1877: Sir James Paget, English surgeon and pathologist, first described PD in a small group of patients who had an "odd overgrowth" of their heads and extremities, often resulting in long bone bowing and fractures[7] (see Figs. 41.3a and 41.4a).
- Together with Rudolf Virchow, Paget is considered to be one of the founding fathers of scientific medical pathology.
- While readers readily recognize Paget's disease of bone, we should also remember Paget's disease of the nipple, extramammary Paget's disease, and Paget's abscess were named for this prominent medical pioneer.
- Oh yes, Sir James's friends included Charles Darwin and Thomas Henry Huxley. Wow!

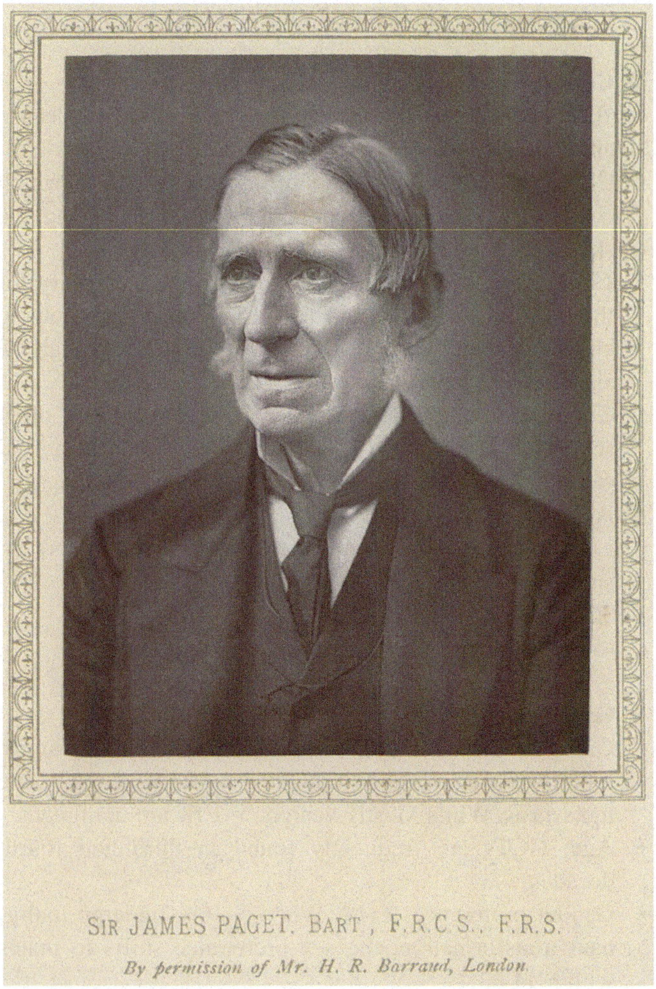

Fig. 41.3 (a) Portrait of Sir James Paget. Ref. Wikimedia

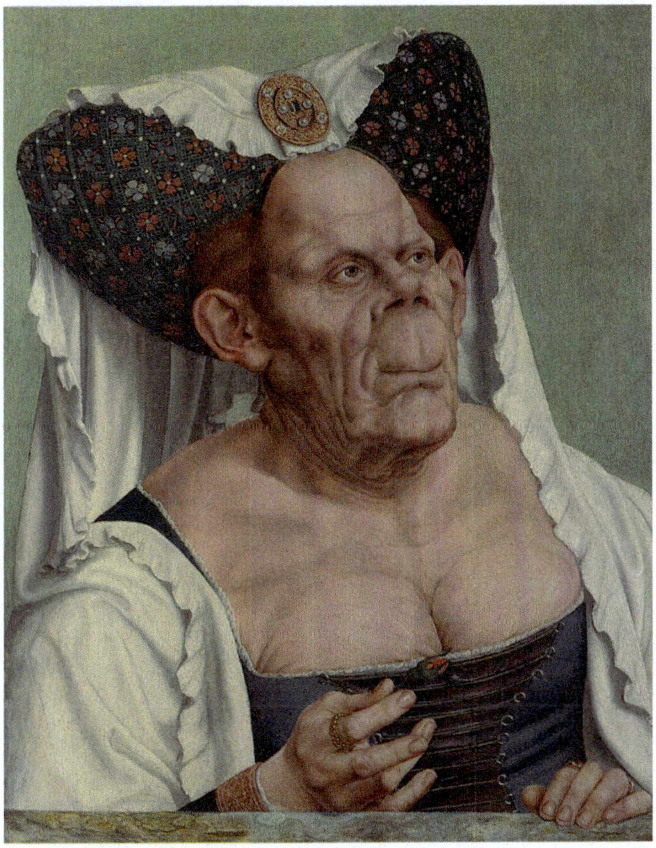

Fig. 41.4 (**a**) Portrait of the "Ugly Duchess". Flemish painter Quinten Matsys, probably intended to satirize older women who try to recreate youth but inadvertently depicted a woman who suffered from Paget's disease of bone in 1513, over three and a half centuries before Sir James Paget described the pathologic process which bears his name. Ref. Wikimedia

Selected References

1. Midyett FA, Mukherji SK. Fibrous dysplasia. Orbital imaging: Elsevier/Saunders; 2015. p. 241–6. ISBN: 978-0-323-34037-3.
2. Ralston SH. Paget's disease of bone. N Engl J Med. 2013;368(7):644–50. https://doi.org/10.1056/NEJMcp1204713.
3. Ralston SH, Langston AL, Reid IR. Pathogenesis and management of Paget disease of bone. Lancet. 2008;372(9633):155–63. https://doi.org/10.1016/S0140-6736(08)61035-1.
4. Whyte MP. Paget's disease of bone and genetic disorders of RANKL/OPG/RANK/NF-kappaB signaling. Ann N Y Acad Sci. 2006;1068:143–64. https://doi.org/10.1196/annals.1346.016. PMID 16831914.
5. Haslam SI, Van Hul W, Morales-Piga A, et al. Paget's disease of bone: evidence for a susceptibility locus on chromosome 18q and for genetic heterogeneity. J Bone Miner Res. 1998;13(6):911 7. https://doi.org/10.1359/jbmr.1998.13.6.911. PMID 9626621.
6. Ryan WG. Treatment of Paget's disease of bone with mithramycin. Clin Orthop Relat Res. 1977;127:106–10.
7. Smith SE, Murphey MD, Motamedi K, et al. From the archives of the AFIP. Radiologic spectrum of Paget disease of bone and its complications with pathologic correlation. Radiographics. 2002;22(5):1191–216.
8. Weinstein RS, Roberson PK, Manolagas SC. Giant osteoclast formation and long-term oral bisphosphonate therapy. N Engl J Med. 2009;360(1):53–62. https://doi.org/10.1056/NEJMoa0802633. PMC 2866022. PMID 19118304.
9. Theodorou DJ, Theodorou SJ, Kakitsubata Y. Imaging of Paget disease of bone and its musculoskeletal complications: review. AJR. 2011;2011:196. https://doi.org/10.2214/AJR.10.7222.
10. Tjon-A-Tham RTO, Bloem JL, Falke THM, et al. Magnetic resonance imaging in Paget disease of the skull. AJNR. 1985;6:879–81.
11. Poncelet A. The neurologic complications of Paget's disease. J Bone Miner Res. 1999;14(2):88–91.
12. Koenigsberg RA, Vakil N, Hong TA, et al. Evaluation of platybasia with MR imaging. AJNR. 2005;26:89–92.

Part VI

Posterior Cranial Fossa [PCF]

42 Posterior Fossa Arachnoid Cyst

Pertinent Points

- *Definition:* Extra-axial cystic posterior fossa mass following CSF on all imaging sequences with *no* restricted diffusion, which can cause conspicuous mass effect on adjacent structures, despite its almost imperceptible wall.
- *Etiology:* True arachnoid cysts arise from unexplained tearing or splitting of an already flimsy spider-like arachnoid membrane [1].
- *Classic Clue*: Non-enhancing fluid-filled posterior fossa mass with an almost imperceptible wall with mass effect on adjacent structures. Fluid follows CSF CT density and CSF MRI intensity with *no diffusion restriction.*
- *AKA*: Intracranial arachnoid cyst, subarachnoid cyst.
- *Gender Preference*: M > F: 3:1 [3, 5, 12, 6].
- *Location:* Intracranial arachnoid cysts (ACs) occur most frequently in the middle cranial fossa. A mere 10% occur in the posterior cranial fossa with the CPA comprising the most common infratentorial site [4]. PFACs fall into an even smaller subset of that group.
- PFACs are frequently found incidental imaging study findings which sometimes enlarge and show symptoms [7].

Imaging

General Imaging Features

- Smooth, cystic, extra-axial posterior fossa lesion exhibiting obvious extrinsic mass effect on adjacent structures.
- Characteristic arachnoid-like, thin, transparent cyst wall is scarcely seen on imaging.
- Classic appearance of midline PFAC displacing normally formed fourth ventricle anteriorly and cranially. (See Fig. 42.1a–f.)
- The fourth ventricle lies anterior to and is separate from the PFAC. (See Fig. 42.1a–f.)
- Nonclassical presentations include lateral locations and sites superior to cerebellum. (See Fig. 42.2a–d.)

CT Features

- See General Imaging Features.
- CT attenuation in Hounsfield units is usually identical to CSF. ↑ attenuation from hemorrhage or protein is rare.
- No postcontrast enhancement of fluid or cyst wall.
- Shows no calcifications.

MRI Features

- See General Imaging Features.
- T1: Usually isointense to CSF. (See Figs. 42.1a–d and 42.2a.)
- T2: Usually isointense to CSF. (See Figs. 42.1e, f and 42.2b, c.)
- T1 Gd: No enhancement.
- FLAIR: Suppresses completely.
- DWI:
  - Shows low signal with *no restricted diffusion.*
  - See Fig. 42.2d.

Clinical Issues

Presentation

- Symptoms:
  - Frequently found as an incidental MRI finding.

F. A. Midyett, S. K. Mukherji, *Skull Base Imaging*, https://doi.org/10.1007/978-3-030-46447-9_42

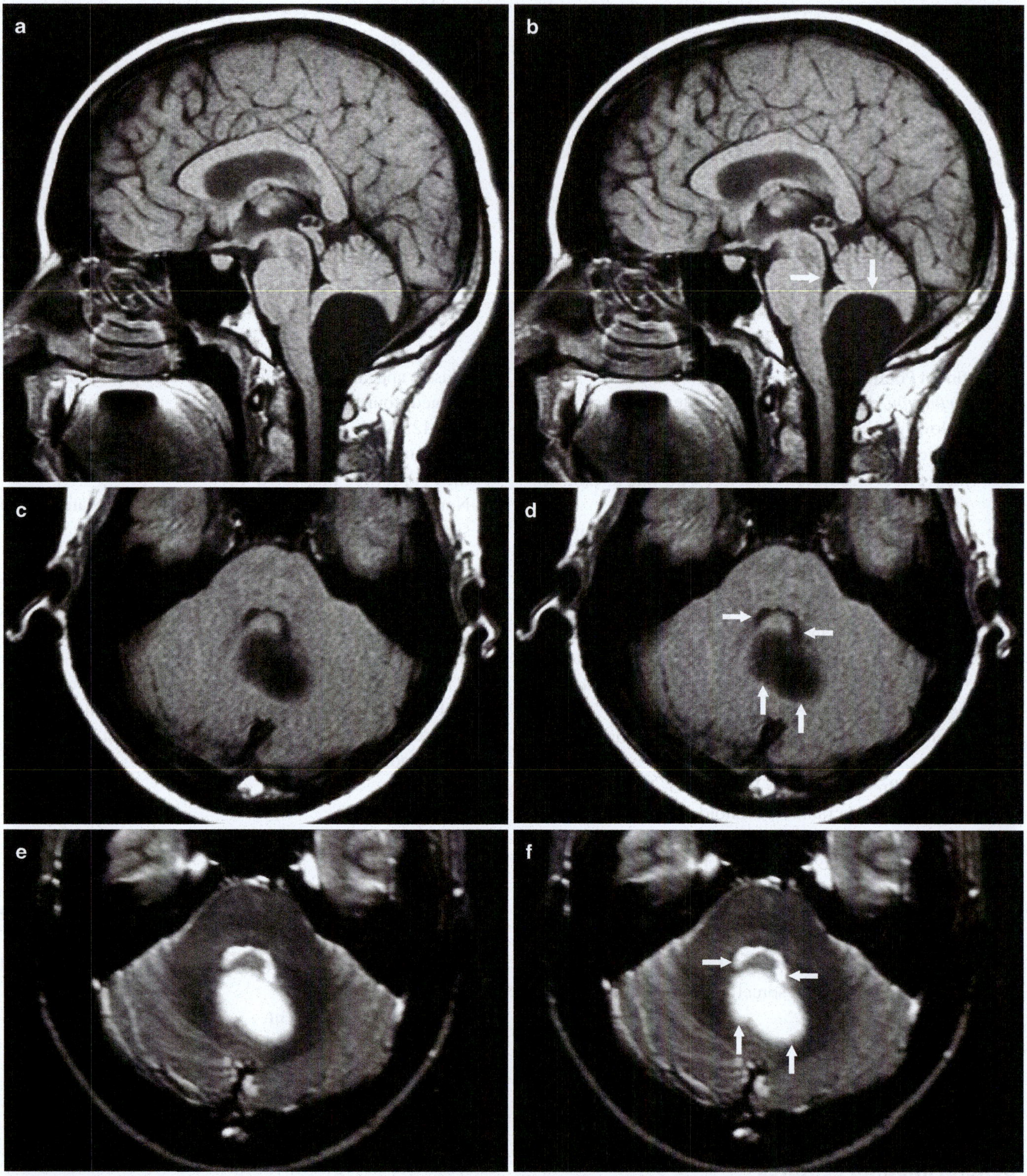

Fig. 42.1 Patient I. (**a**) Sagittal T1 shows classic appearance of midline PFAC displacing normally formed IV ventricle anteriorly and cranially. There is anterior displacement of the medulla and pons. Small incidental pineal region cysts. (**b**) Sagittal T1 with helper arrows shows normally formed IV ventricle (narrow →) with PFAC depicted by (wider ↓) arrow. Axial T1 (**c**, **d**) show fluid in the PFAC follows CSF on all sequences, being low on T1. Fluid in the IV ventricle is anterior to and is separate from the PFAC. [(**c**) Without and (**d**) with helper arrows. Arrows (→←) are on IV ventricle and ↑arrows are on the PFAC]. Axial T2 (**e**, **f**) again show fluid in cyst follows CSF on all imaging sequences. The IV ventricle lies anterior to and is separate from the PFAC. [(**e**) Without and (**f**) with helper arrows. Arrows (→←) on the IV ventricle and (↑) arrows are on the PFAC]

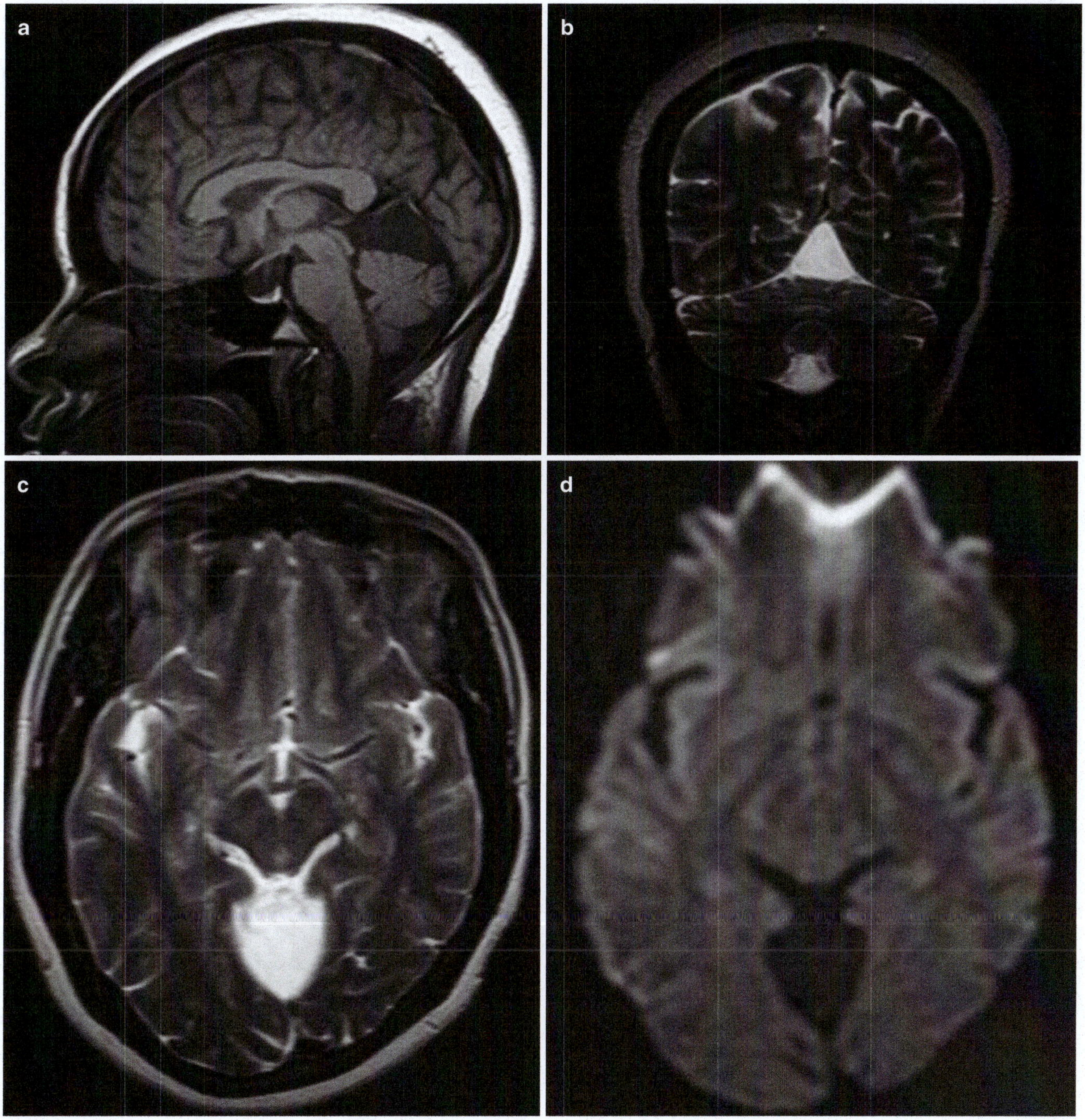

Fig. 42.2 Patient II. (**a**) Sagittal T1 shows low signal PFAC flattening the superior aspect of the cerebellum depressing it inferiorly. Normal-appearing IV ventricle. (**b**) Coronal T2 shows fluid-filled mass located caudal to the tentorium, depressing the cerebellum caudally. The thin arachnoid capsule is virtually invisible on these imaging techniques, but the flattened superior cerebellar hemisphere convinces us it is there. The partially empty sella is an incidental finding. (**c**) Axial T2 shows high-intensity signal fluid-filled mass located above the cerebellum, below the tentorium cerebelli. (**d**) Axial DWI shows *no* restricted diffusion effectively excluding an epidermoid. This is a less common presentation of midline supracerebellar PFAC than Case 1 infracerebellar PFAC (Fig. 42.1a, c, e)

- When symptomatic sometimes, see headache, dizziness, nausea, vomiting, seizures, and hydrocephalus.
- PFACs have been reported to cause hydrocephalus and tonsillar herniation [7].

Natural History

- The reported prevalence of MRI demonstrated intracranial arachnoid cysts in large university studies is 1.4% in adults [6] and 2.6% in children.
- Gender Preference: M > F = 3:1 [3, 5, 6, 12].
- May manifest at any age, but most are found in the first two decades of life [8].
- Only a few patients with arachnoid cysts show symptoms. Those who present without symptoms usually bear out a benign natural history [6].

Epidemiology and Pathology

- Intracranial arachnoid cysts which develop in the arachnoid mater (located between the superficial dura mater covering the skull and the deeper pia mater covering the brain) appear to arise from some strange splitting of this spindly shroud.
- Arachnoid cysts are benign CSF-filled masses enclosed by thin, translucent cyst walls.
- The cyst fluid is consistently clear and colorless, only occasionally having hemorrhage or ↑ protein [2].
- Arachnoid cysts may be congenital or acquired usually beginning in infancy although often not showing symptoms until adolescence or adulthood.
- Microscopically, the cyst wall has a vascular collagenous membrane lined by arachnoid cells [2] appearing histologically indistinguishable from the normal arachnoid membrane [10].
- Progressive enlargement of arachnoid cysts has prompted theories including (1) active cyst wall secretion of fluid, (2) osmotic gradient diffusion of fluid into cyst, and (3) a "ball-valve" mechanism.

Treatment

- Most require no treatment although they enjoy excellent prognosis when treatment is required.
- Surgical therapy is reserved for cases where symptoms are clearly linked to PFAC with ↑ ICP or mass effect [9].
- Surgical options include fenestration, shunting, needle aspiration, and marsupialization [2].
- Endoscopic fenestration offers an option for effective minimally invasive treatment [9].

Differential Diagnosis

The differential for a cystic posterior fossa mass lesion (in addition to PFAC) includes the following:

A. Epidermoid Cyst (EC)

- Epidermoids show *restricted diffusion* and are bright on DWI with dark signal on the corresponding ADC map. This is not a feature of PFACs which follow CSF on all imaging sequences.
- Epidermoids are rare in children [2].
- See Chap. 9, Epidermoid Cyst.

B. Dandy-Walker Malformation (DWM)

- Classic triad: complete or partial vermian agenesis, cystic dilation of the IV ventricle, and enlarged posterior fossa [8].
- DWM shows cystic dilation of the IV ventricle. PFAC shows a midline mass displacing a normally formed IV ventricle anteriorly and cranially. (See Fig. 42.1a–f.)
- DWM contains cystic dilation of the IV ventricle. PFAC has an intrinsically normal IV ventricle anterior to and separate from the offending PFAC. (See Fig. 42.1a–f.)
- Dandy-Walker variant (DWV) is the main moniker used when the anomaly appears to fall short of the complete criteria for DWM.

C. Mega Cisterna Magna (MCM)

- Finding a fully developed cerebellar vermis limits the differential to PFAC and MCM (mega cisterna magna).
- MCM characteristically causes *no* mass effect on the cerebellar vermis. Typically, PFAC causes mass effect.
- Differentiation of MCM from PFAC may be problematic when MCM is asymmetric with "apparent" mass effect [8].

D. Cerebellar Hypoplasia

- Typically shows severely small cerebellum sitting amid a standard-sized fluid-filled posterior fossa [13].
- Habitually have a hypoplastic pons and medulla as well.

E. Neurenteric (NE) Cyst

- Rare benign endodermal lesions which may be mistaken for other more common non-neoplastic cysts or cystic neoplasms.
- AKA: enterogenous cyst, enteric cyst, endodermal cyst, etc.
- Locations: 3:1 = spine: brain; posterior fossa > supratentorial.
- T1: variable – iso- to hyperintense depending on proteinaceous fluid content (which ↑ T1 signal) [1].
- T2 signal is also variable.
- T1 Gd: non-enhancing cystic components; ± partial rim enhancement.

- Neurenteric cysts have been reported to *rarely* cause *partial* diffusion restriction. This suggests we should place this in our differential as a "long shot" when restriction of diffusion is *partial* [1] in a posterior fossa cyst.

F. Cystic Neoplasms

1. Astrocytomas
   - Astrocytomas comprise 1% of CPA masses.
   - Astrocytomas are exophytic exhibiting moderate postcontrast enhancement.
   - Astrocytomas can appear cystic.
     – Usually not a perfectly smooth, thin wall like an AC.
     – Frequently find rim enhancement with astrocytomas [2].
2. Ependymomas
   - Ependymomas can appear cystic.
     – Usually not a perfectly smooth, thin wall like an AC.
     – Usually show rim enhancement [2].
   - Ependymomas pedunculate from the brainstem showing some focus of enhancement.

G. Parasitic Cysts

- Cyst wall usually enhances [2].
- Cysts are usually <1 cm.
- Cysts are usually in subarachnoid space or ventricles.
- Includes:
  A. Neurocysticercosis (NCC)
    - Calcifications are common.
    - Look for scolex.
    - Ependymitis and basilar meningitis are commonly associated.
    - Frequently find multiple lesions within the cisterns and brain parenchyma.
    - Most are <1 cm.
    - They don't typically crop up in clusters.
    - Their cyst walls often enhance.
    - *Imaging finding depends on disease stage:* vesicular, colloidal vesicular, granular nodular, and nodular calcified.

  B. Hydatid Cysts
    - AKA: echinococcosis, hydatid disease, hydatidosis, or echinococcal disease.
    - Uni- or multilocular.
    - Almost all are in children.
    - Daughter cysts are common.
    - Calcification is rare and found in <1%.
    - Typically, exhibit *no* enhancement on CECT.
    - T1 cyst is isointense to CSF.
    - T2 cyst is isointense to CSF with *hypointense rim* and *no peri-lesional edema*.
    - T1 Gd typically shows *no internal enhancement*, ± fine peripheral enhancement.

A Closer Look

I. Fast Facts

- Arachnoid cysts cause ≤2.6% of intracranial space-occupying lesions [6].
- PFACs probably arise from incomplete separation of the endomenix during early embryogenesis [9].

II. Historic Highlights

- In 1831 Richard Bright first described arachnoid cysts [11]. Yes, this is the same Bright we remember for "albuminuric nephritis" as Bright's disease. The brilliance of Bright's pioneering descriptions appears even more amazing when you consider he didn't have the help of a microscope or even formaldehyde for tissue preservation.
- 1958 Starkman reported arachnoid cysts lay between two normal arachnoid layers describing them as "intra-arachnoid" cysts.
- 1907 Placzek and Krause successfully surgically treated an arachnoid cyst.
- 1981 Stein advocated shunting as the primary treatment for arachnoid cysts.

III. *Genetics and Associations*

- The current consensus continues to counsel that arachnoid cysts arise from "unexplained tearing" of arachnoid membranes.
- The precise primary elemental etiology enigmatically endures. Acknowledged associations include agenesis of the corpus callosum, arachnoiditis, mucopolysaccharidosis, and, of course, the Chudley-McCullough and Marfan's syndromes.
- Reports of intracranial arachnoid cysts in siblings suggest some familial cases where inheritance is influenced by an autosomal recessive or polygenic pattern [14–17].

References

1. Preece MT, Osborn AG, Chin SS, Smirniotopoulos JG. Intracranial neurenteric cysts: imaging and pathologic spectrum. Am J Neuroradiol. 2006;27:1211–6.
2. Fischbein NJ, Dillon WP, Barkovich AJ. Teaching atlas of brain imaging. New York: Thieme; 2000. p. 78–81.
3. Osborne AG. Diagnostic neuroradiology. St. Louis: Mosby; 199463-8. p. 639–42.
4. Rengacharry SS, Watanabe I, Brackett CE. Pathogenesis of intracranial arachnoid cysts. Surg Neurol. 1978;9:139–44.
5. Robertson SJ, Wolpert SM, Runge VM. MR imaging of middle cranial fossa arachnoid cysts: temporal lobe agenesis syndrome revisited. AJNR Am J Neuroradiol. 1989;10:1007–10.

6. Al-Holou WN, Terman S, Kilburg C. Prevalence and natural history of arachnoid cysts in adults. J Neurosurg. 2013;118(2):222–31.
7. Kurabe S, Sasaki O, Mitsuhashi D, et al. Growing posterior fossa arachnoid cyst causing tonsillar herniation and hydrocephalus. JAMA Neurol. 2011;68(12):1606–7.
8. Kollias SS, Ball WS, Prenger EC. Cystic malformations of the posterior fossa: differential diagnosis clarified through embryologic analysis. Radiographics. 1993;13:1211–31.
9. Gazioglu N, Kafadar AM, Tanriover N, et al. Endoscopic management of posterior fossa arachnoid cyst in an adult: case report and technical note. Turk Neurosurg. 2010;20(4):512–8.
10. Miyagami M. Tsunokawa: histological and ultrastructural findings of benign intracranial cysts. Noshuyo Byori. 1993;10:151–60.
11. Bright R. Serous cysts in the arachnoid. In: Rees, Orme, Brown, Green, editor. Diseases of the brain and nervous system. Part I. London: Longman Group Ltd; 1831. p. 437–9.
12. Al-Holou WN, Yew AY, Boomsaad ZE, et al. Prevalence and natural history of arachnoid cysts in children clinical article. J Neurosurg Pediatr. 2010;5(6):578–85.
13. Patel S, Barkovich AJ. Analysis and classification of cerebellar malformations. Am J Neuroradiol. 2002;23:1074–87.
14. Handa J, Okamoto K, Sato M. Arachnoid cyst of the middle cranial fossa: report of bilateral cysts in siblings. Surg Neurol. 1981;16:127–130. [PubMed: 7280984, related citations] [Full Text].
15. Helland CA, Wester K. Monozygotic twins with mirror image cysts: indication of a genetic mechanism in arachnoid cysts? Neurology. 2007;69:110–111. [PubMed: 17606888, related citations] [Full Text].
16. Pomeranz S, Constantini S, Lubetzki-Korn I, Amir N. Familial intracranial arachnoid cysts. Childs Nerv Syst. 1991;7:100–102. [PubMed: 1863926, related citations] [Full Text].
17. Wilson WG, Deponte KA, McIlhenny J, Dreifuss FE. Arachnoid cysts in a brother and sister. J Med Genet. 1988;25:714–5. [PubMed: 3225827, related citations] [Full Text].

Posterior Fossa Meningioma

43

Pertinent Points

- *Definition:* Meningiomas are nonglial tumors which arise from arachnoidal cap cells in the arachnoidal membrane. Posterior fossa meningiomas (PFMs) comprise a particularly problematic group of <10% of intracranial meningiomas originating in the posterior fossa.
- *Classic Clue*: Extra-axial, usually solid benign posterior fossa mass with broad base abutting a dural surface. Enhancing "dural tail" is classic but not pathognomonic.
- Usually seen in middle-aged to elderly patients but can be seen in children as well.
- Meningioma's Overall Incidence: F > M = 2:1. Posterior Fossa Meningioma's Incidence: F > M = 3.3:1 [1].
- Meningiomas are the most common nonglial primary brain tumors.
- Meningiomas comprise the most common intracranial extra-axial neoplasms in adults.
- PFMs are slow growing, often becoming large before showing symptoms, and are frequently found on incidental imaging studies.
- Meningiomas constitute 20% of all intracranial tumors. PFMs comprise <10% of all intracranial meningiomas [2–5].
- 20% of meningiomas occur in the posterior fossa most commonly arising from the clivus or petrous temporal bone [2, 6].
- 2% of intracranial meningiomas have no dural attachment, arising from the choroid plexus and tela choroidea as intraventricular masses [6].

Imaging

General Imaging Features

- Sharply circumscribed round or smoothly lobulated extra-axial mass, broad based against the dura, often at an obtuse angle.

CT Features

- See *General Imaging Features*.
- *Density:*
  - *Typically:* About ¾ are hyperdense with most of the rest isodense to adjacent brain.
  - *Potential Pitfall:* A few can be hypodense to brain with the occasional lipoblastic or xanthomatous tumor sometimes showing negative attenuation numbers.
  - *Enhancement:* Exhibit exuberant postcontrast enhancement.
- *Calcifications:*
  - Calcifications are demonstrated in about 25% and may be diffuse or focal.
  - Calcific patterns include rim-like, sandlike (psammomatous), sunburst, or globular.
- *Bony Attachment:*
  - CT shows osseous reaction at the point of tumor attachment in >50% of cases [7].
  - When positive, CT depicts localized hyperostosis and spur formation [7].
  - CT often outperforms MRI for demarcating the tumor's bony attachment. This is a finding important to the neurosurgeon [7].

F. A. Midyett, S. K. Mukherji, *Skull Base Imaging*, https://doi.org/10.1007/978-3-030-46447-9_43

MRI Features

- See *General Imaging Features*.
- T1: Most show heterogeneous low T1 signal (60%) (see Fig. 43.1c).
- T2: Most meningiomas show high signal on T2 (68%) (see Fig. 43.1a, b).
- T1 Gd:
  - All show enhancement with 83% avid and 17% moderate. (See Fig. 43.1d–f.)
  - >50% show a "dural tail" sign. (See Fig. 43.1e, f.)
  - The "dural tail" sign is frequent but nonspecific as it may be seen with any tumor which invades the dura or provokes a dural reaction. Dural tails usually represent hypervascular dural reaction rather than tangible tumor involvement [8].
- FLAIR: Most show high signal on FLAIR 69%.
- DWI:
  - DWI signal is variable and appears to correlate with histologic subtypes.
  - Atypical and malignant meningiomas have less extracellular space for water, reducing ADC values.
  - DWI appears to be a useful tool for separating atypical and malignant meningiomas from the more common benign meningiomas.
  - Most meningiomas are benign and are typically isointense/slightly hyperintense on both DWI and ADC.
  - Restricted diffusion should be a "red flag" when markedly hyperintense (light bulb bright) DW images correspond to hypointense (black hole) ADC maps. This suggests atypical or malignant meningioma [9].
- The most frequent associated findings are *dural tail sign* and *bone infiltration* [9].

Angiographic Features

- Most are dural-based, vascular tumors.
- May demonstrate a radial or "sunburst" pattern of vascular supply.
- Prominent, homogeneous prolonged vascular blush in late arterial and capillary phases.
- Shows Smirniotopoulos' "mother-in-law" sign. The blush "comes early and stays late."
- They sometimes show early draining veins. This is *not* a feature for hemangiopericytoma (HPC). (See DDx/ Section E. Hemangiopericytoma (HPC).

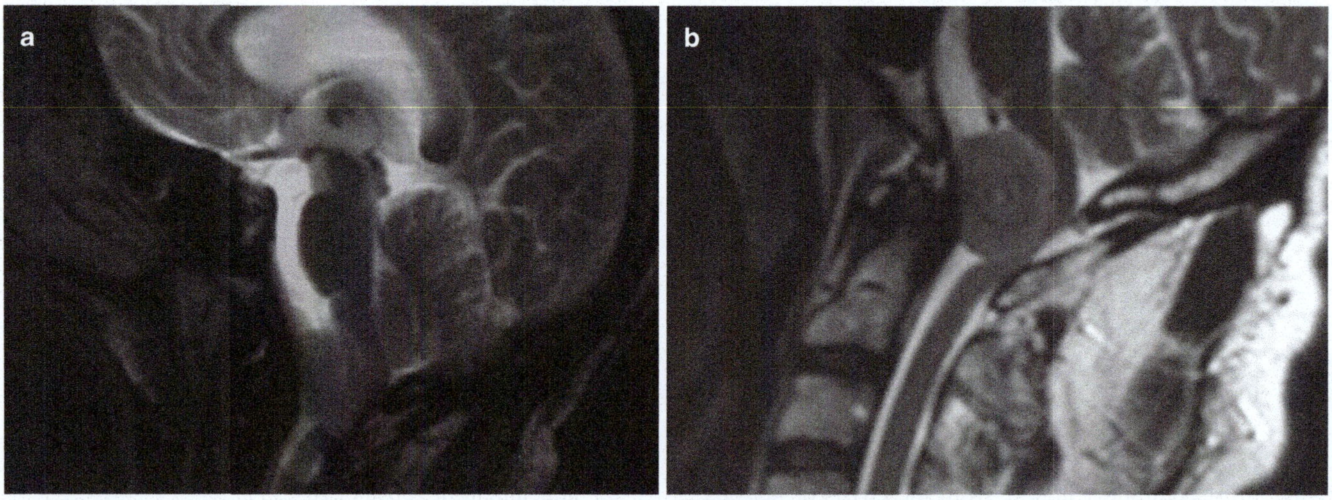

Fig. 43.1 (**a**, **b**) Sagittal T2 shows a large extra-axial craniovertebral junction mass which is relatively isointense to brain. It is relatively heterogeneous with a small area of high signal in its center probably related to necrosis. While well circumscribed and oval in shape, it has a broad base anteriorly which is quite flat. The medulla and cord are deformed and displaced posteriorly. (**c**) Sagittal T1 shows a large tumor causing mass effect on the adjacent medulla and cord displacing and flattening the cord. The mass is relatively isointense to the adjacent pons, medulla, and cord. There is a hint of dural involvement extending superiorly. The (dark) clival cortex appears relatively intact. (**d**) Axial T1 Gd exhibits avid enhancement of the large mass described in prior figures. The mass is fairly well circumscribed although somewhat irregular in outline. It causes significant mass effect on posteriorly displaced neural elements. (**e**) Sagittal T1 Gd shows avid enhancement of a large mass which displaces the adjacent medulla and spinal cord. The demonstrated "dural tail" is thickened and conspicuous with exuberant enhancement extending up the clivus and anteriorly into the sella. (**f**) Coronal T1 Gd shows avid enhancement of the large mass described in prior figures. The mass is well circumscribed and oval with a flattened facade along its left margin where it appears to be attached. Its center shows more enhancement than its periphery. A small "dural tail" extends along the left margin superiorly

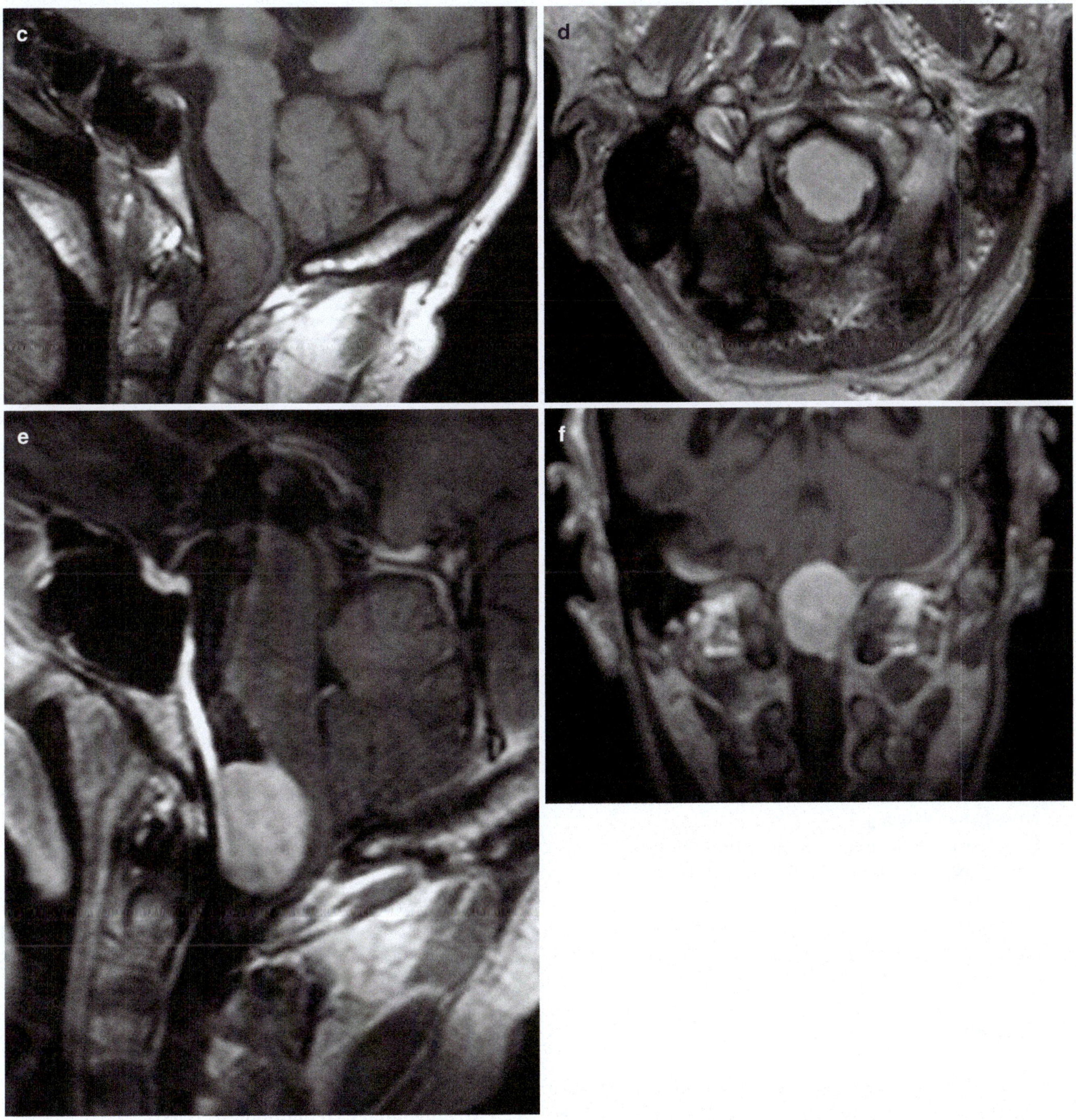

Fig. 43.1 (continued)

Clinical Issues

Presentation

- Frequently find features of ↑ ICP to be presenting symptoms [2].
- Most commonly present with headache [5].
- May demonstrate gait disturbance and cranial nerve dysfunctions.
- The most frequently involved cranial nerves are CN V and CN VIII.

Natural History

- Location, resectability, and histology are major determinants of clinical outcome.

- Posterior fossa meningiomas are generally slow growing and easily compress adjacent structures.
- Meningioma Incidence: F > M = 2:1. PFM Incidence: F > M = 3.3:1 [1].
- More often found in middle-aged patients but can be seen in children as well.
- 1/3 of intracranial meningiomas do not show symptoms.
- There are significant differences in recurrence rates depending on histologic types.
- Using the WHO criteria, the 5-year recurrence rate ranges from 3% for "benign" meningiomas, increasing by more than 10× to 38% for "atypical" tumors and more than 75% for "anaplastic" or malignant meningiomas [6, 10, 11].

Epidemiology and Pathology

- Approximately 1/2 of all primary brain tumors are gliomas.
- The most common nonglial primary brain tumors are meningiomas [6].
- Meningiomas are usually spherical or lobulated but occasionally are flat and carpet-like when "en plaque" lesions infiltrate the dura and occasionally invade underlying bone.
- Posterior fossa meningiomas are sharply circumscribed with well-defined tumor/brain interfaces.
- Often observe distinct "cleft" of arachnoid containing trapped CSF and surrounding vessels.
- Contain hemorrhagic and necrotic foci but usually lack gross hemorrhage.
- Posterior fossa meningiomas arise from the posterior surface of the petrous bone in 3/4 of cases and from the clivus in 10% [7].
- This assigns approximately 15% of posterior fossa meningiomas to other locations.

Treatment

- Surgical results with posterior fossa meningiomas have improved over the last two decades, but radical excision continues to have high morbidity and mortality rates [2, 12, 13]. Proximity to critical neural and vascular structures including cranial nerves causes excision of posterior fossa meningiomas to be challenging even for expert neurosurgeons [2].
- Microsurgical resection is the treatment of choice and total excision is expected in 3/4 of patients [2].
- *CSF Leaks:* One third present postoperative complications with CSF leaks in 12.5% [2].
- *Recurrence:* 16% encounter tumor recurrence with most recurrences following incomplete resection [2].
- While subtotal excision risks fewer complications than radical excision, most authors recommend subtotal resection for older patients and when factors defy complete surgical excision [2, 14, 15].
- Balancing the extent of resection with good functional outcome is the key to managing posterior fossa meningiomas (PFMs) when they are in intimate proximity to critical structures [5].
- *Radiosurgery:* Often a viable alternative for posterior fossa meningioma in patients with significant operative risks or residual or recurrent tumor.

Differential Diagnosis (DDx)

- While the imaging appearance of a posterior fossa meningioma is usually characteristic, many meningiomas "mimic" other entities, and other entities may masquerade as meningiomas [6].
- The differential diagnosis for an atypical appearing meningioma may include the following:

A. Schwannoma

- Vestibular schwannoma is typically rounded and usually extends into and expands the IAC. They often contain hemorrhage or cyst formation. These findings are not common with PFMs.
- Meningiomas tend to be larger than schwannomas when found in the CPA. They usually are more hemispheric than round; have a wide, flat dural base; and often have hyperostosis. They rarely extend into or widen IAC.
- See Chap. 11, Vestibular Schwannoma.

B. Metastasis

- Dural metastases from extracranial primaries like breast or colon may masquerade as meningiomas.
- Metastasis often exhibits multiple foci which encourage edema in adjacent brain parenchyma.
- Rarely, an extracranial primary tumor may metastasize to a meningioma.

C. Extramedullary Hematopoiesis (EH)

- Extramedullary hematopoiesis may appear as multiple contrast-enhancing dural-based masses.
- Extramedullary hematopoiesis may have associated hepatomegaly, splenomegaly, or paravertebral mass.
- Think of extramedullary hematopoiesis in patients who have hematologic abnormities like sickle cell anemia, β thalassemia, etc. [16].
- Can confirm the diagnosis of extramedullary hematopoiesis with Tc^{99m} nuclear scan and avoid biopsy [17]. May treat with radiation therapy [17].

D. DVM (Dural Vascular Malformation) or Tumor

- Cavernous malformations and capillary hemangiomas occurring in the dura or cavernous sinus may mimic meningioma [6, 18].

E. Hemangiopericytoma (HPC)

- WHO classifies hemangiopericytoma as "tumor of uncertain origin."
- Considered by some to be subset of an angioblastic meningioma.
- Hemangiopericytoma is highly vascular with numerous penetrating vessels.
- Hemangiopericytoma comprises 1% of CNS neoplasms.
- Average age of onset 42 years is younger than the older age in most meningiomas.
- M > F predominance as compared to female predominance in most meningiomas.
- Angiography shows hypervascular lesion with prolonged dense but heterogeneous tumor stain.
- Usually does *not* have AV shunting with early draining veins as is occasionally seen with other meningiomas.
- CT is heterogeneous on pre- and postcontrast with strong but inhomogeneous enhancement.
- CT shows areas of low attenuation necrotic or cystic change.
- MRI usually shows extradural mass isointense to cortex on T1, slightly hyperintense on proton density images with heterogeneous T2 signal.
- Avid post gadolinium enhancement is heterogeneous often demonstrating conspicuous serpentine vascular channels [6, 19].

A Closer Look

I. Genetics and Environment

- Ionizing radiation exposure is the environmental risk factor most frequently found with meningiomas although <1% of irradiated individuals develop meningiomas [20].
- Endogenous and exogenous hormones have been implicated in meningioma development, although their precise role requires further study [20].
- The code for tumor suppressor Merlin resides in the NF2 gene and is disrupted in 1/2 of all patients with meningiomas [21].
- Mutation of the NF2 gene with resultant neurofibromatosis type 2 (NF2) is a dominantly inherited disorder where patients commonly present with bilateral vestibular schwannomas, multiple meningiomas, as well as other CNS tumors [21, 22].
- There is hereditary susceptibility for meningioma involving mutations of several other genes in addition to the more commonly recognized NF2 gene.
- Currently impugned genes and locations associated with meningiomas read like an alphabet soup and include chromosomes 1, 9, 10, 14, 17, 18, and 22 and SWI/SNF with subunits SMARCB1 and SMARCE1, and the suspect list grows daily.
- The sonic hedgehog (SHH)-GLI1 signaling pathway gene, SUFU, is clearly the causal culprit for hereditary multiple meningiomas in a Finnish family [23].

II. Fast Facts

- Posterior fossa meningiomas have been classified by Sekhar et al. into six groups:
  - Type I: Cerebellar convexity-lateral tentorial (tentorium, transverse sigmoid sinus)
  - Type II: CPA (petrous ridge, internal acoustic conduit)
  - Type III: Jugular foramen (cerebellomedullary angle, internal jugular vein, extracranial)
  - Type IV: Petroclival (upper 2/3 clivus, cavernous sinus, Meckel's cave, petrous ridge)
  - Type V: Foramen magnum (lower 1/3 clivus, C1-2 region)
  - Type VI: Unclassified (entire clivus, mid and lower clivus, other types) [1, 24, 25]

III. Historic Highlights

- 1922 Harvey Cushing coined the term "meningioma," although this tumor had been known under various other names since the seventeenth century [1, 24].
- 1614 Felix Plater, Professor of Medicine, University of Basel, first reported a lesion most compatible with a meningioma describing a "noble knight" intracranial tumor.
- Plater described "a round flesh tumor like an acorn...hard and full of holes ...as large as a medium sized apple...covered with its own membrane and entwined with veins. It was free of all connections with white matter of the brain."
- 1774 French surgeon Antoine Louis called the tumor "fungus dura matris."
- 1847 Virchow was the first to describe meningiomas as sandlike calling them psammomas.
- Other prior iterations of names include epitheliomas, endotheliomas, and relatives to sarcomas. Thanks Dr. Cushing for bringing order to this colossal confusion [1]!

References

1. Dumitrescu GF, Imndrei A, Husseini ME, et al. Posterior fossa meningiomas: correlation between site of origin and pathology. Rom Neurosurg. 2010;XVII 3:327–38.
2. Velho V, Argarwal V, Mallay R, Palande DA. Asian J Neurosurg. 2012;7(3):116–24.

3. Castellano F, Ruggiero G. Meningiomas of the posterior fossa. Acta Radiol Suppl. 1953;104:1–177.
4. Laird FJ, Harmer SG, Laws ER, Reese DF. Meningiomas of the cerebellopontine angle. Otolaryngol Head Neck Surg. 1985;93:163–7.
5. Javalkar V, Banerjee AD, Nanda A. Posterior Cranial fossa Meningioma. J Neurol Surg B Skull Base. 2012;73(1):1–10.
6. Osborne AG. Diagnostic neuroradiology. St. Louis: Mosby; 1994. p. 579–625.
7. Helie O, Soulie D, Sarrazin JL, Dewrosier C, Cordoliani YS, Cosnard G. Magnetic resonance imaging and meningioma of posterior cerebral fossa, 31 cases. J Neuroradiol. 1995;22:2 52–70.
8. Gasparetto EL, Leite Cda C, Lucato LT, et al. Intracranial meningiomas: magnetic resonance imaging findings in 78 cases. Arq Neurosiquiatr. 2007;65(3):610–4.
9. Filippi CG, Edgar MA, Ulug AM, et al. Appearance of Meningiomas on diffusion-weighted images: correlating diffusion constants with histopathologic findings. *AJNR Am J Neuroradiol.* 2001;22:65–72.
10. Jaaskelainen J, Haltia M, Servo A. Atypical and anaplastic meningiomas: radiology, surgery, radiotherapy, and outcome. Surg Neurol. 1986;25(3):233–42.
11. Maier H, Öfner D, Hittmair A, et al. Classic, atypical, and anaplastic meningioma: three histopathological subtypes of clinical relevance. J Neurosurg. 1992;77:616–23.
12. Hakuba A, Nishimura S, Tanaka K, Kishi H, Nakamura T. Clivus Meningioma,: six cases of total removal. Neurol Med Chir. 1977;17:63–77.
13. Mayberg MR, Symon L. Meningiomas of the clivus and apical petrous bone: report of 35 cases. J Neurosurg. 1986;65:160–7.
14. Saleh EA, Taibah AK, Achilli V, Aristegui M, Mazzoni A, Sanna M. Posterior Fossa Meningioma Surgical Strategy. Skull Base Surg. 1994;4:202–12.
15. Lobato RD, Gonzaáez P, Alday R, Ramos A, Lagares A, Alen JF, et al. Meningiomas of the basal posterior fossa. Surgical experience in 80 cases. Neurocirugia. 2004;15:525–42.
16. Gumbs RV, Higginbotham-Ford EA, Teal JS, et al. Thoracic extramedullary hematopoiesis in sickle-cell disease. AJR Am J Roentgenol. 1987;149(5):889–93.
17. Singer A, Quencer R. Intracranial extramedullary hematopoiesis: a rare cause of headaches. J Neuroimaging. 2014;24(5):524–7.
18. Williams SJ, Faye-Peterson O, Aronin P, Faith S. Capillary hemangioma of the meninges. AJNR Am J Neuroradiol. 1993;14:529–36.
19. Cosentino CM, Poulton TB, Esquerra JV, Sanss SF. Giant cranial hemangiopericytoma: MR and angiographic findings. AJNR Am J Neuroradiol. 1993;14:253–6.
20. Claus EB, Calvocoressi L, Bondy ML, et al. Clinical article. Family and personal medical history and risk of meningioma. J Neurosurg. 2011; https://doi.org/10.3171/2011.JNS11129. Accessed 1/9/2016.
21. Choy W, et al. The molecular genetics and tumor pathogenesis of meningiomas and the future directions of meningioma treatments. Neurosurg Focus. 2011;30:E6.
22. Liu Y, Pang JC, Dong S, Mao B, Poon WS, Ng HK. Aberrant CpG island hypermethylation profile is associated with atypical and anaplastic meningiomas. Hum Pathol. 2005;36:416–25.
23. Semith MJ. Germline and somatic mutations in meningiomas. Cancer Genet. 2015;208(4):107–14. https://doi.org/10.1016/cancergen.2015.02.003. Accessed 1/9/2016.
24. Kaye H. Posterior fossa meningiomas. In: Sindou M, editor. Practical handbook of neurosurgery: from leading neurosurgeons, vol. 2. Berlin: Springer-Verlag; 2009. p. 181.
25. Sekhar LN, Wright DC, Richardson R, Monacci W. Petroclival and foramen magnum meningiomas: surgical approaches and pitfalls. J Neuro-Oncol. 1996;29(3):249–59.

Part VII

Inflammatory

44 Skull Base Osteomyelitis

Pertinent Points

- *Definition*: Skull base osteomyelitis is a potentially life-threatening disorder which is fortunately a relatively rare, although very aggressive, severe skull base infection most frequently found in older diabetics (or immune suppressed of any age) and can cause frequent fatalities in spite of vigorous antibiotic treatment [1].
- *Classic Clue*: While we would all wish our next skull base osteomyelitis patient would present as an elderly diabetic with otalgia, otorrhea, and hearing loss, in a substantial subset of patients, we frequently find them arriving with more obscure headaches, cranial neuropathies, and ↑ ESR (erythrocyte sedimentation rate), with concomitant curious clival imaging findings [1, 3].
- AKA: Central skull base osteomyelitis, malignant otitis externa, skull osteomyelitis.
- *Distributions:*
  - Gender preference M > F = 3:2
  - Age: 26–80 years (mean 58) [2]
  - Locations: Areas more frequently involved include the temporal bone, the occipital bone, the clivus, and the sphenoid bone including body, wings, and pterygoid plates.
- *Best Modality:* Imaging the skull base for infection is best achieved using MRI.
- Progression to skull base foramina can cause cranial neuropathies and is frequently followed by flagrant devastating skull base destruction.
- When the epicenter is near the clival center, the suspected source is most likely paranasal sinus inflammatory disease. When the epicenter involves the sphenoid wings and pterygoid plates, the etiology is most likely otogenic or odontogenic [5].
- Poor prognostic findings include:
  - Fungal infection
  - Dural enhancement involving the middle cranial fossa or foramen magnum [9]

Imaging

General Imaging Features

- Early imaging findings are often subtle and may include signal intensity variations, nonspecific enhancement, and presentation patterns often indistinguishable from infiltrating neoplasm.

CT Features [5]

- *See General Imaging Features.*
- CT exhibits exceptional expertise in detecting the degree of destruction caused by SBO [5] (see Fig. 44.1g, h).
- Involved structures show sclerosis, cortical discontinuity, and medullary expansion [5].
- Frequently affected areas include the pterygopalatine fossa, foramen ovale, and foramen spinosum [5].
- CT often shows area of associated soft tissue involvement (see Fig. 44.1b).
- CT-guided FNA (fine needle aspiration) is often a helpful tissue sampling procedure [3].
- CT findings are generally unhelpful for monitoring treatment response [3].

MRI Features [8]

- *See General Imaging Features.*
- The specific area of involvement is related to the types and subtypes previously described, but in general the MRI signals are similar for all areas of involvement.

F. A. Midyett, S. K. Mukherji, *Skull Base Imaging*, https://doi.org/10.1007/978-3-030-46447-9_44

- Highly sensitive but nonspecific finding includes ↓ T1 and ↑ T2.
- T1:
  - ↓ T1 hypointense clival bone marrow signal [3] (see Fig. 44.1c).
  - Sagittal T1 is most useful for finding abnormalities involving clival marrow [3].
- T2:
  - ↑ T2 signal.
  - Preclival soft tissue infiltration appears almost invariably present with clival involvement.
- T1 Gd:
  - Although abnormal, can see ↑ T1 Gd with both infection and neoplasm [3] (see Fig. 44.1d).
  - Fat saturation is *very helpful* for definitive delineation (see Fig. 44.1e, f).
- DWI:
  - DWI may help to distinguish SBO from lymphoma and NPC [1].
  - Diffusion-weighted imaging (DWI) is a readily available and commonly used MR imaging sequence.
  - DWIs interpretation of intracellular water movement can be used to calculate cellular compactness and nuclear-to-cytoplasm ratios.
  - DWI with ADC is useful in separating SBO from skull base neoplasm, avoiding critical treatment delays which have high morbidity and mortality.
  - In general, malignant neoplasms are hypercellular with enlarged nuclei, ↓ extracellular matrix, and ↓ ADC values. Benign neoplasms have higher ADC values [1].
  - Newer studies, while now small, suggest that SBO ADC values are higher than for the major neoplasms found in this area [1].
  - A noteworthy exception is the presence of fungal disease with ↓ ADC values in a patient with SBO [1].

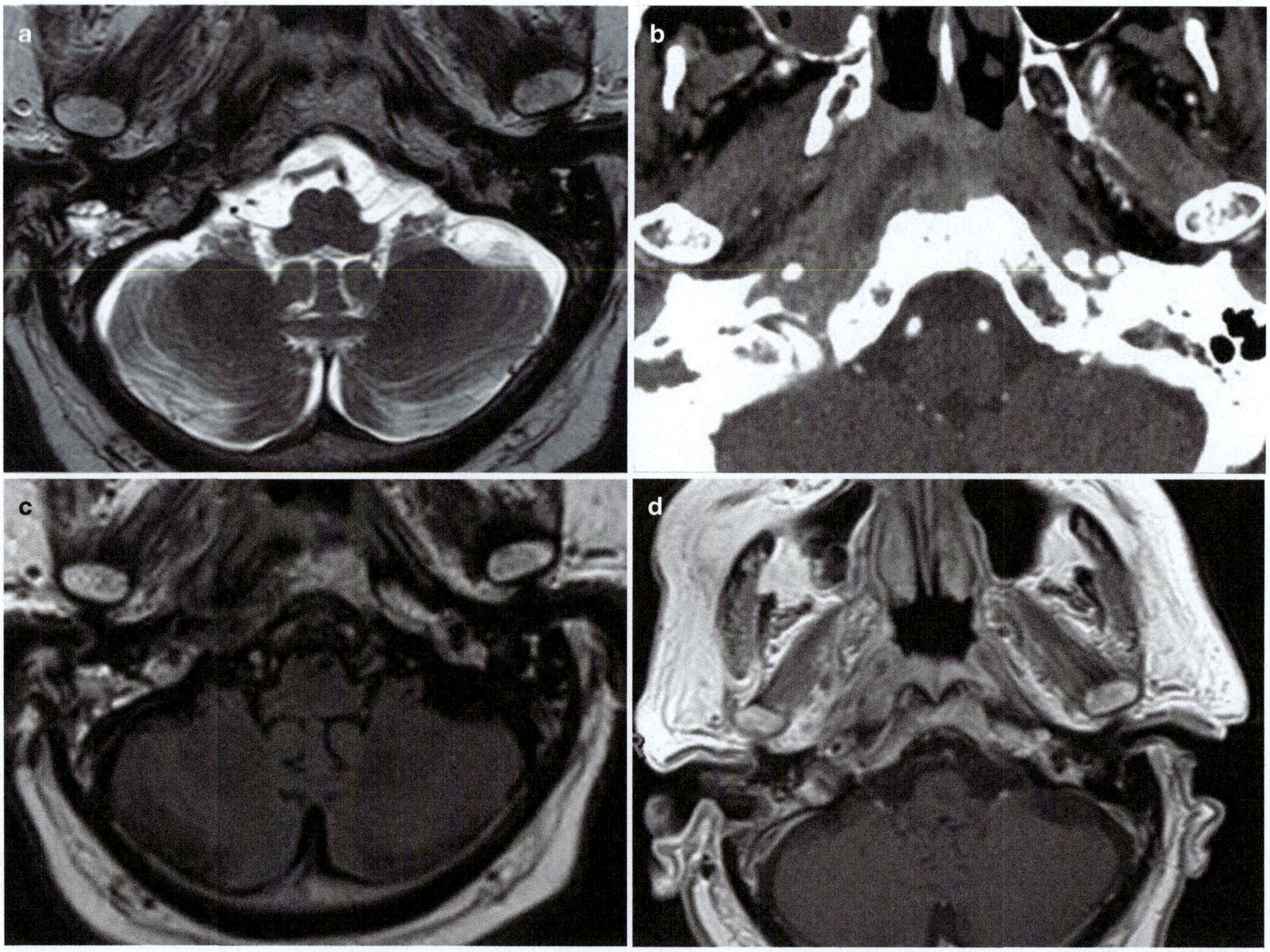

Fig. 44.1 (**a**) Axial T2 shows a bright T2 fluid collection related to a prior right mastoidectomy. (**b**) Axial CECT shows low attenuation phlegmon anterior to the right side of the clivus extending to the midline. (**c**) Axial T1 shows abnormal low signal in the expected location of clival marrow just posterior to phlegmon demonstrated on the prior image. (**d**) Axial T1 Gd exhibits enhancement at the location of the abnormal marrow on the prior image

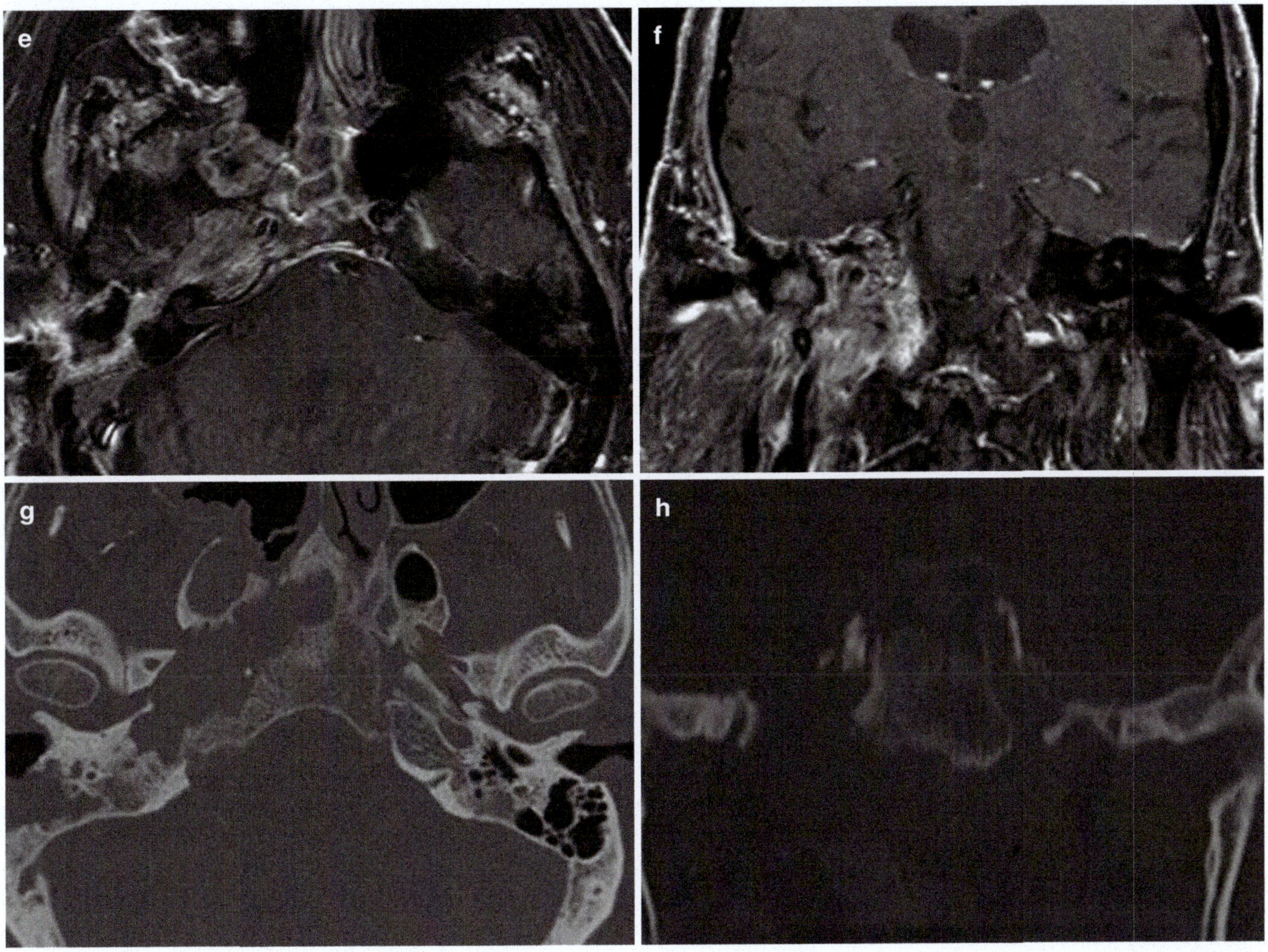

Fig. 44.1 (continued) (**e**) Axial T1 Gd shows large approximately 2.5-cm heterogeneous mass related to right side of the clivus corresponding roughly to the area of abnormal low attenuation in marrow on Figure (**c**). Considerable enhancement surrounds the right mastoidectomy and involves dura anterior to the pons. (**f**) Coronal T1 Gd fat saturation shows huge heterogeneously enhancing central skull base mass containing multiple low attenuation foci. The mass has clearly destroyed the floor of the right central skull base, with conspicuous dural enhancement adjacent the right temporal lobe. Caudally there is no end in sight for the abnormal enhancement. (**g**) Axial NECT depicts flagrant destruction of the central skull base completely destroying most of the structures clearly depicted on the contralateral left. The clival destruction clearly crosses the midline. Gross post-surgical changes in the right mastoid beg us to implicate the ear as the culprit in this case. (**h**) Coronal NECT shows a huge gaping hole in the right skull base and confirms the findings on the coronal MR (**f**)

Nuclear Medicine [6]

- Technetium^{99m} and Ga^{67} gallium citrate are useful in initial diagnosis. Determining when to stop treatment may be more difficult and controversial, as discussed.
- Technetium^{99m}Tc methylene diphosphonate (MDP) scintigraphy:
  - Concentrates in area of ↑ osteoblastic activity.
  - Allows for much earlier diagnosis of SBO than CT although this is not specific for infection.
  - While potentially useful for preliminary diagnosis, positive findings persist months following resolution of infection, so MDP scintigraphy is not a reliable indicator for treatment termination [3].
- Gallium ^{67}Ga citrate:
  - Concentrates in areas of active inflammation attaching to leukocyte containing lactoferrin.
  - Binds to transferrin and bacteria becoming positive for both bone and soft tissue infections.
  - Clinicians tend to repeat this test monthly when used to assess treatment response.
  - Some consider a negative test to be a dependable determinant to discontinue treatment.
  - By contrast, MDP scintigraphy and MRI tend to be persistently positive past this point.
- Indium scintigraphy:
  - Type of white blood cell scintigraphy which is more sensitive than CT for detection of osteomyelitis.

- A grading system proposed by Lee et al. appears helpful in predicting the prognosis for otogenic SBO. This portrays the findings present on ^{99m}Tc SPECT (single-photon emission computerized tomography) at presentation and appears to correlate with final outcomes (with higher grades having a worse prognosis) [7]:
  I. Grade 1 – mild uptake
  II. Grade II – focal mastoid/temporal bone uptake not reaching the midline
  III. Grade III – petrous temporal bone uptake reaching the midline
  IV. Grade IV – uptake crossing midline, involving contralateral temporal bone

Clinical Issues

Presentation

- Symptoms in general vary between type I typical and type II atypical as described earlier in this chapter.
- Even type I "typical" symptoms may be nonspecific subtle symptoms. They include otalgia and otorrhea and are often difficult to diagnose clinically [1].
- Many of these patients possess a predisposition for infection from underlying conditions which include diabetes mellitus, corticosteroid use, HIV infection, and chronic sphenoid sinus inflammatory disease.
- We sometimes subdivide SBO into two groups based on clinical presentation [3]:
  - Type I: Typical Presentation – Usually secondary to malignant or necrotizing external otitis from *Pseudomonas aeruginosa* typically implicating the temporal bones in older diabetics [1].
    Type I SBO typically results from the spread of a soft tissue infection along the floor of the cartilaginous EAC to the skull base. This traverses the fissure of Santorini to the tympanomastoid suture advancing along fascial planes (see Fig. 44.2a–d).
  - Type II: Atypical Presentation – Less frequently found involving the sphenoid or occipital bones in patients without external otitis who have headache as their primary presenting symptom [3].
- Although skull base osteomyelitis is a curable disease, correct diagnosis coupled with prompt treatment is imperative in this often unrecognized and uncommon disease process which frequently flaunts mortality rates >50% [3, 4].
- Radiological evaluation of the pterygopalatine fossa and skull base foramina can provide the critical link between clinicians including dentists, ophthalmologists, as well as maxillofacial and H&N surgeons [5].

Pathophysiology

- Found most frequently complicating malignant otitis externa from *Pseudomonas aeruginosa.*
- Fungal SBO usually involves *Aspergillus or Scedosporium* spp. The latter are increasingly recognized for their role in resistant life-threatening infection in the immunocompromised [12].
- General Pathophysiology: *Pseudomonas aeruginosa* invades vessel walls causing vasculitis, thrombosis, and coagulation necrosis. The pathologic process progresses as follows: cellulitis→ chondritis →osteitis→ osteomyelitis.
- Pathophysiology for type I typical SBO:
  (i) An EAC infection spreads to the skull base through the fissures of Santorini, which are small perforations along the cartilaginous EAC canal floor.
  (ii) Replacement of compact skull base bone by granulation tissue causes bone destruction.
  (iii) Infections spread to skull base foramina causing cranial neuropathies.
  (iv) The close proximity of the stylomastoid foramen to the EAC favors the facial nerve to be the "CN most likely to be involved" (see Fig. 44.2a–d).
  (v) Nerves of the jugular foramen are next to get affected after the facial nerve.
  (vi) More medial spread to the petrous apex can affect the abducens and trigeminal nerves and eventually the *optic nerve*.
  (vii) Spread of infection to the sigmoid sinus can lead to septic thrombosis of the sigmoid sinus and internal jugular vein.
  (viii) Intracranial complications include meningitis and cerebral abscess.

Epidemiology

- Predisposing factors:

Diabetes mellitus	57%
Chronic otitis externa	33%
Chronic sinusitis	29%
Trauma/surgery	30%
Immunosuppression	10%

- Management essentials:
  - Prompt diagnosis
  - Recognizing responsible pathogen
  - Prompt treatment
  - Adequate treatment time

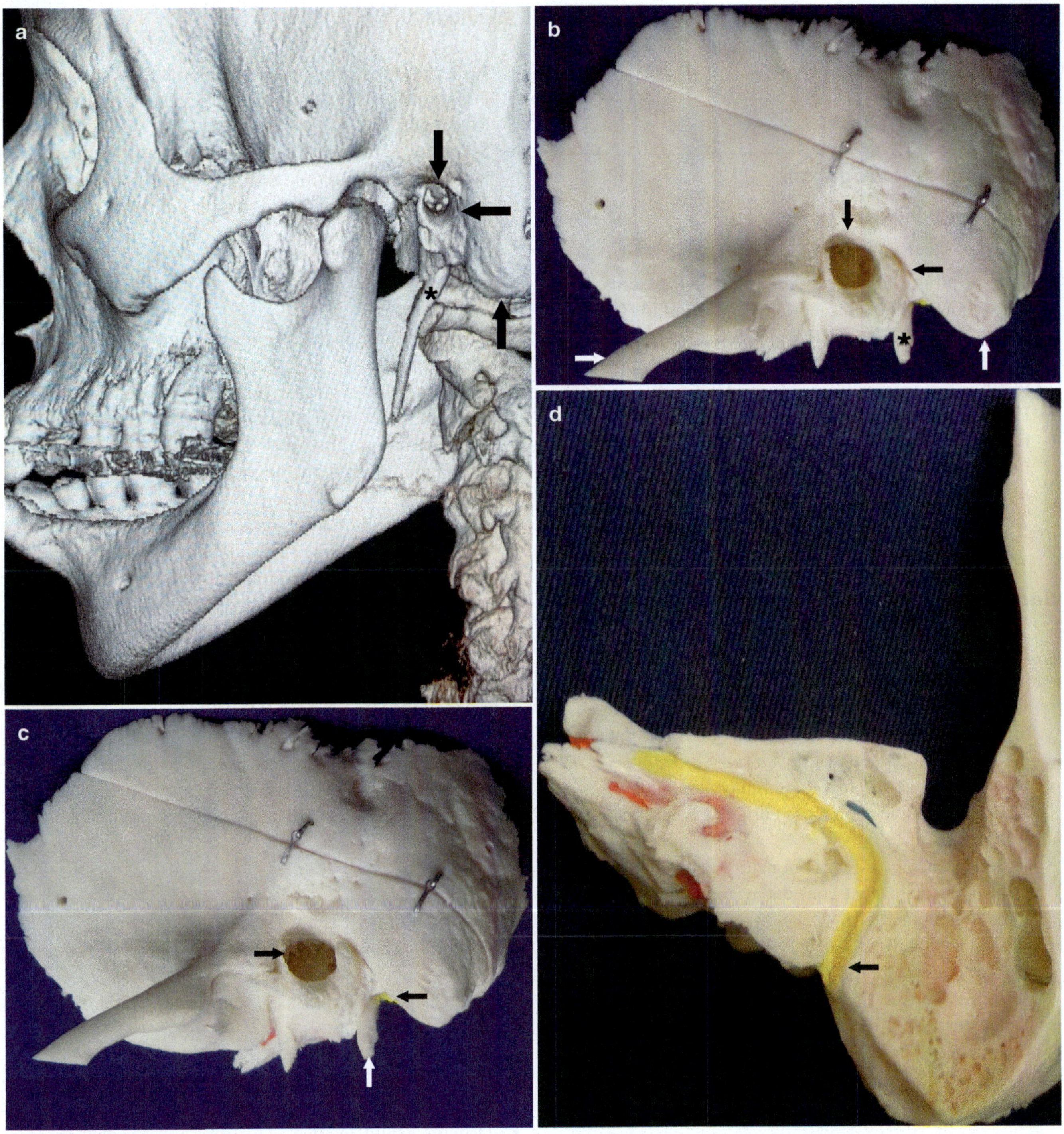

Fig. 44.2 3D NECT (**a**) and disarticulated gross temporal bone (**b**) depict structures in normal patients including ↓ external auditory meatus, ← tympanomastoid fissure, ↑ mastoid process, styloid process (star). The facial nerve resides a mere 5 mm from the tympanomastoid fissure [13]. Disarticulated gross temporal bone from outside (**c**), and inside (**d**) depict structures in a normal patient including → external auditory meatus, ← stylomastoid foramen, ↑ styloid process. For figure (**d**) the temporal bone has been (sagittally) sectioned along the plane of the facial canal which has been highlighted in yellow. This same area (←) seen in yellow on figure (**c**) is mere millimeters away from the tympanomastoid fissure already implicated in the spread of infection from external otitis. There is little wonder why the facial nerve is often the first CN to be involved in patients with otitis externa

- Mean time to presentation:

Bacterial:	26 weeks
Fungal:	8 weeks

Treatment and Prognosis

Medical

- Despite protracted therapy regimes, skull base osteomyelitis shows significant mortality and morbidity in some series show 33.3% and 60%, respectively [1].
- Some studies suggest significant fungal involvement in up to 50%.
- Pending definitive diagnosis prior to isolation of organism, some clinicians assume that there is a 50% chance the process is bacterial and treat for *Pseudomonas aeruginosa* and 50% chance it is fungal secondary to *Zygomycetes* and treat with high-dose amphotericin B.

Surgery

- Early surgical intervention is associated with improved survival with zygomycosis.
- *Debridement:* Vigorous surgical debridement is suggested for *fungal* SBO, but is usually unnecessary, if not contraindicated, for patients with *bacteria*l SBO.
- No one debates the fact that treatment should be started ASAP. Sometimes, the more curious question is when to *stop* treatment.
- In the absence of a persistent neurologic deficit when the ESR is normal, most consider it appropriate to discontinue treatment after 6 weeks.
- With persistently elevated ESR, or the return of symptoms, imaging should be repeated, particularly gallium scanning.
- A negative gallium scan is probably a safe predictor for a treatment end point. By contrast, MRI is known for *showing positive findings past this point.*

Hyperbaric O_2 Therapy (HBO)

- Hyperbaric oxygen (HBO) increases the oxygen tension in infected tissues (including bone) and has been shown to facilitate formation of new capillaries.
- Along with aggressive debridement, hyperbaric oxygen is usually reserved for extensive or unresponsive antibiotic-resistant cases [9].

Survival

- Bacterial: Most patients with bacterial SBO survive.
- Fungal: Most frequently find associated fatalities in the fungal group.
- Mortality is mostly related to intracranial extension and involvement of multiple cranial nerves. Mortality rates do not correlate well with age, sex, or comorbid disease [8].

Complications

- Complications include cranial neuropathy, cavernous sinus thrombosis, septic cavernous sinus thrombosis, meningeal and brain parenchymal involvement, and epidural and petroclival abscess [5, 3].
- Skull base osteomyelitis shows significant morbidity with half of patients having persistent cranial nerve problems.
- Although uncommon, intracranial extension carries a high mortality despite surgical intervention.
- Early diagnosis is indeed imperative to ensure appropriate treatment to prevent intracranial extension, empyema, and even death.

Differential Diagnosis (DDx) [1]

Early imaging findings are sometimes subtle and can include enhancement and altered signal intensity presenting a pattern of infiltration indistinguishable from skull base neoplasms [1].

A. Lymphoma
- Elevation of ESR is not expected in neoplasm [3, 5].
- Lymphoma can appear identical to SBO on imaging studies [3].
- (See Chap. 36, Skull Base Lymphoma)

B. Leukemia
- Displays a more widespread pattern of marrow involvement
- Usually would involve calvarium and cervical spine as well as the clivus [3]

C. Metastatic Neoplasm
- Elevation of ESR not expected with neoplasm [3, 5].
- Metastatic neoplasm can cause a destructive mass anywhere along the skull base.
- Frequently find *multiple metastases* in patients having recognized primary neoplasms.

D. Nasopharyngeal Carcinoma (NPC)

- Elevation of ESR is not expected with neoplasm [3, 5].
- While NPC can be diffusely infiltrating, it usually has an identifiable mass lesion, a feature not usually found with SBO [3].
- (See Chaps. 22, Paranasal Sinus Carcinoma and 26, Sinonasal Undifferentiated Carcinoma)

E. Tuberculosis (TB)

- TB would be expected to be more focally destructive but could cause a similar appearance [3].

A Closer Look

I. Gradenigo's Syndrome (GS)

- In 1958 DeWeese reported three cases of Gradenigo's syndrome (GS) with the warning "Lest we forget that this condition still occurs" [16]. This admonition is true today.
- Pronounced: grah-dā'nē-go
- 1907: First described in a German publication by Italian otologist Giuseppe Conte Gradenigo (1859–1926) [14].
- AKA: Petrous apicitis, apical petrositis, abducens palsy, acute mastoiditis, *Fusobacterium necrophorum*
- The classic Gradenigo's syndrome (GS) triad consists of unilateral periorbital pain, persistent otorrhea, and diplopia.
  – *Unilateral periorbital pain*: Related to pain in the area of the ophthalmic branch of the trigeminal nerve (CN V) when infection extends into Meckel's canal and irritates the trigeminal ganglion.
  – *Otorrhea*: Associated with bacterial otitis media involving the petrous apex.
  – *Diplopia*: Caused by petrositis secondary to epidural abscess at the petrous apex causing the anterior surface of petrous pyramid to compress the abducens nerve (CN VI). The resultant sixth nerve palsy causes diplopia.
  – Other symptoms can include photophobia, epiphora, fever, and ↓ corneal sensitivity.
  – Patients frequently do not portray the full triad [15].
- The classical syndrome is rare but can develop without proper treatment [15].
- Symptoms occur when infection spreads from otitis media to involve the petrous apex where CN VI and the trigeminal ganglion are essentially separated by dura mater.
- The adjacent inflammation causes swelling of the abducens nerve as it passes through Dorello's canal beneath the petroclinoid ligament leaving it nowhere to go and resulting in a sixth nerve palsy [15, 16].
- CT and MRI are helpful in ruling in the diagnosis as well as excluding other entities like leptomeningitis, cerebritis, cerebral abscess, and septic cavernous sinus thrombosis [15].
- *Typical MR signal*: T1 and T2 signals follow fluid; T1 Gd portrays peripheral enhancement.
- MRI shows multiple abnormal findings related to the petrous apex, particularly on T1 Gd images which show extensive enhancement with dural thickening.
- Frequently find fluid signal within the petrous apex with peripheral enhancement.

II. Fast Facts

- 70% of fungal skull base osteomyelitis patients have diabetes, a known risk factor for *Zygomycetes.*
- Fungal skull base osteomyelitis is more likely associated with chronic sinus disease.
- A somewhat sensitive predictor for *fungal* skull base osteomyelitis is the majority of patients with *fungal* skull base osteomyelitis do NOT have purulent ear discharge.
- Failure of antibacterial therapy should suggest a fungal etiology.

III. Historical Highlights

- 1760: Percivall Pott described Pott's puffy tumor [11].
- 1752: French surgeon Sauveur François Morand treated a patient who had developed otitis, mastoiditis, and temporal abscess. Morand drained the patient's pus allowing him to survive. And this was in an era before sterile technique and antibiotics!
- 1959: Meltzer and Kelemen first described skull base osteomyelitis in modern literature [10].

References

1. Ozgen B, Ogua KK, Cila A. Diffusion MR imaging features of skull base osteomyelitis compared with skull base malignancy. AJNR Am J Neuroradiol. 2011;32:179–84.
2. Blyth CC, Gomes L, Sorrell TC, et al. Skull base osteomyelitis: fungal vs bacterial infection. Clin Microbiol Infect. 2011;17(2):306–11.
3. Chang RC, Fischbein NJ, Holliday RA. Central skull base osteomyelitis in patients without otitis externa: imaging findings. AJNR Am J Neuroradiol. 2003;24:1310–6.
4. Chandler JR, Grobman L, Quencer R, Serafini A. Osteomyelitis of the base of the skull. Laryngoscope. 1986;96(3):245–51.
5. Shama SA. Osteomyelitis of the central skull base: otogenic and odontogenic sources. Multidetector CT study. Egypt J Radiol Nuclr Med. 2012;43:519–26.
6. Sharma P, Agarwal KK, Kumar S, et al. Utility of $_{99m}$Tc-MDP hybrid SPECT-CT for diagnosis of skull base osteomyelitis: comparison with planar bone scintigraphy, SPECT, and CT. Jpn J Radiol. 2012; https://doi.org/10.1007/s11604-012-0148-6.
7. Lee S, Hooper R, Fuller A, et al. Otogenic cranial base osteomyelitis: a proposed prognosis-based system for disease classification. Otol Neurotol. 2008;29(5):666–72. https://doi.org/10.1097/MAO.0b013e318179972f.
8. Chen CN. Outcomes of malignant external otitis: survival vs mortality. Acta Otolaryngol. 2010;130(1):89–94.
9. Carfrae MJ, Kessler BW. Malignant otitis externa. Otolaryngol Clin N Am. 2008;41(30):537–49.

10. Meltzer PE, Keleman G. Pyocutaneous osteomyelitis of the temporal bone, mandible, and zygoma. Laryngoscope. 1959;69:1300–16, ISSN 0023-852X.
11. Kim MS. Chapter 3 Skull osteomyelitis. In: Baptista MS, editor. Osteomyelitis: Intech, ISBN: 978-953-51-0399-8;45-88.www.intechopen.com.
12. Cortez KJ, Roilides E, Quiroz-Telles F, et al. Infections caused by scedosporium spp. Clin Microbiol Rev. 2008;21(1):157–97. https://doi.org/10.1128/CMR.00039-07.
13. Bushey A, Quereshy F, Boice JG, et al. Utilization of the tympanomastoid fissure for intraoperative identification of the facial nerve: a cadaver study. J Oral Maxillofac Surg. 2011;69(9):2473–6. https://doi.org/10.1016/j.joms.2010.11.044. Epub 2011 May 7.
14. Gradenigo G. Ueber die paralyse des Nervus abducens bei Otitis. Arch Ohrenheilunde. 1907;774:149–87. https://doi.org/10.1007/BF01930369.
15. Jacobsen CL, Bruhn MA, Yavarian Y, et al. Mastoiditis and Gradenigo's syndrome with anaerobic bacteria. BMC Ear Nose Throat Disord. 2012;12:10. https://doi.org/10.1186/1472-6815-12-10.
16. Gillanders DA. Gradenigo's syndrome revisited. J Otolaryngol. 1983;12(3):169–74.

45 Invasive Fungal Sinusitis

Pertinent Points

- *Definition:* Invasive fungal sinusitis can be divided into acute and chronic varieties. Acute invasive fungal sinusitis (AIFS) is the most aggressive form of fungal sinusitis and is the source of significant morbidity and mortality displaying a dismal survival rate of just 3% when untreated [1]. Because of its more serious nature, the foremost focus of this chapter will be directed to AIFS.
- *Classic Clue*: Poorly controlled diabetic (or immunocompromised individual) presents with fever, facial swelling, and nasal congestion. Imaging studies show signs of sinusitis with mild mucosal thickening and enhancement. However, close inspection frequently demonstrates disruption of periantral fat [3, 7, 12].
- *AKA*: Invasive fungal rhinosinusitis, fulminant invasive fungal sinusitis, zygomycosis.
- *Age*: The mean age is 39 [1].
- *Locations:* Most invasive fungal sinusitis arises from the nasal cavity, predominately at the middle turbinate [4].
- While once regarded as rare, fungal sinusitis is currently reported with rising regularity around the globe [3].
- *Prevalence*: Modern medical marvels have stretched survival for patients having hematologic malignancies and diabetes, with AIDS engendering escalating numbers of immunocompromised hosts consequently increasing the incidence of IFS [4].
- Fungal sinusitis can currently be classified into distinct entities showing separate radiological features by the following five subtypes [3]:
  1. Acute invasive fungal sinusitis (AIFS)
  2. Chronic invasive fungal sinusitis
  3. Chronic granulomatous invasive fungal sinusitis
  4. Allergic fungal sinusitis (AFS) (see Chap. 32)
  5. Fungus ball or fungal mycetoma
- Acute invasive fungal sinusitis (AIFS) is an aggressive, frequently fatal infection having a high mortality with only 50% surviving according to many authors [7]. While many concede an 80% mortality, still others suggest mortality rates can be reduced as low as 18% using currently available treatment methods [5].
- Prompt diagnosis with initiation of optimal therapy can curtail the horrific morbidity and mortality associated with this deadly disease.
- Infection's intracranial spread herald higher morbidity and mortality with 73% succumbing to their disease.
- Treatment and prognosis vary among various subtypes. It is crucial that clinicians and radiologists understand the different subtypes of fungal sinusitis and for radiologists to clearly communicate to clinicians the need for (and findings from) appropriate imaging procedures.
- Radiologists remain obliged to provide patients with optimum imaging studies and interpretations having a high index of suspicion for invasive fungal sinusitis, so early endoscopy, biopsy, and treatment can have a concrete chance to cure this deadly, but potentially curable, disease [11].

Imaging

General Imaging Features

- For detecting early changes of acute invasive fungal sinusitis (AIFS), MRI is more sensitive than CT, although both modalities show similar specificities [9].
- MRI excels in detection of extra-sinus invasion when interpreted by experienced head and neck radiologists [9].

F. A. Midyett, S. K. Mukherji, *Skull Base Imaging*, https://doi.org/10.1007/978-3-030-46447-9_45

- Positive predictive values are high for both MRI and CT. However, negative predictive values are lower showing significant interobserver variation [9].
- When destruction of multiple sinus walls suggests a nonneoplastic etiology, radiologists should suspect IFS [13].
- MRI surpasses CT in depicting disease development and should be employed earlier in this disease process [11].
- Some suggest saving CT for treatment planning purposes and using MRI for acute invasive fungal sinusitis screening could cut costs while concurrently reducing radiation exposure [9].

MRI Features

- See section "General Imaging Features".
- MRI is the modality of choice to access soft tissue extension, particularly when involving intracranial or intraorbital structures.
- Findings within the sinus itself are variable and range from mucosal thickening to complete opacification.
- Inflammatory changes involving orbital fat or EOMs precipitate proptosis and herald intraorbital invasion by this aggressive assailant.
- MRI is more helpful than CT in finding features for early diagnosis including [8, 9]:
  1. Infiltration of periantral fat
  2. Inflammatory changes involving orbital fat and EOMs
  3. Leptomeningeal enhancement [9]
  - Features 2 and 3 foretell advanced involvement [9].
- Infiltration of periantral fat planes may represent the earliest imaging evidence in invasive fungal disease [12].
- In suitable clinical situations, even if encountered as a solitary imaging abnormality, periantral soft tissue infiltration should suggest IFS.
- T1: Intermediate low signal. (See Fig. 45.1a.)
- T2: *Variable* depending on life stage of fungus.
  - Has higher T2 signal than is seen with more chronic fungal sinusitis. The characteristic low T2 signal filling the sinus seen in allergic fungal sinusitis is conspicuously absent.
  - Fungal organisms concentrate various metals including iron, magnesium, and manganese, but these findings are seldom seen in acute IFS. Can sometimes see some component of low T2 signal within the sinus as fungus begins to accumulate minerals. (See Fig. 45.1b.)
  - Sometimes see associated blood or other fluid elsewhere in the paranasal sinuses.
  - If a fungal mass is present, it shows intermediate to low signal.
- T1 Gd
  - When the sinus mucosa exhibits little or no enhancement, it is probably necrotic.
  - Fungal extension outside the sinus causes ↑ enhancement. (See Fig. 45.2c.)
  - The combination of mucosal necrosis and perisinus fungal extension may exhibit an "inside out" or reversed enhancement pattern.

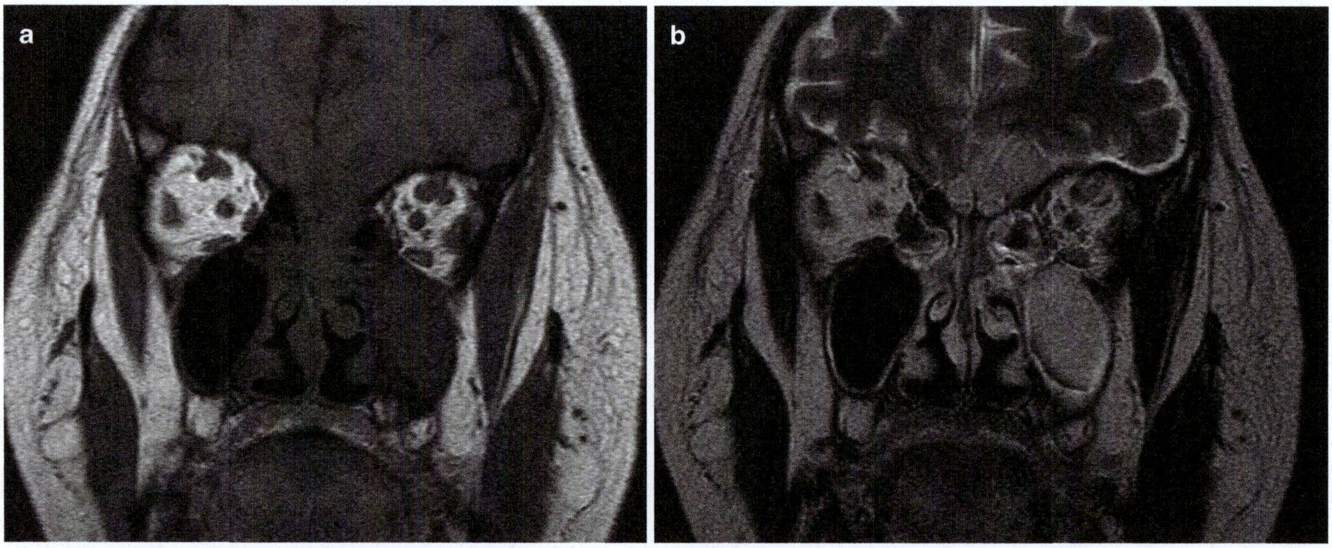

Fig. 45.1 (**a**) Coronal T1 shows abnormal signal in the nasal cavity, as well as the left maxillary and ethmoid sinuses. (**b**) Coronal T2 again shows abnormal signal in the left maxillary and ethmoid sinuses. This signal within the sinus is high and not unlike what we would expect in acute sinusitis. But, there is a peripheral rim of *low* signal inferomedially within the left maxillary sinus. This is a "telltale sign" that there is indeed a fungus among us. And, there is yet another red flag here. There is elevated T2 signal in the frontal lobes (L > R) which corresponds to ↓ T1 signal on the previous images (which we wondered about)

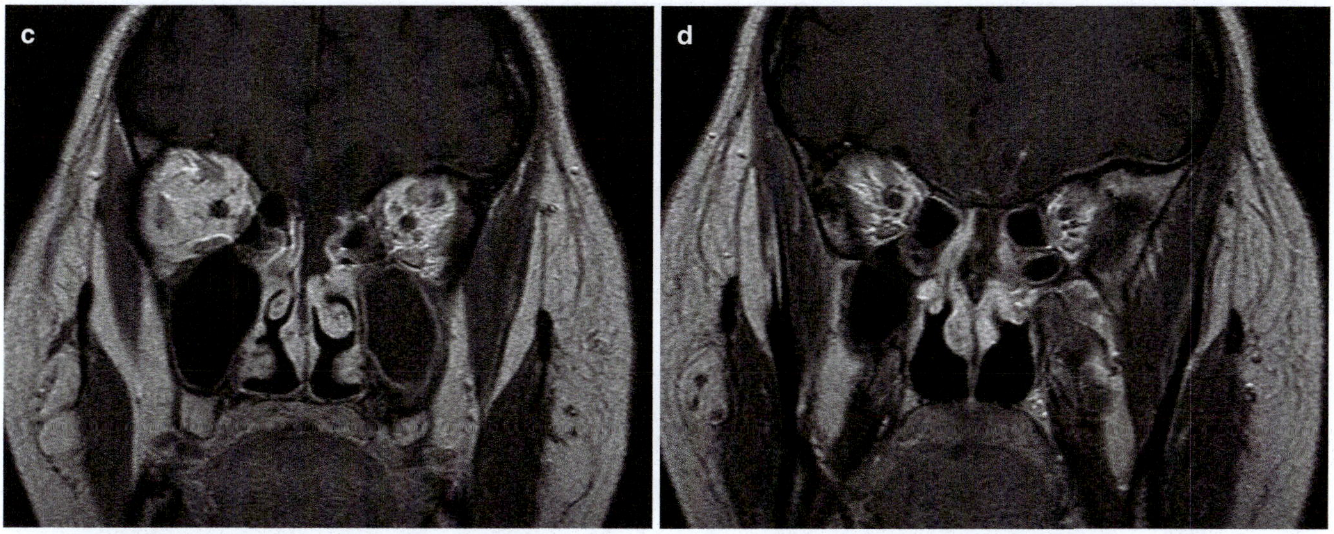

Fig. 45.1 (continued) (**c**) Coronal T1 Gd again shows abnormal signal in the left nasal cavity, the left maxillary and ethmoid sinuses, as well as in the frontal lobes. There is moderate fairly uniform enhancement of mucosa in the left maxillary antrum, again, not unlike what we would expect in acute sinusitis. But the low signal extending intracranially is beginning to be *really worrisome*. The signal above and below the cribriform plate is exactly the same. And we don't need CT to see that the cribriform plate is full of holes! (See Fig. 45.5a, Endocranial Anatomic Skull Base.) (**d**) Coronal T1 Gd depicts enhancement of abnormal vascular structures in the frontal lobes. This shows just how subtle finding can be in acute IFS before patients succumb to this deadly disease and present to pathology for the image displayed in Fig. 45.4a

- Findings suggesting invasion beyond the sinus include:
  - Stranding of periantral fat involving:
    Intraorbital fat
    Masticator space
    Pterygopalatine fossa.
    This "stranding" is best seen on T1 STIR or T2 fat sat.
  - Subtle enhancement on T1 fat sat.
  - Abnormal leptomeningeal enhancement.
  - Intracranial granulomas: T1 and T2 both show low signal.
  - "Inside out" enhancement pattern.
  - Signs of vascular invasion:
    Enlargement of the cavernous sinus (see Fig. 45.2d)
    Loss of vascular "flow voids" (see Fig. 45.2d)
    Vascular involvement on MRA and MRV including thrombosis, stenosis, and occlusion (see Fig. 45.2e)
    Intracranial infarcts

CT Features

- See *General Imaging Features.*
- In the early course of AIFS, most patients do not demonstrate the classic CT findings of bone erosion or extra-sinus extension [10].
- CT findings frequently fall into the following categories:
  1. Sinus opacification:
     - Sometimes shows soft tissue opacification of an involved sinus.
     - Unlike chronic IFS, acute IFS *typically does not* demonstrate hyperdense material on NECT.
  2. Mucosal thickening:
     - Severe *unilateral* nasal cavity mucosal thickening is often the most consistent finding suggesting underlying IFS. While a sensitive finding, it is also nonspecific and frequently found in all forms or rhinosinusitis [10].
     - NECT shows moderate mucosal thickening and/or a soft tissue mass within the nasal cavity and sinus.
  3. Bone destruction:
     - CT excels at assessing bony changes.
     - At earlier stages of this disease, bone erosion and mucosal thickening sometimes seem subtle and insignificant. As the disease progresses, bony destruction often becomes extensive.
     - Aggressive sinus wall destruction progresses rapidly followed by intraorbital and intracranial involvement.
     - In the early course of AIFS, most patients do not demonstrate the classic CT findings of bone erosion or extra-sinus extension [10].
     - See Fig. 45.3a.
  4. Fat stranding outside the sinus involves:
     - Intraorbital fat
     - Masticator space
     - Pterygopalatine fossa

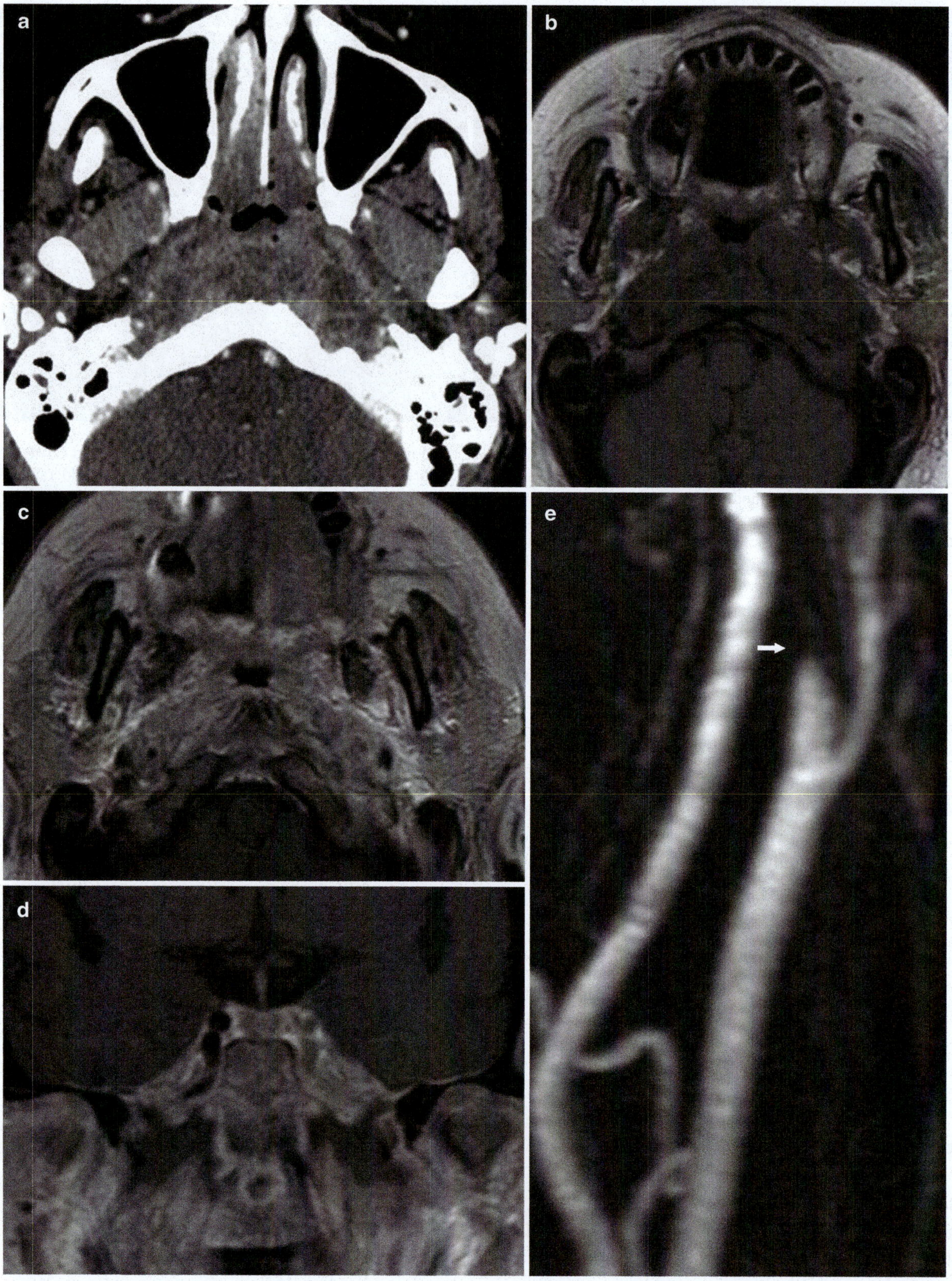

Fig. 45.2 (**a**) Axial CECT showing gross enlargement of the retropharyngeal soft tissues with heterogeneous (but no distinct ring) enhancement to suggest drainable abscess. This phlegmonic pathologic process displaces the airway anteriorly. (**b**) Axial T1 mirrors the findings found on the prior CECT. There is moderate heterogeneity within the enlarged retropharyngeal mass. (**c**) Axial T1 Gd exhibits avid heterogeneous enhancement of the huge process which is predominately retropharyngeal but extends anteriorly and laterally as well. (**d**) Coronal T1 Gd exhibits enlargement of the left cavernous sinus with conspicuous absence of the left carotid siphon flow void. IFS has extended into the left cavernous sinus and invaded and thrombosed the left cavernous sinus. This is clearly cannot be good for intracranial blood flow! (**e**) MRA confirms complete occlusion with no flow above the first 1 cm of the left ICA. The patient had already suffered a serious stroke

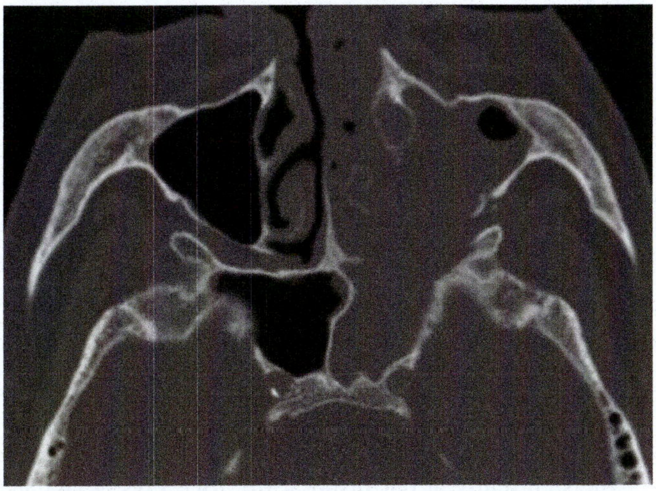

Fig. 45.3 (**a**) Axial bone algorithm CT depicts extensive bony destruction involving the left maxillary and sphenoid sinuses, nasal turbinates, and septum. Soft tissue density fills the involved sinuses and nasal cavity

Clinical Issues

Presentation

- Can demonstrate a capricious clinical course commonly starting with nonspecific nasal congestion followed by dramatic development of fever, facial pain, and epistaxis.
- Frequently find associated involvement of the orbit, cavernous sinus, or calvarium causing visual impairment, proptosis, and neurologic deficits [2, 3].
- Untreated, the disease course typically exhibits evolution over a few days (or at most a few weeks) typically terminating in vascular invasion and systemic dissemination [3].
- Frequently find IFS in *poorly controlled diabetic or immunocompromised individuals* presenting with painless necrotic nasal septal ulcer which when untreated promptly progresses to overwhelming orbital and incurable intracranial involvement [3].
- Symptoms of IFS fall into two general groups:
  I. Acute invasive fungal sinusitis:
    - Fever and cough
    - Facial swelling, pain, or numbness
    - Headache and mental status change
    - Visual disturbances
    - Nasal discharge
    - Ulceration of nasal or oral mucosa
  II. Chronic invasive fungal sinusitis
    - Pressure in forehead, nose, or retroorbital region
    - Post-nasal drainage
    - Nasal and sinus congestion
    - Orbital apex syndrome
      – Characteristic of chronic IFS
      – Decreased vision
      – Ophthalmoplegia

Pathophysiology

- When providing air filtration, the middle turbinates have the highest volume of nasal airflow, putting them at the greatest risk for fungal seeding [4].
- IFS is probably instigated near one of the middle turbinates and subsequently spreads into one or more of the nearby paranasal sinuses [4].
- Frequently found fungal agents include [2, 3]:
  – *Zygomycetes*: Classically in diabetics
    Mucor spp.
    Rhizopus spp.
    Rhizomucor spp.
    Absidia spp.
  – *Aspergillus* spp.: Habitually involving immunosuppressed individuals
- Spread of infection to the sigmoid sinus can lead to septic thrombosis of the sigmoid sinus and the internal jugular vein.
- Intracranial complications include meningitis, cerebral infarction, cerebral abscess, and death.

Epidemiology

- Two distinct populations emerge [3]:
  I. Diabetics
    - Predominately patients with ketoacidosis.
    - 80% have fungi belonging to order of *Zygomycetes*.
      – For example, *Rhizopus*, *Rhizomucor*, *Absidia*, and *Mucor*
      – This group tends to be more virulent, more rapidly progressing, with higher morbidity and mortality.
  II. Immunocompromised individuals with neutropenia
    - AKA: Fulminant invasive sinusitis or neutropenic sinusitis.
    - *Aspergillus* causes 80% of these infections.
    - Patients unable to reverse their neutropenia portend a particularly poor prognosis despite their treatment type [3, 5].
    - Common associations include:
      – Patients having a hematologic malignancy
      – Chemotherapy patients
      – Long-term systemic steroid therapy
      – Bone marrow transplants

  - Immunosuppressive therapy for organ transplants
  - Acquired immunodeficiency.
- Other predisposing factors include renal failure, cirrhosis, and chelating agents (such as deferoxamine).

Treatment and Prognosis

I. Medical

- Prompt diagnosis and treatment of AIFS is imperative. High-dose intravenous antifungal therapy is considered crucial for survival [8].
- While amphotericin B deoxycholate has been the foundation for serious antifungal therapy since 1955, it is well known for severe and potentially lethal side effects. Nephrotoxicity is particularly problematic following intravenous administration.
- In order to lessen the severe side effects, several lipid formulations have been developed including liposomal formulations which lessen its renal toxicity.
- Although antifungal and surgical therapies are absolutely life-saving, in terms of patient outcome, effective treatment of the patients underlying disease process and immunosuppression is equally important [6].

II. Surgery

- Unless the disease is disseminated or widespread, it may be necessary to obtain a surgical biopsy [9].
- Patients who had complete surgical resection survive significantly more often than those who do not.
- Patients undergoing complete surgical resection are more likely to respond to granulocyte colony-stimulating factor [4].
- Early extensive aggressive surgical debridement for AIFS is essential and patients who have not had surgery show a poor prognosis [7, 8].

III. Complications [3]

A. Intraorbital extension

B. Intracranial extension:
- Leptomeningeal enhancement
- Intracranial granulomas
- Epidural abscess and empyema
- Extension through the cribriform plate (see Fig. 45.1a–d)

C. Vascular invasion causes:
- Cavernous sinus thrombosis
- Dural venous sinus thrombosis
- Cerebral infarction
- Cerebral hemorrhage
- Systemic dissemination

- Early diagnosis is indeed imperative to insure appropriate treatment for prevention of intracranial extension, empyema, and even death.
- Outcomes remain poor for patients with uncorrected neutropenia and diabetes who often present late in this fast-moving disease process [3–5].
- AIFS is an aggressive, frequently fatal infection having a high mortality according to many sources with approximately 50% surviving [7]. Although some report mortality rates as high as 80%, still others suggest mortality rates can be brought down to 18% by appropriately using tools currently at our disposal [5]. (See Figs. 45.4a and 45.5a.)
- Surprisingly, diabetics show better overall survival than patients with other comorbidities [7].
- Patients who develop intracranial involvement or those not having surgery show a poor prognosis [7].

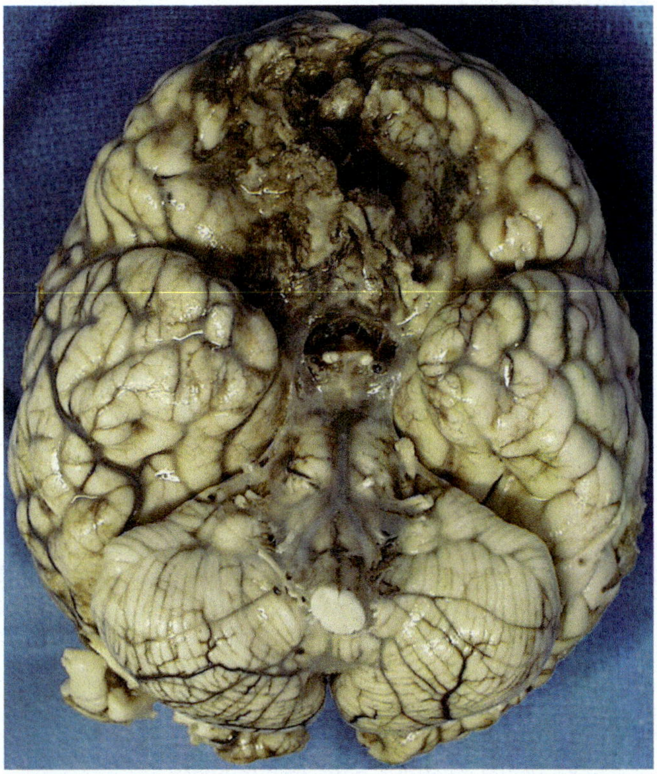

Fig. 45.4 (**a**) Gross image of the brain (from below) of this unfortunate patient with acute IFS. This patient succumbed to mucormycosis and graphically depicts the end result from fungus invading vessels producing vasculitis, thrombosis, infarction, and necrosis. This can (and does) still happen when an early accurate diagnosis is not tied to timely aggressive treatment

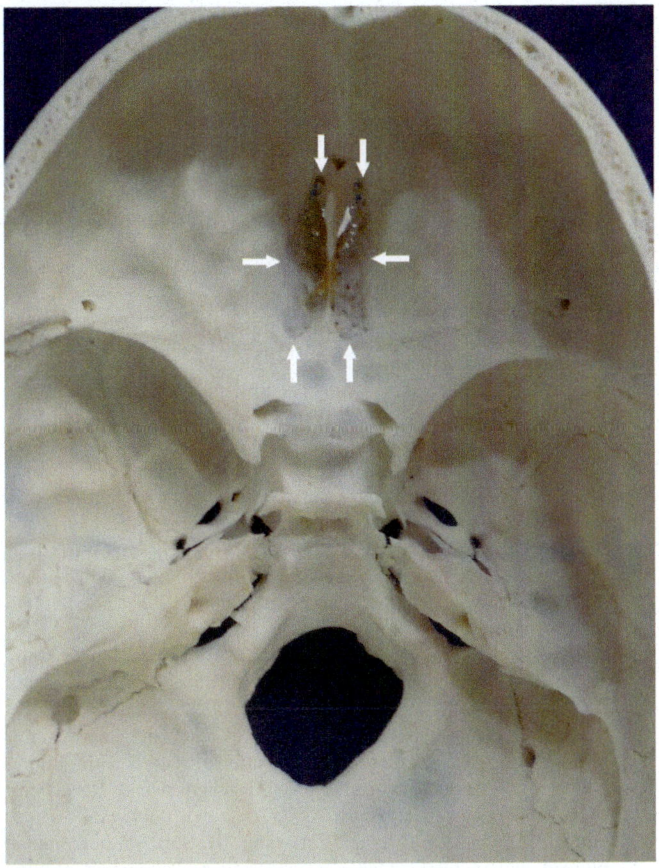

Fig. 45.5 Endocranial gross skull base depicts the cribriform plate (arrows) filled with multiple foramina just waiting to be found by a visiting virulent fungus

Differential Diagnosis [1]

A. Allergic Fungal Sinusitis (AFS)

- Young immunocompetent patient from the Southwestern United States presents with therapy-resistant chronic sinusitis. Hypo-attenuation on T2 MRI corresponds to *characteristically* hyperdense sinus showing *characteristic serpiginous* pattern.
- The *hyperdense* sinus is an *important* finding and may be the ***only*** clue to fungal sinusitis. By contrast this is ***not*** a feature for IFS.
- NECT: The majority of sinuses show near-complete opacification which centrally has hyperdense material surrounded by a peripheral rim of *hypodense mucosa*. The hyperdense central opacification is *characteristically serpiginous*.
- Sinus expansion is typical with 25% having erosion and some exhibiting extension into the surrounding structures.
- T1: Variable, although hypointensity is most common. T1 is optimal for evaluating cortical bone interruption or low signal invasion of high signal fatty skull base bone marrow.
- T2: Hypointense signal or signal voids are secondary to high concentrations of metals, high protein, and low free water in mucin. Fungal organisms frequently concentrate various metals including iron, magnesium, and manganese.
- T1 Gd exhibits enhancement of inflamed mucosa (often corresponding to hypodense rim seen on CT). However, most of the sinus contents *do not* enhance.
- AFS is the most common form of fungal sinusitis and is common in warm, humid climates. It is an immune-modulated disease entity.
- Hypersensitivity reaction to inhaled fungal organisms results in a noninfectious chronic inflammatory reaction.
- Patients often present with a multiyear history of headache, nasal congestion, and chronic sinusitis with allergic rhinitis or asthma.
- AFS usually shows bilateral if not pansinus involvement.
- See Chap. 32, Allergic Fungal Sinusitis.

B. "Average" Acute Sinusitis

- Infiltration of periantral fat planes may represent the earliest imaging evidence in invasive fungal disease [12]. This is *not* a feature of "average" acute sinusitis.
- Inflammatory changes involving the orbital fat and EOMs may be secondary to acute IFS. This is *not* a feature of "average" acute sinusitis.
- Leptomeningeal enhancement may be secondary to acute IFS [9]. This is *not* a feature of "average" acute sinusitis.
- With acute IFS, when the sinus mucosal exhibits little or no T1 Gd enhancement, it is probably necrotic. This is *not* a feature of "average" acute sinusitis and should instead lead to a diagnosis of acute IFS.

C. Paranasal Sinus Cancer

- Malignant tumors arising from paranasal sinus epithelium comprise the most common malignant tumor of the anterior skull base.
- *Classic Clue*: Older male woodworker with moderately enhancing mass destroying the skull base and adjacent paranasal sinus often exhibiting its epicenter near a paranasal sinus.
- NECT shows a solid mass with aggressive bone destruction. CECT exhibits moderate enhancement.
- T1 and T2: Intermediate signal mass.
- T1 Gd: Exhibits moderate tumor enhancement.
- ADCs of malignant tumors are consistently lower than benign tumors and inflammatory lesions.
- ^{18}F FDG PET/CT has high sensitivity with moderate specificity and seems superior to conventional CT and MRI for assessing residual/recurrent tumor.

- Squamous cell carcinoma is the most common malignant sinonasal tumor (80%), followed by adenocarcinomas.
- See Chap. 22, Paranasal Sinus Cancer.

D. Metastatic Neoplasm

- Elevated ESR (erythrocyte sedimentation rate) is not expected in neoplasm, but is frequently found with infection.
- Metastatic neoplasm can cause a destructive mass anywhere along the skull base.
- Frequently find *multiple metastases* in patients having recognized primary neoplasms.

E. Leukemia

- Displays a more widespread pattern of marrow involvement.
- Usually involves the calvarium and cervical spine as well as the skull base.

A Closer Look

I. Fast Facts

While many papers dealing with IFS develop their statistics from relatively small patient populations, they must also be interpreted in view of their various time frames. However, one sizeable study which reviewed 929 mucormycosis cases published in the English language between 1885 and 2005 provided the following interesting and somewhat sobering statistics [1]:

- Associated infections were present [1]:

Sinus	39%
Pulmonary	24%
Cutaneous	19%

- Dissemination developed in 23%.
- Mortality rates varied with infection sites:

Disseminated disease	96%
GI infections	85%
Pulmonary infections	76%

- 92% of patients with malignancy had pulmonary disease.
- 66% of patients with diabetes had sinus disease.
- Rhinocerebral disease was seen in 33% of patients with diabetes compared to 4% of patients with malignancy.
- Treatment-based survival:

No treatment:	3%
Amphotericin B deoxycholate:	61%
Surgery alone:	57%
Surgery with antifungal medications:	70%

References

1. Roden MM, Zaoutis TE, Buchanan WL, et al. Epidemiology and outcome of Mucormycosis: a review of 929 reported cases. Clin Infect Dis. 2005;41(5):634–53.
2. Momeni AK, Roberts CC, Chew FS. Imaging of chronic and exotic sinonasal disease: review. AJR Am J Roentgenol. 2007;189(6):S35–45. https://doi.org/10.2214/AJR.07.7031.
3. Aribandi M, McCoy VA, Bazan C. Imaging features of invasive and noninvasive fungal sinusitis: a review. Radiographics. 2007;27(5):1283–96. https://doi.org/10.1148/rg.275065189.
4. Gillespie MB, O'Malley BW, Francis HW. An approach to fulminant invasive fungal rhinosinusitis in the immunocompromised host. Arch Otolaryngol Head Neck Surg. 1998;124(5):520–6. https://doi.org/10.1001/archotol.124.5.520.
5. Parikh SL, Venkatraman G, DelGaudio JM. Invasive fungal sinusitis: a 15-year review from a single institution. Am J Rhinol. 2004;18(2):75–81.
6. Kasapoqlu F, Coskun H, Ozmen OA, et al. Acute invasive fungal rhinosinusitis: evaluation of 26 patients treated with endonasal or open surgical procedures. Otolaryngol Head Neck Surg. 2010;243(5):614–20.
7. Turner JH, Soudry E, Nayak JV, Hwang PH. Survival outcomes in acute invasive fungal sinusitis: a systematic review and quantitative synthesis of published evidence. Laryngoscope. 2013;123(5):1112–8. https://doi.org/10.1002/lary.23912. Epub 2013 Jan 8.
8. Liu M, Zhou B, Liu HC, et al. Acute fulminant invasive fungal sinusitis. Zhonghua Er Bi Yan Hou Ke Za Zhi. 2003;28(4):251–4.
9. Groppo ER, El-Sayed IH, Aiken AH, Glastonbury CM. Computed tomography and magnetic resonance imaging characteristics of acute invasive fungal sinusitis. Arch Otolaryngol Head Neck Surg. 2011;137(10):1005–10. https://doi.org/10.1001/archoto.2011.170.
10. DelGaudio JM, Swain RE, Kingdom TT, et al. Computed tomography findings in patients with invasive fungal sinusitis. Arch Otolaryngol Head Neck Surg. 2003;129(2):235–40.
11. Howells RC, Ramadan HH. Usefulness of computed tomography and magnetic resonance in fulminant invasive fungal rhinosinusitis. Am J Rhinol. 2001;15(4):255–61.
12. Silverman CS, Mancuso AA. Periantral soft-tissue infiltration and its relevance to the early detection of invasive fungal sinusitis: CT and MR findings. AJNR Am J Neuroradiol. 1998;19(2):321–5.
13. Addleston RB, Baylin GJ. Rhinocerebral mucormycosis. Radiology. 1975;115(1):113–7.

Part VIII

Sarcomas

46 Skull Base Chondrosarcomas

Pertinent Points

- *Definition:* Chondrosarcomas are chondroid malignancies which commonly select a synchondrosis when they rarely involve the skull base.
- *Classic Clue*: Skull-based mass exhibiting an affinity for the POF (petro-occipital fissure) sometimes showing chondroid matrix, characterized by low T1 and high T2 signal.
- *AKA:* Cranial chondrosarcoma
- *Distributions and Incidence:*
  - Gender Preference: M < F = 1:1.3 [1]
  - Age: 10–79 years (mean 39) [1]
  - Incidence:

    Most skull base chondrosarcomas (SBCs) arise de novo comprising <1% of intracranial tumors but 6% of skull base tumors [1, 2].

    Chondrosarcomas can occur de novo or from preexisting conditions including enchondromas, exostoses, and osteochondromas, as well as from Ollier's and Paget's disease [1].
- DWI:
  - Diffusion-weighted imaging (DWI) is a readily available and commonly used MR imaging sequence.
  - DWI interpretation of intracellular water movement can be used to calculate cellular compactness and nuclear-to-cytoplasm ratios.

    DWI with ADC values is sometimes useful in separating SBC from chordoma [3].

    DWI is certainly significant since several prior studies showed "no reliable MRI or CT features to definitely distinguish chordoma from chondrosarcoma" [3, 4].

    SBCs have a markedly more favorable prognosis than chordoma and exhibit fewer recurrences [5].

Imaging

General Imaging Features

- Most skull base chondrosarcomas (SBCs) occur off midline while most chordomas are midline.
- Local extension of SBC is common and they often invade paranasal and cavernous sinuses.

CT Features [6]

- *See General Imaging Features.*
- SBCs appear as well-circumscribed, often scalloped, or lobulated lytic lesions exhibiting chondroid calcifications.
- Low attenuation may make them subtle on brain soft tissue algorithms. (See Fig. 46.1i.)

MRI Features [7]

- *See General Imaging Features.*
- T1: ↓ hypointense (to intermediate) signal intensity [7, 8]. (See Fig. 46.1a, c, e, g.)
- T2: Very high T2 signal [7, 8]. (See Fig. 46.1b, d.) Areas with inhomogeneity commonly correspond to calcifications [1].
- T1 Gd:
  - Exhibits exuberant enhancement [7, 8]. (See Fig. 46.1f, h.)
  - Usually heterogeneous enhancement in ~60% caused by matrix mineralization and/or fibrocartilaginous elements [7].
  - Fat saturation is very helpful for definitive delineation. (See Fig. 46.1f, h.)
- DWI: Shows a spectrum of diffusion values [3]:
  - Chondrosarcoma has the highest mean ADC at 2051.

F. A. Midyett, S. K. Mukherji, *Skull Base Imaging*, https://doi.org/10.1007/978-3-030-46447-9_46

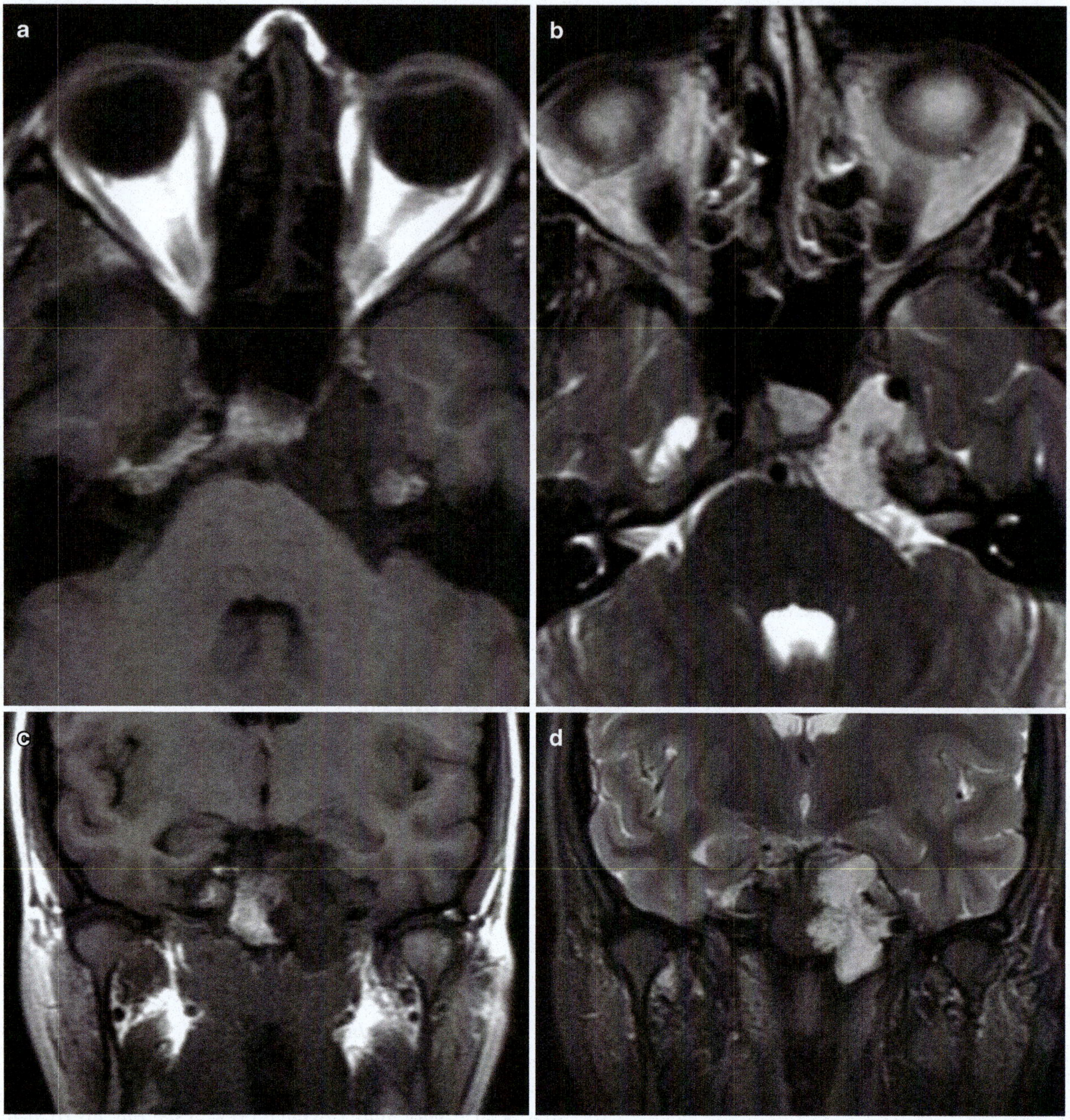

Fig. 46.1 (**a**) Axial T1 shows a large (~ *2.5 cm*) mass involving the left central skull base. It is relatively homogeneous and conspicuously hypointense to brain and adjacent fatty marrow. The left carotid (black flow void) has been displaced anteriorly and laterally. (**b**) Axial T2 more convincingly confirms the position of the mass described on prior T1. The mass has ↑ T2 signal roughly isointense to CSF and globes. It contains multiple focal foci with ↓ T2 signal. There is fluid in adjacent sphenoid and ethmoid sinuses. Such dramatic anterior displacement of the left carotid (black flow void) would not be expected from a fluid-filled mass. Figures, Coronal T1 (**c**) and T2 (**d**) demonstrate that the mass depicted on prior images was really the "tip of the iceberg" and its craniocaudal size is even larger than perceived on axial planes. Many of its margins are curiously irregular appearing to actually invade clival marrow [bright on T1 (**c**)] medially

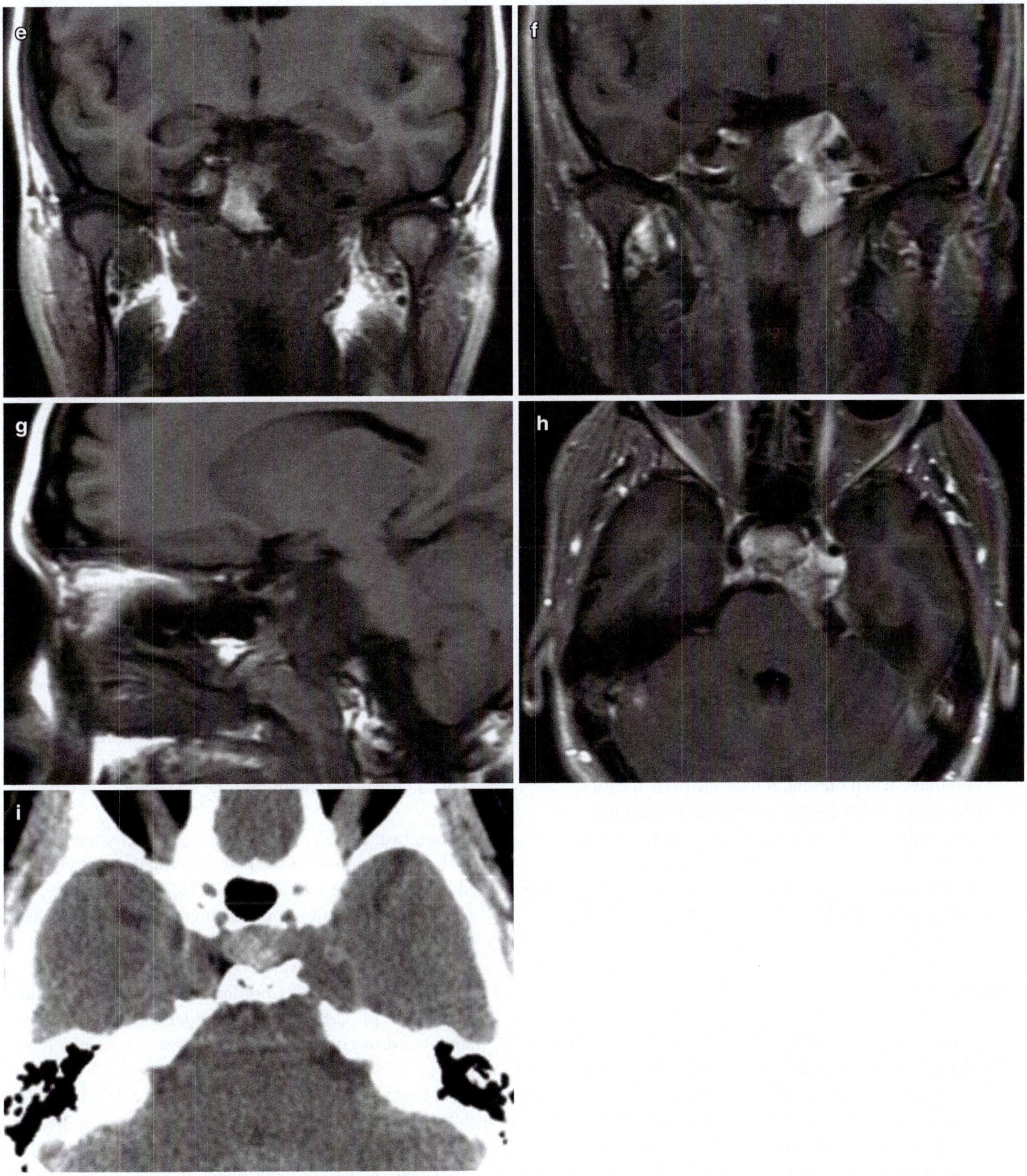

Fig. 46.1 (continued) Coronal T1 without (**e**) and with Gd and fat saturation (**f**) clearly separate enhancing tumor from clival marrow and other adjacent structures. [Clival marrow is bright on (**e**) and dark on (**f**), whereas tumor is dark on (**e**) and bright on (**f**).] (**g**) Sag T1 shows a large low attenuation mass has destroyed the clivus replacing most of the high T1 signal marrow displacing the pons posteriorly. Little high signal marrow remains just below the sella and at the clival tip. (**h**) Axial T1 Gd shows heterogeneously enhancing central skull base mass containing multiple foci of low attenuation, with some representing vascular flow voids. The mass has clearly invaded the cavernous sinuses surrounding and displacing the carotid siphons. The mass extends asymmetrically toward the left petro-occipital fissure displacing the adjacent pons and temporal lobe. (**i**) Axial CECT depicts relative hypo-attenuation presented by this same huge central skull base tumor. This image is shown *only* to depict how subtle some findings can be with CT as compared to the flagrant findings depicted on MRI

- Classic chordoma has a lower mean ADC at 1474.
- Poorly differentiated chordoma has the lowest mean ADC at 875.
- Chondrosarcoma is associated with statistically higher ADC values compared to classic chordoma.
- Therefore, DWI may be useful in distinguishing classic chordoma from chondrosarcoma. DWI is probably not helpful, however, in distinguishing the more favorable chondroid chordoma.

Angiography

- Sometimes shows a distinct tumor stain.
- May observe occlusion of arteries or cavernous sinus [9].

Plain Films

- 50% show lytic lesions.
- 60% contain calcifications.
- Included for historic note. Alas, not used much anymore having fallen from favor, as clinicians currently order CT and/or MRI.

Clinical Issues

Presentation

- Symptoms, when present, mirror the mass location.
- Most present with diplopia and/or headache [10].
- Sometimes see decreased visual acuity or symptoms involving the eighth and lower cranial nerves [9].
- The duration of symptoms shows slow growth ranging from 1.5 to 14 years.

Pathology

- Gross Features: Grayish-white, lobulated, scalloped, irregular, destructive, mass containing calcifications.
- Microscopic Features: Chondrosarcomas are composed of atypical chondrocytes having enlarged hyperchromatic nuclei embedded in copious cartilaginous stroma. Higher-grade chondrosarcomas show ↑ cellularity, ↑ nuclear size, ↑ mitotic activity, ↑ nuclear hyperchromasia, and ↑ aggressiveness [3, 11].
- Locations: SBCs commonly crop up along synchondrosis, particularly at the petro-occipital fissure [1, 8]. (See Fig. 46.2a–c Anatomic Skull.)

Treatment and Prognosis

- Skull base chondrosarcomas are slow growing but locally aggressive.
- Gross total resection is the favored regimen and is more often possible because of newer lateral skull base techniques including the infratemporal fossa approach [2].
- Complete tumor extirpation, however, is not always possible.
- Proton beam radiation is preferred for residual or recurrent SBC tumors, despite their propensity for low sensitivity to radiation [4, 9].
- For well-resected, low-grade chondrosarcomas, some say the benefit-to-risk ratio does not support radiotherapy [5].
- Characteristic slow growth often makes assessment of treatment outcome difficult [2].

Differential Diagnosis (DDx) [3]

A. Clivus Chordoma
- Chordoma is the classic contender in the skull base chondrosarcoma (SBC) differential.
- Chordomas lack coarse chondroid calcifications frequently found in SBCs.
- While chordomas and SBCs often have common locations and cause similar symptoms, *recurrence and survival rates are considerably better for SBC than for chordoma* [3].
- Since chordomas arise from notochordal remnants, they typically display a more midline epicenter near clivus [3, 12].
- By contrast, chondrosarcomas are mesenchymal in origin with a predilection for the petro-occipital fissure and tend to arise in a more lateral location [3, 13].
- Unpredictable patterns of origin, growth, and invasion combine to dash any real hope that the prior discussed features could be considered pathognomonic [3, 14].
- Microscopic Features: Chordomas are somewhat cellular, composed of vacuolated *physaliferous cells* (situated singly and in *cords*) surrounded by a mucus-like matrix [3, 6].
- DWI (with ADC) is useful in separating SBCs from chordomas as well as portraying the presence of the rare poorly differentiated chordoma.
- See Chap. 30, Clivus Chordoma.

B. Plasmacytoma/Myeloma
- Plasmacytomas are usually more midline than SBCs.
- Plasmacytomas have low to intermediate T2. SBCs characteristically show ↓ T1 and ↑ T2.

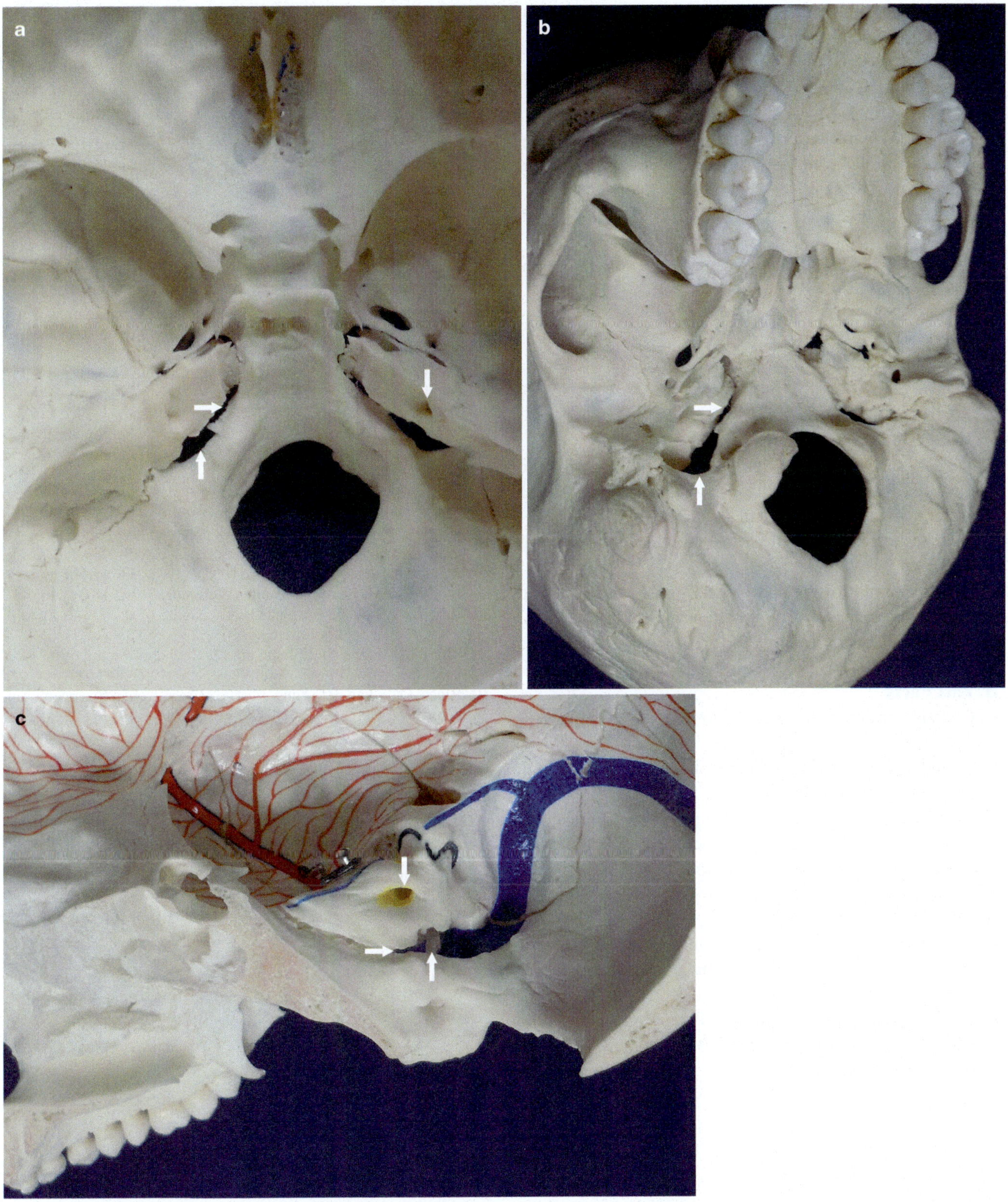

Fig. 46.2 (**a**) View of endocranial anatomic skull base specimen. Key: → petro-occipital fissure, ↑ jugular foramen, ↓ IAC. (**b**) Oblique view of extracranial anatomic skull base specimen. Key: → petro-occipital fissure, ↑ jugular foramen. (**c**) Sagittal view of anatomic skull base specimen from inside. Depicts sigmoid sinus entering jugular foramen in blue with IAC in yellow. Key: → petro-occipital fissure, ↑ jugular foramen, ↓ IAC

- > 50% of patients with plasmacytoma have coexisting multiple myeloma.

C. Metastatic Neoplasm

- Metastatic neoplasm can cause a destructive mass anywhere along the skull base. Although they can occur elsewhere in the skull base, chondrosarcomas show a predictable predilection for the POF (petro-occipital fissure).
- Frequently find *multiple metastases* in patients having recognized primary neoplasms.

A Closer Look

I. Genetics and Associations

- Most skull base chondrosarcomas (SBCs) are sporadic; however, reported predisposing conditions include Ollier's disease and Maffucci syndrome.
- Genetic aberrations increase as chondrosarcomas progress from low to high grade.
- Overexpression of the p53 protein plays some role with 17p1 alterations and TP53 mutations present in almost all high-grade chondrosarcomas [15].

II. Fast Facts

- Chondrosarcomas are thought to arise from embryonic rest cells.
- Chondrosarcomas are uncommon, usually low grade showing sluggish growth.
- *Recurrence:* In a large study composed of 2000 patients with cranial chondrosarcoma (including 560 nonduplicated patients), the overall recurrence rate was 22% [10].

III. Historical Highlights

- 1993 Stapleton et al. reported eight skull base chondrosarcomas (SBCs) treated surgically at London's Atkinson Morley Hospital between 1985 and 1991.
- 2001 Crockard et al. reported 17 patients with SBCs treated surgically at London's St Bartholomew's Hospital between 1986 and 1998.
- 1995 Gay et al. reported 60 patients with SBCs and chordomas treated surgically at the University of Pittsburgh between 1984 and 1993. Five-year survival for the 14 SBC patients was 90%.

References

1. Mendenhall WM, Lewis SB, Villaret DB, Mendenhall NP. Skull base chondrosarcoma. Cancer Ther. 2004;2:519–24.
2. Brachmann DE, Teufert KB. Chondrosarcoma of the skull base: long-term follow up. Otol Neurotol. 2006;27(7):981–91.
3. Yeom KW, Lober BC, Mobley BC, et al. Diffusion-weighted MRI: distinction of skull base chordoma from chondrosarcoma. AJNR Am J Neuroradiol. 2013;31:1056–61. https://doi.org/10.3174/ajnr.A3333.
4. Ott RF, Melville GE, New PF, et al. The role of MR and CT in evaluating clival chordomas and chondrosarcomas. AJR Am J Roentgenol. 1988;151(3):567–75.
5. Almefty K, Pravdenkkova S, Colli BO, et al. Chordoma and chondrosarcoma: similar but quite different, skull base tumors. Cancer. 2007;110(11):2457–67.
6. Mirra JM, Nelson SD, Della Rocca C, et al. Chordoma. In: Fletcher CDM, Unni KK, Mertens F, editors. World Health Organization classification of tumours: pathology and genetics of tumours of soft tissue and bone. Lyon: IARC Press; 2002. p. 315–7.
7. Myers SP, Hirsch WL Jr, Curtin HD, et al. Chondrosarcomas of the skull base: MR imaging features. Radiology. 1992;184(1):103–8.
8. Raut AA, Naphade PS, Chawla A. Imaging of skull base: pictorial essay. Indian J Radiol Imaging. 2012;22:305–16.
9. Morimoto T, Sasaki T, Takakura IT. Chondrosarcoma of the skull base: report of six cases. Skull Base Surg. 1992;2(4):177–85.
10. Bloch OG, Jian BJ, Yang I, et al. Cranial chondrosarcoma and recurrence. Skull Base. 2010;20(3):149–56.
11. Bertoni F, Bacchini P, Hogendoorn PC. Chondrosarcoma. In: Fletcher CDM, Unni KK, Mertens F, editors. World Health Organization classification of tumours: pathology and genetics of tumours of soft tissue and bone. Lyon: IARC Press; 2002. p. 247–51.
12. Burrow JF, Stewart MJ. Original papers: malignant spheno-occipital chordoma. J Neurol Psychopathol. 1923;15:205–17.
13. Heffelfinger MJ, Dahlin DC, MacCarty CS, et al. Chordomas and cartilaginous tumors of the skullbase. Cancer. 1973;32:410–20.
14. Pamir MN, Ozduman K. Analysis of radiological features relative to histopathology in 42 skull-base chordomas and chondrosarcomas. Eur J Radiol. 2006;58:461–70.
15. Kim MJ, Cho KJ, Ayala AG, Ro JY. Chondrosarcoma: with updates on molecular genetics. Sarcoma. 2011, 2011:Article ID 405437, 15 pages. https://doi.org/10.1155/2011/40537. Accessed 02/15/2016

47 Ewing's Sarcoma of the Skull Base

Pertinent Points

- Definition: Ewing's sarcoma (ES) is an aggressive malignant tumor of childhood and adolescence which contains small round blue cells and predominately presents in the second decade of life.
- *Classic Clue*: Caucasian child or adolescent presenting with pain, fever, and ↑ ESR found on imaging to have an extra-axial mass extending cranially and caudally from its skull base epicenter. On examination the patient demonstrates orbital or cranial nerve symptoms.
- *AKA:* Ewing sarcoma, Askin's tumor, peripheral primitive neuroectodermal tumor, or pPNET.
- *Tumor Family:* Ewing's sarcoma belongs to a group of entities which share a common EWS gene translocation taken together to compose the "Ewing family of tumors."
- Most likely to see on board exam or high-level neuroradiology panel.
- *Distributions:*
  - Gender preference: M > F = 1.6:1 [1].
  - Age: Childhood or adulthood. Peak 10–20 years. However, one case has been reported in a 54-year-old man.
  - Incidence:

    Primary Ewing's sarcoma of the skull base is a rare entity [1].

    Rare among Asians and African-Americans.

    ESs comprise 16% of primary bone sarcomas.

    <4% of ES occur in the skull.

    ES accounts for 10–15% of childhood malignant bone tumors being second only to osteosarcoma [8].
  - Ewing's sarcoma may occasionally present as a second cancer, particularly in patients treated with radiation therapy.
- Locations:
  - When Ewing's sarcoma does involve the skull, it is more often found in temporal, followed by parietal and occipital bones. The sphenoid and ethmoid bones are less commonly involved [9].

Imaging

General Imaging Features

- Primary Ewing's sarcoma is usually extradural, but dural invasion has been documented [7, 8].
- (See Fig. 47.1a–d.)

CT Features

- *See* Section "General Imaging Features".
- Usually demonstrate destructive, permeative bone involvement with soft tissue components showing *no* soft tissue calcifications [7].
- Depending on the tumor stage, Ewing's sarcoma can cause cortical erosion with rarefaction and "moth-eaten" permeative destruction [7]:
  - The classic "onion peel" appearance observed with extracranial Ewing's sarcoma is *frequently not found with cranial involvement* [7].
  - Ewing's has high attenuation secondary to sheets of densely packed cells [8].
  - CECT shows moderate heterogeneous enhancement.

F. A. Midyett, S. K. Mukherji, *Skull Base Imaging*, https://doi.org/10.1007/978-3-030-46447-9_47

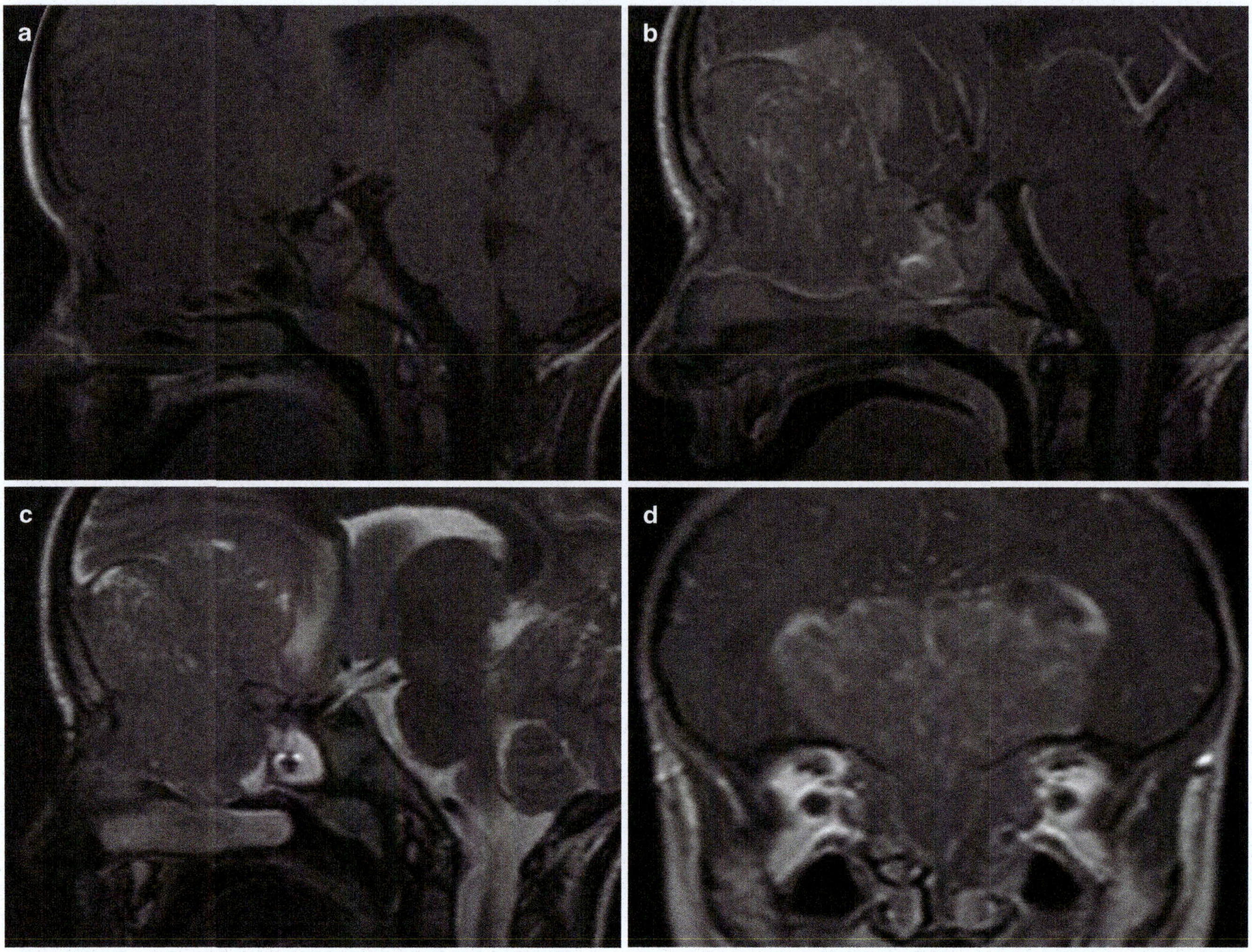

Fig. 47.1 Sagittal T1 (**a**) without and (**b**) with Gd depict a huge anterior skull base mass extending caudally into the nasal cavity and cranially creating a huge intracranial extradural component. The anterior cranial fossa floor has clearly been destroyed showing absence of the normal low signal dark black line. The tumor is low signal before and mildly enhancing after Gd. Multiple enhancing vascular channels are seen in and around the tumor. The conspicuous clival synchondrosis (wide dark black line) alerts us to the fact that this is a child. (**c**) Sagittal T2 shows a huge mass involving the anterior skull base depicted on prior images. Clearly, the floor of the anterior cranial fossa is absent with tumor extending intracranially and into nasal cavity. Signal is relatively isointense to brain with multiple focal fluid collections. (**d**) Coronal T1 Gd, shows moderate heterogeneous enhancement of the huge extradural intracranial mass. The floor of the anterior cranial fossa (depicted by a thick dark black line) has been clearly breached by this dumbbell shaped tumor extending above and below the now demolished skull base. A great clue as to site of origin! The tumor has invaded both orbits showing ↓ signal compared to orbital fat

MRI Features

- *See General Imaging Features.*
- T1: Low to intermediate signal, isointense to brain and EOMs. (See Fig. 47.1a.)
- T2: Heterogeneous signal, relatively isointense to brain with focal fluid collections which show high T2 signal. (See Fig. 47.1c.). Low signal striations sometimes show "hair on end" appearance.
- T1 Gd:
  - *Mild heterogeneous enhancement.* (See Fig. 47.1b, d.)
  - *Fat saturation* techniques are very helpful.
- DWI:
  - Bony involvement by ES may be more conspicuous on DWI than other MRI sequences particularly when they are small and metastatic.
  - Since the 30 seconds required to perform the DWI sequence is so short, it should be included in *all* patients having (or suspected of having) cancer [10].

Nuclear Medicine Features

- Ewing's sarcoma exhibits increased uptake on ^{67}galium citrate and all three phases of ^{99m} technetium MDP (methyl diphosphonate) bone scans.

Clinical Issues

Presentation

- Diagnostic Delay: Most patients present with headache and papilledema, but some show symptoms 2 weeks to 2 years before presenting for diagnosis and treatment [7].
- Patients may also have proptosis, painful ophthalmoplegia, ↓ visual acuity, epistaxis, and nasal bridge broadening [7].
- Patients progressing to intracranial spread sometimes show signs of increased intracranial pressure [9].
- May show ↑ ESR, low-grade fever, soreness, or swelling in the tumor region.

Pathology

- *Gross Pathology*
  – Well-circumscribed with gelatinous cut surface showing yellow to grayish-white cut surface [9]
- *Microscopic Features*
  – Most show sheets of monotonous monomorphic round tumor cells containing sparse vacuolated cytoplasm, round nuclei, inconspicuous nucleoli, and atypical mitosis [11]

Treatment and Prognosis

Surgery

- With most Ewing's sarcoma patients, when surgery is performed, it frequently follows chemotherapy by weeks or months.
- However, patients with cranial Ewing's sarcoma may require urgent surgical intervention to control ↑ intracranial pressure, or impending neurologic deficits.
- For skull base Ewing's sarcoma, total excision is often not possible without substantial surgically induced morbidity [11].

Chemotherapy

- Almost all patients with Ewing's sarcoma exhibit micrometastases at the time of diagnosis, so chemotherapy is routinely recommended.
- Currently, combination chemotherapy with vincristine, adriamycin, cyclophosphamide, and actinomycin D appears superior to other regimens [1, 3].

Radiotherapy

- *Radiosensitive:* Ewing's sarcoma is relatively *radiosensitive* [7].
- Radiotherapy along with aggressive multidrug chemotherapy is touted by some to have a significant role in preventing local or systemic recurrences, particularly pulmonary [3].

Treatment Trials

- Current treatment trials include:
  – SBRT1 – Stereotactic radiation therapy for pediatric sarcomas
  – SJGD2 – Monoclonal antibody therapy in treating younger patients with relapsed or refractory neuroblastoma, osteosarcoma, or melanoma. Phase I also includes Ewing's sarcoma.

Prognosis

- With radical surgery, aggressive multidrug chemotherapy and radiotherapy clinicians can expect a 57% 5-year survival for all cases of cranial Ewing's sarcoma [2].
- Despite aggressive treatment, 20–40% of patients with localized disease and 80% of patients who have metastasis at presentation succumb to their disease [4].
- Children with all types of Ewing's can currently expect a cure rate of approximately 70%. Children with metastasis at presentation show survival rates of <30%.
- Teens aged 15–19 have a lower survival rate of approximately 56%.

Differential Diagnosis

A. Chondrosarcoma

- Chondrosarcomas are chondroid malignancies which commonly select a synchondrosis when rarely involving the skull base.
- *Classic Clue*: Skull base mass exhibiting an affinity for the POF (petro-occipital fissure) sometimes showing chondroid matrix, characterized by low T1 and high T2 signals.
- Appear as well-circumscribed, often scalloped, or lobulated lytic lesions exhibiting chondroid calcifications. In contrast, skull base Ewing's usually *do not* show calcifications.
- Age: 10–79 years (mean 39). In contrast, Ewing's is usually found in children mostly <20 years of age.

- Low attenuation may make them subtle on brain soft tissue algorithms. (See Chap. 46, Fig. 46.1i.) In contrast ES typically has high attenuation.
- T2: Very high T2 signal. (See Chap. 46, Fig. 46.1b, d.) In contrast, ES shows low T2 signal secondary to sheets of densely packed cells [8].
- See Chap. 46, Skull Base Chondrosarcoma).

B. Clivus Chordoma

- *Classic Clue*: Midline lobular tumor with bony destruction arising in or near the clivus which on MRI T2 imaging is hyperintense to nearby intervertebral discs.
- Chordomas and ES both typically lack coarse chondroid calcifications frequently found in SBCs.
- CT: Destructive lytic bone lesion usually with hypodense soft tissue mass.
- T1: Heterogeneous hypo- to isointense signal compared to marrow.
- T2: Hyperintense to intervertebral discs and CSF.
- T1 Gd: Heterogeneous enhancement with honeycomb pattern varies from barely blushing to avid light bulb bright.
- Gradient Echo: If hemorrhage is present sometimes see "blooming".
- Microscopic Features: Chordomas are somewhat cellular, composed of *vacuolated physaliferous cells* (situated singly and in *cords*) surrounded by a mucus-like matrix.
- (See Chap. 30, Clivus Chordoma)

C. Esthesioneuroblastoma (ENB)

- Rare neuroendocrine malignancy of neural crest origin arising from olfactory epithelium.
- AKA: Olfactory neuroblastoma.
- ENB is more often found in middle-aged patients but can be seen in children. In contrast, ES is usually found in children mostly <20 years of age.
- Classically shows avidly enhancing dumbbell-shaped mass with "waist" at the cribriform plate.
- May involve the anterior cranial fossa, skull base, and orbit.
- ENBs show intermediate signal on T1 and T2 with avid enhancement on T1 Gd.
- Cystic areas (with foci of ↑T2) at the tumor/brain interface are diagnostic and may be pathognomonic.
- DWI demonstrates moderate restricted diffusion.
- ENB exhibits an epicenter near the cribriform plate.
- ENB displays no gender preference.
- (See Chap. 28, Esthesioneuroblastoma)

D. Neuroendocrine Carcinoma (NEC)

- Neuroendocrine tumors (NETs) comprise a vast variety of tumors which may exhibit either epithelial or neural origins. NETs arising from neural origin are paragangliomas, and those arising from epithelial origin are neuroendocrine carcinomas (NECs).
- The median age of presentation for NEC is 56 years. In contrast, Ewing's are usually found in children, and most are <20 years of age.
- With NEC, skull base involvement is a frequent finding.
- Ewing's show marked heterogeneous enhancement on CECT; not a feature for NEC.
- See Chap. 16, Neuroendocrine Carcinoma.

E. Metastatic Neoplasm

- Metastatic neoplasm can cause a destructive mass anywhere along the skull base.
- Frequently find *multiple metastases* in patients having recognized primary neoplasms.
- In children, metastatic neuroblastoma should be considered [9].

F. Langerhans Cell Histiocytosis (LCH)

- LCH is the modern moniker bestowed on a rare, ill understood but significant, pathologic process related to proliferation of macrophages and dendrites (formerly dubbed histiocytes).
- *Classic Clue*: Pediatrics refers for MRI a child who has a history of diabetes insipidus. This child is found to have an enlarged avidly enhancing infundibular stalk and an absent posterior pituitary bright spot.
- LCH predominately involves age 1–5 of pediatric population, typically appearing during the first decade. This is a similar age group to Ewing's sarcoma.
- Sometimes see lytic lesions involving the calvarium and/or temporal bones.
- CNS manifestations of LCH occur in ≤50% and are more frequent in patients with multisystem disease. Patients *rarely present* with isolated CNS involvement.
- See Chap. 8, Langerhans Cell Histiocytosis.

A Closer Look

I. Genetics and Associations

- While not a single entity, Ewing's sarcoma consists of connected maladies showing similar clinical and biologic features [4].
- One thing these entities do have in common is an EWS gene translocation which results in the "Ewing family of tumors" [4].
- At presentation, these destructive tumors have clinically apparent metastases in almost 25% [4].
- 90–95% have a consistent cytogenetic abnormality, t (11;22) (q24;p12).

II. Fast Facts

- Ewing's sarcoma is the second most common tumor primarily presenting in long bones.
- Ewing's sarcoma is most frequently found in children, 75% of whom are <20 years old.
- Only 1% of Ewing's sarcoma commences in cranial bones [5].
- The Ewing's sarcoma family of tumors includes:

Ewing's sarcoma, involving bone	87%
Extra-osseous Ewing's sarcoma, involving soft tissues	8%
Peripheral PNET	5%
Askin's tumor	

III. Historical Highlights

- 1921: James Ewing described this tumor as diffuse endothelioma of bone [4, 6].

References

1. Cugati G, Singh M, Pande A, et al. Isolated skull base primary Ewing's sarcoma: an extremely rare location. J Cancer Res Ther. 2013;9(4):141–2.
2. Desai KI, Nadkarni TD, Goel A, Muzumdar DP, Naresh KN, Nair CN. Primary Ewing's sarcoma of the cranium. Neurosurgery. 2000;46:62–8.
3. Agrawal A, Dulani R, Mahadevan A, Vagaha SJ, Vagha J, Shankar SK. Primary Ewing's sarcoma of the frontal bone with intracranial extension. J Cancer Res Ther. 2009;5:208–9.
4. Thacker MM, Temple HT, Scully SP. Current treatment for Ewing's sarcoma. Expert Rev Anticancer Ther. 2005;5:319–31.
5. Seckin H, Varan A, Demirhan B, et al. Primary Ewing's sarcoma of the cranium. Turk Neurosurg. 2001;11:130–3.
6. Ewing J. Diffuse endothelioma of bone. Proc N Y Pathol Soc. 1921;21:17–24.
7. Shukla D, Rao VS, Rajesh A, et al. Neglected primary Ewing's sarcoma of ethmmoid presenting as surgical emergency. Asian J Neurosurg. 2013;8(1):51–3. https://doi.org/10.4103/1793-5482.110281.
8. Li WY, Brock P, Saunders DE. Imaging characteristics of primary cranial Ewing's sarcoma. Pediatr Radiol. 2005;35:612–8.
9. Gupta A, Bansal S, Chaturvedi S. Primary Ewing's sarcoma of frontoparietal bone with major soft tissue extension: an unusual presentation and review of the literature. Case Rep Pathol. 2012:Article ID 713836, 3 pages. https://doi.org/10.1155/2012/713836.
10. Nemeth AJ, Henson JW, Mullins ME, et al. Improved detection of skull metastasis with diffusion-weighted MR imaging. AJNR Am J Neuroradiol. 2007;28:1088–92.
11. Kadar AA, Hearst MJ, Collins MH, et al. Ewing's sarcoma of the petrous temporal bone: case report and literature review. Skull Base. 2010;20(3):213–7.

48 Skull Base Fibrosarcoma

Pertinent Points

- *Definition*: Sarcomas are spindle cell malignancies of mesenchymal origin named and classified for their predominant cell line which for fibrosarcoma is the fibroblast. As the second most common H&N sarcoma, fibrosarcomas comprise ≤10% of all H&N sarcomas, sometimes involving the skull base and paranasal sinuses.
- *Classic Clue*: An unfortunate patient presents with a destructive skull base mass containing a large soft tissue component and has a history of having a prior pituitary adenoma treated by radiation therapy many years earlier. The large soft tissue component contains foci of collagen which have high T2 signal.
- *Incidence and Distributions:*
  - Incidence: Fibrosarcomas comprise <5% of all primary bone sarcomas [2].
  - Age: Mean age at diagnosis is 35 years (range 2–76).
  - Gender: Slight male predominance.

Imaging

General Imaging Features

- Classically shows a large soft tissue mass demonstrating erosion and destruction of bone.

CT Features

- *See General Imaging Features.*
- Although typically osteolytic, depending on tumor stage, fibrosarcomas *can range from ragged and moth-eaten to well defined.*
- Periosteal reaction progresses to cortical destruction and commonly extends into the soft tissues.
- Tumor attenuation is similar to nearby muscle.

MRI Features

- *See General Imaging Features.*
- MRI is the premier method for evaluating skull base fibrosarcoma.
- Most are well-circumscribed with 50% showing internal fibrous septae.
- Fibrosarcomas may be homogenous or heterogeneous.
- T1: Isointense to muscle.
- T2: Quite heterogeneous signal with solid component isointense to brain but filled with multiple foci of high T2 signal probably caused by collagen collections. (See Fig. 48.1.)
- T1 Gd:
  - Demonstrates avid enhancement which may be homogeneous or heterogeneous depending on the number of collagen collections,
  - DWI:

    ADC values are potentially useful in separating various benign and malignant tumors.

    Low ADC:

    - ADC values range from high in benign lesions to low for fibrosarcoma.
    - Among soft tissue malignancies, chondrosarcoma has the highest ADC value, followed by liposarcoma, with fibrosarcoma showing the lowest ADC value [7].

Nuclear Medicine Features

- Fibrosarcoma exhibits increased uptake on bone scans.

F. A. Midyett, S. K. Mukherji, *Skull Base Imaging*, https://doi.org/10.1007/978-3-030-46447-9_48

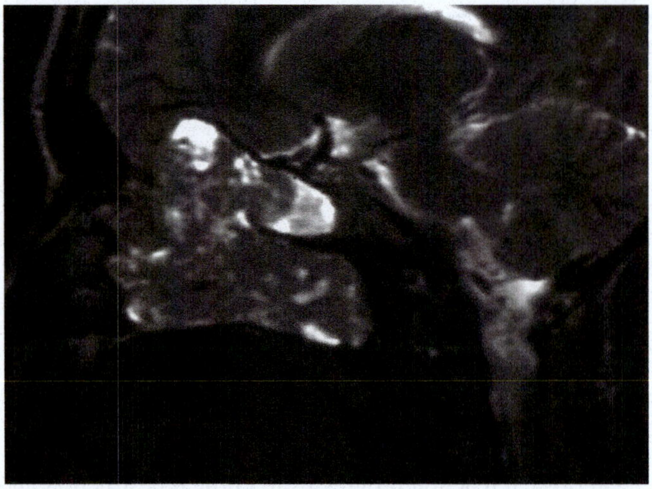

Fig. 48.1 Sagittal T2 shows a huge anterior skull base mass extending caudally into the nasal cavity and cranially creating a large intracranial extradural component causing mass effect on the adjacent frontal lobes. The floor of the anterior cranial fossa is absent with the tumor "waist" near the breached floor. MRI signal shows the solid tumor is predominately isointense to brain but contains multiple high signal collagen-filled foci scattered throughout

Clinical Issues

Presentation

- Most patients present with pain, sinusitis, nasal obstruction, epistaxis, and/or hypoesthesia.
- Patients occasionally demonstrate diplopia.

Pathology

- *Gross Features*:
  - Periodically portrays a polypoid appearance resembling ordinary nasal polyps.
  - Fibrosarcomas are unencapsulated, sometimes ulcerated, and can appear well-circumscribed or invasive.
  - The tumor is tan to grayish with a rubbery consistency.
  - Larger lesions have hemorrhagic and necrotic foci.
- *Microscopic Features*:
  - The cellular appearance varies widely among these tumors.
  - Spindle cells separated by keloid-like collagen are often arranged in compact bundles at acute angles showing a "chevron" or "herringbone" pattern.
  - Invagination of the surface epithelium can be prominent enough to imitate an inverted papilloma.
  - Most sinonasal tract fibrosarcomas are low-grade.
  - Lichtenstein emphasized that some FSs may be so well differentiated that the "uninitiated" may mistake them for benign processes [3, 4].
  - David Dahlin throughout his long luminary career continued to emphasize the need for correlating radiologic and pathologic findings when making a bone tumor diagnosis [3]. While Dr. Dahlin, a pathologist, was clearly a better "bone" radiologist than the average radiologist, he consistently consulted with the best "bone" radiologist available before finalizing many of his pathologic diagnoses.
- Immunohistochemical Staining:
  - Fibrosarcomas stain positive for vimentin and sometimes focally positive for actin [1].

Treatment and Prognosis

Surgery

- Radical surgical excision is the treatment of choice with adjuvant chemotherapy.
- When located in the skull base, the extent of surgery is often limited.

Chemotherapy

- Since they tend to metastasize early, prompt chemotherapy is suggested.

Radiotherapy

- Not used to treat fibrosarcomas, although radiotherapy has been incriminated in its etiology.

Prognosis

- When found in children <4 years, fibrosarcoma has better prognosis with less local recurrence and distant metastasis.
- Prognosis is distinctly better than osteosarcoma [3].
- Following treatment for pituitary adenomas, schwannomas, and skull base meningiomas, radiation-associated sarcomas (RAS) possess a particularly poor prognosis [5].
- Prognosis is primarily dependent on tumor grade.

Differential Diagnosis

A. Chondrosarcoma (CS)

- Chondrosarcomas are chondroid malignancies which commonly select a synchondrosis when involving the skull base.
- *Classic Clue*: Skull base mass exhibiting an affinity for the POF (petro-occipital fissure) sometimes showing chondroid matrix, characterized by low T1 and high T2 signals.
- Chondrosarcomas appear as well-circumscribed, often scalloped, or lobulated lytic lesions exhibiting chondroid calcifications. In contrast, skull-based fibrosarcomas (FSs) usually *do not show calcifications*.
- Age: 10–79 years (mean 39).
- Low attenuation may make them subtle on brain soft tissue algorithms. (See Chap. 46, Fig. 46.1i.)
- T2: *Exhibit exceptionally high T2 signal.* (See Chap. 46, Fig. 46.1b, d.)
- (See Chap. 46, Skull Base Chondrosarcoma)

B. Clivus Chordoma

- Chordomas typically lack coarse chondroid calcifications.
- CT: Destructive lytic bone lesion usually with *hypoattenuating* soft tissue mass.
- T1: Heterogeneous hypo- to isointense signal compared to marrow.
- T2: Hyperintense to intervertebral discs and CSF.
- T1 Gd: Heterogeneous enhancement with honeycomb pattern varies from barely blushing to avid light bulb bright.
- Gradient Echo: If hemorrhage is present sometimes shows "blooming."
- Microscopic Features: Chordomas are somewhat cellular, composed of *vacuolated physaliferous cells* (situated singly and in *cords*) surrounded by a mucus-like matrix.
- (See Chap. 30, Clivus Chordoma)

C. Ewing's Sarcoma (ES)

- Ewing's sarcoma is an aggressive malignant tumor of *childhood and adolescence* containing small blue round cells which usually presents in the second decade.
- *Classic Clue*: *Caucasian child or adolescent* presenting with pain, fever, and ↑ ESR found on imaging to have extra-axial mass extending cranially and caudally from its skull base epicenter. At presentation, the patient exhibits orbital or cranial nerve complaints.
- Ewing's accounts for 10–15% of childhood malignant bone tumors and is second only to osteosarcoma.
- Ewing's is rare among Asians and African-Americans.
- Ewing's usually demonstrates destructive, permeative bone destruction with soft tissue components showing *no* soft tissue calcifications.
- Depending on the tumor stage, Ewing's can cause cortical erosion with rarefaction and "moth-eaten" permeative destruction.
- T1: Low to intermediate signal, isointense with brain and EOMs. (See Chap. 47, Fig. 47.1a.)
- T2: Heterogeneous signal, relatively isointense to brain with focal fluid collections which show high T2 signal. (See Chap. 47, Fig. 47.1c.) Low signal striations sometimes suggest "hair on end" appearance.
- T1 Gd:
  - *Mild heterogeneous enhancement.* (See Chap. 47, Fig. 47.1b, d.)
  - *Fat saturation* techniques are very helpful.
- DWI:
  - Bony involvement by ES may be more conspicuous on DWI than other MRI sequences particularly when they are small and metastatic.
  - (See Chap. 47, Ewing's Sarcoma)

D. Esthesioneuroblastoma (ENB)

- Rare neuroendocrine malignancy of neural crest origin arising from olfactory epithelium.
- AKA: Olfactory neuroblastoma.
- ENB is more often found in middle-aged patients but can be seen in children.
- Classically exhibits avidly enhancing dumbbell-shaped mass with "waist" at the cribriform plate.
- May involve the anterior cranial fossa, skull base, and orbit.
- ENBs show intermediate signal on T1 and T2 exhibiting enthusiastic enhancement on T1 Gd.
- Cystic areas (with foci of ↑T2) at the tumor/brain interface are diagnostic and may be pathognomonic.
- DWI reveals moderate restricted diffusion.
- ENB exhibits an epicenter near the cribriform plate.
- ENB displays no gender preference.
- (See Chap. 28, Esthesioneuroblastoma)

E. Neuroendocrine Carcinoma (NEC)

- Neuroendocrine tumors (NETs) comprise a vast variety of tumors which may exhibit either epithelial or neural origins. NETs arising from neural origin are paragangliomas, and those arising from epithelial origin are neuroendocrine carcinomas (NECs).
- The median age of presentation for NEC is 56 years.
- With NEC, skull base involvement is a frequent finding.
- (See Chap. 16, Neuroendocrine Carcinoma)

F. Metastatic Neoplasm

- Metastatic neoplasm can cause a destructive mass anywhere along the skull base.
- Frequently find *multiple metastases* in patients having recognized primary neoplasms.
- In children, metastatic neuroblastoma should be considered.

A Closer Look

I. Genetics and Associations

- While most fibrosarcomas develop de novo, some arise in areas of prior irradiation, burn scars, or implanted synthetic material such as grafts.
- In older patients fibrosarcoma has been thought to arise from "transformation" of benign lesions including enchondroma, fibrous dysplasia, giant cell tumor, chronic osteomyelitis, Paget's disease, bone infarct, surgically treated fracture, and low-grade chondrosarcoma.

II. Fast Facts

- Fibrosarcomas comprise $\leq$10% of all H&N sarcomas.
- Fibrosarcomas comprise <5% of all primary bone sarcomas [2].

III. Historic Highlights

- 1948: Cahan et al. reported 11 cases of sarcomas arising in previously irradiated bone [6].

References

1. Wasserzug O, Leider-Trejo L, Fliss DM, Gil ZR. Malignant tumours of the paranasal sinuses. In: Gil Z, Fliss DM, editors. Tumours of the skull base and paranasal sinuses. New York, NY: Springer.
2. Dorfman HD, Czerniak B. Bone cancers. Cancer. 1995;75(1 Suppl):203–10.
3. Dahlin DC, Ivins JC. Fibrosarcoma of bone: a study of 114 cases. Cancer. 23:35–41. https://doi.org/10.1002/1097-0142(196901)23:1<35:AID-CNCR2820230104>3.0.CO;2-V4.
4. Lichtenstein I. Bone tumors. 3rd ed. St. Louis: C. V. Mosby Company; 1958. p. 298. 1965; p. 229
5. Sedney CL, Morris JM, Giannini C, et al. Radiation-associated sarcoma of the skull base after irradiation for pituitary adenoma. Rare Tumors. 2012;4(1):e7.
6. Cahan WG, Woodard HQ, Higginbotham NL, et al. Sarcoma arising in irradiated bone; report of 11 cases. Cancer. 1948;1:3–29.
7. Khedr SA, Hassan MA, Abdelrazek NM, et al. Diagnostic impact of echo planar diffusion-weighted magnetic resonance imaging (DWI) in musculoskeletal neoplastic masses using apparent diffusion coefficient (ADC) mapping *as a quantitative assessment tool*. Egypt J Radiol Nucl Med. 2012;43(2):219–26.

49 Skull Base Rhabdomyosarcoma

Pertinent Points

- *Definition*: Although relatively rare, rhabdomyosarcoma (RMS) is the most common childhood soft tissue sarcoma caused by primitive mesenchymal cells retaining their capacity for skeletal muscle differentiation [1]. Rhabdomyosarcoma is most frequently found in children <10 years and currently comprises 5% of childhood cancers [2].
- *Name Origin:* Rhabdomyosarcoma originates from the Greek words *rhabdo* meaning rod shape and *myo* meaning muscle. Sarcomas are uncommon malignant neoplasms which develop from connective tissues with RMS developing from primitive muscle cells called "rhabdomyoblasts."
- *Classic Clue*: Child presents with headache showing signs of cranial nerve involvement with imaging depicting a large homogeneous well-circumscribed skull base mass *without hyperostosis or calcification*. It is similar to muscle on NECT and T1 and reveals rampant *restricted diffusion*.
- Distributions and Incidence:
  - *Age:* Peak incidence is 1–5 years old.
  - *Gender:* Slight M > F = 1.5:1 prevalence.
  - *Race:* First recognized race predilection for RMS is *Maori* [3].
  - *Incidence:* Incidence in the United States is 6 cases per 1,000,000 per year in children <15 years.
- Common Type: The embryonal type is most common and is the most likely to involve the skull base.

Imaging

General Imaging Features

- Classically appears as a homogeneous well-circumscribed non-calcified soft tissue mass with irregular margins isodense to muscle. Rarely resembles a cystic mass having hemorrhagic foci [4, 5].

CT Features

- *See General Imaging Features.*
- NECT shows a homogeneous mass isodense to muscle. CECT shows *mild enhancement* with the mass appearing slightly hyperdense to surrounding muscle [6].
- RMS classically erodes and destroys adjacent bone but usually does not contain calcifications or provoke hyperostosis from adjacent bone [4–6].
- CT and FDG PET/CT play primary roles in assessing metastatic disease.

MRI Features

- *See General Imaging Features.*
- MRI is the preferred modality for assessment of skull base rhabdomyosarcoma.
- T1: Isointense to muscle but hypointense to orbital fat.
- T2: Heterogeneous, hyperintense to muscle with multiple foci of high T2 signal. (See Fig. 49.1b.)
- FLAIR: Heterogeneous, isointense to brain with multiple high signal foci. Signal is iso- to hyperintense to EOMs. (See Fig. 49.1a.)

F. A. Midyett, S. K. Mukherji, *Skull Base Imaging*, https://doi.org/10.1007/978-3-030-46447-9_49

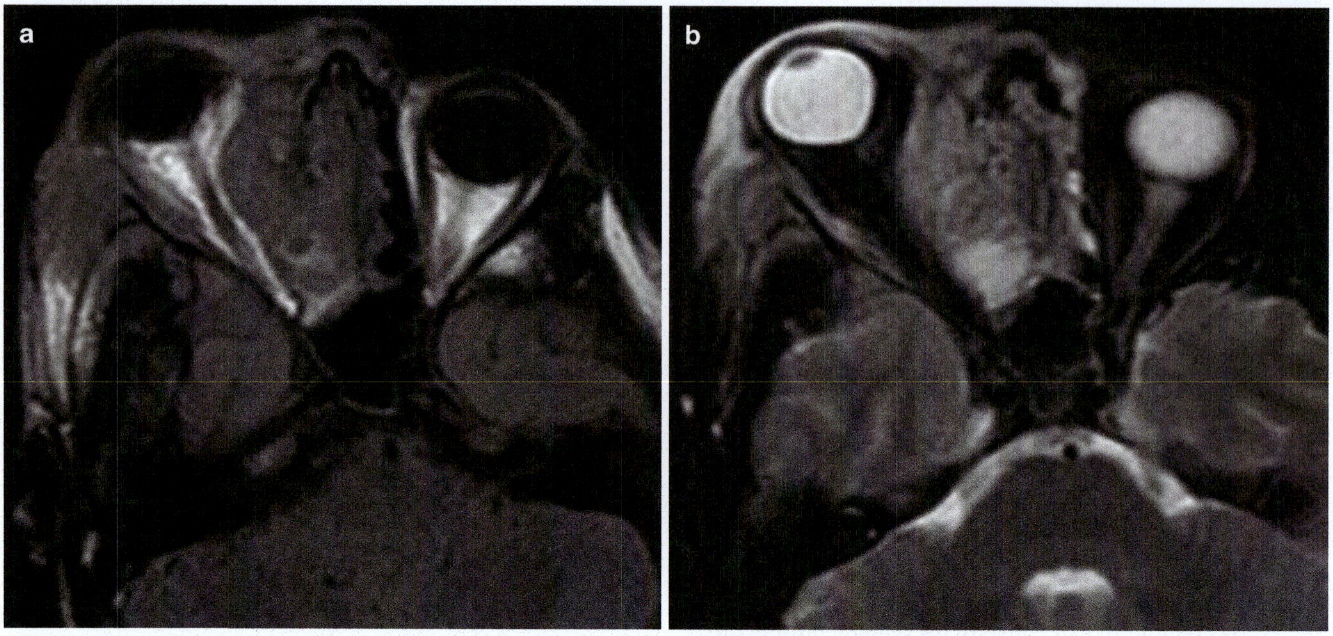

Fig. 49.1 (**a**) Axial FLAIR shows a large anterior skull base mass extending laterally into the right orbit, displacing orbital contents. It fills the right ethmoid air cells, crossing to involve the contralateral ethmoids. Signal is predominately isointense to brain but contains foci of higher signal. Signal is mildly hyperintense to the EOMs. (**b**) Axial T2 Fat Sat shows a large anterior skull base mass extending laterally into the right orbit, displacing orbital contents. Tumor fills the right ethmoid air cells, crossing to involve the contralateral ethmoids. Signal is heterogeneous and hyperintense to brain but contains foci of higher signal

- T1 Gd:
  - Exhibits avid heterogeneous enhancement.
- DWI:
  - ADC values are potentially useful in separating various benign and malignant tumors.
  - Demonstrates *restricted diffusion* with *bright DWI* images and corresponding *dark ADC* images.

Nuclear Medicine Features

- Scintigraphy shows increased uptake by tumor.

Clinical Issues

Presentation

- Patient presentation is related to tumor location varying from proptosis and diplopia with orbital involvement to chronic otitis media, facial nerve palsy, headache, hearing impairment, and bleeding when the ear is involved [7].
- More central skull base involvement solicits symptoms related to sinuses or other cranial nerves.
- A history of trauma can clearly confound the diagnosis [8].

Epidemiology

- *Rare:* Rhabdomyosarcoma is a rare childhood sarcoma showing a predilection for the H&N with an estimated 300 new cases per year.
- *Location:* While 10% of new cases involve the orbit, 90% are H&N and sometimes seen in the skull base.

Pathology

- Rhabdomyosarcoma is the most common childhood soft tissue cancer caused by primitive mesenchymal cells which have retained their capacity for skeletal muscle differentiation [1].
- *Tumor Types*: Although some overlap, major tumor types tend to manifest as follows [9]:
  - Embryonal RMS: Infants and young children
  - Alveolar RMS: Adolescents and young adults
  - Pleomorphic RMS: Older adults
  - Spindle cell and sclerosing RMS: Children and adults
- *Gross Features:*
  - Tumors of the skull base are rare in children but when they occur can be very large and extensive.
  - Rhabdomyosarcoma is typically highly heterogeneous [2].

   - Gross appearances vary with location. Sinonasal and nasopharyngeal RMS are often multinodular, grape-like "sarcoma botryoides."
- *Microscopic Features*:
   - Microscopic features vary with subtype:
      I. The embryonal subtype is most common (>70%) showing small round spindle cells and lymphocytes with elongated nuclei surrounded by eosinophilic cytoplasm.
      II. Alveolar RMS displays alveolar spaces lined by round or oval cells. Interspersed solid areas are filled with fibrous tissue and multinucleated giant cells.
      III. Pleomorphic rhabdomyosarcomas are least common, but they are more frequently found in older patients. Large pleomorphic rhabdomyoblasts predominate.
- Immunohistochemical Staining:
   - Myogenin is a specific marker for rhabdomyosarcomas [10].
   - The recommended panel of positive stains currently includes myogenin (sensitive and specific), sarcomeric actin (90%), desmin (95%), and myoglobin (specific but only found in more differentiated tumors).
   - Glycogen-containing tumor cells are positive to PAS and myofibrils stain positive with phosphotungstic acid.

Treatment and Prognosis

Surgery

- Skull base tumors present some of the most complex and technically difficult problems confronting surgeons, often limiting the extent of their excision.
- Image guided needle biopsy is often obtained to confirm cytology.
- Relatively recent advancements in skull base surgery have improved the prognosis for these unfortunate patients.

Chemotherapy

- Since they tend to metastasize early, prompt chemotherapy is suggested.

Radiotherapy

- Alveolar subtypes are almost always treated with irradiation.
- Most feel that all children with rhabdomyosarcomas should have radiation and chemotherapy.

Prognosis

- Skull base rhabdomyosarcomas has historically been a devastating disease, but enhanced surgical and other treatment techniques combine to make this a more curable disease.
- Variations in prognosis are primarily related to histologic subtypes.
- Patients with local (nonmetastatic) rhabdomyosarcoma have a 70% long-term survival when given multimodality therapy comprised of chemotherapy, surgery, and radiation [2].
- Leptomeningeal involvement portends a particularly poor prognostic finding [3].
- 30% of rhabdomyosarcoma patients present with metastasis most commonly involving liver, lungs, and bones [7].

Differential Diagnosis

A. Chondrosarcoma (CS)

- Chondrosarcomas are chondroid malignancies which commonly select a synchondrosis when involving the skull base.
- *Classic Clue*: Skull base mass exhibiting an affinity for the POF (petro-occipital fissure) sometimes showing a chondroid matrix, characterized by low T1 and high T2 signals.
- Gross: Chondrosarcomas appear as well-circumscribed, often scalloped, or lobulated lytic lesions exhibiting chondroid calcifications.
- Age: 10–79 years (mean 39).
- Low attenuation may make them subtle on brain soft tissue algorithms. (See Chap. 46, Fig. 46.1i.)
- T2: Very high T2 signal. (See Chap. 46, Fig. 46.1b, d.)
- (See Chap. 46, Skull Base Chondrosarcoma)

B. Juvenile Nasopharyngeal Angiofibroma (JNA)

- Rare, highly vascular, locally invasive benign nasopharyngeal neoplasm occurring almost entirely in adolescent and young adult males displaying a distinct tendency for recurrence.
- *Classic Clue*: Adolescent male presenting with epistaxis exhibiting an avidly enhancing, heterogeneous posterior nasal mass with MRI showing *characteristic salt and pepper appearance* from presence of prominent flow voids.

- Typically have the Holman-Miller sign with archetypical anterior bowing of posterior maxillary sinus wall:
  - T1: Heterogeneous intermediate signal
  - T2: Heterogeneous signal with dark flow voids.
  - T1 Gd: Exhibits avid enhancement. Axial and coronal fat saturation images are essential to define involvement of skull base, sphenoid, and cavernous sinuses.
- Most sequences show *characteristic salt and pepper appearance* from presence of prominent flow voids.
- Catheter angiography illustrates a plethora of dilated tortuous vessels and depicts an intense characteristic capillary blush.
- (See Chap. 15, Juvenile Nasopharyngeal Angiofibroma)

C. Ewing's Sarcoma (ES)

- Ewing's sarcoma is an aggressive malignant tumor of *childhood and adolescence* containing small blue round cells and usually presenting in the second decade.
- *Classic Clue*: *Caucasian child or adolescent* presenting with pain, fever, and ↑ ESR found on imaging to exhibit an extra-axial mass extending cranially and caudally from its skull base epicenter. On examination the patient demonstrates orbital or cranial nerve symptoms.
- Ewing's accounts for 10–15% of childhood malignant bone tumors and is second only to osteosarcoma.
- Ewing's is rare among Asians and African-Americans.
- Usually demonstrates destructive, permeative bone destruction with soft tissue components showing *no* soft tissue calcifications.
- Depending on tumor stage, Ewing's can cause cortical erosion with rarefaction and "moth-eaten" permeative destruction.
- T1: Low to intermediate signal, isointense with brain and EOMs. (See Chap. 47, Fig. 47.1a.)
- T2: Heterogeneous signal, relatively isointense to brain with focal fluid collections which show high T2 signal. (See Chap. 47, Fig. 47.1c.) Low signal striations sometimes suggest "hair on end" appearance.
- T1 Gd:
  - *Mild heterogeneous enhancement.* (See Chap. 47, Fig. 47.1b, d.)
  - *Fat saturation* techniques are habitually helpful.
- DWI:
  - Bony involvement by ES may be more conspicuous on DWI than other MRI sequences particular when small and metastatic.
- (See Chap. 47, Ewing's Sarcoma)

D. Esthesioneuroblastoma (ENB)

- Rare neuroendocrine malignancy of neural crest origin arising from olfactory epithelium.
- AKA: Olfactory neuroblastoma.
- Esthesioneuroblastoma is more frequently found in middle-aged patients but can be seen in children.
- Classically shows avidly enhancing dumbbell-shaped mass with "waist" at the cribriform plate.
- May involve anterior cranial fossa, skull base, and orbit.
- Esthesioneuroblastomas show intermediate signal on T1 and T2 with avid enhancement on T1 Gd.
- Cystic areas (with foci of ↑T2) at the tumor/brain interface are diagnostic and may be pathognomonic.
- DWI shows moderate restricted diffusion.
- Esthesioneuroblastoma exhibits an epicenter near the cribriform plate.
- Esthesioneuroblastoma displays no gender preference.
- (See Chap. 28, Esthesioneuroblastoma)

E. Metastatic Neoplasm

- Metastatic neoplasm can cause a destructive mass anywhere along the skull base.
- Frequently find *multiple metastases* in patients having recognized primary neoplasms.
- In children, metastatic neuroblastoma should be considered.

F. Langerhans Cell Histiocytosis (LCH)

- Rare lesion of pediatric skull base temporal bone.
- Imaging characteristics similar to rhabdomyosarcoma.
- The lesion's location may be helpful in making correct diagnosis.
- Langerhans cell histiocytosis more frequently involves the mastoid.
- Rhabdomyosarcoma is typically confined to the anterior temporal bone [11].
- (See Chap. 8, Langerhans Cell Histiocytosis)

A Closer Look

I. Statistical Soup

- Sarcomas account for 1% of all malignancies with <5000 new sarcomas occurring per year in the United States.
- 80% of sarcomas occur in adults.
- 80% of sarcomas arise from bone while 20% arise from soft tissues.
- 20% of all sarcomas occur in the head and neck.
- RMS accounts for >50% of soft tissue sarcomas in children.
- RMS currently comprises 5% of childhood cancers [2], most frequently found in children < age 10.
- 40% of pediatric RMS occur in the H&N with 40% of those involving the anterior skull base [12].
- 90% of RMS occur <16 years of age (mean onset 5–7 years). Odd outlier cases have been documented in newborns as well as the elderly [13].

II. Fast Facts

- A New Zealand series of skull base and craniofacial rhabdomyosarcomas portrayed a predominance for Maori [3].
- Rhabdomyosarcoma is a rare childhood sarcoma with an estimated 350 new cases in the United States annually.
- Because rhabdomyosarcoma shows a H&N predilection, orbital rhabdomyosarcoma should be considered in any child exhibiting progressive unilateral proptosis.
- Rhabdomyosarcoma probably arises from primitive pluripotential mesenchymal cells, which possess the ability to differentiate into striated muscle. Rhabdomyosarcoma *does not arise directly from the EOMs* [14].

III. Genetics and Associations

- While a clear-cut cause for rhabdomyosarcoma remains unknown, we currently recognize a number of associated genetic syndromes and environmental factors.
- Associated genetic syndromes include neurofibromatosis type I, Li-Fraumeni (germline p53 mutation), Rubinstein-Taybi, Gorlin basal cell nevus, Costello, and Beckwith-Wiedemann syndromes.
- Associated environmental factors include fetal intrauterine exposure to radiation, marijuana, and cocaine, as well as other prior radiation and alkylating agent exposure.
- Some studies have shown a link between rhabdomyosarcoma and tungsten alloy from shrapnel imbedded in muscle. That actual alloy of tungsten contained 6% nickel which is known to be carcinogenic [15].
- While there is currently no known gene responsible for rhabdomyosarcoma's transmission, there are associated genetic mutations including the RB1 gene on chromosome 12q14, as well as NF1 [16].

References

1. Rubin E, Farber EL, editors. Pathology, vol. 1. Philadelphia: J.B. Lippincott Company; 1994. p. 1343–4.
2. McCarville MB, Spunt SL, Pappo AS. Rhabdomyosarcoma in pediatric patients the good, the bad, and the unusual. AJR Am J Roentgenol. 2001;176(6):1563–9. https://doi.org/10.2214/ajr.176.6.1761563.
3. Yang A, Wickremesekera A, Parker, et al. Surgical management of craniofacial and skull base rhabdomysarcomas. J Craniofac Surg. 2009;20(5):1388–93. https://doi.org/10.1097/SCS.0b013e3181b187bb.
4. Sohaib S, Moseley I, Wright J. Orbital rhabdomyosarcoma-the radiological characteristics. Clin Radiol. 1998;53:357–62.
5. Scotti G, Harwood-Nash D. Computed tomography of rhabdomyosarcomas of the skull base in children. Comput Assist Tomogr. 1982;6:33–9.
6. Lee JH, Lee MS, Lee BH, et al. Rhabdomyosarcoma of the head and neck in adults: MR and CT findings. AJNR Am J Neuroradiol. 1996;17:1923–8.
7. Durve DV, Kanegaonkar RG, Albert D, Levitt G. Pediatric rhabdomyosarcoma of the ear and temporal bone. Clin Otolaryngol Allied Sci. 2004;29(1):32–7.
8. Gandhi P, Fleming J, Haik B, Wilson M. Ophthalmic complications following treatment of paranasal sinus rhabdomyosarcoma in comparison to orbital disease. Ophthal Plast Reconstr Surg. 2011;0:1–6.
9. Parham DM, Ellison DA. Rhabdomyosarcomas in adults and children: an update. Arch Pathol Lab Med. 2006;130(1):1454–65.
10. Kumar S, Perlman E, Harris CA, et al. Myogenin is a specific marker for rhabdomyosarcoma: an immunohistochemical study in paraffin-embedded tissues. Mod Pathol. 2000;13(9):988–93.
11. Chevallier KM, Wigging RH, Quinn NA, Gurgel RK. Differentiating pediatric rhabdomyosarcoma and langerhans cell histiocytosis of the temporal bone by imaging appearance. AJNR Am J Neuroradiol. 2016;37:1185–9.
12. Deutsch M. Radiation therapy in the treatment of tumors of the cranial base. In: Sekhar LN, Schramm VL, editors. Tumors of the cranial base. New York: Futura; 1987. p. 163.
13. Wharam M, Beltangady M, Hays D, et al. Localized orbital rhabdomyosarcoma. An interim report of the Intergroup Rhabdomyosarcoma Study Committee. Ophthalmology. 1987;94:251–4.
14. Karcioglu Z, Hadjistilianou D, Rozans M, et al. Orbital rhabdomyosarcoma. Cancer Control. 2004;11:328–33.
15. Kalinich JF, Emond CA, Dalton TK, et al. Embedded weapons-grade tungsten alloy shrapnel rapidly induces metastatic high-grade rhabdomyosarcomas in F344 rats. Environ Health Perspect. 2005;113(6):729–34.
16. Shields J, Shields C. Rhabdomyosarcoma: review for the ophthalmologist. Surv Ophthalmol. 2003;48:39–57.
17. Saboo SS, Krajewski KM, Ziltumslo K, et al. Imaging features of primary and secondary adult rhabdomyosarcoma. *Am J Roentgenol.* 2012;199(6):W694–703.
18. Newton WA, Gehan EA, Webber BL, et al. Classification of rhabdomyosarcomas and related sarcomas. Pathologic aspects and proposal for a new classification – an Intergroup Rhabdomyosarcoma Study. Cancer. 1995;6(6):1073–85.
19. Weiss SW, Goldblum JR, Enzinger FM. Enzinger and Weiss's soft tissue tumors. Maryland Heights, Missouri: Mosby Inc; 2001.
20. Cooper S, Munk P, Downey D, et al. Findings of magnetic resonance and colour-flow Doppler imaging of orbital embryonal rhabdomyosarcoma. Can Assoc Radiol J. 1994;45:217–20.
21. Schaffler GJ, Simbrunner J, Lechner H, et al. Idiopathic sclerotic inflammation of the orbit with left optic nerve compression in a patient with multifocal fibrosclerosis. AJNR Am J Neuroradiol. 2000;1:194–7.
22. Erly WK, Carmody RF, Dryden RM. Orbital Histiocytosis X. AJNR Am J Neuroradiol. 1995;16:1258–61.
23. Zafar MA, Waheed SS, Enam SA. Orbital aspergillus infection mimicking a tumour: a case report. Cases J. 2009;2:7860.
24. Primeggia J, Cyriac G, Kumar P. Invasive orbital aspergillosis in an apparently immunocompetent host without evidence of sinusitis. J Microbiol Infect Dis/JMID. 2012;2(3):113–6.
25. Duan F, Smith LM, Gustafson DM, et al. Genomic and clinical analysis of fusion gene amplification in rhabdomyosarcoma: a report from the Children's Oncology Group. Genes Chromosomes Cancer. 2012;51(7):662–4.
26. Midyett FA, Mukherji SK. Chapter 23, Rhabdomyosarcoma. In: Orbital imaging: Elsevier/Saunders; 2015. p. 99–102. ISBN : 978-0-323-34037-3.

Skull Base Osteosarcoma

50

Pertinent Points

- *Definition*: Osteosarcoma is an aggressive malignant mesenchymal spindle cell neoplasm in which tumor cells directly *produce osteoid* or immature bone [1, 15]. Osteosarcoma is the most common primary bone tumor found in children and young adults [1].
- *AKA:* Osteogenic sarcoma (OGS).
- *Classic Clue*: White male patient presents with new skull base symptoms several years following *prior radiotherapy* for a different problem.
- Development of neoplasm following radiation therapy is unusual but has been reported. [5–7]
- De novo spontaneous sarcomatous transformation by fibrous dysplasia is rare with most of its sarcomas following former radiation therapy.
- RIOS
  – These secondary radiation induced osteosarcomas (RIOS) tend to have a higher tumor grade than their primary (de novo) counterparts and they behave more aggressively [11].
  – RIOS (radiation-induced osteosarcoma) is the modern-day equivalent of Frankenstein, having been created by science but belligerently behaving to resist current medical marvels. As if de novo osteosarcomas were not bad enough, radiation-induced osteosarcomas are doggedly determined to be worse!
- Incidence, Preferences, and Distributions
- Incidence
  – Osteosarcoma is most prevalent in children and young adults where it is the *most common non hematologic primary malignant bone tumor* [12, 15].
  – Osteosarcomas occurrence is second only to multiple myeloma, relegating it to the *second most common of all primary malignant bone tumors* [4].
  – Osteosarcoma is the eighth most common childhood cancer causing 2.4% of pediatric malignancies and 20% of all primary bone cancer [12].
  – While <7% of osteosarcomas occur in the H&N, skull base osteosarcomas are fortunately rare [2, 3].
- *Age Prevalence*
  – Large osteosarcoma series show bimodal peaks [16].
  – Osteosarcoma is more prevalent in the second and third decades with 75% of cases encountered in patients 15–25 years of age [1].
  – Primary osteosarcomas <6 or >60 years of age are unusual, but a second incidence peak does exist for the over 60 crowd [16].
  – More frequently found in white males but can occur in other ethnic groups.
- *Gender Preference*: F > M. Female incidence is slightly higher than males in all age groups, and this ↑ incidence *occurs earlier for females* [16].
- *Locations*: 95% arise in the metaphysis. Primary involvement of the diaphysis is unusual showing a longer duration of symptoms prior to diagnosis. While very rare, cases exhibiting epiphyseal origin occur in <1% [1].

F. A. Midyett, S. K. Mukherji, *Skull Base Imaging*, https://doi.org/10.1007/978-3-030-46447-9_50

Imaging

General Imaging Features

- Osteosarcomas radiologic facade fluctuates across an assorted gamut [1].
- Frequently find a large *lytic or blastic* mass portraying *permeative destructive* margins.
- Osteosarcoma can breach its cortex with periosteal elevation.
- Osteosarcoma sometimes shows a *sunburst pattern* portraying new bone formation in the soft tissues.

CT Features

- *See Section General Imaging Features.*
- Characteristically exhibits aggressive bony destruction with tumor matrix mineralization of soft tissue components
- Extraordinary exceptions involve predominately lytic lesions with little mineralized material apparent on plain film or MRI.
- CT's current role is basically for biopsy and staging abdicating the role of thorough tumor evaluation to MRI.

MRI Features

- *See Section General Imaging Features.*
- T1 Signal
  – Shows *very heterogeneous* signal intensity (SI) portraying a plethora of characteristic components:

Non-mineralized soft tissues:	Intermediate SI.
Mineralized (or ossified) soft tissue:	Low SI.
Peritumoral edema:	Intermediate SI.
Hemorrhage:	Sprinkled spots of hemorrhage have variable SI

- T2 Signal
  – Shows *very heterogeneous* signal intensity (SI) portraying a plethora of vcharacteristic components:

Non-mineralized soft tissue:	High SI.
Mineralized (or ossified) soft tissue:	Low SI.
Peritumoral edema:	High SI.
Hemorrhage:	Sporadic spots of hemorrhage have variable SI.

- T1 Gd
  – Solid components exhibit moderate enhancement.

Nuclear Medicine Features

- Scintigraphy shows marked ↑ uptake on blood flow, blood pool, and delayed images [1].
- Currently the chief role for nuclear scintigraphy is searching for secluded metastasis [1].
- May observe osseous and extraosseous metastatic foci [1].

Clinical Issues

1. Signs and Symptoms
   - Osteosarcoma involving the skull base may present in myriad manners.
   - Osteosarcoma can compromise any cranial nerve causing clinical findings similar to those exhibited by Paget's disease. [See Chap. 41, CVJ 2, Paget's Disease/ Complications.]
   - Clival involvement by osteosarcoma can cause a painful presentation with lower cranial nerve palsies [2].
2. Pathology
   - *Gross Features*
     – The gross appearance of osteosarcoma varies with matrix type.
     – ~75% of osteosarcomas arise in the intramedullary cavity and are considered "classical" or "conventional" osteosarcoma [15].
     – See Baron Dupuytren classic 1847 gross description [in A Closer Look/IV. Historic Highlights/1847].
   - *Microscopic Features*
     – The microscopic appearance of osteosarcoma varies with the matrix type.
     – Most osteosarcomas show a common pleomorphic anaplastic cell population producing a disorganized immature bone, cartilage, or fibroblastic matrix [17].
     – RIOS reveals more aggressive features than primary osteosarcoma [13].

Treatment and Prognosis

RIOS is a distressing difficulty for radiation therapy earning it the epithet for being a "double-edge sword" [18]. It is critical that patients have long-term posttreatment follow-up. Secondary RIOS is more aggressive, more difficult to excise, and more apt to recur showing shorter survivals than primary osteosarcoma.

Treatment

I. Surgery

- The conventional foundation for treatment is extensive excision of the offending malicious malignancy [14].

- Skull base tumors present some of the most complex and technically difficult problems confronting surgeons, often limiting the extent of excision [4].
- Image-guided needle biopsy is often obtained to confirm cytology.
- Complete surgical excision is the treatment of choice for radiation-induced osteosarcoma, although this is often difficult when there is skull base involvement [11].

II. Chemotherapy

- Most advocate chemotherapy as micrometastasis is found in 80% of patients at the time of diagnosis [6, 14].
  - Most skull base osteosarcoma receives adjuvant chemotherapy [11].
  - Chemotherapy is routinely recommended for tumors >5 cm [11].

III. Radiotherapy

(a) Sometimes supplementary radiotherapy is performed. [11]

(b) *However*, patients with radiation-induced osteosarcoma are often *not considered* candidates for further radiation treatment of a formerly irradiated field [11].

  (a) Radiation-induced osteosarcomas (RIOS)
    - Usually occur 10–15 years after exposure to 40–60 Gy for various conditions.
    - Unfortunately, most RIOS are higher in grade than primary osteosarcomas and behave differently [11].
    - RIOS, with their cantankerous character and propensity for local recurrence, pose particularly problematic treatment challenges [11].
    - Five-year disease-free survival for patients with RIOS is ~17% and is in sharp contrast to 70% for patients with primary H&N osteosarcomas [11].
    - Median overall survival time is 29 months for RIOS vs. 46 months for primary osteosarcoma.
    - The incidence for RIOS is <0.03% of all irradiated patients, accounting for 5.5% of osteosarcoma [11, 13].

  (b) Metastasis
    - Metastasis frequently involves the lungs, bones, pleura and heart. Rarely involves nodes, GI tract, and the brain.
    - Excision of metastatic lung nodules may prolong patient's survival.

Radiotherapy choices include:

1. Conventional radiotherapy
2. Gamma knife therapy
3. Cyber-knife therapy advantages
   (a) Can focus on target via multi-angled planes.
   (b) 3D tumor size and shape can be accommodated by CT or MRI during treatment.
   (c) Does not require cumbersome equipment as with proton beam and gamma knife treatment [13].
   (d) When coupled with endoscopic resection appears initially to significantly extend survival of RIOS [13].

Prognosis

- Tumor size >10 cm and advanced presentation stage significantly prejudice patient outcome [1]
- The 5-year survival for craniofacial RIOS is only 17% compared to 70% for primary osteosarcoma [13].
- This prognostic disparity demonstrates the difficulty of total surgical resection as well as the consequence of the more hostile histology for RIOS [13].

Differential Diagnosis

A. Fibrous Dysplasia [FD] [1]

- Fibrous dysplasia is a slowly progressing tumor-like process in which normal cancellous bone is replaced by immature woven bone and fibrous tissue.
- Fibrous dysplasia's fondness for the cranium can cause serious skull base and orbital problems.
- Fibrous dysplasia falls into in three basic types: sclerotic, lytic, and mixed.
- Sclerotic lesions dominate the skull base with lytic lesions least likely.
- Fibrous dysplasia's matchless medullary cavity expansion conserves original bone shape while simultaneously sparing its cortex.
- Classically fibrous dysplasia displays a "ground-glass" appearance. Conversely, cystic degeneration is a "red flag" which when near the orbit heralds a high incidence of visual impairment.
- While the cortex is classically preserved, severe expansion may cause the cortex to virtually "vanish."
- Periosteal reaction raises a "red flag" for a pathological fracture or underlying malignant metamorphosis.
- Progressive lytic lesions suggest malignant degeneration.
- Tc^{99m} bone scans show ↑ uptake.

CT:

- Fibrous dysplasia expands the bone keeping the original shape while the sparing cortex.
- Ground glass appearance is "classic." When not classic, "ground-glass" lesions may appear quite heterogeneous.
- Clinicians frequently find 3D CT reconstructions provide useful presurgical planning roadmaps.

MRI:

- T1 shows heterogeneous low to intermediate signal often isointense to the brain.
- T2 is heterogeneous, usually low, often isointense to the brain but may have regions of higher signal.
- T1 Gd exhibits avid enhancement.
- Cysts and hemorrhage can cause heterogeneous signals which vary depending on protein content and age of blood products.
- See Fig. 50.1a–e featuring concomitant FD and RIOS.
- See Chap. 25, ACF 13, Fibrous Dysplasia.

B. Chondrosarcoma (CS)
- Chondrosarcomas are chondroid malignancies which, when involving the skull base, studiously start in a synchondrosis.
- *Classic Clue*: Skull based mass exhibiting an affinity for the POF (petro-occipital fissure) sometimes showing chondroid matrix, characterized by low T1 and high T2 signals.
- Chondrosarcomas appear as well-circumscribed, often scalloped, or lobulated lytic lesions exhibiting chondroid calcifications.
- Age: 10–79 years (mean 39).
- Low attenuation may make them subtle on brain soft tissue algorithms. [See Chap. 46, Fig. 46.1I.]
- T2: Exhibit exceptionally *high T2* signal.
- See Chap. 46 (SBC, Skull Base Chondrosarcoma).

C. Juvenile Nasopharyngeal Angiofibroma (JNA)
- Rare, highly vascular, locally invasive benign nasopharyngeal neoplasm occurring almost entirely in adolescent and young adult males displaying a distinct tendency for recurrence.
- *Classic Clue*: Adolescent male presenting with epistaxis exhibits an avidly enhancing heterogeneous posterior nasal mass with MRI showing a *characteristic salt and pepper appearance* from the presence of prominent flow voids.
- Typically have a Holman-Miller sign with archetypical anterior bowing of the posterior maxillary sinus wall.
- T1: Heterogeneous intermediate signal.
- T2: Heterogeneous signal with dark flow voids.
- T1 Gd: Exhibits avid enhancement. Axial and coronal fat saturation images are essential to define involvement of the skull base, sphenoid, and cavernous sinuses.
- Most sequences show *characteristic salt and pepper appearance* from the presence of prominent flow voids.
- Catheter angiography illustrates a plethora of dilated tortuous vessels illustrating an intense characteristic capillary blush.
- See Chap. 15, ACF 3, Juvenile Nasopharyngeal Angiofibroma (JNA).

D. Ewing's sarcoma (ES)
- Ewing's sarcoma is an aggressive malignant tumor of *childhood and adolescence* containing small blue round cells which usually presents in the second decade.
- *Classic Clue*: *Caucasian child or adolescent* presenting with pain, fever, and ↑ ESR found on imaging to have an extra-axial mass extending cranially and caudally from its skull base epicenter. On assessment, the patient portrays orbital or cranial nerve symptoms.
- Ewing's accounts for 10–15% of childhood malignant bone tumors and is second only to osteosarcoma.
- Ewing's is rare among Asians and African-Americans.
- Usually demonstrates destructive, permeative bone destruction with soft tissue components showing *no* soft tissue calcifications.
- Depending on the tumor stage, Ewing's can cause cortical erosion with rarefaction and "Moth-eaten" permeative destruction.
- T1: Low to intermediate signal, isointense with the brain and EOMs. [See Chap. 47 Fig. 47.1a.]
- T2: Heterogeneous signal, relatively isointense to the brain with focal fluid collections which show high T2 signal. [See Chap. 47, Fig. 47.1c.] Low signal striations sometimes suggest "hair on end" appearance.
- T1 Gd:
  - *Mild heterogeneous enhancement.* [See Chap. 47, Fig. 47.1b, d.]
  - *Fat saturation* techniques are very helpful.
- DWI
  - Bony involvement by ES may be more conspicuous on DWI than other MRI sequences particularly when small and metastatic.
- See Chap. 47, Ewing's Sarcoma (ES).

E. Esthesioneuroblastoma (ENB)
- Rare neuroendocrine malignancy of neural crest origin arising from olfactory epithelium.
- AKA: Olfactory neuroblastoma.
- ENB is more often found in middle-aged patients but can be seen in children.
- Classically show avidly enhancing dumbbell-shaped mass with "waist" at the cribriform plate.
- May involve anterior cranial fossa, skull base, and orbit.
- ENBs show intermediate signal on T1 and T2 exhibiting avid enhancement on T1 Gd.
- Cystic areas (with foci of ↑T2) at the tumor/brain interface are diagnostic and may be pathognomonic.
- DWI shows moderate restricted diffusion.
- ENB exhibits an epicenter near the cribriform plate.
- ENB displays no gender preference.
- See Chap. 28, Esthesioneuroblastoma (ENB).

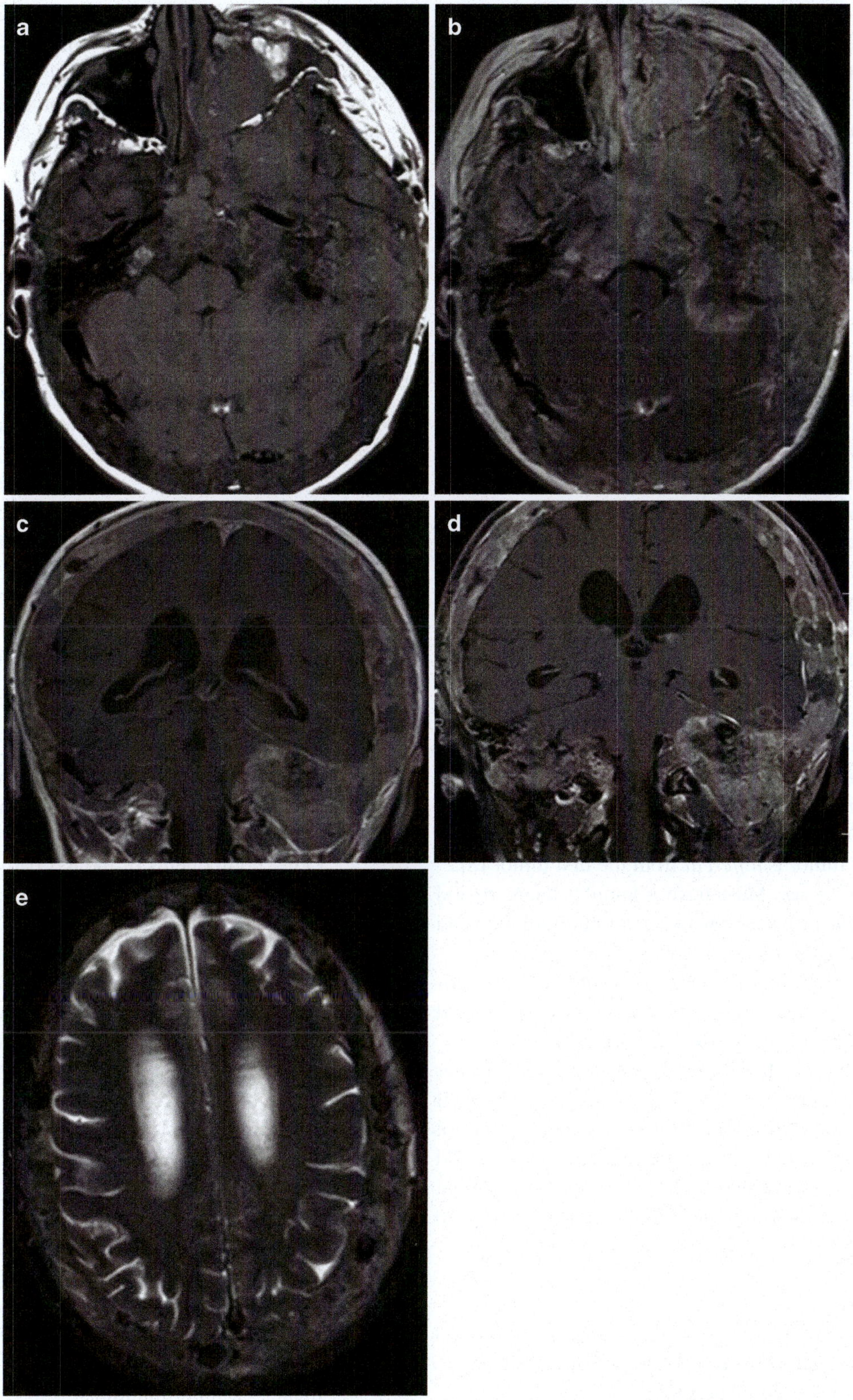

Fig. 50.1 Axial T1 without (**a**) and with Gd (**b**) show a huge skull base mass isointense to the brain showing moderate heterogeneous post-Gd enhancement. This extensive pathologic process involves the central skull base extending into the anterior and posterior fossae as well as the left maxillary sinus. One component compresses the left cerebellar hemisphere, and the calvarium shows expansive diploic changes which look familiar. Coronal T1 Gd without (**c**) and with (**d**) fat saturation demonstrate generalized intradiploic marrow widening of the visualized calvarium and skull base. These images depict an asymmetrical lesion involving the left skull base extending up to the tentorium. This represents osteosarcoma which developed years after the patient received radiation therapy for an osseous abnormality. And on second look, the right skull base doesn't look too good either. (**e**) Axial T2 shows uniform but heterogeneous intradiploic calvarial marrow expansion. Most of the signal is isointense to the brain but there are multiple hypointense foci. There is no hint of the OS at this more cephalic imaging level

F. Metastatic Neoplasm

- Metastatic neoplasm can cause a destructive mass anywhere along the skull base.
- Frequently find *multiple metastases* in patients having recognized primary neoplasms.
- In children, metastatic neuroblastoma should be considered.

A Closer Look

I. Fast Facts

- *RIS*
  - Many radiation-induced sarcomas (RIS) mirror the host's genetic alterations and provide support, but not proof, that a given malignancy is a consequence of prior radiation therapy [5].
  - AKA: RIM (radiation-induced malignancy) [18].
- Cahan's Criteria [8, 18]
  - Even in today's era of modern molecular genetics, a problem persists to aver absolute proof that radiation therapy triggered a certain malignancy, and therefore, Cahan's criteria continue to be crucial. [5]
  - In 1948 Cahan et al. proposed the now familiar *four criteria* for consideration in recognizing RIS, modified as follows:
    1. *Previously Irradiated Field:* The new neoplasm arose in a previously irradiated field.
    2. *Histologic Proof:* There is *histologic proof* that the second tumor is *different* from the first tumor [8].
    3. *Latent Period:* Must have a lengthy latent period (preferably >4 years) between initial irradiation and occurrence of the second neoplasm.
    4. *Previously Normal:* There is radiologic and histologic evidence that the area in which the alleged tumor arose was "normal" prior to irradiation.

    Comment: The first three criteria are certainly easier to reconcile than the fourth, particularly with skull base sarcomas. Often the entire irradiated area was not originally biopsied or was not "normal," or it would not have been irradiated in the first place. This should not constrain us from considering prior irradiation to be the cause of new malignancies.

II. Statistical Soup

- Sarcomas account for 1% of all malignancies with <5000 new sarcomas occurring per year in the United States.
- 80% of sarcomas occur in adults.
- 80% of sarcomas arise from bone while 20% start in soft tissues.
- 20% of all sarcomas occur in the head and neck.
- The first recognized case of radiation-induced malignancy occurred in an unfortunate x-ray tube tester in 1902 [11].
- One of the most devastating complications of therapeutic radiation exposure is the formation of new malignancies [11].
- The most frequent RIS is fibrosarcoma, with radiation induced osteosarcoma (RIOS) being extremely rare [13].

III. Genetics and Molecular Biology

- In addition to the now familiar Cahan's criteria for consideration in recognizing radiation-induced sarcomas (RIS), new genetic mutations documented daily seem to support induction of malignancy [5].
- Several genes have been implicated including various tumor suppressor genes, oncogenes, and genes coding growth factors.
- Inactivation of the P53 and RB pathways appear central to creation of osteosarcoma [15].
- RB1
  - The retinoblastoma protein pRb is a tumor suppressor protein which is dysfunctional in several major cancers. Its gene name is abbreviated RB or RB1.
  - Alterations in the RB gene pathway include:

    Patients with hereditary RB increase their incidence of Osteosarcoma (OS) by 1000 times.

    70% of sporadic osteosarcoma show RB gene alterations.

    LOH (loss of heterozygosity) at 13 q, (gene site for RB) is found in ≤70% of osteosarcomas.

    LOH at the RB locus is proposed as a poor prognostic factor for osteosarcoma.

    Other components of the RB pathway gene subject to alterations include INK4, p16, CDK 4, and cyclin D1.

    The INK4A gene located on chromosome 9p21 is inactivated in 10% of osteosarcomas.

    Loss of p16 expression is found in ≤15% of OS and correlates with ↓ survival in pediatric osteosarcoma.

    Amplification of 12q13–15 chromosomal region containing CDK4 and MDM2 is found in 10% of osteosarcomas [15].
- TP53
  - Alterations in the TP53 pathway include the following:

    Inactivation of the p53 pathway is the pivotal point for numerous neoplasms including osteosarcomas.

    The p53 gene resides on chromosome 17p13.

    P53 abnormalities are found in 50% of OS.

    Alterations can cause allelic loss, gene rearrangements, or point mutations.

    Patients with Li-Fraumeni syndrome with germline mutations of p53 have a high risk of osteosarcoma.

    Germline p53 mutations are found in 3% of patients with sporadic OS.

MDM2 gene on chromosome 12q13 encodes a protein which (binds to and) negatively modulates p53 function. MDM2 is ↑ in ≤10% of OS.

The INK4 gene produces the p14 protein which exerts a protective effect on p53. INK4A deletion or 12q13 amplification can inactivate two separate pathways of cell cycle control.

These provide at least three possible pathways for induction of osteosarcoma [15].

- DCC
  - The DCC (deleted in colon cancer) gene is located at chromosomal region 18q22.
  - Abnormalities of chromosomal regions 18q22 and 3q26 are found in Paget's disease where OS risk is ↑ [15].
- Other Oncogenes
  - C-fos is expressed in >60% of osteosarcoma and is frequent in patients with metastasis.
  - c-myc is overexpressed in patients with metastatic osteosarcoma.
  - Her 2/neu is found in 40% of osteosarcoma and ↓ survival.
  - SAS gene located on 12q13 is amplified in 1/3 of osteosarcoma and *all* parosteal osteosarcoma [15].

IV. Historic Highlights

- In 1804 English surgeon John Abernathy introduced the term sarcoma, from the Greek root meaning "fleshy excrescence" [9].
- In 1805 Napoleon's personal surgeon, French surgeon Alexis Boyer, coined the term "osteosarcoma." [9, 10]
- In 1847 noted French anatomist, pathologist, and military surgeon Baron Guillaume Dupuytren described osteosarcoma as "a white or reddish mass, lardaceous and firm at early stage of disease and later showing softening, extravasating blood and viscid straw-colored fluid."
- In 1921 Ernest Amory Codman, James Ewing, and Joseph Bloodgood created the Registry of Bone Sarcoma. This was a significant step forward in studying these rare and threatening tumors [10].
- The mid-1900s showed significant strides in bone pathology. Pathologists Henry L Jaffe (1896–1979) and Louis Lichtenstein (1906–1977) established virtually all key histologic criteria used to diagnose most commonly encountered bone tumors.
- In 1948 Cahan et al. proposed *four criteria* for recognizing radiation-induced sarcoma (RIS).

Selected References

1. Murphey MD, Robbin MR, McRae GA, et al. From the archives of the AFIP: the many faces of osteosarcoma. Radiographics. 1977;17:1205–31.
2. Chennupati SK, Norris R, Dunham B, Kazahaya K. Osteosarcoma of the skull base: case report and review of literature. Int J Pediatr Otorhinolaryngo. 2008;72(1):115–9.
3. Hadley C, Gressot LV, Patel AJ, et al. Osteosarcoma of the cranial vault and skull base in pediatric patients. J Neurosurg Pediatr. 2014;13(14):380–7.
4. Meel R, Thulkar S, Sharma MC, et al. Childhood osteosarcoma of greater wing of sphenoid: case report and review of literature. J Pediatr Hematol Oncol. 2012;34(2):59–62.
5. Hansen MR, Moffat JC. Osteosarcoma of the skull base after radiation therapy in a patient with McCune Albright syndrome: case report. Skull Base. 2003;13(2):79–83. https://doi.org/10.1055/s-2003-820562.
6. Mock D, Rosen IB. Osteosarcoma in irradiated fibrous dysplasia. J Oral Pathol. 1986;15:1–4.
7. Ruggieri P, Sim FH, Bond JR, Unni KK. Malignancies in fibrous dysplasia. Cancer. 1994;73:1411–24.
8. Cahan WG, Woodard HQ, Higginbotham NL, et al. Sarcoma arising in irradiated bone: report of eleven cases, 1948. Cancer. 1998;82:8–34.
9. Peltier LF. Tumors of bone and soft tissues. Orthopedics: a history and iconography. San Francisco: Norman Publishing; 1993. p. 264–91.
10. Rutkow IM. The nineteenth century. Surgery: an illustrated history. St Louis: Mosby-Year Book; 1993. p. 321–504.
11. Patel AJ, Rao VY, Fox BD, et al. Radiation-induced osteosarcomas of the calvarium and skull base. Cancer. 2011;117:2120–6. https://doi.org/10.1002/cncr.25734.
12. Ottaviani G., Jaffe N. (2009). The epidemiology of osteosarcoma. In: Jaffe N, et al. Pediatric and adolescent osteosarcoma. New York: Springer. doi:https://doi.org/10.1007/978-1-4419-0284-9_1. ISBN 978-1-4419-0283-2. PMID 20213383.
13. Yamada SM, So Yamada YI, Kuribayashi S, et al. Advanced therapeutic strategy for radiation-induced osteosarcoma in the skull base: a case report and review. Radiat Oncol. 2012;7:136.
14. Kim SY, Helman LJ. Strategies to explore new approaches in the investigation and treatment of osteosarcoma. Cancer Treat Res. 2010;152:517–28.
15. Capodano AM. Bone: osteosarcoma. Atlas genet and cytogenet. Oncol Hematol. 2003;7(1):44–7.
16. Mirabello L, Troisi RJ, Savage SA. Osteosarcoma incidence and survival rates from 1973 to 2004: data from the surveillance, epidemiology and end results program. Cancer. 2009;115(7):1531–43.
17. Bullough PG. Chapter 16, Bone forming tumors and tumor like conditions. In Orthopedic pathology, 5th ed. 2009. New York, NY: Elsevier; 382.
18. Singh GK, Yadav V, Singh P, Bhowmik KT. Radiation-induced malignancies making radiotherapy a "two-edged sword": a review of literature. World J. Onco. 2017; 8(1): 1–6; Accessed on line 2/15/2015.

Part IX

Anatomy

Skull Base and Facial Foramina

51

Pertinent Points

A foramen is an opening which potentially permits passage of structures between anatomic areas. The collective group of skull foramina *(plural)* characteristically conveys nerves, arteries, and veins. Most cranial foramina are related to the skull base and are considered *skull base foramina* with many containing critical cranial nerves. Another adjacent group of associated apertures includes the *facial foramina*. It is particularly important for neuroradiologists to be fluent in foraminal anatomy in order to evaluate pathologic processes which could commandeer these pathways for deadly disease disbursement. This is particularly problematic when we evaluate patients for possible perineural tumor spread. In addition to the usual structures which traverse these foramina, most contain fat which has been found to be the imager's friend. Consistent careful evaluation of skull base and facial foramina is essential for contemporary head and neck imaging.

Just as no two humans have identical fingerprints, skull base and facial foramina are similarly unique with foramina pairs frequently varying between sides. These bountiful breaches may be bilateral, unilateral, or supernumerary. Countless crevasses we commonly encounter are everyday emissary foramina. This chapter characterizes the most common presentations for 65 foramina which we regularly review on imaging studies.

While various foramina are clearly connected to more than one bone, for ready reference please consult Table 51.1 SBFF to examine these foramina codified according to their primary bony origin.

Table 51.1 Skull Base & Facial Foramina

Bone	#	Foramen	SBFF figure
A. Frontal bone.	1	Supraorbital foramen	51.1
	2	Supratrochlear foramen	51.1
	3	Foramen cecum	51.2
B. Ethmoid bone.	1	Olfactory foramina	51.2, 51.3, 51.4, 51.5a
	2	Anterior ethmoidal foramina	51.4, 51.5a, b, 51.6a
	3	Posterior ethmoidal foramina	51.4, 51.5b, 51.6a
C. Sphenoid. D. Bone	1	Optic foramen	51.1, 51.6a, b, 51.26a
	2	Foramen rotundum	51.6b, 51.7
	3	Foramen ovale	51.8, 51.9, 51.12
	4	Vidian canal	51.6b, 51.10
	5	Foramen spinosum	51.9, 51.12
	6	Foramen lacerum	51.11
	7	Foramen of Vesalius	51.12
	8	Sphenopalatine foramen	51.10
D. Temporal bone.	1	Carotid canal	51.10
	2	Jugular foramen	51.13a–d
	3	Internal auditory canal	51.10, 51.11, 51.13a, d
	4	Vestibular aqueduct	51.15
	5	Dorello's canal	51.16
	6	Petromastoid canal	51.17
	7	Stylomastoid foramen	51.18a, b
	8	Petrotympanic fissure	51.19
E. Occipital bone.	1	Foramen magnum	51.2, 51.4, 51.12, 51.11, 51.13b, d
	2	Hypoglossal canal	51.20a, b
	3	Condylar canal	51.21
F. Maxilla.	1	Incisive foramina	51.3
G. Mandible.	1	Mandibular foramen	51.22
	2	Mental foramen	51.23
H. Zygoma.	1	Zygomaticofacial foramen	51.24
	2	Zygomaticotemporal foramen	51.25
I. Orbit.	1	Superior orbital fissure (SOF)	51.1, 51.26–c, 51.27
	2	Inferior orbital fissure (IOF)	51.1, 51.28
	3	Lacrimal foramina	51.28

F. A. Midyett, S. K. Mukherji, *Skull Base Imaging*, https://doi.org/10.1007/978-3-030-46447-9_51

Skull Base Foramina

A. Frontal Bone

A1. Supraorbital Foramen

- *Location:*
  - The supraorbital foramen is a small groove or notch situated just below the eyebrow near the frontal bones superomedial orbital margin.
  - The supraorbital foramen is lateral to the supratrochlear foramen.
- *Contents:* The supraorbital foramen transmits the supraorbital nerve, artery, and vein.
- *Variants*: A wide anatomic positional variation has been noted, and brow lift surgeries show rates of >40% forehead paresthesia following deep dissection near the supraorbital notch and foramen [1].
- *Images*: See Fig. 51.1.

A2. Supratrochlear Foramen

- *Contents:* The skull's small paired supratrochlear foramina adorn the superomedial orbital margins conveying the supratrochlear nerve, artery, and vein *medial* to the supraorbital foramina.
- *Variants*: Development spans a spectrum from an intact foramen, a notch, or even complete absence. When the foramen is absent, the neurovascular bundle slyly slinks beneath the medial orbital margin and is potential prey to an unsuspecting surgeon. It behooves the radiologist to at least flag visible anomalies in this region.
- *Images:* See Fig. 51.2.

A3. Foramen Cecum

- *Name Origin: Latin* – foramen caecum ossis frontalis.
- *Origin:* Foramen cecum is the bony remnant of a primitive midline tract between the anterior cranial fossa and the nasal cavity.
- *Location:* Foramen cecum is situated just anterior to the cribriform plate within the frontoethmoidal suture.
- *Variants:* It varies in size and is often obstructed.
- *Contents and connections:* When patent, foramen cecum transmits an emissary vein from the nasal cavity to the superior sagittal sinus.
- *Clinical Significance:* Intracranial spread of infection from the facial danger triangle can cause calamitous complications including cavernous sinus thrombosis, meningitis, and brain abscess.
- *Images:* See Fig. 51.2.

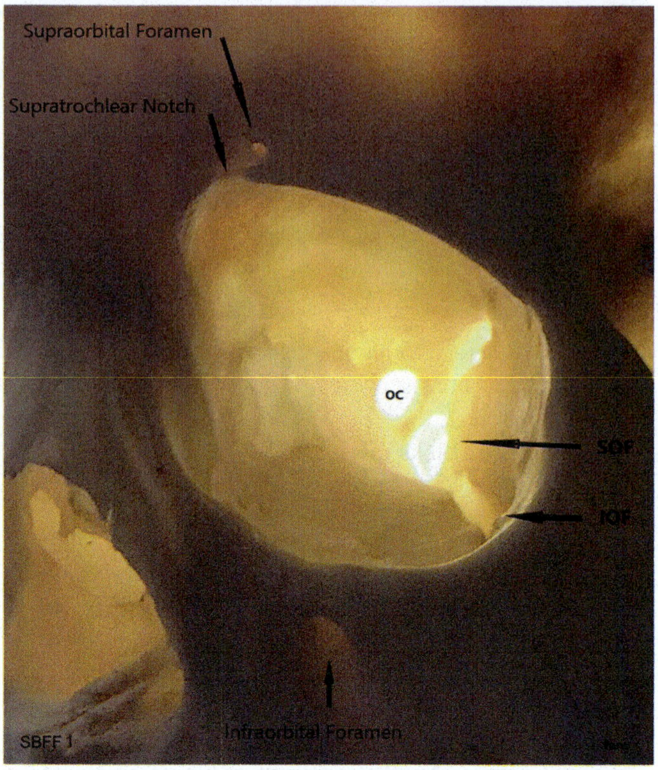

Fig. 51.1 Frontal oblique osseous left orbit shows OC (optic canal), SOF (superior orbital fissure), IOF (inferior orbital fissure), supraorbital foramen, infraorbital foramen, and supratrochlear notch

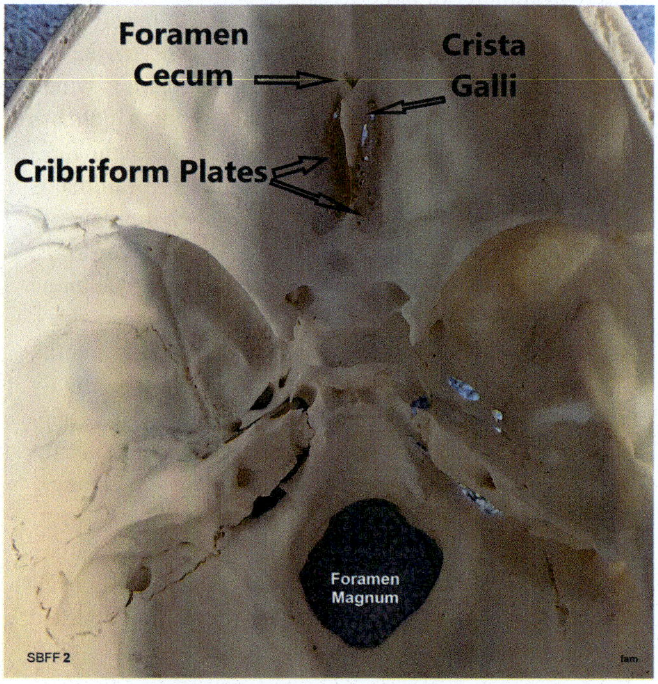

Fig. 51.2 Osseous endocranial skull base from above shows the foramen cecum anterior to the crista galli and the cribriform plates with multiple olfactory foramina

B. Ethmoid Bone

B1. Olfactory Foramina

- *Name Origin:*
  - *Latin* – foramina cribrosa ossis ethmoidalis.
  - *Greek*: cribr is sieve. Its sieve-like appearance from above prompted this Greek name.
  - Cribriform classically connotes an anatomical structure pierced by copious chasms, i.e., the cribriform plate.
  - The olfactory foramina, also known as the cribriform foramina, consist of a cluster of crevasses in the cribriform plate.
- *Connections:* Links the anterior cranial fossa to the nasal cavity.
- *Contents*: Branches of CN I from the olfactory bulb pass through the olfactory foramina to nasal mucosa.
- *Anatomy*:
  - The cribriform plate constructs the nasal cavity's roof with multiple tiny olfactory foramina found beside the central crista galli (*Latin*) which juts cranially like the "roosters crest" affording an anterior attachment for the falx.
  - The olfactory bulbs bask on top of the cribriform plate contiguous to the crista galli.

Clinical Significance: This is the premier example where a mere millimeter of bone separates the nasal cavity from the intracranial space. See Chapters 13–16 for specific examples.

Images: See Figs. 51.2, 51.3, and 51.4.

B2,3 Anterior and Posterior Ethmoidal Foramina

- *Connections:* The anterior and posterior ethmoidal foramina form critical conduits *connecting* the orbit to the anterior cranial fossa.
  - *Orbital Entrance:* The ethmoidal canals *enter* the medial orbital wall along the frontoethmoidal suture at the junction of the orbital roof and medial wall. See Figs. 51.4c and 51.8.
  - *Intracranial Exit:* The ethmoidal canals *exit* along the frontoethmoidal suture near the 12′ and 6 o'clock positions of the cribriform plates. See Fig. 51.4.
- *Contents*: The ethmoidal canals convey the anterior and posterior ethmoidal nerves, arteries, and veins.
- *Anatomy:*
  - The ophthalmic artery gives rise to the anterior and posterior ethmoidal arteries along the medial orbital wall where they enter the ethmoidal canals.

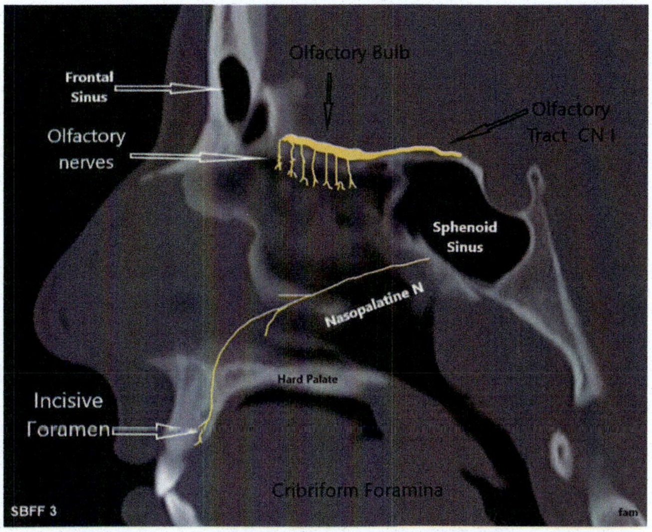

Fig. 51.3 Midline sagittal CT shows the olfactory tracts relationship to the cribriform plate and foramina. The nasopalatine nerve traverses the incisive foramen emerging as the anterior palatine nerve to provide parasympathics for the oral cavity particularly pain sensation to six front teeth. Ref. [2] Jones

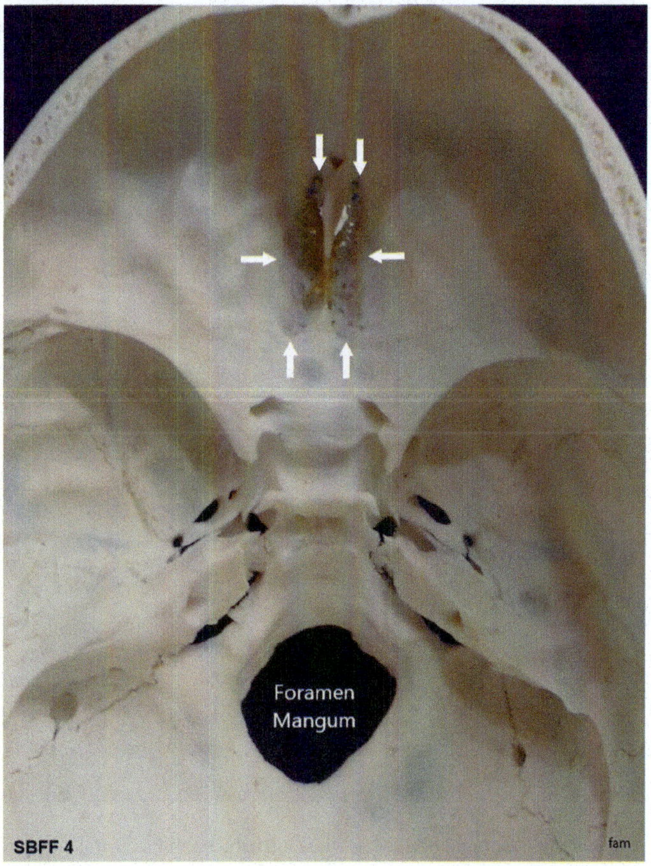

Fig. 51.4 Shows an anatomic endocranial skull base depicting the cribriform plate (horizontal → ← arrows) filled with myriad foramina. Down ↓ arrows elucidate the paired anterior ethmoidal foramina. The up ↑ arrows show the approximate locations for the posterior ethmoidal foramina although obscured by the overlying cantilevered sphenoid lamina

- The tiny (0.5–1 mm) anterior ethmoidal artery *exits* the ethmoidal canal as the *anterior meningeal artery* furnishing frontal dura and forming an anterior falcine artery.
- Upon reaching the anterior cranial fossa, the anterior ethmoidal nerve inclines into the nasal cavity through a crevasse between cartilage and the nasal bone supplying sensation to the anterior septum, lateral nose, and nasal tip.

• *Clinical Significance:* Posttraumatic nasal numbness suggests anterior ethmoidal nerve injury [3].
• *Images:* See Figs. 51.4, 51.5a, b, and 51.6a.

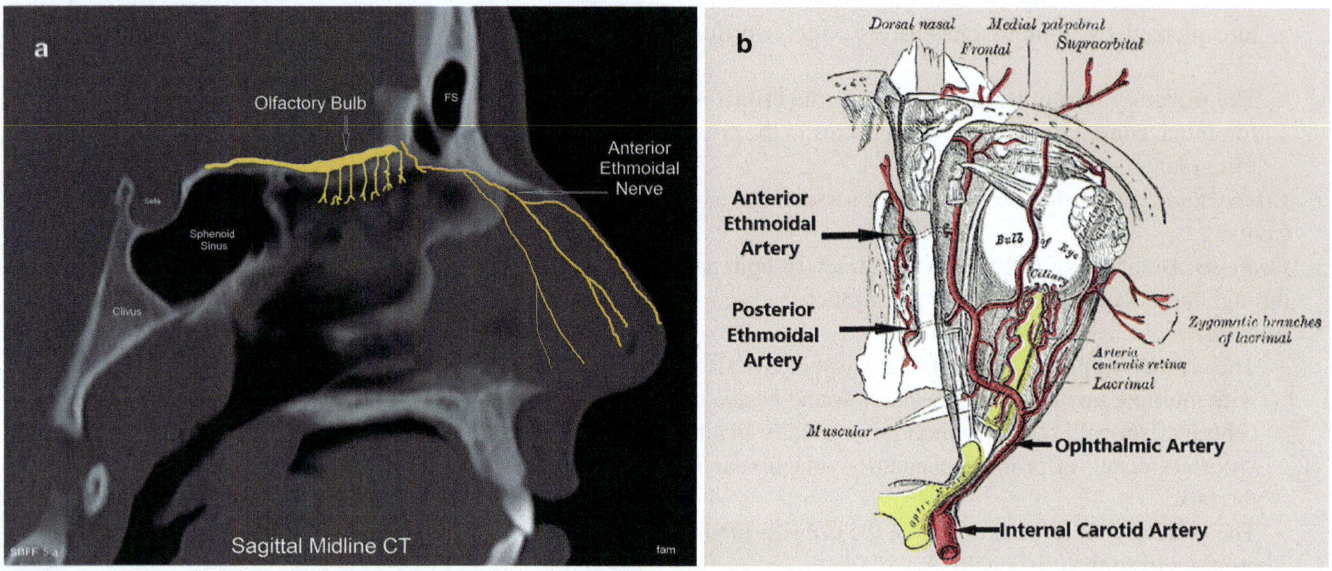

Fig. 51.5 (**a**) Sagittal midline CT depicts the anterior ethmoidal nerve after it *exits* from the anterior ethmoidal foramen just anterior to the cribriform plate. It slyly slips through a nasal bone cartilage crevasse supplying sensation to the anterior septum, lateral nose, and nasal tip. (**b**) Axial drawing demonstrates the ophthalmic artery arising from the ICA giving rise to the posterior and anterior ethmoidal arteries which traverse the medial orbital wall through the posterior and anterior ethmoidal foramina into the anterior cranial fossa adjacent the cribriform plate. Ref. Gray's Anatomy Public Domain/Wikimedia

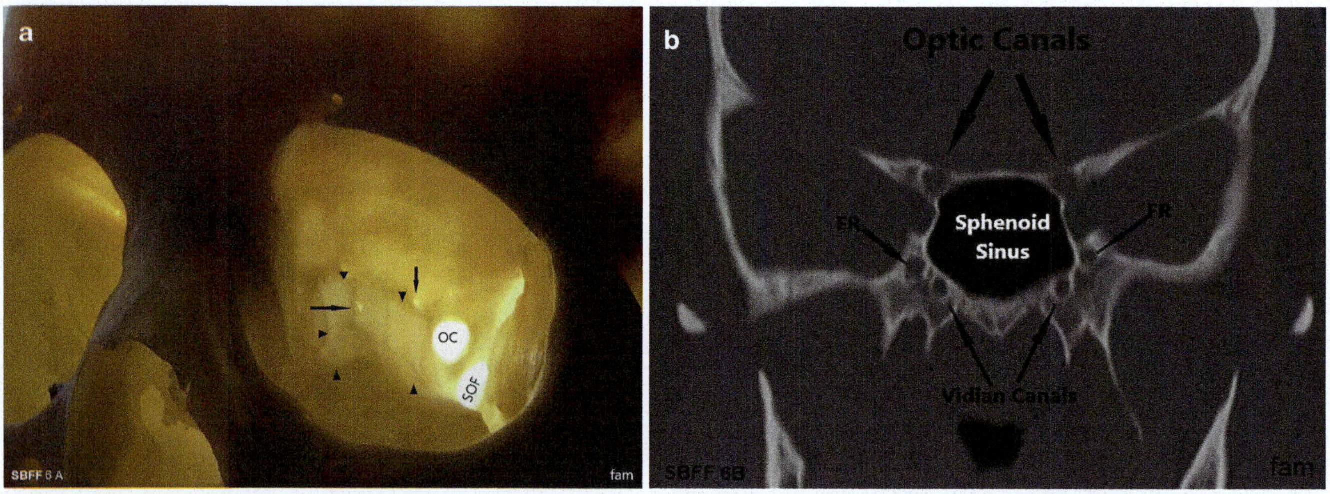

Fig. 51.6 (**a**) Frontal oblique osseous left orbit exhibits orbital entrance to the anterior (right arrow→) and posterior (down arrow↓) ethmoidal foramina located near the superior margins of the ethmoid bone (arrowheads◀▶▼▲). The optic canal (OC) and the superior orbital fissure (SOF) are observed in the orbital apex. (**b**) Coronal CT clarifies the conventional relationships of foramen rotunda (FR), optic and Vidian canals through the plane of the pterygoid plates

C. Sphenoid Bone

C1. Optic Foramen

- *Name Origin:* Latin – canalis opticus, foramen opticum ossis.
- *Connections*: The optic foramen forms the funnel shaped skull base opening to the cylindrical *optic canals* which run obliquely through the sphenoid bone connecting the middle cranial fossa to the orbit.
- *Contents*: The optic canals convey the *ophthalmic artery* and the *optic nerve* (CN II) with supplementary sympathetic fibers. Within the optic canal, the ophthalmic artery lies inferolateral to the optic nerve.
- *Anatomy:* The optic canals create approximately a 45^0 angle to the skull's mid-sagittal plane. They are bounded medially by the sphenoid body, superiorly by the superior root of the lesser wing, laterally by the anterior clinoid, and inferolaterally by the optic strut. The optic strut is the inferior root of the lesser wing and separates the optic canal from the superior orbital fissure inferolaterally [4].
- *Images:* See Figs. 51.1, 51.6a, b and 51.26a.

C2. Foramen Rotundum (FR)

- *Name Origin: Latin* – round passage or opening.
- *Plural*: Foramina rotunda.
- *Connections*: It connects the middle cranial fossa to the pterygopalatine fossa.
- *Contents*: Its crucial contents include:
  - Maxillary nerve (*CN* V_2).
  - Artery of foramen rotundum.
  - Emissary veins.
- *Anatomy*.
  - Located in the middle cranial fossa (MCF), in the base of the greater wing is a parasagittal trough-shaped canal, just posterior and inferior to the medial margin of the superior orbital fissure (SOF).
  - Size: In adults, the foramen rotundum averages 3.55 mm diameter.
- *Anomalies*.
  - Although the foramen rotundum classically shares its medial margin with the lateral wall of the sphenoid sinus, modern imaging has shown significant variation related to sphenoid sinus pneumatization.
  - While various classifications for anatomic variants have been proposed, from a practical standpoint, these foramina either are in the usual location protected by bone or they are in an unusual location and/or are not protected by bone.
  - It is important for the modern imager to announce anatomic anomalies particularly when the contents of FR or the VC could be compromised during endoscopic surgery.
- *Images*: See Figures 51.5b, 51.6b, and 51.7.

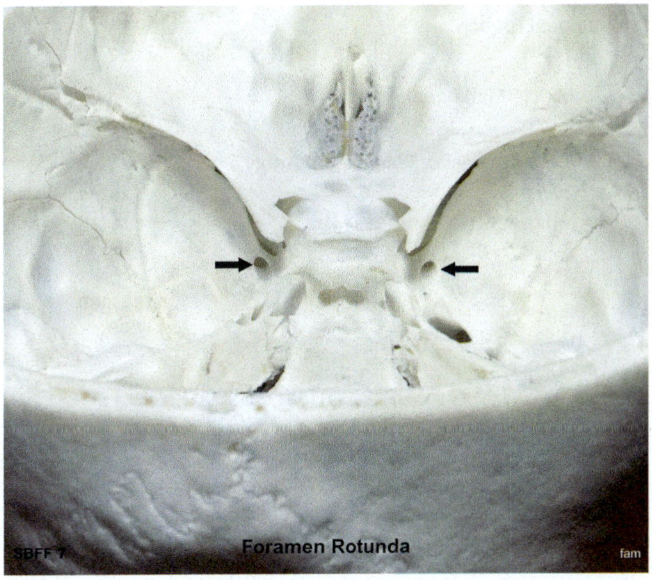

Fig. 51.7 Osseous endocranial skull base exhibits middle cranial fossa entrances to foramina rotunda (horizontal arrows→←)

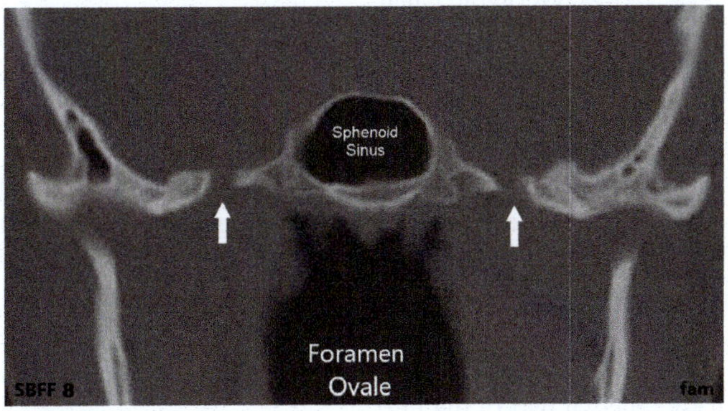

Fig. 51.8 Coronal CT cavorts foramen ovale forming a formidable fissure through the skull base

C3. Foramen Ovale (FO)

- *Name Origin:* Latin – oval opening or passage.
- *Connections:* Foramen ovale connects the middle cranial fossa to the infratemporal fossa.
- *Contents*: Foramen ovale opens into the infratemporal fossa classically conveying the following:
  - *Mandibular nerve (CN* V_3*).*
  - *Accessory meningeal artery.*
  - *Lesser petrosal nerve* (sometimes passes through canalis innominatus between FO and FS).
  - *Emissary veins* (connecting the cavernous sinuses to the pterygoid plexus).
- *Boundaries*: Foramen ovale is one of the larger skull base foramina and is located at the posterior base of the greater sphenoid wing posterolateral to foramen rotundum and lateral to the sphenoidal lingula (i.e., a bony ridge along the lateral margin of the carotid groove).
- *Images*: See Figs. 51.8, 51.9, and 51.12.

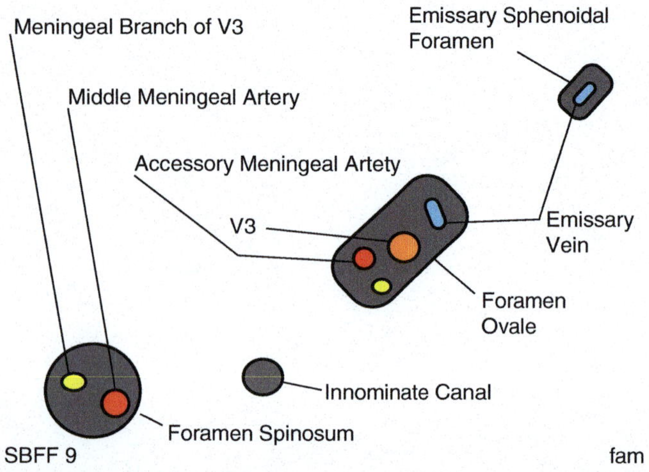

Fig. 51.9 Color cartoon showing several significant structures spanning foramen ovale and foramen spinosum

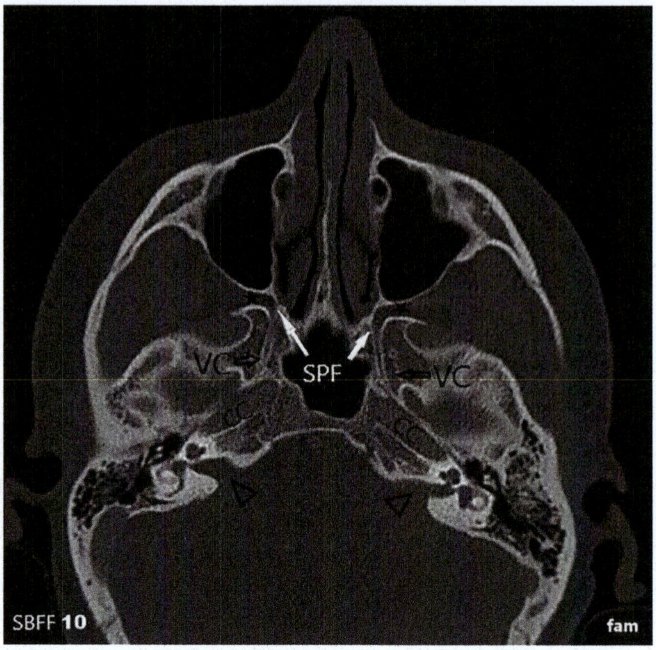

Fig. 51.10 Axial CT through the caudal pterygopalatine fossa (PPF) branded by a black star shows connection to the Vidian canals (VC). Also displayed are the carotid canals (CC), the internal auditory canals [(IAC) black triangles ▲], and the medial sphenopalatine foramen (SPF)

C4. Vidian Canal (VC)

- *Name Origin.*
  - AKA: Pterygoid canal.
  - The Vidian canal is named after Italian anatomist and surgeon, Guido Guidi [*Latin*: Vidus Vidius 1509–1569].
- *Location.*
  - The paired Vidian canals are positioned inferomedial to foramina rotunda below the sphenoid sinus floor at the junction of the sphenoid body and pterygoid process.
  - The canal begins posteriorly at the anterolateral edge of foramen lacerum extending anteriorly into the medial part of the PPF.
- *Contents.*
  - The Vidian canal provides a pathway for the Vidian nerve and artery from the MCF to the PPF where the nerve joins the pterygopalatine ganglion.
  - The Vidian nerve is created by convergence of the greater and deep petrosal nerves within the Vidian canal.
- *Variants*: Approximately 60% of Vidian canals protrude into the sphenoid sinus, and its fairly frequent bony dehiscence should be pointed out to endoscopic surgeons as the nerve may await defenseless just beneath the mucosa [5].
- *Images:* See Figs. 51.6b and 51.10.

C5. Foramen Spinosum

- *Name Origin.*
  - Latin – spina means thorn.
  - *Plural*: foramina spinosa.
  - First described by Danish anatomist Jakob Benignus Winslow in the eighteenth century.
  - So-named because of its relationship to spinous process of greater sphenoid wing. Literal meaning is “hole full of thorns.” Purists profess the correct name would be *foramen spinae* [6].
- *Boundaries*: Located posterolateral to foramen ovale, in the greater sphenoid wing.
- *Connections*: Foramen spinosum connects the middle cranial fossa to the infratemporal fossa.
- *Contents*: Foramen spinosum permits passage of the middle meningeal A, V, and the nervus spinosus. The nervus spinosus is the recurrent or meningeal branch of V_2 which usually re-enters the calvarium through FS (or occasionally FO).
- *Nervus Spinosus*: The nervus spinosus supplies sensation to the cartilaginous eustachian tube, the trigeminal ganglion, and the MCFs posterior dura. Distally it supplies the mastoid antrum and air cells.
- *Pertinent anatomic variant*: When the middle meningeal artery originates directly from a persistent stapedial artery, the foramen spinosum is absent or small.
- See Figs. 51.9 and 51.12.

C6. Foramen Lacerum (FL)

- *Name Origin.*
  - Latin – lacerated piercing.
  - *Plural*: foramina lacera.

- First described in the literature by anatomist Wenzel Gruber in 1869 [7]
- *AKA*: sphenopetroclival synchondrosis.

- *Connections*: Connects the pterygoid venous plexus in the infratemporal fossa to the cavernous sinus and middle cranial fossa.
- *Boundaries*: Triangular skull base opening at the base of greater sphenoid wing, petrous apex and basiocciput. Like several other foramina discussed in this chapter, the foramen lacerum is basically a breach between bones rather than an actual bony foramen formed from a single bone.
- *Contents*.
  - Foramen lacerum contains connective tissue and meningeal branches from the ascending pharyngeal artery and emissary veins conveyed from the cavernous sinus to the pterygoid plexus.
  - Foramen lacerum contains the artery and nerve of the pterygoid canal (Vidian) and some venous drainage.
  - The deep and greater petrosal nerves join to form the Vidian nerve in foramen lacerum.
- *Clinical Significance*: Foramen lacerum has been shown to be a significant port of entry for neoplasm including melanoma, lymphoma, adenoid cystic carcinoma, nasopharyngeal carcinoma, and juvenile angiofibroma [7, 8].
- *Images*: See Fig. 51.11.

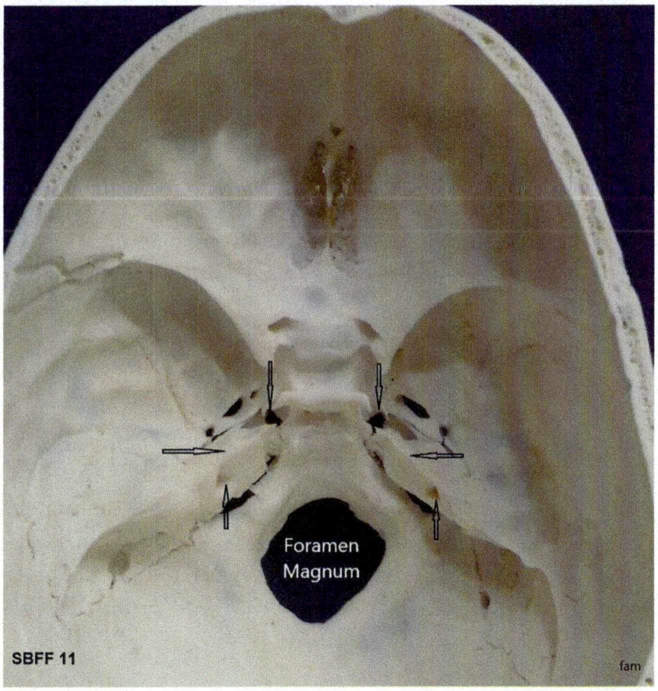

Fig. 51.11 Osseous endocranial SB portrays foramen lacerum (down arrows↓↓), IACs (up arrows↑↑), and petrous apices (horizontal arrows→←)

C7. Foramen of Vesalius

- *Plural*: Foramina Vesalii.
- *AKA*: Sphenoidal emissary foramen, foramen venosus, or canaliculus sphenoidal.
- *Location*: Tiny, variably present, sphenoidal foramen anteromedial to foramen ovale, lateral to foramen rotundum and the Vidian canal.
- *Connections and Contents*: Transmits a sphenoidal emissary vein linking the pterygoid venous plexus in the infratemporal fossa to the cavernous sinus.
- *Clinical Significance:* While the incidence of unilateral and bilateral foramina of Vesalius varies widely, some suggest that asymmetric foramina of Vesalii on high resolution CT more likely represents a pathologic process than an anatomic variation [9].
- *Name Origin.*
  - Perhaps, however, the real significance of these tiny skull base foramina is that they serve to remind us of their namesake, Andreas Vesalius.
  - Andreas Vesalius (1514–1564), a sixteenth-century Flemish anatomist, physician, and author, has been called the creator of contemporary anatomy who published the earliest sweeping study of the sphenoid bone almost 500 years ago. His alluring anatomic plates were painstakingly carved into wood before being printed on paper. And you thought some publishing programs were tedious. One of his texts *De Humani Corporis Fabrica* is currently considered to be among history's most influential books [10].
- *Image:* See Fig. 51.12.

C8. Sphenopalatine Foramen (SPF)

- *Location:* The opening for the sphenopalatine foramen (SPF) on the lateral nasal wall is created by the confluence of the inferior sphenoid and vertical palatine bones [10].
- *Connections:* The sphenopalatine foramen (SPF) forms the medial connection of the pterygopalatine fossa (PPF) to the nasal cavity at the superior nasal meatus.
- *Contents*: The sphenopalatine foramen typically transmits the sphenopalatine artery and vein, the nasopalatine nerve, and the posterior superior nasal nerves.
- *Clinical Significance.*
  - Probably more noteworthy than normal structures this foramen carries, it possesses the potential for significant spread of pathologic processes, particularly perineural tumor spread and dissemination of infection.
  - The SPF is probably best known for the straightforward skull base access it provides to juvenile angiofibromas which possess a predilection for the neighboring nearby nasal cavity.
- *Image:* See Fig. 51.10.

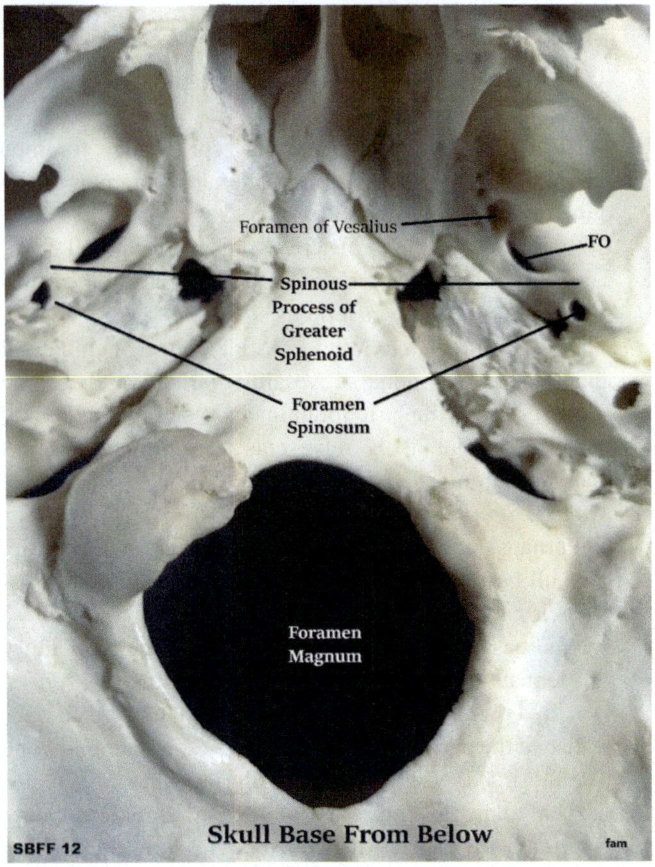

Fig. 51.12 Osseous exocranial skull base reveals the relationship of the foramen spinosum to its namesake, the small spinous process of the greater sphenoid and foramen ovale (FO). The foramen of Vesalius is frequently unilateral as shown in this specimen

D. Temporal Bone

D1. Carotid Canal

- *Connections:* The temporal bone's carotid canal permits passage of the internal carotid artery along with its associated carotid plexus passing from the neck into the middle cranial fossa (MCF) with subsequent orbit extension.
- *Location:* The carotid canal commences at the *carotid foramen* in the petrous portion of the inferior temporal bone just cephalic to the jugular fossa. It ascends superiorly before bending anteromedially.
- *Contents.*
  - It conveys the ICA which exits the carotid canal coursing cranially over foramen lacerum into the cavernous sinus.
  - The carotid plexus comprises a system of sympathetic fibers arising from the superior cervical ganglion stretching superiorly along the lateral aspect of the ICA.
  - The following nerve fibers furnish multiple motor implications including:
    1. The superior tarsal muscle which raises the eyelid.
    2. The pupillary dilator muscle which dilates the pupil.
    3. Innervation of facial and scalp sweat glands.
    4. Innervation of intracranial vasoconstrictors.
- *Image*: See Fig. 51.10.

D2. Jugular Foramen (JF)

- *Connections:* The jugular foramen is a significant skull base foramen situated posterior to the carotid canal between the petrous temporal bone anteriorly and the occipital bone posteriorly. Although paired, it is regularly asymmetrically larger on the right.
- *Contents.*
  - Anatomically the JF is best known for several significant structures it conveys including: CN IX (glossopharyngeal n.), CN X (vagus n.), and CN XI (accessory n.) which exit the skull base to enter the neck.
  - The intracranial sigmoid sinus becomes the internal jugular vein and traverses the JF along with the inferior petrosal sinus and some meningeal branches of the occipital and ascending pharyngeal arteries. See SBFF 14, Sagittal MRV.
- *Anatomy.*
  - Anatomic aficionados sometimes subdivide the JF into three compartments, each containing characteristic contents.

    The *anterior* compartment contains the inferior petrosal sinus.

    The *intermediate* compartment contains CN IX, X, and XI.

    The *posterior* compartment contains the sigmoid sinus (becoming the internal jugular vein) and some meningeal branches from occipital and ascending pharyngeal arteries.
  - However, most neuroradiologists and neurosurgeons use an alternative image-based subclassification set out by the jugular spine, which splits the jugular foramen into two compartments.

    I. Pars Nervosa CN IX.
    - "Pars Nervosa" is the smaller, anteromedial compartment containing *CN IX*, the *tympanic nerve* (a branch of CN IX), and the *inferior petrosal sinus*.

    II. Pars Vascularis CN X, CN XI, Jugular bulb.
    - "Pars Vascularis" is the larger, posterolateral compartment contains *CN X, CN XI, Arnold's nerve* (auricular br. of CN X), the *jugular bulb*, and the *posterior meningeal branch of the ascending pharyngeal artery*.
- *Images: See Fig. 51.13a–d.*

D3. Internal Auditory Canal

- *AKA*: Internal auditory meatus, internal acoustic meatus, internal acoustic canal, meatus acusticus internus.

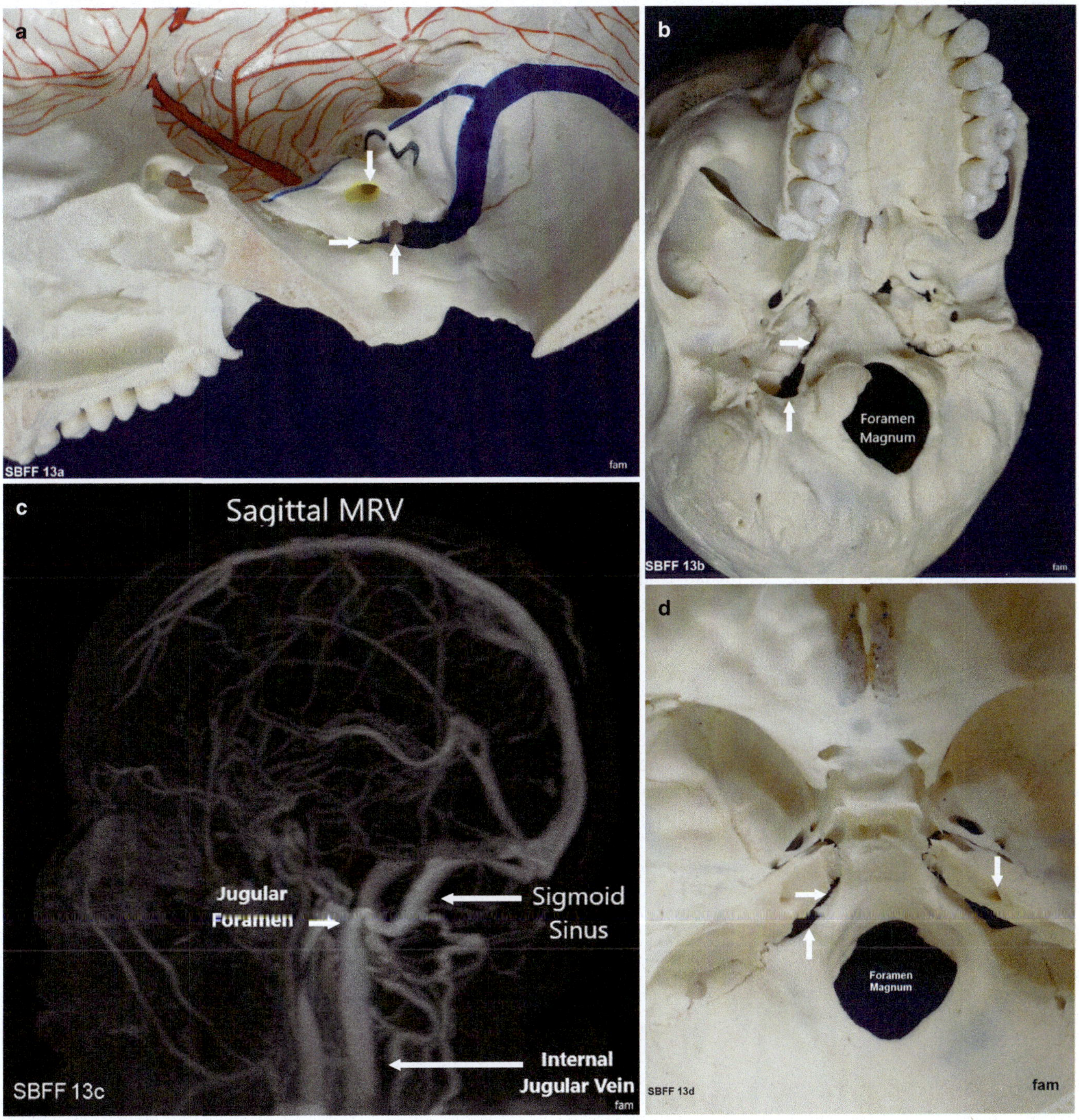

Fig. 51.13 (**a**) Sagittal section of endocranial anatomic skull shows the (blue) sigmoid sinus traversing the jugular foramen (↑ arrow) before exiting the skull base as the internal jugular vein. The IAC (↓ arrow) is highlighted in yellow. Adjacent petro-occipital fissure (→). (**b**) Oblique osseous exocranial skull base shows the jugular foramen (up arrow ↑) adjacent to the petro-occipital (POF) fissure (horizontal arrow→). (**c**) Sagittal MRV illustrates the intracranial sigmoid sinus spanning the skull base through the jugular foramen to exit as the extracranial internal jugular vein. (**d**) Anatomic endocranial skull base specimen shows petro-occipital fissure (→), jugular foramen (↑), IAC (↓), and foramen magnum

- The IAC opens into the posterior cranial fossa, near the center of the posterior petrous temporal bone.
- The meatus progresses laterally approximately 1 cm into the temporal bone.
- The lateral portion of the canal called the fundus is divided by bony spicules into separate channels containing facial and vestibulocochlear nerve branches.

- The horizontal falciform crest divides the meatus into superior and inferior sections.
- A slim vertical stalactite splits the superior section into anterior and posterior portions. This vertical spike is named for notable otologist William F. House and is commonly called "Bill's bar."
- While bony crests definitely divide the fundus into three segments, contemporary anatomists apportion the fundus into four quadrants based on major nerve branches. These are depicted in the next color cartoon Fig. 51.15 as:
  - Anterior superior – Facial nerve area containing CN VII and the NI (nervus intermedius).
  - Anterior inferior – Cochlear nerve area containing the cochlear Nerve ($VIII_{c)}$.
  - Posterior superior – Superior Vestibular Area containing the Superior Division of CN VIII.
  - Posterior inferior – Inferior Vestibular Area Containing the Inferior Division of CN VIII.
- CN VIII terminates in the inner ear.
- CN VII travels through the facial canal eventually exiting the skull at the stylomastoid foramen. [See Fig. 51.15e, f.]
- The IAC also provides passage for the labyrinthine artery and the vestibular ganglion.
- *Images:* See Figs. 51.10, 51.11, 51.13a, d, 51.14, and 51.16.

D4. Vestibular Aqueduct

- *Contents:* The vestibular aqueduct contains the endolymphatic duct, a tubular extension of the membranous labyrinth, which ends blindly as the endolymphatic sac.
- *Connections:* The vestibular aqueduct extends from the inner ear's endolymphatic space posterolaterally to the petrous portion of the temporal bone.
- *Anatomy:* Vestibular aqueducts are narrow, bony canals with 1.0 to 1.5 mm considered "normal."
- *Clinical Significance:* Aqueductal enlargement >2 mm is associated with enlarged vestibular aqueduct (EVA) syndrome. EVA is the most common inner ear malformation associated with hearing loss [11].
- *Imaging:* While the vestibular aqueducts are most frequently found in axial planes, current scanners sanction reformatting source images into any plane without real resolution loss. Comparison of axial, sagittal, coronal, and 45° oblique Pöschl planes has shown the Pöschl plane to be the most reliable as it parallels the vestibular aqueduct's long axis predictably portraying the entire canal [12].
- *Image*: See Fig. 51.15.

D5. Dorello's Canal (DC)

- *Location:* Dorello's canal is a bow-shaped structure near the temporal bone tip which surrounds CN VI and the inferior petrosal sinus at the confluence with the cavernous sinus.
- *Contents:* Dorello's canal advances the abducens nerve (CN VI) and the inferior petrosal sinus from the pontine cistern to the cavernous sinus.
- *Name Origin:* First described by Gruber in 1859 and later in 1905 by Italian Anatomist and ENT Chair Primo Dorello whose critique caused this clandestine canal to carry his eponym.
- *Boundaries.*

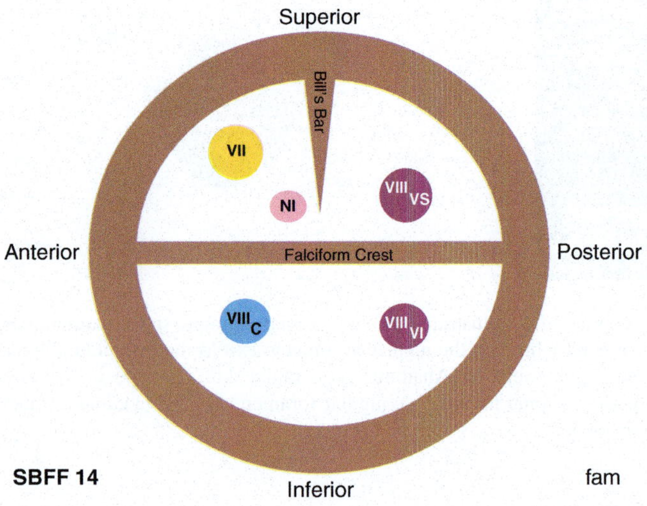

Fig. 51.14 Color cartoon portrays a transverse section through the IAC revealing important relationships of the facial nerve (CN VII), nervus intermedius (NI), cochlear nerve (CN VIII_c), superior vestibular nerve (VIII_{Vs}), and inferior vestibular nerve (VIII_{VI}) delineated by the horizontal falciform crest and vertical Bill's bar

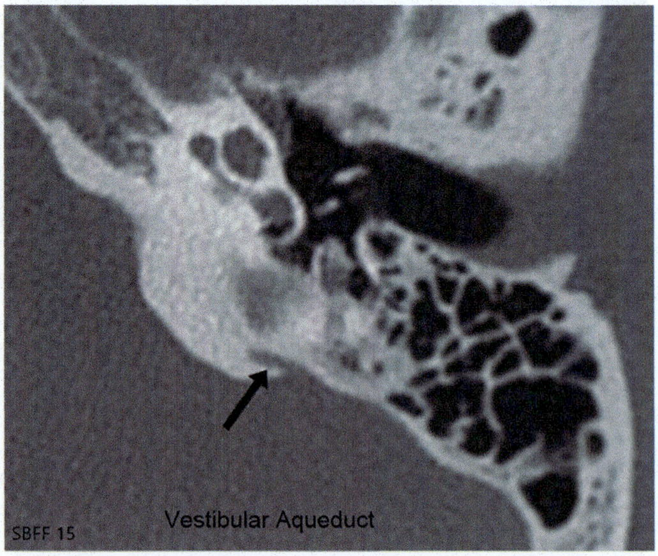

Fig. 51.15 Axial CT through the left temporal bone at the level of the vestibular aqueduct (↑). A diameter of 1 to 1.5 mm is considered normal. If in doubt, this can be further evaluated using axial, coronal, sagittal, and Pöschl (45° oblique) planes

- Classic compositions define Dorello's canal as a small space between Gruber's ligament and the petrous apex. More recent anatomists conceive a statelier space between two dural leaves extending from the dural entrance of CN VI to the cavernous sinus.
- The literature has been choked with complex descriptions of Dorello's canal for more than a century. Most neuroimagers welcome the "new concept in Dorello's canal microanatomy: the petroclival venous confluence" depicting Dorello's canal as the CSF invagination into the petroclival dura surrounding CN VI [13].
- No matter which boundaries anatomists definitively decide, Dorello's canal will doubtless be discovered near the superior clivus, *immediately beneath the posterior clinoid*, adjacent the *medial margin of the petrous ridge* and the petrosphenoidal suture.

- *Clinical Significance*: We shouldn't forget about it especially when confronted with entities like Gradenigo's syndrome [14].
- *Image:* See Fig. 51.16.

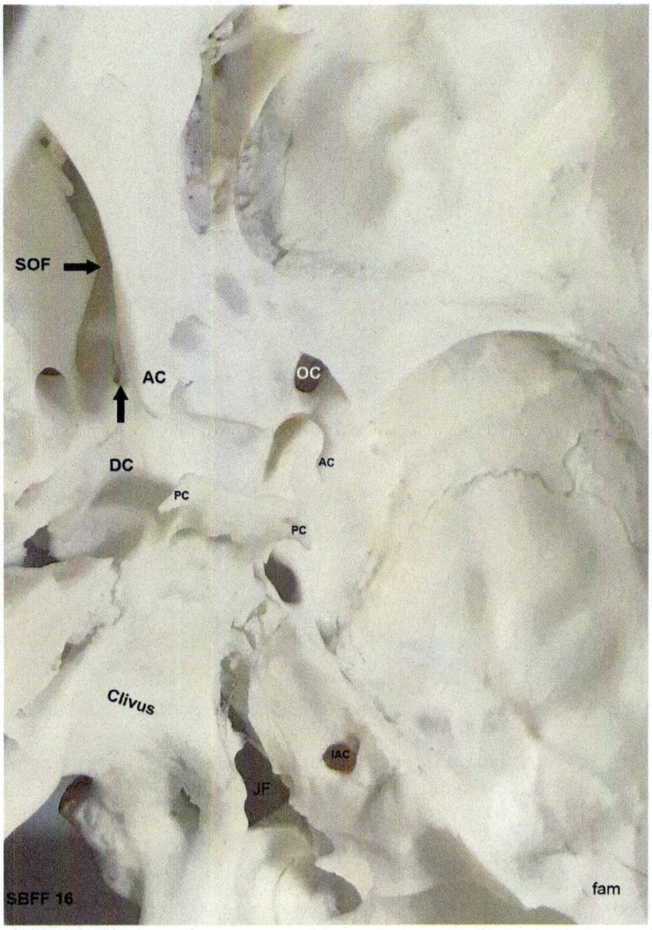

Fig. 51.16 Oblique osseous endocranial skull base shows the left Dorello's canal (DC up arrow ↑) located just caudal to the anterior clinoid (AC), along the medial margin of the superior orbital fissure (SOF). The optic canal (OC), superior orbital fissure (SOF), internal auditory canal (IAC), clivus, jugular foramen (JF), and posterior clinoids (PC) are pridefully portrayed

D6. Petromastoid Canal

- *AKA*: Subarcuate canal.
- *Connections:* Links the mastoid antrum to the posterior cranial fossa.
- *Contents:* Surrounds the subarcuate artery and vein.
- *Clinical Significance.*
  - The petromastoid canal can conduct middle ear infections into the posterior fossa.
  - The narrow, elongated adult appearance is attained by age 5 but varies considerably before that and should not be mistaken for pathology. For example, under five, a wide canal >2 mm is a normal variant [15].
  - Various variations may be significant when considering children for cochlear implants [16].
- *Image*: See Fig. 51.17.

D7. Stylomastoid Foramen

- *Location*: Rounded opening on the inferior surface of the petrous temporal bone, between the styloid and mastoid processes, deep to the digastric belly.
- *Contents:* It is the termination of the facial canal and transmits the facial nerve (CN VII) and the stylomastoid artery.
- *Images*: See Fig. 51.18a, b.

D8. Petrotympanic Fissure (PTF)

- *AKA:* Squamotympanic fissure or Glaserian fissure is named for noted Swiss Anatomist Johann Glaser (1629–1675).
- *Contents.*
  - The petrotympanic fissure is the medial continuation of the tympanosquamosal suture which runs from the TMJ's mandibular fossa to the temporal cavity conveying connections of cranial nerves VII and IX.
  - It contains the chorda tympani, the anterior tympanic artery, and tympanic veins which cross this crevice into the infratemporal fossa.
  - A branch of CN VII, the *chorda tympani* joins the lingual nerve to provide taste sensation to the tongue.
  - The petrotympanic fissure (PTF) contains a few fibers from the Casserio's ligament (anterior ligament of the malleus) which extend from the neck of the malleus just above its anterior process and eventually attaches to the sphenoidal spine.
- *More Neuroanatomy.*
  - Frequently forgotten murkier neuroanatomic nuances include a branch of CN IX, the *tympanic nerve* traverses the PTF as the lesser petrosal nerve, transiting

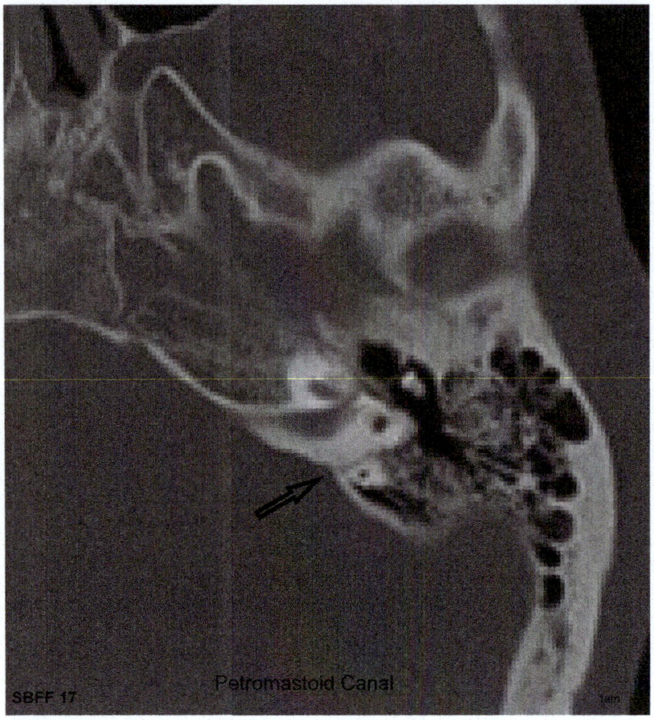

Fig. 51.17 Axial CT through the left temporal bone portrays the petromastoid canal extending from the mastoid antrum to the posterior cranial fossa

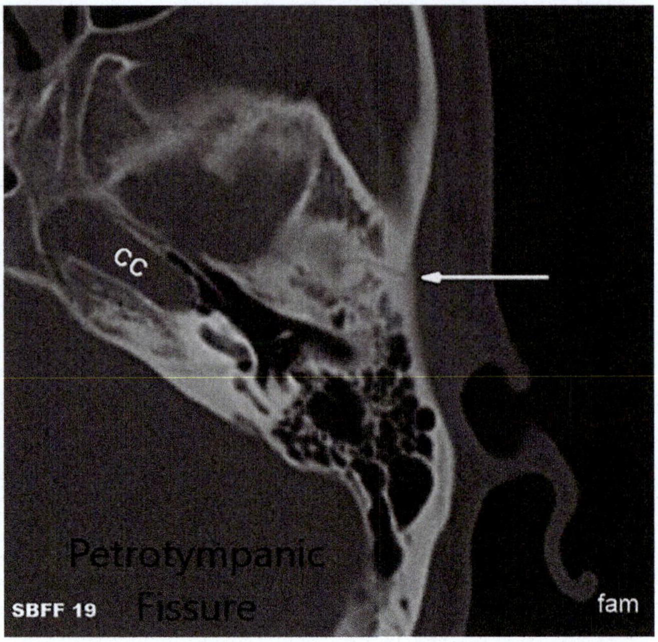

Fig. 51.19 Axial CT through the left TB at the level of the carotid canal (CC) portrays the petite petrotympanic fissure (white arrow ←) whose size belies the sum of significant structures it conveys

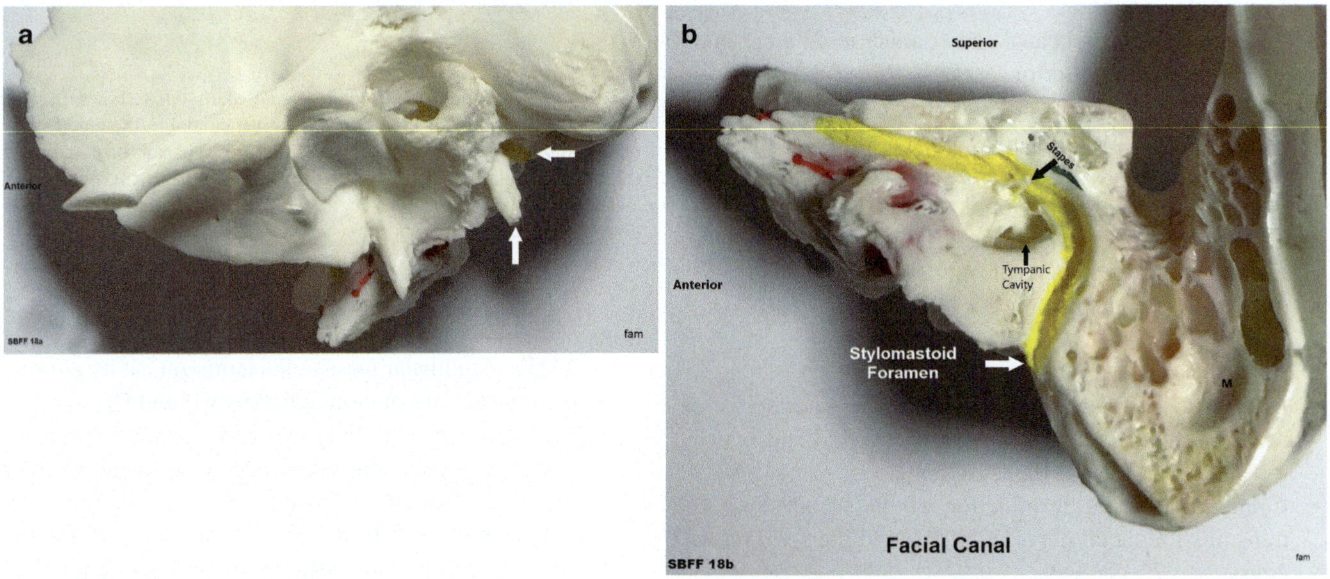

Fig. 51.18 (**a**) Oblique osseous exocranial skull base shows the stylomastoid foramen (yellow highlights with ← arrow) just posterior to the temporal bone's styloid process (up arrow ↑). (**b**) Sagittal section of the left mastoid (M) and petrous portion of the temporal bone through the facial canal (yellow) which opens caudally through the stylomastoid foramen (white → arrow). The tympanic cavity shows the stapes in place at the oval window. Multiple air cells fill the left mastoid (M). The (red) internal carotid artery (ICA) enters the carotid canal anterior to the caudal aspect of the skull base

foramen ovale joining V3, synapsing in the otic ganglion to provide parotid parasympathetics.
  - At the very least, the petrotympanic fissure should not be mistaken for a fracture.
- *Image:* See Fig. 51.19.

E. Occipital Bone

E1. Foramen Magnum

- *Great Hole:* The ~3 × 3.5 cm oval occipital opening is uncontested as the chief cranial foramina definitely deserving its Latin name connoting the *great hole.*

- *Connections:* The foramen magnum merges the posterior cranial fossa to the spinal canal.
- *Contents*: Its critical contents include the medulla oblongata, meninges, the spinal cord, vertebral arteries, anterior and posterior spinal arteries, spinal root of the accessory nerve (CN XI), the tectorial membrane, and the alar ligaments.
- *Anatomy.*
  - Pertinent midline landmarks include the basion anteriorly, the occipital condyles laterally, and the opisthion posteriorly.
- Clinical Significance.
  - While the foramen magnum normally facilitates pulsatile CSF flow through the spinal canal, pathologic processes sometimes sanction spread of infection, hemorrhage, or tumor through this crucial chasm.
  - Under certain conditions, normal intracranial structures descent into the foramen magnum proves perilous.
- *Images*: Figs. 51.2, 51.4, 51.11, 51.12, 51.13b, d, and 51.26b.

E2. Hypoglossal Canal

- *Name Origin: Greek* – hypo (under) glossal (tongue).
- *Connections*: Paired canals link the posterior cranial fossa to the nasopharyngeal carotid space.
- *Contents.*
  - The hypoglossal canal commences hosting the hypoglossal nerve (CN XII) near its anterior medullary origin to its skull base exit adjacent the jugular foramen.
  - A branch of the ascending pharyngeal artery.
  - Sometimes a persistent hypoglossal artery.
  - An ample venous plexus.
  - A small variable emissary vein [17]
- *Anatomy.*
  - The hypoglossal canals are located between the occipital condyle and the jugular tubercle running anterolaterally allowing the hypoglossal nerves to exit the posterior cranial fossa.
  - These paired occipital foramina which previously seemed somewhat obscure now proclaim their presence with their enigmatic eagle's profile providing dependable discernable landmarks for CT and MRI.
- *Anatomic Variants.*
  - Hypoglossal canal enlargement suggests the possibility of a persistent hypoglossal artery.
  - A frequently ossified fibrous septum separates two hypoglossal nerve roots before they merge within the hypoglossal canal.
  - Supernumerary hypoglossal canals are frequent with a recent Japanese study showing double hypoglossal canals in 16.9% of which 2.2% were bilateral [17].
- *Images:* See Fig. 51.20a, b.

E3. Condylar Canal

- AKA: Condyloid canal, posterior condylar canal.
- The condylar canal is located in the posterior cranial fossa and although small is the largest of the skull's emissary foramina.
- *Contents:* The condylar canal transmits the posterior condylar vein and a meningeal branch of the occipital artery [18].
- *Connections:* The condylar canal connects the *extracranial* condylar fossa to the *intracranial* jugular bulb. The occipital emissary vein allows anastomosis of the *extracranial* suboccipital venous plexus to the *intracranial* dural venous sinuses including the jugular bulb and the sigmoid sinus [19].
- *Incidence:* It is confirmed on CT in 80% of cases with 31% bilateral, 50% unilateral [19], and is sometimes supernumerary.
- *Image:* See Fig. 51.21.

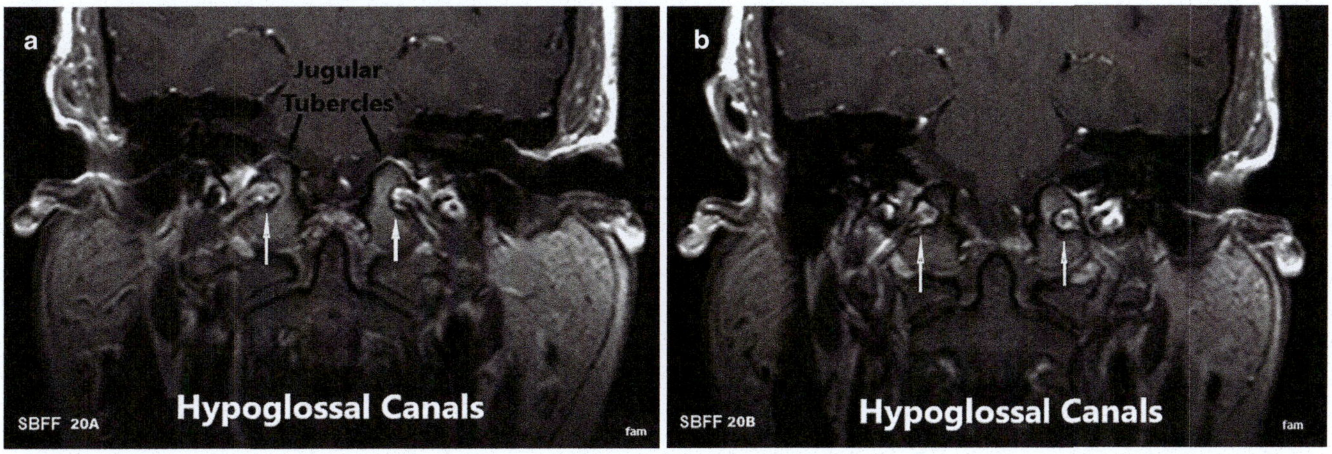

Fig. 51.20 (**a**, **b**) Depict the hypoglossal canals (white ↑ arrows) filled with fat containing low signal CN XII rootlets distinctly displayed as internal filling defects. The emblematic eagle shaped jugular tubercles are admirably appreciated

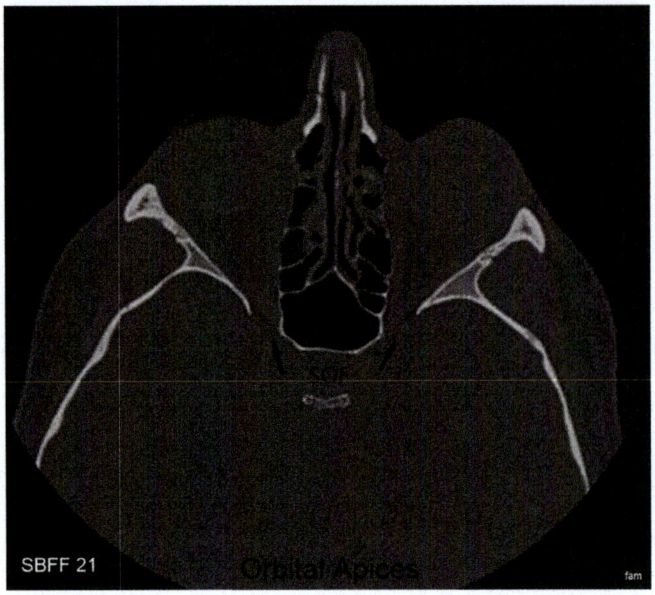

Fig. 51.21 Axial CT with bone windows through the orbital apices show bony openings for the superior orbital fissures (white ↑ arrows)

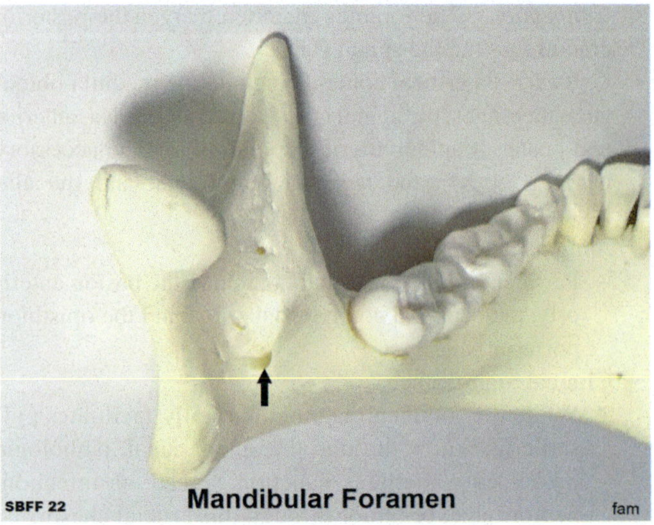

Fig. 51.22 *Medial* mandibular surface near the junction of the vertical and horizontal rami is home to the *mandibular foramen* which effects entrance for the inferior alveolar nerve and artery into the *mandibular canal*

Facial Foramina

F. Maxilla

F1. Incisive Foramina

- The incisive foramen Latin: foramen incisivum. (aka nasopalatine or anterior palatine foramen) outlines the oral opening for the nasopalatine canal.
- The incisive foramen forms a funnel shaped opening in the oral hard palate posterior to the incisors at the junction of the medial palatine and incisive sutures.
- It conducts the nasopalatine nerve and the sphenopalatine artery from the nasal cavity floor supplying mucous membrane over the oral cavity hard palate [20].
- See Fig. 51.3.

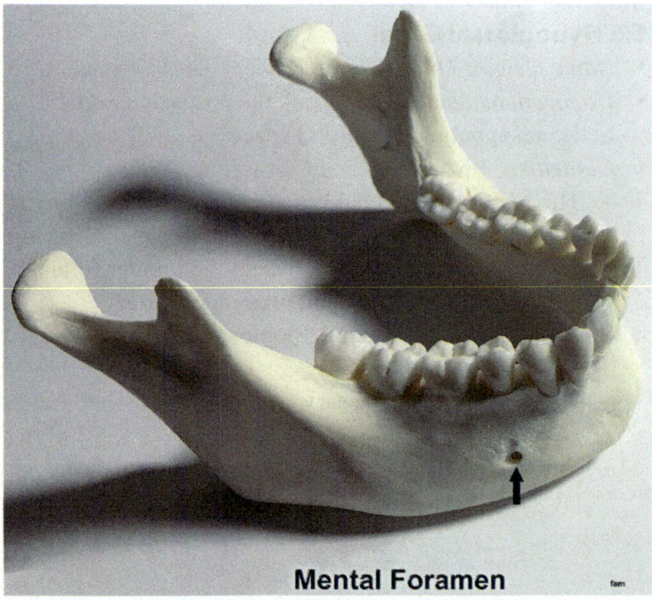

Fig. 51.23 *Lateral* surface of the anterior horizontal ramus where the *mental foramen* (up arrow ↑) affords *exodus* for the inferior alveolar nerve from the mandibular canal as the *mental nerve*

G. Mandible

G1. Mandibular Foramen

- Small mandibular canal opening on the *medial* aspect of the mandibular ramus.
- The inferior alveolar n. enters the mandibular foramen following the mandibular canal to exit through the mental foramen antero*laterally* as the mental nerve along with the artery.
- See Fig. 51.22.

G2. Mental Foramen

- One of two foramina on the antero*lateral* buccal aspect of the mandible where the terminal branch of the inferior alveolar nerve exits the mandibular canal as the mental nerve and associated artery.
- See Fig. 51.23.

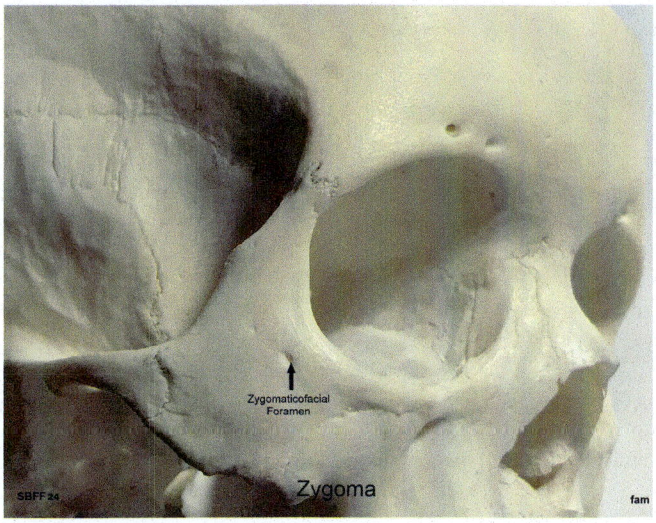

Fig. 51.24 Oblique face and orbit shows the zygomaticofacial foramen (up arrow ↑) in the mid zygoma infero*lateral* to the orbital rim conveying the zygomaticofacial nerve and vessels

H. Zygoma

H1. Zygomaticofacial Foramen

- Latin: Foramen zygomaticofaciale.
- The zygomaticofacial foramina pierces the *lateral* surface of the mid zygoma inferolateral to the orbital rim conveying the zygomaticofacial nerve and vessels.
- See Fig. 51.24.

H2. Zygomaticotemporal Foramen

- The small zygomaticotemporal foramen is situated on the *medial* margin of the zygoma anteriorly and transmits the zygomaticotemporal nerve and vessels.
- See Fig. 51.25.

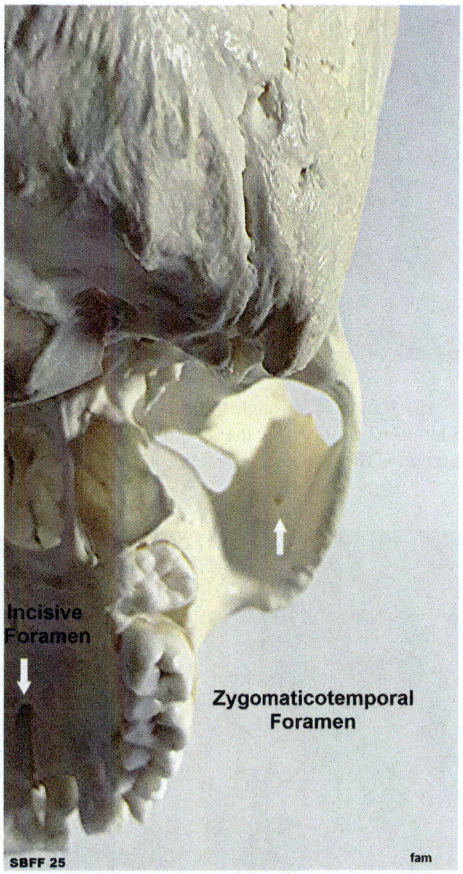

Fig. 51.25 Oblique view of the exocranial skull base shows the zygomaticotemporal foramina (up arrow ↑) along the *medial* margin of the mid zygoma. Down arrow (↓) annotates the intraoral opening of the incisive foramen

I. Orbit

I1. Superior Orbital Fissure (SOF)

- Conveys CN III, CN IV, CN V1, CN VI.
- Located lateral and caudal to the optic canal, the SOF is a craggy cleft at the orbital apex formed by the medial margin of the greater and the caudal surface of the lesser sphenoid wing. Its teardrop (or comma) shape widens inferomedially with its bulbous bottom located just anterior to the cavernous sinus [4].
- The SOF divides the roof and lateral orbital wall and provides a pathway between the orbit and the middle cranial fossa (MCF).
- The SOF contents are related to the annulus of Zinn as follows:
  - Outside annulus of Zinn.
    CN IV (trochlear nerve).
    Ophthalmic vein.
    lacrimal and frontal nerves (divisions of V_1).
  - Through the annulus of Zinn.
    CN VI (abducens).
    Nasociliary n. (branch CN II).
    - The optic strut separates the SOF from the optic canal [4].

    Superior and inferior divisions of CN III (oculomotor).
- See Figs. 51.1, 51.26a–c, and 51.27.

I2. Inferior Orbital Fissure (IOF)

- The IOF enters the orbit caudal to the SOF opening onto posterolateral orbital floor.
- It is bounded superiorly by the greater sphenoid wing, laterally by the zygoma, and inferiorly by the maxilla and orbital process of the palatine bone.
- The IOF transmits the infraorbital and zygomatic nerves, the infraorbital artery (and vein), orbital ganglionic branches of the pterygopalatine ganglion, a branch of the inferior ophthalmic vein, and various venous emissaries to the pterygoid plexus.

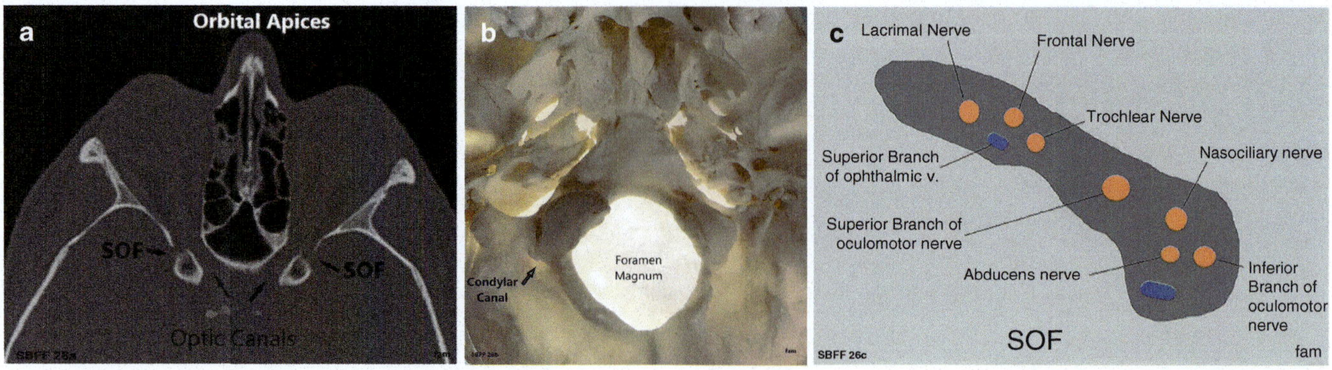

Fig. 51.26 (**a**) Axial CT through the orbital apices demonstrates the more medial optic canals and the laterally located cranial superior orbital fissures (SOF) at the level of the anterior clinoids (AC). (**b**), Axial CT through the orbital apices, caudal to prior image, at the level of the mid superior orbital fissures (SOF). (**c**) Color cartoon conveys crucial contents of the superior orbital fissure (SOF)

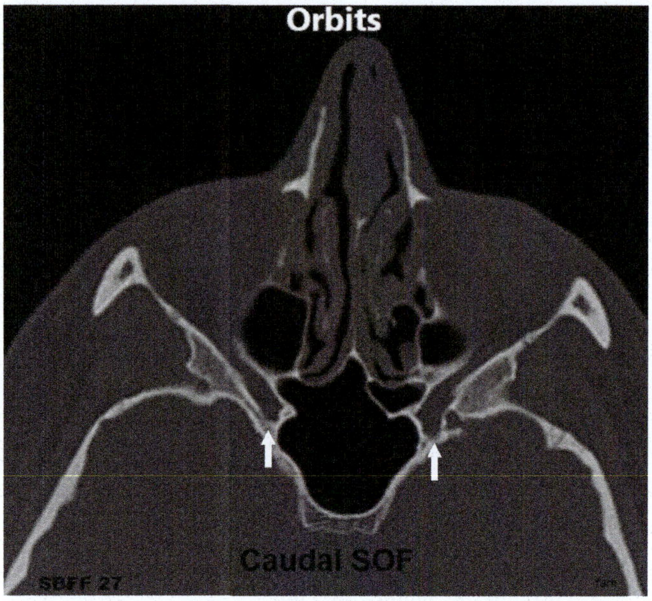

Fig. 51.27 Axial CT through the orbits caudal to the prior image, showing the caudal aspect of the superior orbital fissures (SOF)

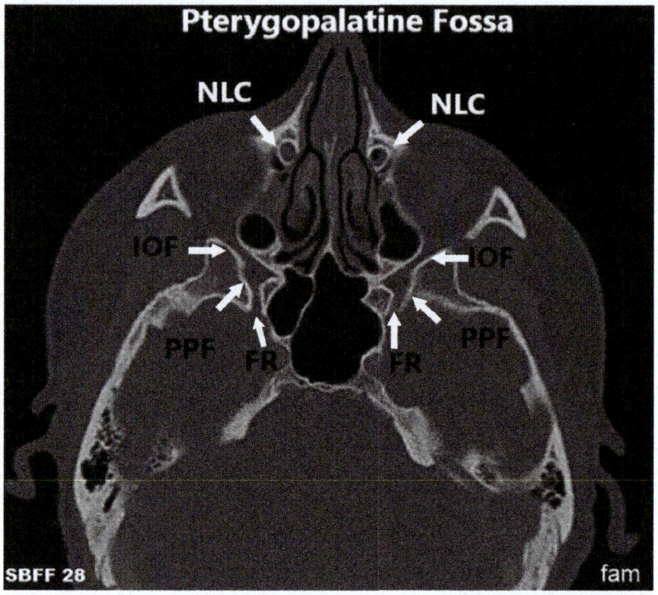

Fig. 51.28 Axial CT, caudal to the prior image, through the level of the pterygopalatine fossa (PPF), reveals relationship of the inferior orbital fissures (IOF) and foramen rotundum (FR). The paired nasolacrimal canals (NLC) are well demonstrated just posterior to the nasal bones

- The long axis of the IOF forms a 45^0 angle to the skull's sagittal plane and is perpendicular to the pterygomaxillary fissure.
- See Figs. 51.1, 51.27, and 51.28.

13. Lacrimal Foramina

- The lacrimal foramina are the bony openings to the nasolacrimal canals.
- The paired nasolacrimal canals are nestled in the anteromedial orbital walls created by collaborative contributions from the inferior nasal conchae, the maxilla, and the lacrimal bone. The nasolacrimal canals pitch posteriorly as they descend caudally.
- The nasolacrimal canals contain the nasolacrimal ducts which transport tears from the orbit to the nasal cavity where they drain through the inferior meatus, beneath the inferior nasal turbinate.
- The caudal aperture of the nasolacrimal duct drains beneath the inferior nasal concha and is fitted with a flap-like mucosal fold, called the lacrimal fold, or valve of Hasner.
- The lacrimal bone is one of our tiniest and most fragile bone roughly, the size of a small fingernail. It contains a depression along its anterior inferior aspect forming the lacrimal fossa which houses the membranous lacrimal sac.
- Lacrimal fluid flows from the lacrimal glands with excess fluid flowing into the nasolacrimal duct through the upper and lower puncta into the superior and inferior canaliculi.

- Human nasolacrimal ducts vary between 13 and 28 mm in length and 1–4 mm AP and oblique diameter with average AP and oblique diameters of 2.3 and 2.8 mm [21].
- Progressing from superior to inferior the nasolacrimal drainage system contains multiple valves named after medical historic notables including Rosenmueller, Bochdalek. Foltz, Huschke, Krause, Teillefer, and Hasner.
- These various valves regulate tear flow fostering constant fluid reabsorption.
- See Fig. 51.28.

References

1. Barker L, Naveed H, Adds PJ, Uddin JM. Supraorbital notch and foramen: positional variation and relevance to direct brow lift. Ophthalmic Plastic Reconstr Surg. 2013;29(1):67–70.
2. Jones JE, Dean JA. Local anesthesia and pain control for the child and adolescent. In: Dean J, editor. McDonald and Avery's dentistry for the child and adolescent, 10th ed. ISBN: 9780323287456; Elsevier's Imprint: Mosby; 2015. Published: 22 September 2015.
3. Singh DJ, Lenhart DE, Dolezal RF. Chapter 45-Fractures of the Nose. In: Plastic surgery secrets plus, 2nd ed. Weinzweig, Jeffrey, editor. 2019, Mosby, pp. 295–298; ISBN 978-0-323-03470-8,. https://doi.org/10.1016/B978-0-323-03470-8.00045-4.
4. Daniels DL, Leighton PM, Mafee MF, et al. Osseous anatomy of the orbital apex: anatomic moment. AJNR. 1995;16(9):1929–35.
5. Osawa S, Rhoton AL, Seker A, et al. Microsurgical and endoscopic anatomy of the Vidian canal. Neurosurgery. 2009;64(5 Suppl 2):385–411. discussion 411–2
6. Krayenbuhl NI, Isolan GR, Al-Mefty O. The foramen spinosum: a landmark in middle fossa surgery. Neurosurg Rev. 2008;31(4):397–402.
7. Tauber M, van Lovern HR, Gallo G, et al. The enigmatic foramen lacerum. Neurosurgery. 1999;44(2):391–3.
8. Christodouleas JP, Hristov B, Lin SH. Radiation oncology: a question-based review. Lippincott Williams & Wilkins. p. 138. ISBN 1608314448.
9. Lanzieri CF, Duchesneau PM, Rosenbloom SA, et al. The significance of asymmetry of the foramen of Vesalius. AJNR Am J Neuroradiol. 1988;9(6):1201–4.
10. Kim JH, Oka K, Jin ZW, et al. Fetal development of the incisive canal, especially of the delayed closure due to the nasopalatine duct: a study using serial sections of human fetuses. Anat Rec (Hoboken). 2017;300(6):1093–103.
11. Ogura Y, Clemis JD. A study of the gross anatomy of the human vestibular Aquduct. Ann Otol. 1971;80
12. Juliano AF, Ting EY, Mingkwansook V, Hamberg LM, Curtin HD. Vestibular aqueduct measurements in the 45° oblique (Pöschl) plane. AJNR. 2016;37(7):1331–7.
13. Destrieu C, Velut S, Kakou MK, et al. A new concept in Dorello's canal microanatomy: the petroclival venous confluence. J Neurosurg. 1998;87:67–72.
14. Dorello P. Considerazioni sopra la causa della paralisi transitoria dell'abducente nelle flogosi dell'orecchio medio. In: Atti della Clinica Oto-Rino-Laringoiatrica della R. Università di Roma, 1905.
15. Leung JY, Ishak GE. Prominent subarcuate canal in children: a normal variant. Pediatr Radiol. 2020;40(supplement 1):161.
16. Migirov L, Kronenberg J. Radiology of the petromastoid canal. Otol Neurotol. 2007;27(3):410–3. Pubmed citation.
17. Kanda T, Kiritoshi T, Osawa M, Toyoda K, Oba H, Kotoku J, et al. The incidence of double hypoglossal canal in Japanese: evaluation with multislice computed tomography. PLoS One. 2015;10(2):e0118317. https://doi.org/10.1371/journal.pone.0118317
18. Kavitha S, Anand A. A study of the condylar canal and its incidence, morphology and clinical significance. IJCRR. 2013;5:66–70.
19. Ginsberg LE. The posterior Condylar Canal. AJNR Am J Neuroradiol May. 1994;15:969–72.
20. Kim JH, Oka K, Jin ZW, et al. Fetal development of the incisive canal, especially of the delayed closure due to the nasopalatine duct: a study using serial sections of human fetuses. Anat Rec (Hoboken). 2017;300(6):1093–103.
21. Maliborski A, Rozycki R. Diagnostic imaging of the nasolacrimal drainage system. Part I. Radiologic anatomy of lacrimal pathways. Physiology of tear secretion and tear outflow. Med Sci Monit. 2014;20:628–38.

Index

F. A. Midyett, S. K. Mukherji, *Skull Base Imaging*, https://doi.org/10.1007/978-3-030-46447-9

I

J

P

R

S

T

The manufacturer's authorised representative in the EU is Springer Nature Customer Service Centre GmbH, Europaplatz 3, 69115 Heidelberg, Germany. If you have any concerns regarding our products, please contact ProductSafety@springernature.com

Printed and bound by CPI Group (UK) Ltd, Croydon, CR0 4YY
30/09/2026
02225476-0004